WHAT TO EXPECT

THE

SECOND YEAR

FROM 12 TO 24 MONTHS

Heidi Murkoff
and Sharon Mazel

Foreword by Mark D. Widome, M.D., M.P.H., Professor of Pediatrics,
The Pennsylvania State University

SIMON &
SCHUSTER

London · New York · Sydney · Toronto · New Delhi

A CBS COMPANY

To Erik, my everything
To Emma, Wyatt and Russell, my greatest expectations
To Arlene, with so much love, always and forever
To my WTE family – and the mums, dads, babies, and toddlers everywhere

First published in Great Britain by Simon & Schuster, 2012
A CBS COMPANY

Book design: Rae Ann Spitzenberger & Lisa Hollander
Interior illustrations: Karen Kuchar

1 3 5 7 9 10 8 6 4 2

Simon & Schuster UK Ltd
1st Floor
222 Gray's Inn Road
London WC1X 8HB

www.simonandschuster.co.uk

Simon & Schuster Australia, Sydney
Simon & Schuster India, New Delhi

A CIP catalogue record for this book is available from the British Library

ISBN 978-0-85720-670-1

Printed and bound in Finland by Bookwell

Note: All children are unique and this book is not intended to substitute for the advice
of your doctor or health visitor, who should be consulted on toddler matters,
especially when a child shows any sign of illness or unusual behaviour.

Thanks
(Or, Ta-Ta)

....

I NEED HELP. There, I've said it . . . I need help, and lots of it. And as luck would have it, I've not only got that help in spades, I've got the best a girl could hope for. Starting, as always, with the man I've been blessed to wake up beside for 29 years – my partner in love, life, business, and pleasure, my DH and my BFF, Erik (though occasionally that man is a six-pound chihuahua named Harry, who manages to snuggle his way to the sweet spot between Erik and me – just like Emma used to do back in the toddler day . . . though she didn't shed).

And there's more help where that comes from . . . plenty more. The WTE family of books has grown, but happily so has the number of wonderful, talented, committed WTE family members who have pitched in to help it grow. Some have come, helped, and moved on (and when they do, I try not to take it personally), others have stuck by me since WTE's conception. Thanks a lot, or as the toddlers say, "ta-ta" to:

Arlene Eisenberg, my first partner in WTE and my most important one. Your legacy of caring and compassion lives on forever – you'll always be loved and always be remembered.

Sharon Mazel, you're the wind in my sail, the answer to my questions, the chocolate on my peanut butter – and always, the yin to my yang. How could I live (or work) without you? Love to you, your ever-patient doctor husband, Jay, and the four girls who've somehow raised themselves (really well): Daniella, Arianne, Sophia, and Kira.

Suzanne Rafer, true friend, exceptional editor, awesome author advocate, whose critiques are always as sharp as her pencils (and hey, I've even stopped erasing some of them!). Not surprisingly – after all these years of passes, we're both wearing glasses.

Peter Workman, for his dedication, passion, and commitment, and for creating the house that became WTE's home.

Everyone else at Workman who has helped deliver my latest baby (I guess that makes you my doulas): Bob Miller, new fearless leader, for your finesse with facilitating and your excellence in expediting. David Matt, for always going, well, to the mat for me – and for sharing an artistic vision that, let's face it, definitely doesn't come cheap. Lisa Hollander and Rae-Ann Spitzenberger, my two favourite designing women, for your talent – and patience. Painting genius Tim O'Brien for bringing the world's cutest toddler, Gigi, to life (and to Gigi, for the smile you bring to my face every time I see yours), and to Anne Kerman for finding Gigi. Lynn Parmentier for your crazy beautiful quilt. Karen Kuchar, for capturing perfectly that quintessential toddler cuteness (and for your astonishing grace under deadlines). Peggy Gannon for always going with the flow and keeping the flow going. And my other phenomenal friends at Workman, including Suz2 (Suzie Bolotin), Erin Klabunde, Beth Rees, Walter Weintz, Page Edmunds, Jenny Mandel, James Wehrle, Joe Ginis, Steven Pace, Marilyn Barnett, Jodi Weiss, Emily Krasner, Beth Wareham, Barbara Peragine – and the entire sales and marketing team.

Dr Mark Widome, for your vast wealth of medical expertise, your deep pockets of wisdom, your endless reservoir of patience, passion, and good humour – plus, can you write a fabulous foreword, or what? I'm not sure who's luckier – the students you teach, the children you care for, the parents you counsel, or me (I'm just glad there's enough of you to go around!).

Steven Petrow (MG), Vince Errico (Dimples), Mike Keriakos, Ben Wolin, Jim Curtis (CSOB), Sarah Hutter, and all my wonderful friends and partners at Everyday Health, for making our vision of WhatToExpect.com a reality. Thanks, also, to the amazing WTE community of moms – not only for making our site the special place that it is, but for sharing your bellies, babies, and toddlers with me every day. With a special shout (and XO) out to my Facebook and Twitter family – thanks for always being there for me.

Two other men I don't wake up with but couldn't face a day without: Marc Chamlin, for your keen legal eagle eye, your business smarts, your unflagging friendship and support; and Alan Nevins, for your masterful management, phenomenal finessing, endless patience, persistence, and handholding (we'll always have Cairo). And to the newest member of the WTE team, someone who has a great name and even a greater gift of communication: Heidi Schaeffer – thanks for getting the word out!

The mamas of my other baby: The What to Expect Foundation, Lisa Bernstein (mama, also to Zoe and Oh-that-Teddy) and Ruth Turoff (mama, also to the beautiful Bluebell), for spreading mom power to those who need it most.

Emma (the toddler who started it all), Wyatt (the toddler who followed), and my newest son, Russell – you've made me one lucky mama, and I love you all so much.

And speaking of family that I adore: Sandee Hathaway, my sweet sister and friend; my endlessly adorable father Howard Eisenberg; my treasured in-laws, Abby and Norman Murkoff. And Victor Shargai, for your love, support, and DNA.

To AAP, for being tireless advocates for children and their parents, and to all of the practitioners who work every day to make little lives happier, healthier, and safer.

And most of all, to all moms, dads, and toddlers everywhere. Big hugs to you all!

Contents

....

CHAPTER 3

CHAPTER 4

CHAPTER 7

Disciplining Your Toddler 244

CHAPTER 8

Talking 256

CHAPTER 9

Learning 270

CHAPTER 13

Second Year Safety

Treating Toddler Injuries

Developmental Disorders

A Road Map

WHAT HAPPENS ON the morning of the first birthday? Does yesterday's infant awake a fully formed toddler? Does child development pay some special respect to the Gregorian calendar? And, more to the point, must parents one day put aside their infant parenting skills, and open a new toolbox of skills for parenting a toddler?

The answer, of course, is "no". Biologically, the first birthday is a non-event. The day of and the days after the birthday celebration are not noticeably different than those before. From the standpoint of a child's growth and development – physical development, intellectual development, emotional development – you might as well have held the party at the end of the eleventh month or the thirteenth. Milestones happen on their own schedule, with wide variation and with disregard for the calendar. As before, your child's growth and development will progress in fits and starts. Viewed over months, rather than days, developmental progress appears smooth. Things move mostly in the right direction.

Yet there is some biological and developmental rationale for thinking about the second year of life as a discrete phase. Entering the second year, the child has grown to roughly three times his or her birthweight, and has gained half again his or her birth length. From now on, the growth trajectory will largely depend on some combination of genetics and environment, rather than factors left over from pregnancy and birth. Babies born prematurely – or otherwise small – have mostly caught up to their peers. Likewise, babies who were large at birth have now found a growth path consistent with genetics and family patterns. Most 1-year-olds are capable (or near capable) of taking their first steps, and even those who still need to hold on to furniture or a hand, do so mostly out of a lack of bravery rather than a lack of balance.

And, it is right around that arbitrary first birthday that most children achieve what is perhaps the most surprising of milestones: the ability to appreciate and use symbols. Symbols with consistent meanings make possible much more efficient communication and the seemingly exponential learning curve of the second year. First evidence of this is when a toddler points to things. Finger-pointing is code. It has one of two meanings: either indicating a want or drawing attention to something interesting. Finger-pointing has these same meanings, whether the toddler is doing the pointing, the parent is doing the pointing, or an older sibling is doing the pointing.

Words are also symbols. One-year-olds enter toddlerhood with a first vocabulary. That small handful of words – perhaps just two or three at first – also have specific and consistent meanings. Mama and Dada are specific words for the right people, and those almost-words for the dog, for a sibling, for the bottle or the teddy bear consistently mean the same things to both you and your toddler. Pretty amazing.

Socially, it is at or around the first birthday that a child really becomes his own person. Toddlers finally see themselves as separate from their mothers and fathers, no longer extensions or appendages of their parents. Of course, they show this newly realized independence in both welcomed and unwelcomed ways. The first brave steps are as often away from the parents as towards them. The word "no" develops an edge, often becoming decidedly defiant: "Pay attention, I have thoughts of my own." Temper tantrums are just around the corner. It is almost as if a little teenager has moved in.

I'll say less about how that second year ends: how your toddler will become a preschooler. But, suffice it to say, by two years, children have acquired a much more complex emotional and imaginative life. They have acquired communication tools and skills that will soon have them talking in sentences – sentences good enough for conversation. Imagination and creativity, supported by advanced motor skills, keep parents on their toes. Making friends, developing empathy, and wanting to please others are developmental tasks and hallmarks for the stage of development just beyond the purview of this book.

Coming on the heels of a series of successful and well-received *What to Expect* books, *What to Expect the Second Year* is a testament to how much we benefit from road maps in navigating pregnancy and child-rearing. Constructing one looks particularly easy when it is done well. But consider constructing a road map for travellers when you know that each of them will take a slightly different route to get to that same destination: becoming a grown-up. Figure out how to suggest paths for travellers who have widely differing needs as well as differing strengths, competencies, and challenges. Faced with a complex journey, convince the driver (the parent) that routes are navigable, that most judgements and intuitions are correct, and that it is okay to make an occasional wrong turn. Do all that without dampening a parent's enthusiasm and excitement, or their appreciation of the rewards for the effort. That is what this book sets out to accomplish.

Heidi Murkoff has stamped this book with her familiar trademarks. First, is her reassuring and optimistic tone. She reminds us that minor deviations from the expected course of behaviour, growth, nutrition, or development are usually of little consequence. She reminds us that the range of normal is wide, and that things, in most cases, usually turn out all right. She gives us permission to be less than perfect, and reminds us that course corrections are routine. She is both a coach and a cheerleader.

The Second Year is authoritative – when it needs to be. Like its predecessors, it relies heavily on professional guidelines and recommendations, particularly in areas such as immunisation, nutrition, safety, and management of common illnesses. Even complicated recommendations (such as those for CPR) are made clear and compact without cutting corners. Yet, Heidi knows when to go out on a limb. Some of her suggestions about probiotics, herbal remedies and other nutritional supplements, for example, will be of interest to readers even if they do not enjoy full consensus among the experts. Rather, she calls on emerging research and thought. She labels this material appropriately; her policy is "full disclosure".

Heidi's voice is familiar. It's not quite your mum's voice, nor is it your best friend's, nor is it the voice of your favourite school teacher – but neither is it the voice of a stranger. This voice recognises and acknowledges your frustrations and sleep deprivation. It also recognises how, on some days, some little thing your toddler says or does creates such surprise and pleasure. Such days, the world is good.

The Second Year offers frequent insights – frequently with a smile. It reminds us that "the fashion police do not fine toddlers." And, "If there is a law of toddler physics, it is that little bodies in motion stay in motion." Heidi reminds parents repeatedly to stay calm and to stick to routines. Set limits, but sometimes go with the flow. When you reach an impasse, change the subject. When you run out of parenting steam, take a break, read an adult book, go to the gym, don't ever turn down help when you need it.

Medical students learn early *Primum non nocere:* "First, do no harm." It becomes a mantra for those who choose paediatrics. So what might sometimes seem an excess of caution in these pages, really is not. You will detect this caution in the discussion of environmental toxins, response to fever, and management of injuries. Read

labels, use medicines only when needed, store things safely. Seek layers of protection, whether the potential hazard is poison, sunlight, or deep water. If you are not sure your child is feeling well, if it seems like something is not right, or if you are just plain worried, seek medical advice.

Beyond the opinions of experts, *Second Year* relies on experience and common sense. It favours what works in practice over what works in theory. It favours the middle ground over extremes. In discussing discipline, Heidi reminds us that excessive permissiveness leads to children who are often "rude, selfish, quick to argue, slow to comply". Beyond that, discipline is about preparation for the real world: "where rules rule". She reminds us that there is no one best way to discipline. Be fair, avoid extremes, let consequences teach when you can, especially natural and relevant consequence. Above all, dispense discipline with love.

This practical approach extends to discussion of nutrition (eat sensibly), promoting early learning (don't raise a "techno-tot"), treating illness (medicate, but only when necessary), and much else. It is an approach that has weathered well. It is the zone where most parents, with good reason, feel comfortable.

Mark D. Widome, M.D., M.P.H.
Professor of Pediatrics
The Pennsylvania State University

Bye-Bye Baby, Hello Toddler

NOT LIKE YOU haven't noticed, but in just 12 short months, your baby has come a long, long way. Yesterday's bundle of joy is today's bundle of energy . . . a snuggly armful turned into a wriggly handful. Content to coo, cuddle, and stay put? Reliably pliable, simple to satisfy, and easily totable? That's so last year.

Bye-bye baby, hello toddler . . . and welcome to the wonder year: the second year. Twelve jam-packed (and jam-smeared) months of fabulous firsts (first steps, first words . . . first tantrum), mind-boggling growth and develop-ment, lightning-speed learning, and end-less explorations and discoveries driven by insatiable curiosity.

Not to mention, monumental chal-lenges – both for your toddler ("How do I get those bricks to stack without falling over?" "How can I turn that puzzle piece so it fits?" "How can I get my hands on mummy's laptop?") and for you ("How do I get my toddler to eat/sleep/play nicely/separate at nursery drop-off/put on a coat/leave the play-ground – without a struggle? Or get through a supermarket trip without a meltdown on the frozen foods aisle?").

Toddlers, like babies, don't come with an owner's manual, and yet they're at least as difficult to figure out . . . and to operate safely. Happily, help is here. Picking up the action where *What to Expect the First Year* leaves off (and as the action really starts to pick up), *What to Expect the Second Year* is a complete why, when, and how-to guide to your fledgling toddler, from 12 months to 24 months.

It's all here, in a brand-new, easy-to-access, fast-to-flip-to, topic-by-topic format – everything you need to know to decode, cope with, and fully enjoy the fascinating, complicated, sometimes maddening, always adorable little person last year's baby has suddenly become. You'll find the facts – along with realistic solutions, strategies, and tips – on feed-ing (including how to get a head start on healthy eating habits without picking food fights with a picky eater). Sleeping (how to help your toddler get the sleep he or she needs – but without the battles – at bedtime and naptime). Playing and making friends (how to promote shar-ing and turn-taking, how to keep play-dates from turning into boxing matches). Getting your toddler talking . . .

and listening. Cultivating creativity, encouraging curiosity, and nurturing your little one's natural love of learning-by-doing. Taking on tantrums (at home and in public), and tackling those first glimpses of the "terrible twos" in your terrific 1-year-old. Making sense of every conceivable (and inconceivable) toddler behaviour – from the predictable to the seemingly random. Teaching (and enforcing) right and wrong, setting age-appropriate expectations, and disciplining effectively. Keeping your toddler safe and healthy as he or she takes on the world . . . or at least the local park.

Wondering about where your toddler stacks up in the growth department? It's in here. Developmentally?

A milestones timeline – and milestone boxes throughout the book – have you covered. Thinking of travelling with your toddler in tow? There's a chapter for that, too. Need a parental pep talk (and what parent of a toddler doesn't)? You'll get plenty of those.

It's the next step in *What to Expect* – and the next step in your parenting adventure. So take a deep breath, lace up your running shoes, and whatever you do, don't blink: The wonder year is here.

Here's to a happy second year!

heidi

What to Expect the Second Year

The Second Year at a Glance

YOUR CHILD, like every child, is one of a kind. Not like any other. In other words, incomparable. That, of course, probably doesn't stop you from comparing your little one's development to that of other kids the same age. Or comparing it against developmental timelines, like the one that follows.

Sometimes comparisons are helpful, even reassuring – as when you scan a list of skills considered age-appropriate to make sure your toddler's development is on target. Or when you compare your toddler's rate of development one month to a previous month's – to see if it's keeping steady, lagging a little, or racing ahead. And you won't be the only one who's making comparisons as your toddler grows. Your child's doctor will look for certain milestones at each checkup, to be sure that your toddler's development fits within the (very) wide range of normal for his or her age.

Sometimes, though, comparisons to an "average" pace of development can be misleading. After all, there are few "average" kids, or kids who develop at a uniform pace, or kids who develop at the same rate in all areas

across the board. Some 1-year-olds may be zooming around the playground, while others haven't even taken their first steps yet. Some may be running circles around others when it comes to verbal skills. Some may speed ahead early in most departments, while others may get a bit of a late start, eventually catching up or even whizzing past. Some are relatively consistent in their pace of development, others develop in fits and starts. Illness or a major disruption or change in a child's life (a new childcare situation, a parent who's sick or away, the arrival of a baby sibling, a move to a new home, even an extended holiday) can temporarily throw development off course altogether. That's why comparing your toddler to other toddlers the same age isn't really very helpful, and why you should always compare with care when it comes to developmental timelines.

Your unique toddler may hang out pretty consistently in the average-for-age category for months – or even for the full year. Or maybe his or her overall development won't ever fit a predictable pattern – it's slow one month, jumping ahead the next. Most kids will also go through frustrating, disorganized periods of no apparent progress – weeks in a row without a single new accomplishment. That's usually because a giant step – like taking first steps – is just around the corner. A developmental drought, and then, bingo – your toddler's walking or talking up a storm.

Remember: most rates of development are just right. As long as your toddler is reaching the majority of milestones on time, his or her development is on target – which means you can sit back and marvel at those amazing achievements, instead of analysing them. If, on the other hand, you notice that your toddler is consistently missing milestones or seems to be suddenly slipping significantly in development – or if you have a gut feeling that something isn't right – go and see the doctor. Most likely there's no problem at all (some children keep moving forward, just on a slower-than-average developmental timetable), and you'll get the reassurance you're looking for. If a lag is identified, your toddler will be able to get help maximising his or her developmental potential.

Something else you'll need to keep in mind: developmental timelines are a quick and easy way to check on developmental progress every once in a while, but they're not predictive of your child's future. No words yet? It doesn't mean there isn't a law career on the cards later on. Not the most coordinated tot on the street? It doesn't mean your little one won't one day be tearing up the tennis court or the football pitch. Something else timelines aren't: a must-do for parents. Are you happy letting your child's development take its course without wondering if he's on track or she's where she should be? That's completely fine. Take a timeline time-out, let your toddler do the developing, and leave the screening to the doctor.

Developmental Milestones in the Second Year

12 to 13 Months

Most toddlers will probably be able to . . .

- Pull up to standing

- Get into sitting position

- Cruise from place to place holding on

- Clap hands (play Pat-a-Cake)

- Pick up an object from the floor while standing (and holding on)

- Communicate needs without crying (at least, sometimes)

- Say 1 word

Half of all toddlers will be able to . . .

- Stand without help

- Take a few solo steps

- Drink from a cup

- Put an object into a container

- Say 2 words

- Point to something they want

Some toddlers may be able to . . .

- Walk well

- Scribble

It's Cumulative

Toddlers gather lots of new skills every month but typically hold on to last month's achievements (and the month before last, and so on). So assume that your toddler's skill set will incorporate those "will be probably able to" items from previous months in addition to brand-new ones acquired this month. Just keep in mind that once a skill has outgrown its age-appropriateness, your toddler will drop it from his or her repertoire (clearly, once walking is mastered, for instance, there's no need to keep up crawling).

- Hold out an arm or leg to help with getting dressed
- Play games like peek-a-boo
- Look in the right direction when asked to locate something ("Where's Mummy?" or "Where's the light?")

A few toddlers may be able to . . .

- Roll a ball back and forth
- Attempt to lift heavier items
- Use a fork or spoon to eat, once in a while
- Undress
- Identify a body part when asked, by pointing to it

13 to 14 Months

Most toddlers will probably be able to (see box, this page) . . .

- Stand alone
- Cruise

- Walk with help
- Take a few steps unassisted
- Wave bye-bye
- Put an object into a container (and then dump it out again)
- Eat with their fingers
- Say "mama" and "dada" intentionally
- Follow a 1-step direction ("Pick up the doll, please")
- Imitate others (clap hands when someone else claps hands, for instance)

Half of all toddlers will be able to . . .

- Walk well
- Push a toy with wheels while walking
- Pick up an object from the ground while standing (without holding on)
- Point to a body part when asked ("Where's your nose?")

Some toddlers may be able to . . .

- Pull a toy while walking
- Imitate with an object (use a phone to "talk", a cloth to "clean")
- Use a spoon or fork to eat, once in a while
- Drink from a cup independently
- Say 3 words

A few toddlers may be able to . . .

- Run
- Climb steps
- Build a tower of 2 bricks
- Match shapes in a shape sorter

- Say 6 words or more
- Follow a 2-step direction ("Pick up the teddy and give it to me, please")

14 to 15 Months

Most toddlers will probably be able to . . .

- Take a few solo steps
- Point to a desired object
- Say at least 1 word

Half of all toddlers will be able to . . .

- Walk well
- Bend over and pick up an object while standing
- Play with a ball
- Scribble with a crayon
- Drink independently from a cup
- Say at least 2 words
- Laugh at something funny or silly
- Recognise what objects are used for (a hairbrush, a hat, a broom)

Some toddlers may be able to . . .

- Run
- Stack 2 bricks to build a tower
- Point to a few body parts when asked
- Turn paper pages in a book
- Point to a picture in a book when asked
- Say at least 3 words
- Say the word "no" often

A few toddlers may be able to . . .

- Walk backwards
- Walk up stairs (but not down yet)
- Say 5 or more words
- Draw lines with a crayon
- Sing

15 to 16 Months

Most toddlers will probably be able to . . .

- Climb (on things, out of the pushchair, and so on)
- Walk well
- Imitate activities
- Scribble
- Turn paper pages in a book
- Carry objects in each hand
- Understand simple directions ("no", "look", "come", "please give me")

Half of all toddlers will be able to . . .

- Stack 3 bricks
- Imitate with an object (use a phone to "talk", a broom to "sweep")
- Use a spoon or fork
- Throw a ball
- Say 3 words
- Recognise self in mirror or picture

Some toddlers may be able to . . .

- Run
- Walk backwards

- Dance to music
- Say 6 words

A few toddlers may be able to . . .

- Kick a ball forward
- Brush teeth, with help
- Take off one piece of clothing without help
- Say 15 words or more

16 to 17 Months

Most toddlers will probably be able to . . .

- Play on riding toys
- Drink from a cup
- Say 2 to 3 words
- Enjoy saying "no"
- Point to a desired object

Half of all toddlers will be able to . . .

- Run
- Throw a ball underarm
- Point to body parts when asked
- Say 6 to 10 words regularly
- Play pretend games

Some toddlers may be able to . . .

- Walk up steps
- Kick a ball
- Take off one piece of clothing without help
- Sort toys by shape or colour
- Follow a 2-step verbal command (without gestures)
- Say 10 to 20 words regularly

A few toddlers may be able to . . .

- Throw a ball overarm
- Build a tower of 4 bricks
- Identify 2 items in a picture by pointing
- Identify 1 picture by naming ("dog", "cat", and so on)
- Combine words
- Speak and be understood half the time
- Say 50+ words

17 to 18 Months

Most toddlers will probably be able to . . .

- Run
- Drink from a cup
- Point to something they want
- Pull off mittens, hat, socks
- Look at board books independently
- Enjoy finger play ("Incy Wincy Spider", for instance)
- Say 10 words
- Play alone on the floor
- Recognise themselves in mirror or pictures
- Laugh at something funny or silly

Half of all toddlers will be able to . . .

- Dance to music
- Drag things around
- Crawl backwards down stairs
- Brush teeth with help

- Drink with a straw
- Start showing a preference for one hand over the other
- Stack 4 bricks
- Say 20+ words
- String 2 words together in phrases
- Ask for something by name

Some toddlers may be able to . . .

- Jump
- Throw a ball overarm
- Identify 2 pictures by naming
- Combine words
- Be understood when speaking, about half the time
- Sing
- Remember where things belong
- Show off to get attention or repeat sounds (or actions) that make people laugh
- Recognise emotion/show empathy (hugging someone who is sad, for instance)

A few toddlers may be able to . . .

- Take toys apart and put them back together
- Help put toys away
- String large wooden beads
- Blow bubbles
- Take off clothes
- Draw circles

18 to 20 Months

Most toddlers will probably be able to . . .

- Run
- Bend over to pick up a toy and not fall
- Climb
- Play pretend games
- Imitate behaviours (such as feeding a doll)
- Feed themselves with a spoon and fork
- Say 10 to 20 words

Half of all toddlers will be able to . . .

- Walk up steps
- Kick a ball
- Take off clothes without help
- Draw a straight line
- Brush teeth with help
- Say 20 to 50 words
- Combine words
- Identify 2 pictures by naming

Some toddlers may be able to . . .

- Balance on one foot while holding on
- Take off clothes
- Name 6 body parts
- Identify 4 pictures by naming
- Say 50+ words
- Form short sentences
- Ask "why" and "what's that" questions

A few toddlers may be able to . . .

- Walk down stairs, holding on
- Wash and dry hands
- Build a tower of 6 bricks
- Show some signs of potty readiness (for example, announce a poo in progress)
- Speak in full sentences

20 to 22 Months

Most toddlers will probably be able to . . .

- Run well
- Squat
- Throw a ball underarm
- Take off an article of clothing
- Enjoy playing with clay, musical instruments, and other manipulative toys
- Follow 2-step directions
- Say 10 to 20 words
- Set simple goals (such as deciding to fill a bucket with water and bring it to the sandpit to wet the sand)

Half of all toddlers will be able to . . .

- Open doors
- Walk down stairs with assistance
- Play with simple puzzles
- Understand (though not use) as many as 200 words, or just about everything said to them
- Say 50+ words
- Recognise when something is identified incorrectly (like when a "cat" is called a "car")

Some toddlers may be able to . . .

- Wash and dry hands
- Understand opposites (hot vs. cold, for instance)
- Name family members (or other familiar people) in pictures
- Know when a picture book is upside down
- Say 50 to 100 words
- Follow 3-step directions

A few toddlers may be able to . . .

- Play tag
- Put on an article of clothing
- Put on shoes (though not always on the correct feet)
- Fold a piece of paper in imitation

22 to 24 Months

Most toddlers will probably be able to . . .

- Kick a ball
- Walk backwards
- Take off an article of clothing
- Build a tower of 4 bricks
- Imitate adult behaviour (sweep, feed a doll, talk on a telephone, and so on)
- Identify 2 items in a picture by naming
- Combine words
- Say close to 50 words
- Show awareness of parental approval or disapproval

Half of all toddlers will be able to . . .

- Balance on one foot (while holding on)

- Put on an article of clothing

- Brush hair, wipe nose, or perform other basic hygiene skills with help

- Show signs of potty readiness

- Be understood when speaking, about half the time

- Say 50 to 70 words

- Ask "why" and "what's this" questions

- Talk about themselves ("Me want milk", "Jack go on swing")

- Sing simple tunes

- Take interest in playing with other children

Some toddlers may be able to . . .

- Build a tower of 8 bricks

- Use prepositions ("on", "under", "next to")

- Carry on a conversation of 2 to 3 sentences

- Say 100+ words

A few toddlers may be able to . . .

- Pedal a tricycle

- Arrange things in categories (balls, dolls, animals)

- Understand the concept of adjectives (sticky, funny, soft)

- Take turns

- Say 200 words

- Use adjectives

- Answer "What is your name?"

CHAPTER 1

Your Toddler On the Grow

H OW BIG IS YOUR TODDLER? So big . . . and growing bigger . . . and even bigger, seemingly every day. (Can you remember when your once-upon-a-time newborn was tiny enough to fit neatly cradled in one arm? Try pulling that off with your strapping – and squirming – 1-year-old.) Still, a tot's growth can keep you guessing, especially because it can be so all over the place – and all over the charts. It can come at a pretty consistently average (or slower-than-average, or faster-than-average) rate – or in unpredictable fits and starts. For most toddlers, normal growth is what's normal for them, not for the kid on the swing next to them. That, of course, won't keep you from wondering, and sometimes worrying, about your growing toddler's growth. Is he too short? Is she too chunky? Too skinny? Gaining inches faster than pounds – or the other way around? The likely answer: Nope, your toddler's growth is just right.

What You May Be Wondering About

Growth Charts

"My son is in the 15th percentile on the weight and length charts. What does that mean?"

I t means your little boy's on the little side, but still within the normal range for his age – good news, since normal (whether it's big-normal, little-normal, or average-normal) is the name of the game.

By plotting measurements of height and weight at each checkup (and until age 2, head circumference as well), the doctor can see how your toddler stacks up percentile-wise against other children of the same age and gender. Your little man is in the 15th percentile for weight and height, which means 85 per cent of other children his age are taller and weigh more than he does, and 15 per cent are shorter and weigh less.

But comparing your toddler to the general toddler population only tells part of the growth story. Even more important is comparing your toddler to himself. That's why the doctor will be focused on your son's growth trends over time rather than which percentiles he falls into at a given time. If your little one has been consistently hovering around the 15th percentile for most of his life, then he may be destined to be on the small side (or he may be predisposed to a dramatic growth spurt later on in childhood). If, however, he'd always been in the 60th percentile and abruptly dipped to the 15th percentile, that sudden deviation from his accustomed growth rate might raise questions: has he been sick? Under stress? Is there another underlying medical reason for his growth slowdown? Or is he just moving towards a genetically programmed small stature after starting off on the bigger side? Likewise, a child who had hovered around the 45th percentile since birth, but then shot up to the 90th percentile in just a few months, might need a closer look. Is he eating too many calories? Getting too little physical activity? Or just catching up, after a slower start, to the specs on his genetic blueprint?

Assessing how your toddler grows isn't just a simple numbers game. To get a really clear big picture of growth, the doctor will also consider the extremely significant relationship between weight and length. While the height and weight percentiles plotted on separate growth charts don't have to match up precisely (a 40th percentile for height and a 50th percentile for weight is perfectly normal, as is an 80th percentile for height and an 85th percentile for weight), they should be within a 10 to 20 per cent range of each other. If height is at the 30th percentile but weight is at the 85th percentile,

TWINS

Different Growth for Different Folks

Got twins (or more) and wondering how their growth will likely stack up against other children or against each other? If your twins are identical, they'll probably (though not always) follow the same patterns of growth – with growth spurts and growth lags coming at approximately the same time, especially as they get older. If they're fraternal, you may notice some differences in those patterns – differences that can be anywhere from slight to significant. Have fraternals of the opposite sex? Chances are your son will grow larger and faster than your daughter (just as singleton boys outpace singleton girls, on average). Of course, averages don't always tell the story – especially when it comes to your unique twins. A lot of their growth this year will depend on their weight at birth. Were they small for their gestational age? Did they arrive prematurely? Was one twin much larger than the other? All those factors will come into play when assessing their growth curve. The good news is that even twins (or higher-order multiples) born prematurely or low in weight for gestational age catch up to their peers growth-wise by the time they reach school age. All systems grow!

you've got an overweight toddler on your hands. The other way around? Your toddler might be underweight. While doctors usually judge this weight–length relationship intuitively, in the US they sometimes turn to yet another chart: the weight-for-length chart. This chart measures the weight-to-length relationship

---

Measuring Your Wiggly Worm

Wondering why your toddler looks taller – but seems to have "lost" several centimetres since the last doctor visit? It's probably because measuring a toddler's length is a very imprecise science. Between all that wriggling and squirming, it's hard even for a professional to get an accurate reading. It won't be until your child is measured in an upright position (standing still) that you'll be able to count on reliable results.

(it's similar to a BMI – Body Mass Index – measurement) and is used most often to help a doctor determine whether a child is undernourished or overnourished.

Also worth a look before leaping to any conclusions about where your toddler falls on any growth chart are patterns of growth on his family tree. Did Mum, Dad, or siblings follow a similar pattern (are they also tall and large, for instance, or short and skinny)? Did they start out plump and then slim down? Were they petite as toddlers and then filled out and shot up as they got older? If so, that could explain why your toddler's growth is trending a certain way. Say your little one's really little (only hitting the 5th percentile for height and weight) – that might be right on target if he's following in tiny footprints.

Wondering where your tot plots on a growth chart? You can fill in your own on pages 16 to 19.

The Tubby Toddler

"I think my toddler's chubby thighs are so cute, but my mother says my daughter is too fat. Is that even possible at this age?"

Those typical toddler trademarks – ready-for-pinching chubby cheeks, a rub-worthy round belly, and kissable dimpled elbows and knees – are definitely signs of cuteness, but they're not automatically signs of overweight. Sometimes, a pleasantly plump 1-year-old starts to thin out closer to the end of the second year, as her growth in height overtakes her increase in weight. Or maybe she hasn't started walking yet, so her level of activity (or lack of it) is keeping her pudgy for now, and you may start to see her slim down when she gets up and goes – walking, running, climbing.

But sometimes those roly-poly cheeks and thighs can indeed be signs of overweight. If you suspect your toddler is more tubby than just plain chubby, talk to the GP at the next visit about your concerns. If your tot is within an average percentile for both height and weight, you can put aside your weighty worries for now – your toddler's rotund physique is likely to eventually slim down to more appropriate proportions. If your toddler is truly overweight (she's placing in the 85th percentile or higher for age and gender), getting a hold on eating and activity habits now will be important. That's because experts say the critical period for preventing childhood obesity may be during the first two years of life. So now is the time to begin to weigh the scales in your toddler's favour. The goal won't be to put your toddler on a weight-loss diet – instead, it will be to balance the calories-in, calories-out equation so weight gain slows down and, as your toddler grows, stops outpacing height. Here's how:

- Check with the doctor. Before you take any action to regulate your toddler's weight, make sure you've checked in with your GP for advice and a sensible eating game plan that won't affect

Height and Weight

During the second year, your growing toddler will actually slow down in the growth department. Until his or her next big growth spurt (which usually happens during the tween years), you can expect your toddler's growth to be slow and steady. Here's how, on average, you can expect it to stack up (keeping in mind that most tots will fall somewhat higher or lower than these numbers):

12 to 15 months. By 15 months, the average little girl will weigh approximately 10.4 kg, with a height of about 77.5 cm. The average 15-month-old boy will weigh about 11.1 kg and stand 78.7 cm tall.

15 to 18 months. By 18 months, the average girl will weigh 11.1 kg and measure about 80 cm in height. By 18 months, the average boy will weigh in at 11.7 kg and measure approximately 81.3 cm in height.

18 to 24 months. The average 24-month-old girl will be 12.2 kg and 86.4 cm tall; the average 24-month-old boy will be 12.7 kg and 87.6 cm tall.

Be on the lookout: If your toddler's weight jumps more than 30 percentile points from one visit to the next (say, from the 40th to the 70th percentile), if your child's weight is more than 20 percentile points greater than his or her height (for instance, 30th percentile for height and 80th percentile for weight), or if your child is less than the 3rd percentile for weight and declining at each visit, talk to your toddler's doctor about what may be causing these growth issues.

growth or development. (It won't be a "diet" – toddlers need a wide range of nutrients and sufficient calories.)

- Focus on the right foods. Helping your little one acquire a taste for whole grains, fruits and vegetables, and lean protein – with only the occasional sugary treat – will go far in preventing future weight problems (and a host of health problems as well). Since too much dietary fat is usually the major culprit in the accumulation of too much body fat, it makes sense to limit excessive amounts of fat in her diet, too – particularly unhealthy fats, like the saturated fat in fries. But the operative word is *limit*. A young toddler shouldn't have her fat or cholesterol intake restricted (unless her doctor has advised this due to a family history of heart disease and/or high cholesterol).

- Focus on the right drinks. Many toddlers, especially those who still get most of their fluids from a bottle – or those who carry a beaker wherever they go – guzzle a lot of unneeded calories. Most often the fluid at fault is apple juice (which, incidentally, provides little nutrition for the calories). Weaning to a regular cup, if you haven't already, and diluting juices, particularly apple and apple-based juices, with water will help to cut calories safely.

- Have snack smarts. Tiny tummies – and busy, on-the-go bodies – can't go the four or five hours between meals without refuelling. But too many snacks can be a pitfall for a child who's gaining weight at too quick a pace – especially if those snacks are calorie-packed. Provide your toddler with a nutritious snack between breakfast and lunch, another between lunch and dinner, and a light bite before bed. But that should be it – all-day grazing (and an open-cabinet snack policy) can tip the scales fast.

- Put your toddler in control. Toddlers who are still being spoon-fed often consume more than they want or need. So give your toddler plenty of opportunity to self-feed – and when she loses interest in the meal, end it. No pushing to finish last bites, and no selling memberships in the clean-plate club.

- Feed for the right reasons. There's only one good reason for eating: hunger. Children who learn this important lesson at an early age rarely have eating problems of any kind later in life. Avoid the biscuit to stop the snivels, the chocolate to buy quiet in the supermarket aisles, the car-seat compliance treat. Instead, offer a kiss for the tears, engage in a supermarket game, sing a car-seat song. If you don't offer food for the wrong reasons (as a reward or bribe, as comfort, in place of attention, to banish boredom), your toddler won't eat for the wrong reasons.

- Model healthy eating habits. Don't look now, but your toddler's watching your every move, including your eating moves. If you're always chomping on chips or digging into ice cream, your toddler will follow your lead (to the biscuit tin). Instead, let your toddler catch you savouring your salad or snacking on fruit.

- Get moving. For toddlers who exercise little but their appetite, weight will soon become a problem. Structured classes aren't necessary, but plenty of opportunities to run, climb, jump, and walk are. And don't forget to join in – the family that gets a move on together stays healthy and fit together.

- Say no to TV. While exercise is proven to prevent obesity, television viewing has been proven to encourage it. If your little one spends a lot of time in front of the screen, nip that habit in the bud now – before it (and your toddler's waistline) expands. Limit electronic games, too, if your little one has already been bit by the computer bug.

- Watch the labels. Food labels, yes, but also the labels you put on your toddler. Don't say "You can't have a biscuit because you're too fat." Though the concept will likely still be well out of your little one's cognitive reach, it'll slowly start to sink in – and with it, possible negative body image issues that can stick. Instead of talking about dieting, talk about healthy eating: "Let's share a yummy peach because that will make us big and strong!"

Remember, no matter how concerned you might be about your toddler's weight, a weight-loss diet is never appropriate for a young child who's still growing. The goal, once again, will be to slow down the rate of gain while maintaining healthy growth. For more on healthy eating, see Chapter 4.

The Thin Toddler

"My son is so skinny, there's not an ounce of toddler chubbiness on him. Is he underweight?"

Thinking thin when you look at your little one? Thinness, like chubbiness, is often a matter of perception – usually a parent's perception. So what you might perceive as too thin may be just right for your toddler. Rather than trusting your eyes, check with the doctor to see if the numbers match up on the growth chart. Though toddlers are renowned for their central-casting dimples, some are naturally on the slim side – either because they're tall, very active, or just genetically predisposed. Bottom line: if the doctor is satisfied with your toddler's growth and general health, then you should be, too.

If the numbers do come up short (or underweight), it will be important for you to work together with the doctor to understand why, and what to do about it. Happily, most factors that can contribute to a toddler being underweight can be easily resolved. Here are some possible reasons for underweight:

- Too much fluid. Maybe your toddler is sucking down too much liquid, leaving too little room for solids. Cutting out the bottle and limiting access to a beaker can step up appetite and food intake (a regular cup isn't as easy to guzzle from).

- Too few calories. Maybe your super-busy bee isn't taking in enough calories to compensate for those that are being burned by all that running around. Or maybe the foods you're offering your tot are too low in fat or calories (some diet-conscious parents do this without realising it), or are so low in nutrition that they don't adequately fuel growth and weight gain. Take a look at your toddler's diet, and see if there's room for more calories in healthy forms (in other words, not in a cupcake).

- Too much pushing. Your job is to provide healthy food, his job is to eat enough to satisfy his appetite. Pushing your slim Jim to eat up will only lead him to push back (as in, "You can't make me eat!").

- Stress or illness. Sometimes, a stressed-out child doesn't eat well. If there's an obvious source of stress in your toddler's life (or yours – little ones are super sensitive to a parent's stress, too), try to remedy it, or offer extra attention and comfort to compensate for it. If your child's not eating well and is otherwise out of sorts, check in with the doctor to see if there could be an illness that needs treating.

Potbelly

"Our little girl is average weight for her size, but she has a big potbelly. Is that normal?"

A tubby tummy is as normal on a toddler as it is adorable. It's not until age 3 or 4, when the abdominal muscles gain maturity and strength, that most children start sporting a slimmer profile. And most do – that is, unless they start overdoing the junk food or underdoing the exercise. In the meantime, your toddler doesn't need any tummy tightening exercises or advice on sucking in her Buddha belly (definitely don't comment on it in a teasing way, since that could set up future body image problems). All she needs is a healthy diet and plenty of opportunities for fun physical activity.

If your toddler's tummy seems distended and is associated with discomfort or constipation, check with the doctor.

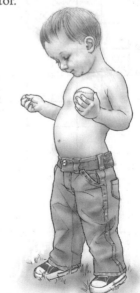

A tubby tummy is a toddler trademark.

Growth Charts

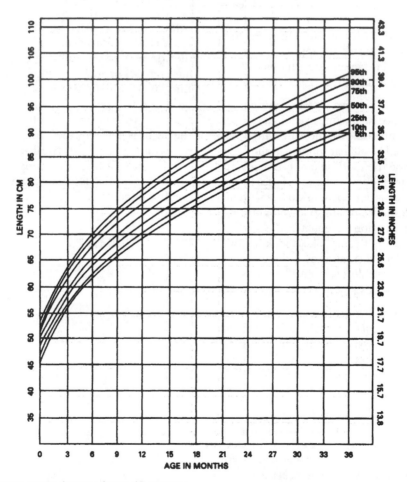

Girl's Height Chart

Percentiles: Birth To 36 Months

Source: National Center for Health Statistics

How does your little one measure up? You can plot that progress on these charts. The growth charts on these pages keep track of height and weight separately. There are separate charts for boys and girls. That's because even at this young age, boys tend to be taller, heavier, and grow faster than girls do.

Girl's Weight Chart

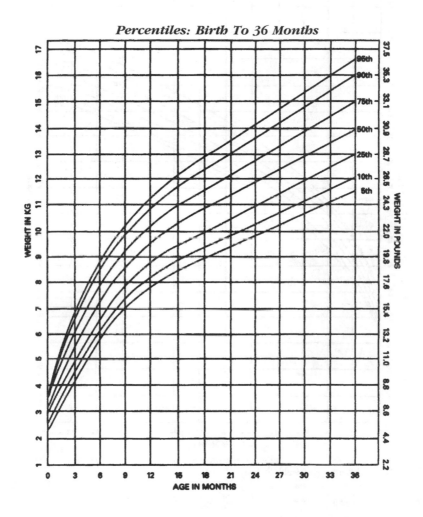

Percentiles: Birth To 36 Months

Boy's Height Chart

Percentiles: Birth To 36 Months

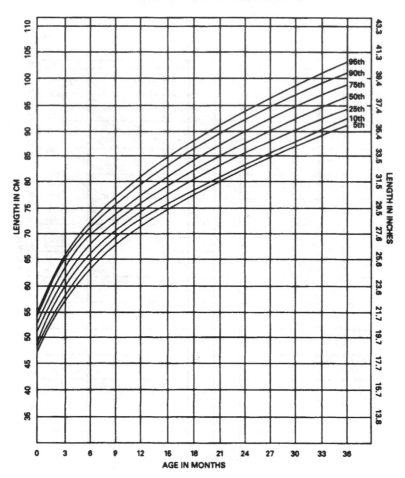

Source: National Center for Health Statistics

Boy's Weight Chart

Percentiles: Birth To 36 Months

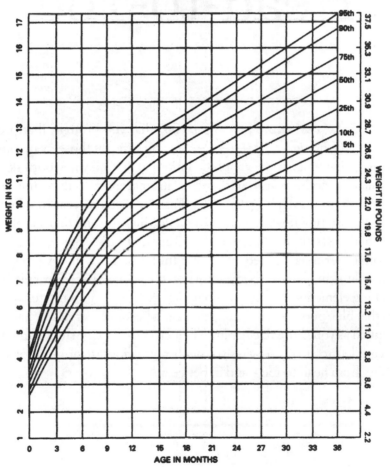

CHAPTER 2

Your Toddler, Head-to-Toe

....

I T WAS ONLY YESTERDAY, or so it seems, that you brought that precious little bundle home – only yesterday that you gazed at those teeny-tiny feet, changed that first nappy, smoothed lotion on that silky newborn skin, witnessed that first toothless grin, and watched in amazement as those numbers on the scale crept up at each baby weigh-in. Fast-forward one year (my, how time flies!) and those tiny feet are now a whole lot bigger, sometimes look a little funny (what's up with that tiptoeing?), and are in need of some walking shoes. That toothless grin has turned into a mouthful of teeth that have to be cared for. That silky skin, part of a body always on the go, is exposed to a plethora of skin-chafing elements. And nappy contents are a little more mysterious these days (is that blue poo?), even as nappy changes become ever more challenging. But as much as your little one has grown (all too fast), he or she still has plenty of growing left to do . . . leaving you with a growing list of questions about everything from head to toe – and in between.

Hair

HAIR CARE

Whether it's a mass of ringlets or a fine coating of down, every toddler's hair needs some daily care, if only to remove lunch from it. Here's what you need to know:

- Shampoo only as needed. Since oil glands on the scalp, like oil glands elsewhere on the body, don't become fully functional until puberty, daily shampoos are rarely necessary – except for toddlers who tend to get a lot of food, sand, or dirt in their hair, or those who have particularly oily scalps. Many toddlers – especially those with Afro-textured hair, or those with very dry hair or scalps – are best off with just a weekly shampoo (they may benefit from a little oil rub every now and then, too). Others require a shampoo every other day or even every third day – though more frequent shampooing is often needed in hot weather, when hair gets sweaty and sticky faster. Be sure to rinse well – a soapy residue can become a magnet for grime.

- Choose the right tools. Think gentle when you select brushes and combs. A brush should be flat, rather than curved, and have bristles with rounded ends. If your child has tight, curly hair, the bristles should be long, firm, and widely spaced. A comb – very useful for detangling, and a must have for children with extra-thick, frizzy, or Afro-textured hair – should have widely spaced, nonscratchy teeth.

- Brush up. Brushing helps to bring oil to the surface of the scalp, and that can be especially helpful if your toddler's scalp or hair is dry. It can also remove much of the food and dirt that works itself into toddler hair. But use a light touch when brushing or combing your toddler's hair, avoiding tugging or yanking. See the question that follows for detangling tips.

- Don't share when it comes to hair. As far as hair care implements are concerned, sharing isn't a virtue. Each member of the family should have his or her own comb and brush, and, to prevent transmission of head lice or other problems, should keep these styling tools to themselves. Combs and brushes should occasionally be washed in suds made with a dash of shampoo and warm water.

A Sticky Situation

You just shampooed your toddler last night, but now there's a blob of porridge stuck in her locks? Or maybe there's no time for a shampoo, but your little cauliflower cheese maniac has highlighted his hair with Cheddar sauce. The best way to deal with these bad hair days: use a spritz of detangling spray and carefully work those remnants of breakfast, lunch, and dinner out with a wide-tooth comb.

Hair-Brushing Hijinks

"My daughter puts up a fight whenever I try to brush her hair. But when I don't brush it, the tangles just get worse and worse."

Getting the brush-off when you try to brush your toddler's hair? Few toddlers like to sit still for styling, or even for the most cursory comb-out – and some start screaming and struggling the moment they spy a hairbrush headed their way.

Even though many 1-year-olds don't have a whole lot of hair to contend with, the hair they do have is often fine, delicate, and sometimes fragile – making the daily chore of brushing even more challenging. Multiply the hairs (some tots have a headful), and multiply the challenges.

To take the trauma (for both of you) out of detangling:

Open a salon. Set up your toddler on a chair or high chair in front of a mirror and play "hairdresser". While you're primping your client, allow her to primp one of her own: supply her with a favourite long-haired doll or stuffed animal and a hairbrush to style with.

Time for a Trim?

You may look forward to the hairdresser (if only for the scalp massage that comes with the shampoo), but toddlers often aren't such fans. A more likely scenario: your toddler starts squirming or bawling the minute the hair stylist (a perfect stranger) approaches with the scissors (an implement you've probably warned is dangerous) and a plastic bottle (whoa . . . what's that for?). And if you think about it, isn't that shear anxiety perfectly reasonable? Is it really any wonder that your tot's a moving target?

Even so, if your toddler has a fair amount of hair, the time will come for a trim. These tips may help keep haircutting from getting too hairy:

- Choose a hairdresser that aims to please kids. Bright smocks, fun-shaped chairs or boosters, balloons, toys, and videos to distract children while their hair is getting snipped are a big plus. But even more important is a hair stylist who's patient, experienced with squirming children, and willing to entertain and trim at the same time.

- Choose your words carefully. You're probably better off calling it a "trim" or "style" instead of a "cut". After all, your very literal little one associates cuts with pain, bleeding, and crying.

- Skip the suds. A few spritzes of water can dampen hair enough so the stylist can cut right to the trim, without the added trauma of shampooing.

- Be your toddler's booster chair. If your toddler balks at sitting alone on that big, high seat, ask if your lap is an option. Sitting on your lap may not be easy for you or for the stylist, but it may make this first experience more comfortable for your toddler. Hold your child on your lap facing the mirror while the front's being cut, then turn him or her around so he or she is facing you for the back trim. (You'll need a smock, too.)

- Try a trick. When you get to the hairdresser, put stickers on your toddler's shoes, so that there will be something interesting to look at when the stylist says "look down". Make funny faces in the mirror when it's time for your toddler to look straight ahead. What to do if he's fidgeting? Play "statue" (try practising in advance for best results) – you'll both get a giggle out of watching your images freeze in the mirror. And, of course, don't forget to bring toys – especially the ones your toddler loves clutching.

- Follow a trim with a treat. Remember, the haircut is your idea, not your toddler's. To make it a win-win, tie the haircut in with a favourite destination or special activity ("Today we're going to the playground, but first we'll stop to get your hair trimmed."). This may help take your toddler's mind off any anxiety – hopefully he or she will be too busy anticipating the fun. If your toddler hesitates at the hairdresser, offer a reminder: "Let's hurry, so we can get to the playground before it closes!"

Take two to untangle. Your toddler will be less likely to resist hair brushing if she's participating in it. When she gets tired of brushing her doll's hair, let her brush her own. You take the left side, and let her take the right. Then switch sides so you can go over what she's done. Or simply take turns ("Now it's my turn to brush"). Just be sure you get last licks. If you're brave enough, you can even let her tackle your hair with a comb or brush (but be ready to do some major detangling afterward).

Tackle tangles gently. A toddler's scalp – like all of her skin – is tender, especially if it isn't protected by much in the way of hair. So have an extra-gentle touch. Use a wide-tooth comb (fine-tooth ones can tug and tear) or a brush that has bristles with rounded tips. To reduce pulling, hold the hair at the roots while you work on the ends. For longer hair, try a spray-on detangler to help untangle between shampoos.

Curtail tangling. Sometimes the easiest way to deal with a problem is to get rid of it. If your toddler's tresses are on the long side, consider a short, low-maintenance haircut – it'll make untangling a breeze. Or try plaits (but don't pull too tightly – it can cause hair loss) or putting it up in pigtails. Hair that's worn loose isn't just vulnerable to tangles, but to sticky blobs of food, mud, paint, and more – all of which can dry into major roadblocks for the comb and brush.

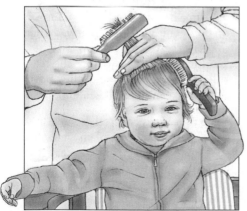

Allowing your toddler to brush her hair while you work on the tangles may make the job easier.

No matter what your child's hairstyle, combing out tangles before each shampoo will make combing out after the shampoo less of a trial. So will smoothing suds through the hair (instead of vigorously working hair up into a snarl when lathering), and using a tangle-reducing conditioner (or a shampoo-conditioner combo) that's designed for babies and toddlers.

Take bows (or hair slides) when it's over. Do her hair up with pretty accessories (let her choose them) as the reward for sitting through the brushing. And don't forget to reward your toddler's "client" the same way. Do be sure, however, that your tot can't take off any small (and potentially chokeable) accessories from her hair on her own. For safety's sake, remove small hair slides or bows from your toddler's hair before putting her to bed, and store them safely out of her reach.

Shampoo Struggles

"To say washing our son's hair is a struggle is an understatement. Is there any way to make it less of a hassle?"

Hair washing can be hair-raising when you're trying to shampoo and rinse a toddler. But you can minimise the struggles if you keep these shampoo-surviving techniques in mind:

- Keep your cool. If you anticipate a struggle, you're sure to get one – so approach hair washing calmly. You may get the struggle anyway, but the more unflappable you are, the less flap you'll get.

- Keep it streamlined. Have everything at the ready when you begin (water at the perfect temperature, shampoo and a towel nearby) so that neither of you needs to endure the shampooing

Chemicals in Shampoo?

Yes, of course there are chemicals in shampoos . . . in fact there are chemicals everywhere (in the air, in the foods you eat, on products you touch). Some are bad, most are benign, and others are controversial or still being studied. One chemical that falls into the latter category is phthalate. Found in soft plastics (like food packaging and plastic wrap) as well as in shampoos, lotions, and powders, phthalate has generated a lot of questions about safety – and it's still too early for definitive answers. One study suggests that phthalates absorbed through the skin could have effects on the endocrine and reproductive systems of infants. Others in the scientific community are not convinced – they maintain that the amount of phthalates children are exposed to isn't enough to be harmful. In other words, the jury is still out.

Should you toss your toddler's baby shampoo? Never moisturise those chapped cheeks again? It probably isn't necessary to go that far, at least not until that jury comes back in. But with demand growing for phthalate-free products, the selection's growing, too – which means it's getting easier to limit your toddler's exposure. When you have the option, look for products that are labelled "phthalate-free." Since the scent in a product is often the component that contains the phthalate, you can also reach for products labelled "fragrance-free", or products that contain natural fragrance. Keep in mind, however, that greener products typically carry a steeper price tag. If you can't afford the extra cost, don't stress. Don't hesitate to use a product that contains phthalate, either, if it's medically necessary.

ordeal any longer than necessary. To reduce the number of hair-washing steps, use a one-step conditioning shampoo instead of shampoo plus separate conditioner. Or spray on a no-rinse detangler after you've rinsed out the shampoo.

- Keep it short. The shorter the hair, the shorter the shampoo. If your toddler's hair is long or hard to deal with, consider an easy-care cut.

- Keep it gentle. Always choose a shampoo that won't irritate skin or eyes (most baby and toddler shampoos are gentle, but sensitivities vary from child to child).

- Keep it fun. To minimise the struggles, maximise the fun. Choose foaming shampoo with appealing natural aromas (always offer a sniff) or a brand with favourite characters on the bottle to keep your tot diverted.

- Stay tangle-free. There'll be less tangling if you "pat" the shampoo through the wet hair gently, rather than fiercely working up a lather. Working out tangles before the bath will also facilitate a smoother post-shampoo comb-out.

- Keep those eyes covered. Even a "no-tears" shampoo (even plain water, for that matter) can produce tears if it gets into your toddler's eyes. Protect his peepers by having him hold a flannel across his forehead to protect his eyes. Or use a shampoo visor or child-size swimming goggles to keep his eyes dry.

- Control the rinse. A handheld spray nozzle offers more control, and less risk of a misdirection mishap. If you don't have one, use a child's plastic watering can or cup. After shampooing, your toddler can play with it in the bath.

- Give him a turn. Your toddler may feel less victimised if he's allowed to shampoo a waterproof doll or other water-friendly toy.

- Let him watch. Mount an unbreakable mirror in the bath so shampooing can become a spectator sport. Making "suds sculptures" with your toddler's hair can also be diverting.

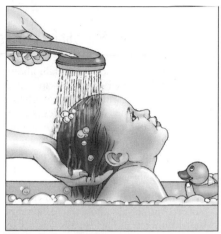

When rinsing out shampoo, lean your toddler's head back so the soap doesn't get into his or her eyes.

Eyes

EYE CARE

From the moment they pop open in the all-too-early morning until the moment they finally, reluctantly, close at night, your toddler's eyes are busy soaking up – and learning about – the world around him or her. To protect your little one's precious peepers for a lifetime of sight, start now with:

- Regular checkups. It's important to catch vision or eye problems early, so be sure your toddler's eyes are checked at all regular checkups, and call between checkups if you have any vision or eye concerns at all (Do his eyes appear crossed? Does she seem to have a hard time recognising small objects from across the room?). If the doctor turns up anything out of the ordinary, your little one may be referred to an eye specialist, or ophthalmologist, for evaluation. In general, children

who were born prematurely are more vulnerable to vision problems, so they may need more frequent eye examinations. Check with the doctor.

- Protection from the sun. Even if you've applied sunscreen to vulnerable skin, your little one's still not sun-ready. Those adorable eyes need to be protected from the sun, too. Get your toddler used to wearing a wide-brimmed hat when outdoors in strong midday sun. Sunglasses can also be a good option, and wearing them is a great habit to get into early, though it may be difficult to get your toddler to keep them on (you'll have a better shot at it if you wear a pair, too – toddlers love to copy their parents). When buying sunglasses, be sure to choose ones with UV-blocking lenses, which block 99 per cent of both UVA and UVB light. Unlabelled or toy sunglasses may be cheap, but they're probably worse

Spotting Vision Problems

Since toddlers can't complain about not being able to see well – and have no way of knowing that their vision isn't normal – vision problems that aren't discovered at a regular checkup can easily go undiagnosed. That's why it's so important for you to keep an eye out for symptoms of vision problems in your little one, especially if eye issues run in your family. But even if they don't, you should know the behaviours and symptoms that can tip you off to a vision problem that needs checking out. Call the doctor if you notice any of the following in your toddler:

- An obvious inability to see well: your toddler is extremely clumsy or stumbles a lot (beyond normal toddler clumsiness; see page 73), or seems not to notice or recognise objects or people, either close up or at a distance.

- Frequent squinting unrelated to bright sunlight, or face scrunching when trying to perform a visual task. (Either of these can also be a temporary habit that has nothing to do with vision – many toddlers go through experimental squinting and scrunching phases.)

- Apparent sensitivity to light (your toddler seems to squint in discomfort when a light is turned on in a dimly lit room or when stepping outside into bright sunlight) or frequent staring at lights.

- Eyes that bulge or seem to "bounce" in rapid, rhythmic movements.

- Frequent tilting of the head to one side, as though trying to see better.

- Holding the body rigid or at an angle when trying to look at distant objects.

- Repeated covering or shutting of one eye in apparent discomfort (as opposed to covering or shutting an eye periodically to see how the world looks with just one eye open, which is just a sign of normal toddler curiosity).

- Holding books, toys, and other objects close to the face in order to see them better, or consistently sitting or standing too close to the TV (though this, too, can just be a toddler's fascination with the world from different perspectives, not necessarily a vision issue).

- Entirely avoiding activities that require good vision (such as looking at books – though some toddlers just can't sit still long enough for these activities, anyway).

- Eyes that look crossed or wandering, or that don't move in unison.

- Pupils (the small black spot in the centre of the eye) that are sometimes or always unequal in size (they should work simultaneously: getting larger in dim light, smaller in bright light) or that appear white instead of black.

than no sunglasses at all, since they can provide a false sense of protection. Keep sunglasses from sliding off during play by attaching them with a specially designed child's glasses band (see the illustration, page 30).

- Protection from injury. So your toddler's always prone to bumps and bruises – but eyes can also be injured at play. Never allow your child to play with toys that have sharp points or rods, with sticks, or with pencils and pens, except under close supervision (never allow these items in a moving car); cushion sharp corners on furniture (especially tables that are eye-level for your toddler); teach your toddler never to run with toys in hand; keep all toxic substances (such as cleaning supplies, dishwasher detergent, and garden products, many of which can cause eye damage on contact) out of your toddler's reach; and keep your child away when the grass is being mowed or leaves are being blown.

■ Protection from television. While (contrary to your mother's warnings) no amount of TV watching will actually damage a child's eyes, prolonged viewing can cause temporary eyestrain. If you let your toddler watch TV, keep the viewing to no more than 30 minutes a day to minimise the strain on those beautiful little eyes. For more reasons to skip TV entirely or limit viewing to a lot less than those 30 minutes, see page 281.

For information on eye injuries and infections, see page 448.

Blinking

"My toddler has been blinking a lot lately. She doesn't seem to be in any discomfort, but should I have her eyes checked?"

Most toddlers go through a brief blinking phase at some point. Often, it starts when a tot notices that opening and shutting her eyes quickly makes for an interesting visual perspective. Sometimes, it's a copycat behaviour – picked up (like so many other habits) from siblings or nursery peers. Either way, when it's not accompanied by other symptoms, blinking is nothing to worry about – generally, the behaviour runs its course within a month or two, as it loses its fascination. Nagging or

otherwise calling attention to your little one's blinking will only give it longer-lasting appeal.

If the blinking is virtually nonstop or seems to bother your child, or if she's blinking and doing a lot of eye rubbing that's not related to sleepiness, check with the doctor. Occasionally, blinking is a sign of a tic. These repetitive muscle twitches are common in children, generally benign, but worth mentioning at the next checkup. If you think your toddler is blinking because there's something wrong with her eye, see the box on the facing page.

VISION PROBLEMS

Like eye colour and shape, vision problems are also often passed down from Mum and Dad – so if you wear glasses or contacts, you'll want to watch your toddler even more closely for signs that he or she isn't seeing clearly (see facing page for symptoms to look out for). While abnormal sight is often difficult to spot in a toddler (who not only can't complain about having a vision problem, but has no way of knowing it's a problem in the first place), early diagnosis and treatment can keep a condition from getting worse. Here are the vision problems that occur most commonly among toddlers:

Shortsightedness (myopia). More common in children who have a shortsighted parent or parents, myopia is the inability to see objects clearly when they're more than a short distance away. Though some children become shortsighted in the second or third year of life, the condition more often develops later. Signs and symptoms include squinting, holding books and other objects very close, and having difficulty identifying distant objects. If your child is shortsighted, he or she will need glasses (see page 29).

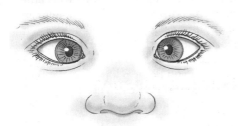

Cross-eyes: When one eye (or both) wanders inward. You may only notice this in photos.

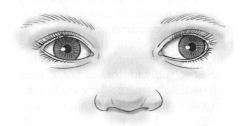

Walleyes: When one eye (or both) wanders outward.

Longsightedness (hyperopia). All babies and young children tend to be somewhat longsighted (unable to see objects clearly when they're very close), but in most, vision normalises by age 5. Kids who remain longsighted usually have a family history of the condition. Signs and symptoms are difficult to detect in younger children (since they all have some trouble with up-close vision). Glasses aren't necessary unless longsightedness is extreme, interfering with play and other activities.

Astigmatism. Astigmatism causes vision that is blurred or wavy (it's sort of like looking in a fun-house mirror). Children who are either shortsighted or longsighted are the most likely to have astigmatism, which is usually present at birth. Like shortsightedness, the signs and symptoms of astigmatism are squinting, holding books and objects close to the face, and sitting close to the TV. Glasses can usually correct astigmatism.

Cross-eyes (strabismus). Strabismus is when the eyes can't focus in unison, and it's more common in children with a family history of the condition and in those who are longsighted. Infants often appear cross-eyed for the first few months of life for a variety of reasons (including that cute newborn puffiness),

and sometimes their eyes seem not to work as a coordinated pair. But by the middle of the first year, the eyes should be able to move right and left and up and down in tandem, and focus together all of the time. In about 4 per cent of children, however, the lack of eye coordination persists. The wandering eye (or eyes) may drift inward towards the nose (cross-eye), or outward (walleye), or up or down – some of the time or all the time. The condition may be subtle, and in some cases it's only noticeable in photos. If your toddler rubs or covers one eye frequently, tilts his or her head to try to coordinate vision, or is reluctant to play games that require judging distances (such as catching a rolling ball), mention it to the doctor. Treatment may include medicated eye drops to blur vision in the stronger eye or placing a patch over it (for short periods each day) to force the use of the weaker one, glasses to equalise vision, and sometimes, exercises to strengthen the eye muscles.

Lazy eye (amblyopia). Lazy eye is when vision is lost in one eye because it's being chronically underused (or not used). The condition is the most common cause of vision loss in children and can go unnoticed by both child and parent. It can happen in one of three ways:

- Cross-eyes (strabismus). In this case, a toddler's eyes don't move or focus in unison because of a slight muscle imbalance. To avoid seeing double, he or she subconsciously opts to use only one eye. The brain eventually loses the ability to recognise images sent from the unused (or seldom used) eye.

- Longsightedness (or astigmatism) in one eye. The toddler uses only the eye with the clearer picture. The brain eventually stops accepting signals from the unused eye.

- A condition that blocks vision (such as ptosis; see below), if it just affects one eye.

At this age, lazy eye – no matter what's triggering it – is nearly always correctable, usually with an eye patch, eye drops, and/or glasses. By the time a child has reached school age, however, it may be too late to correct the condition, because the brain has already decided that it isn't ever going to pay attention to the images produced by the affected eye. That's why it's so important to get a vision screening for your toddler if you even suspect lazy eye or another vision problem.

Droopy eyelids (ptosis). Some children are born with ptosis (which is often inherited), while others develop it later. Signs and symptoms include an enlarged, heavy, or drooping eyelid, though occasionally both eyelids are affected. In some cases, the lid totally covers the eye, inhibiting vision, or it distorts the cornea, causing astigmatism. Ptosis requires evaluation and treatment by an ophthalmologist to prevent the development of lazy eye (when the child and the child's brain learn to depend on the eye with the normal lid and ignore the images from the droopy-lidded eye). When the problem

is weak eyelid muscles, surgery (usually performed when the child is 3 or 4) can strengthen them and give the lid a normal appearance.

Getting Glasses

"We just got word that our 20-month-old needs glasses. He's so active, it's hard to imagine him wearing them."

While it might be hard to imagine those baby blues, browns, or greens covered up by glasses – or those glasses staying put on a toddler who never does – corrective lenses will make a remarkable difference in how your little one sees the world, and can have a major impact on all developmental fronts. And the logistics aren't as tricky as you might think, either. In fact, getting used to glasses as a 1-year-old is generally easier than acclimatising to them later.

Given your toddler's on-the-go, likely collision-prone lifestyle, you're best off with lenses made of regular plastic or of polycarbonate (a lightweight, strong, and shatterproof plastic, which reduces the risk of accidental eye injury). When selecting glasses, consider, too, how they'll stay in place. For infants and young tots, elastic straps are usually substituted for the earpieces. They hold the glasses in place and will allow your little one to lie on his side, roll around, and otherwise act his age without knocking the glasses off. Another age-appropriate option is comfort cables (also called cable temples), which secure glasses with earpieces that curl around the ears rather than pressing against the head (see illustration on the following page). Flexible hinges are also a good idea, since they tolerate more abuse (which they'll get).

Be patient but persistent while your toddler adjusts to wearing glasses. If the glasses are whipped right off, try again a little later. But don't allow too much wiggle room. Your toddler needs to understand that wearing the glasses isn't optional or negotiable. And while it's likely to be several years before you'll be able to count on him to care responsibly for his glasses, it's never too early to begin the training process. Teach your toddler how to take off the glasses with two hands, without touching the lenses, and show him how they should stay in their case when they're not being worn.

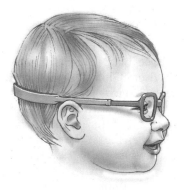 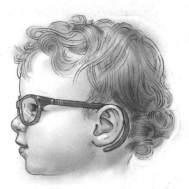

On infants and young toddlers, glasses are generally kept in place by an elastic strap (left) in place of ear pieces. Some toddlers do well with comfort cables, which curve around the ears (right).

Ears

EAR CARE

They come in all shapes and sizes (though they're uniformly cute) – and like that pair of peepers, your toddler's two standard-issue ears must last a lifetime. Though genetics and other factors can also play a part, how well those ears will function over that lifetime depends a lot on the care they get in the early years of life. To keep your toddler's ears in the best working order possible:

- Be alert to signs of hearing loss (see box, facing page) and report any concerns to your child's doctor. It's likely your toddler was tested for hearing issues as a newborn, but many problems aren't present at birth – they develop over time. That's why a parent's observations are extremely important, too, and can often detect an as yet undiagnosed hearing deficit. The next formal hearing tests will be when your child starts primary school (unless a hearing problem is suspected earlier).

- At bath time, clean the outside crevices of your toddler's ears with a damp, soft cloth or cotton swab, and check ears carefully for foreign objects (toddlers are known to stick

Signs of a Hearing Problem

Many toddlers may seem not to hear at least half of what their parents say, but in most cases, it's just a matter of selective listening or inattention. The child who truly doesn't hear well usually exhibits one or more of the following signs of hearing loss (although some of these may also be exhibited by a child with normal hearing):

- An apparent inability to hear what is said by others, all or part of the time.

- Difficulty hearing when a sound comes from the side or the rear, or when the child is not directly facing the person who's speaking. Many hearing-impaired children instinctively learn some rudimentary lip-reading and understand more when they can see the speaker's lips.

- A consistent lack of response when spoken to quietly.

- A consistent inattentiveness to any verbal or other auditory cues.

- An apparent inability to follow any directions (more so than is age-appropriate).

- A vocabulary – both receptive (the words that are understood) and spoken – that is more limited than it should be for the child's age.

- A lack of response to music – a child doesn't clap, sing along, or move rhythmically to music, or enjoy or recognise frequently played tunes, even those designed especially for children.

- Lack of response to the nuances of language (can't seem to tell from the tone of your voice whether you're angry, sad, excited, and so on).

- Lack of response to sounds in the environment (the ring of the telephone or doorbell; the sound of the garage door opening, signalling Mum or Dad's arrival home; the buzzer on a timer; the rain on the roof; the howling of the wind).

- A tendency to favour one ear when turning towards a sound.

If you have the slightest suspicion that your little one has a hearing problem, get it checked out quickly with the doctor – even if routine testing at birth was completely normal. Sometimes, a hearing deficit that shows up in the second year is a result of persistent fluid in the ears (due to repeated infections), in which case treatment can resolve it; see page 384. In other cases, it's due to another type of infection or syndrome, an injury, a medication, or a previously undiagnosed congenital defect. See page 401 for more on hearing impairment.

items into their ears). Do not probe the inside of the ear with a finger, a cotton swab, or – as the expression goes – anything smaller than your elbow. Probing, even in the name of cleaner ears, could puncture the eardrum and/or push wax farther into the ear (where it can encourage infection or interfere with hearing).

- Wax, though icky to look at, isn't usually something that needs removing. Secreted by glands in the ears, that gooey gunk actually serves an important purpose – helping to protect the sensitive ear canals by trapping potentially harmful dirt and debris that would otherwise find its way in, then working its way out, taking that

Sound Defence

While your little one's ears can handle most day-to-day sounds, exposure to excessive noise is linked to hearing loss. So it makes sense to keep your toddler's environment as free of extraneous, loud noise as possible. Here's how:

- Steer clear of toys that make loud sounds (you should be able to speak normally over the noise).

- Monitor the volume of television and music in your home and in the car. Maximum volume should never be louder than normal speech – and if you can't talk easily over it, it's too loud.

- When buying new appliances or power tools, look for those that are quieter.

- Limit your toddler's exposure to very noisy situations where you need to shout in order to be heard (at a fireworks display or football match, around drilling, lawn mowing, vacuuming, and so on). When it's unavoidable, have him or her wear soundproofing ear muffs.

- Teach your child to cover his or her ears when hearing a loud noise, like a passing fire engine's siren. Make this more fun by covering your ears, too, and calling your hands "ear muffs".

- Teach your child never to shout in anyone else's ears or to let someone shout in his or her ears. And practise the sound control you preach. Don't scream loudly, at least not in or near your toddler's ears.

If you think your toddler may be exhibiting signs of hearing loss, see page 31, and check with the doctor.

---

rubbish with it. It is possible, however, to have too much of this good thing – excessive amounts of earwax can occasionally build up in the ear canal. If you're concerned about a waxy buildup that you've noticed in your toddler's ears, check with the doctor, who may remove it, recommend drops to help loosen it up, or suggest you ignore it. Never try to remove wax yourself, even with a cotton swab. Not only could you push the goo up farther into the ear canal, but there's a very real risk of puncturing your toddler's eardrum (yes, with a cotton swab). As for wax that's hanging around the outer ear, wipe it away gently with a wet flannel.

- If you suspect an ear infection (see page 382), check with the doctor.

Ear Piercing

"I'd like to pierce my daughter's ears. Is she too young?"

Technically, a girl's never too young – or too old – to join the pierced ear club. Still, whether you're eager to pierce for cultural or family tradition reasons, for the fashion statement, or for the gender announcement (as in, "I'm a girl, people!"), there are some issues to consider before letting the piercing gun near your little one's lobes:

- The possibility of infection. Infections are common in the first few months after a piercing (for people of any age), and because your toddler probably won't have the words to tell you that her ear is itchy, sore, or tender, an infection can get out of hand pretty quickly – and before you're even aware of it.

- The danger of small parts. Your toddler could manage to take off her earrings to play with (look at this cool toy!), or they could accidentally fall off and wind up in her hands. The potential problem? She could prick herself with a stud or swallow (or choke on) one or more of the parts.

- The possibility of allergy. Some people are allergic to the metals in earrings, though it's often possible to avoid this problem by using only 14-carat gold or surgical steel studs and butterflies.

- In some toddlers, scarring. If your little one tends to get lumpy scars (a.k.a. keloids), she may be prone to them after piercing, too.

For these reasons, most doctors recommend holding off on piercing until a child is at least 4, and preferably closer to 8 years old (about the age she can take care of her pierced ears herself). Still, it's a perfectly safe procedure for young children – as long as it's done under sterile conditions by someone who is qualified (there are many beauty salons that offer ear piercing) and – here's the biggie – if you can get your toddler to sit still long enough to get them done. Keep in mind, too, that piercing hurts (remember that day at the salon?).

If you choose to pierce now, be extra careful to follow the normal post-piercing protocol: clean her lobes daily by dabbing them with a cotton ball saturated with surgical spirit or the solution given to you by the piercing place and rotate the earrings each morning and evening (to keep them from sticking to the holes), using clean fingers. If you notice any signs of infection (redness, swelling, pus or crusting, tenderness, or bleeding) call your child's doctor.

One last caveat: save dangling and hoop earrings until your tot is grown up – they can be pulled by other children (or by your child herself), possibly tearing the earlobe. If your little one starts trying to remove her earrings or play with them, stop inserting the earrings and let the holes close up. You can always have her ears repierced when she's a little older and more responsible.

Teeth

TOOTH CARE

The second year is a busy, busy time in a child's mouth. By the time they turn 2 to 2½ years old, most tots will sport a full set of 20 primary teeth. Though these baby teeth aren't for keeps, they'll take your child through the next 5 to 10 years – in fact, the last of them won't be replaced by permanent teeth until somewhere between ages 12 and 13. And since each tooth is vulnerable to decay from the moment it breaks through the gum (in fact, decay is most common in the first 6 months after a tooth erupts), it's definitely important to make good dental hygiene a priority early on.

So, if you haven't already done so, get your toddler into the habit of brushing – and being brushed – regularly each morning (after breakfast)

Tooth Problems Don't Fall Far from the Tree

Have a mouthful of strong, healthy teeth – or rows of fillings and crowns? Oral hygiene, diet, and overall health all play a significant role in your child's dental future, but so do genetics. Check your immediate family tree, and if you discover a pedigree of problem mouths, be especially proactive when it comes to your toddler's oral care. Also, let the dentist know about a strong family history of dental issues so he or she can help maximise prevention. One treatment shown to prevent cavities in young teeth: a fluoride varnish that the dentist can easily paint on once a year.

and evening (after any bedtime snack). Here's how:

- Select a toothbrush designed for young children, with a small head and soft, rounded bristles. To make toothbrushing more palatable for your tot, choose a brush that's decorated with favourite characters or with lights that flash and/or music that plays for 2 minutes (the recommended amount of time to spend brushing). Keep in mind, however, that bells, whistles, and a hefty price tag don't make a toothbrush inherently more effective. The secret to a thorough tooth cleaning is in the brushing technique, not the brush.

- Be the designated brusher. Until your child is up to the challenge of thorough brushing (which can happen any time between ages 5 and 10, depending on the child), you'll be in charge of brushing. Working one tooth at a time, use a gentle back and forth motion across the chewing and inner surfaces (finish one side first before going on to the other so you don't lose track). Switch to a circular motion along the sides and the outer gum lines (with the brush at a 45-degree angle). Lightly brush the gums where teeth haven't yet erupted, or wipe them with a gauze pad, baby finger brush, or facecloth, and also do a gentle once-over on the tongue (where a lot of bacteria can hang out). If your toddler resists brushing altogether or your help with brushing (and most will), see the next question.

- Start teaching your little one how to rinse after brushing (most toddlers master the rinse and spit around age 2). As always, it's easiest to teach through example: show him or her how you lean over the sink and say "ptooe". Rinsing is important not only because it removes the toothpaste before it's swallowed, but it also eliminates bits of loosened food that would otherwise resettle on the teeth.

- Consider skipping the toothpaste until your toddler can be relied on to rinse and spit. Though it can definitely make brushing more appealing (a major plus, for sure), it doesn't necessarily make it more effective. If you use toothpaste earlier on, choose an infant/toddler formula that's fluoride-free to avoid ingesting too much fluoride (overdosing can lead to teeth that are permanently stained). Once rinsing and spitting are mastered, you can begin to put a pea-size or smaller amount of fluoridated toothpaste on the brush, but watch out for toothpaste eaters. Some kids will gobble the stuff when you're not looking.

- Once any two teeth have grown in side by side – even if they're not exactly touching – it's time to start flossing. Yes, really, flossing. Flossing is as essential to good dental health as brushing and rinsing – and a really important habit for your tot to get into. Once again, you'll be on floss duty until your child's much older, at least 7 or 8. Which is easier said than done, both because it's difficult to manoeuvre large adult hands around such a tiny toddler mouth, and because most tots will not sit long enough to be fully flossed. Realistically, unless you have an unusually cooperative toddler, you probably won't get through the entire mouth every day, and that's okay – it's more about getting into the habit than it is about getting the job done. Focus first on molars – if there are any – and work your way back to front. Gently does it.

- Don't forget to explain. No, toddlers aren't always motivated by messaging, but it's good to build the benefits of good oral hygiene into the conversation anyway. When you're brushing and flossing, remind him or her that keeping those teeth clean helps them stay strong and healthy, so they won't get "sore". Also point out that strong teeth will let him or her eat yummy food. When your little one drinks milk or eats cheese or yogurt, reinforce: "Healthy foods make your teeth healthy, too!"

Toothbrushing Tussles

"My toddler clamps his mouth shut when I try to brush his teeth. I'm tempted to give up trying."

The tussle of the toothbrush is just another skirmish in your toddler's stubborn struggle for autonomy – in this case, autonomy over his mouth (which, he's discovered, is a cinch to control). Since surrender on his side is unlikely, and surrender on yours isn't smart – after all, even baby teeth need to be protected from cavities – a little creative compromise is called for:

Brush in style. Let your toddler choose two or three colourful child-size toothbrushes at the shop (be sure the bristles are soft and of good quality). Then let him select the one he wants to use at brushing time. This helps defuse the control issue (even though he can't decide whether or not to brush, he can decide what to brush with) and may distract him enough so that he'll forget to protest.

Strike the right position. It'll be easier to manoeuvre around your toddler's mouth if you're positioned right. Cradle his head in one arm while you brush

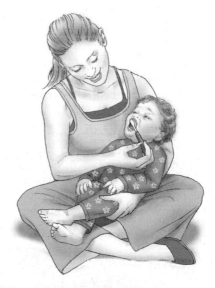

Approaching your tot from behind and tilting his or her head back slightly may give you the best visibility and manoeuvrability for toothbrushing. Or you can sit on the floor, seat your child in your lap, and have him or her lean back against you.

Time for Fluoride Toothpaste?

Of course you're eager to prevent tooth decay in your poppet's pearly whites, especially if you've had your share of cavities. But don't reach for the fluoride toothpaste just yet. Although a tiny amount of fluoride helps strengthen a child's teeth and reduces the risk of decay, large amounts can actually stain teeth permanently, a condition called "fluorosis". The British Dental Health Foundation recommends children under 3 use a toothpaste with a fluoride level of around 1000 ppm (parts per million). Ask the dentist if your toddler should be taking a fluoride supplement and at what dose. The answer will depend on how much fluoride is in your local water, and how much water your little one takes in from the tap, assuming he or she drinks tap water or consumes drinks or food prepared with tap water.

In any case, it really isn't the tooth-paste that cleans your toddler's teeth – it's the technique. Most dentists agree that water does the job just as well as, if not better than, paste. Still, the flavour kick that toothpaste offers can be motivating to many reluctant brushers. If your toddler is one of them, use a pea-size or smaller dab of toothpaste on his or her brush. Spread it out and press it into the bristles so that it can't be easily licked off. Explain that toothpaste is for cleaning, not for eating. And don't forget to start teaching the fine art of rinsing and spitting.

with the other, or for even more control (and a better view of what you're doing), have him lie on the floor with his head in your lap. Or sit on the floor with him on your lap, his head leaned against you (see illustration on the previous page).

Let him do it himself. Though you're the brushing boss, you'll get more cooperation if you team up. First, give your toddler his own brush to do some preliminary brushing. Or, if you find he cooperates better with the promise of a reward ahead, reverse the order: you start, he finishes. Don't worry about his technique or the condition of his toothbrush (the bristles will soon become flattened and misshapen from being chewed on) – just let him get the job done the best way he knows how. Praise his efforts, even if the toothbrush doesn't really make its mark. As he becomes a more skilled (and thorough) brusher, you may be able to let him take over the morning brushing completely, while you continue to help out at bedtime. But don't expect really proficient, independent brushing for many years to come.

Letting your toddler "brush the teeth" of a stuffed animal or doll (using a toothbrush reserved for play) or even brush yours may make him more amenable to having the brush wielded on him.

Then do it yourself. After you've told your toddler what a great job he's done on his teeth, take your turn – using a different brush. Letting him hold the toothbrush along with you will let him maintain some control over the process, as will giving him a complete brush-by-brush as you go ("These two teeth look nice and clean, let's try the next two"). Injecting a little levity may also loosen your toddler up a bit. Pretend to go for the wrong body part: "It's time to brush your tummy!" Or try the old favourite: "I see a giraffe (or an elephant, or a turtle) in there – let's see if I can get it out with the toothbrush."

Check each other. When the brushing's done, it's time to check your work and his. Challenge him to open his mouth as wide as he can so you can inspect his teeth for lingering bits of food (an older toddler may enjoy checking his teeth in the mirror, too). You can also have him check after you've brushed your own teeth, or after other family members have brushed theirs. Make him the official tooth checker.

Teething, Round Two

"Our 15-month-old seems to be getting molars now. He's a lot more miserable with them than he was with his other teeth."

He's miserable for good reason. Because of their large size and double edge, first molars (which usually make their appearance some time between 13 and 19 months) are at least twice as hard to cut as incisors – and for many children that means at least twice as much ouch.

To soothe your toddler's pain, turn to some of the same standbys that helped him through earlier teething episodes, like rubbing his gums with a clean finger or letting him chomp on a refrigerator-chilled teething ring. Chilled yogurt or frozen banana may also soothe those sore gums, as may a cup of icy cold water (don't leave ice in it, though). Other old teething relief favourites should be shelved now that your tot has teeth (a chilled carrot, for instance, because he's capable of biting

off a chokable chunk, or teething biscuits, because their high carbohydrate content could lead to tooth decay if they're mouthed all day long). A topical teething soother (like Bonjela) can numb gums briefly (usually for about a half hour), but probably shouldn't be applied more than four times a day – which means it won't provide around-the-clock relief. Your child's doctor might also recommend an ibuprofen or a paracetamol suspension when the pain is at its worst, probably at bedtime, and especially if teething pain interferes with your little one's eating and sleeping.

Teeth and Sweets

Brushing and flossing, along with the right amount of fluoride (from water, toothpaste, or supplements), are a great first line of defence against tooth decay. But unless you're planning to follow your toddler around with a toothbrush and a spool of floss, there are other protective measures you should be taking, too. First, skip sugary drinks and limit even 100 per cent fruit juice to no more than 120 ml to 180 ml ounces a day, and always water juice down before serving it to your toddler. Second, stick mainly to complex carbs, since refined carbs (bread, crackers, and teething biscuits made with white flour) quickly turn into sugar on your toddler's pearly whites, posing as much of a cavity risk as a boiled sweet. And most important, never put your little one to sleep with a bottle or beaker of anything but water (pooled liquids increase the risk of tooth decay as well).

Tooth Timetable

There's a wide range of normal when it comes to tooth eruptions – some babies and toddlers start cutting their teeth very early, while others take their own sweet tooth time. Here's when you can expect your tot's teeth to appear – on average:

12 to 15 months. By now, most tots will already be sporting some teeth in their adorable little mouths, including the upper and lower central incisors. The upper and lower lateral incisors should also be making their debut about now if they didn't already erupt during the first year. First (or front) molars begin to appear early in the second year, though some late tooth eruptors may not start cutting those molars until age 2½.

15 to 18 months. Watch out, Dracula – here come your toddler's fang teeth (better known in dental circles as canines). The upper canines usually make their appearance a few months before the lower ones do.

18 to 24 months. Second (or back) molars can start appearing at the end of the second year, but many toddlers don't get that extra set of chompers until after they bite into their second birthday cake.

Be on the lookout: If your toddler hasn't cut a single tooth by 16 to 18 months, talk to the GP or a dentist. Also bring to the attention of your toddler's doctor or dentist any discoloured teeth, or chipping or softening of the teeth.

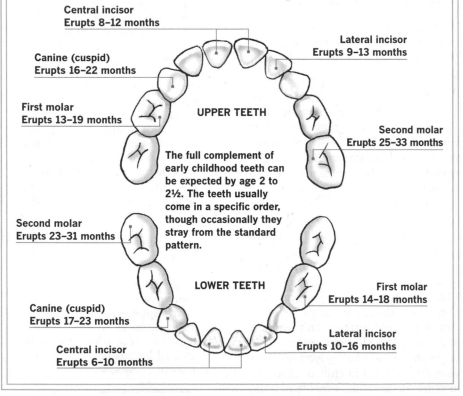

Central incisor
Erupts 8–12 months

Lateral incisor
Erupts 9–13 months

Canine (cuspid)
Erupts 16–22 months

First molar
Erupts 13–19 months

UPPER TEETH

Second molar
Erupts 25–33 months

The full complement of early childhood teeth can be expected by age 2 to 2½. The teeth usually come in a specific order, though occasionally they stray from the standard pattern.

Second molar
Erupts 23–31 months

LOWER TEETH

First molar
Erupts 14–18 months

Canine (cuspid)
Erupts 17–23 months

Central incisor
Erupts 6–10 months

Lateral incisor
Erupts 10–16 months

Speaking of sleeping, often a toddler who's cutting molars may start waking during the night (or may wake up more frequently). While you'll want to provide comfort, keep in mind that this kind of waking can become chronic – continuing long after the pain has left the building – so try to minimise those midnight comfort runs.

While teething can definitely trigger grumpiness, lack of appetite, even a slightly elevated temperature, report any symptoms of illness that warrant a call to the doctor. They could be completely unrelated to teething and may need treatment.

Gaps Between Teeth

"I'm guessing our daughter is going to need braces because there is so much space between her teeth."

Often, the front primary teeth debut with big gaps between them – and that could actually be a good thing as far as a perfect smile is concerned. That's because the front adult teeth are bigger than baby teeth, and they'll need the extra space when they eventually move in. Those primary front teeth are also apt to shift closer together as adjacent baby teeth erupt, pushing their way into place. The comforting

Preparing for the Dentist

Taking your toddler to the dentist for the first time? A little prep can go a long way in making sure that first visit goes off without a hitch (like a toddler tantrum or a fear fest). Start by reading or looking at the pictures in children's books about dentists (such as *What to Expect When You Go to the Dentist*). Explain that dentists are "tooth doctors", and their job is to help teeth stay healthy and strong. Point out that everyone goes to see the dentist (including you). Role-play to reinforce that message on a basic level. You can play the dentist first, then let your toddler play dentist on you or on dolls and stuffed animals. Especially worthy of practice: "Open up wide – like a lion!" Also call the dentist's surgery to find out if little rewards (toys, stickers, toothbrushes) are offered after a visit. This way your toddler will know going in what's in it for him or her at the end.

When making that first appointment, get as many details up front as possible. Will it be just a get-acquainted session, with some friendly conversation, an introduction to the dentist's surgery, and a quick checkup? Or will there be a cleaning or other treatment (like a fluoride varnish) performed? Will the dentist allow you to stay in the room? Some dentists find that children are more cooperative and less fearful without a parent present, but most are open to either scenario, especially when it comes to a 1-year-old.

Worried your little one will lose it big time at the dentist's surgery? Don't anticipate a meltdown, but do be prepared for one (it's been known to happen). Lots of reassurance and support (see the tips for minimising doctor anxiety, a similar experience, on page 342) will make that leap into the dentist's chair easier all around and set the tone for a lifetime of happier visits.

bottom (and top) line: there's no direct correlation between irregularly spaced baby teeth and a smile that needs fixing later.

Visiting the Dentist

"Do I need to take my 1-year-old to a dentist? I can't imagine he'll ever sit still in the chair."

Your toddler definitely doesn't need a full set of gnashers to qualify for the dentist's chair. In fact, the British Dental Health Foundation suggests scheduling a first dental visit at about 6 months old, when his or her teeth start to appear. The GP or health visitor may also perform basic dental examinations checking for problems that require a referral to a dentist, and counselling you about keeping your toddler's teeth healthy.

Why is it so important that a dentist or doctor is on tap for tooth duty this early on? Besides getting your toddler into the dental hygiene habit early, professional attention to those tiny teeth can prevent or identify decay (which could lead to premature loss of baby teeth) and diagnose mouth irregularities that may interfere with speech development. The dentist or doctor can also be an excellent backup authority when it comes to convincing your toddler to cooperate with brushing, or to give up the bottle, thumb, or dummy. Plus, either one can answer the questions you may have on teething, brushing and flossing (you can even ask for a demo), fluoride intake, and all those sucking habits.

Opting out of the dentist for now? Definitely make sure your toddler sees a dentist by his third birthday, if not before (the sooner the going-to-the-dentist habit is established, the better). Most first visits are basic – more like an introductory icebreaker than a full-fledged dental visit. The dentist will count your little one's pearly whites, examine his jaw, bite, and gums, and do a gentle tooth cleaning.

See the box on the previous page for tips on preparing your toddler for the dentist.

Skin

SKIN CARE

Keeping a baby's skin baby soft and protected is child's play (a little after-bath lotion and judicious care in the nappy area and an infant is cuddle-ready). Keeping a toddler's skin soft and protected, however, can be, well, a little rougher. Toddlers are constantly on the go, indoors and out (meaning more exposure to skin-chafing elements) and they have a knack for getting dirty (both dirt and dirt cleaning can irritate tender skin), giving their skin a tough time. And because the sebaceous glands, which will eventually lubricate and protect the skin, don't kick in until the hormones start flowing just before puberty, young skin is especially prone to dryness and irritation. To keep your toddler's skin clean but as soft and touchable as a baby's, treat it with care. Look for very gentle soaps or cleansers that promise not to irritate your little one's sensitive skin (hands off your body wash, bubble

Keeping Clean . . . By Myself

So your toddler's only interest in hygiene is avoiding it? Toddlers aren't exactly known for being clean freaks – or grooming fanatics. Even if the interest is there, the follow-through and technique definitely won't be. Which is why you'll have to keep handling most of your tot's grooming needs (from bathing and hair brushing to toothbrushing and hand washing). Still, now's the perfect time to start teaching some basic (really basic) hygiene skills that will one day allow your little one to proudly proclaim: "I did it all by myself!" at washing time. Your toddler will learn best from your example, which is a good reason to soap up at the sink, but encouragement (when she tries to brush her hair – even when she uses the wrong side of the brush), praise (when you see him reaching for the sink to soap up his dirty hands), and patience (when the brush gets tangled up in her locks or a puddle of water forms at his feet) will also help spur on the development of self-grooming abilities. That, and a whole lot of practice. Here's what you can expect this year on the self-grooming front:

12 to 15 months. Your toddler still has plenty of progress to make in the coordination and dexterity department before he or she can be put on hygiene detail – but baby steps towards self-care are already being taken. Early in the second year toddlers begin to recognise the tools of the hygiene trade and their uses: a brush neatens hair, a towel dries wet hands, soap washes away grime. Along with that

awareness comes the strong desire to mimic "grown-up" activities – so he'll reach for the brush and go through the motions of brushing hair, and she'll point to the soap next to the sink when she's got dirt on her hands.

15 to 18 months. By the middle of the second year, most toddlers have developed a burning desire to flex their independence muscle. To that end, your wanna-do-it-myselfer might try a power grab for the comb or toothbrush or rebuff your offers of help when you try to step in. Celebrate these early attempts at self-grooming and surreptitiously finish the job when your toddler is otherwise distracted.

18 to 24 months. By age 2 your toddler will have a better handle on personal hygiene – but most grooming tasks will still require a good deal of adult supervision until age 4 to 6, at least. A 2-year-old may be able to brush her hair or wipe his nose with a tissue – but you'll still need to follow up (tackling tangles, wiping away crusted snot, and so on). Taking an I'll-start/you-finish approach (or the other way around), or offering an option of "You wash my hands, I'll wash yours" can often coax cooperation – as can putting your little one in charge of a doll's hygiene (a little control can go a long way).

Be on the lookout: If your toddler hasn't shown any interest in doing anything for him- or herself by the end of the second year, tell the GP or health visitor about it at the next visit.

bath, or soap bars unless they're extra mild). Also avoid antibacterial soaps because they can be unnecessarily irritating (and also aren't necessary). Use

even the gentlest of soaps sparingly, soaping up only as needed (where dirt is most obvious, and around the nappy area). And when it comes to toddler skin care, less is more. There's no need to smooth on lotions or creams (unless your little one has very dry skin; see page 44).

Bath Rejection

"My son has always loved his bath, and he isn't afraid of water at all. So I can't understand why he's suddenly refusing to get into the bath."

As you've probably already noticed, refusals of every kind are big in the second year. A toddler may refuse to eat, refuse to wear a coat, refuse to go outside, refuse to come back in – simply for refusal's sake, without apparent rhyme or reason. The truth is, however, there is a reason – a very good one: his struggle for independence. Here's how to get your toddler back in the bath – or, at least, help you find other ways to clean up his act:

Bring on the toys. Like the fleet of plastic boats. And the funnels and cups. And the bath books. And colourful soaps. And any other waterproof diversion you can come up with. Let the toys and fun – and not the washing – be the focus of the bath experience. Instead of announcing bath time with "Time to get in the bath", announce it with "Look at all these boats you can play with!" or "Let's paint tiger stripes on you with this funny soap!"

Schedule a change. If bath time comes at an unexpected hour, rather than at the accustomed battle time, it's possible that your toddler's surprise may ease his opposition. Admittedly, a change in schedule may mean that your child won't be getting clean when he's his dirtiest (if bath has been switched to mid-morning instead of after dinner, for instance), but in the short run that's better than not getting

clean at all. Until he becomes more amenable to bathing, and bath time can return to a more sensible time slot, a quick session with a flannel on the more glaringly grimy areas can get him passably clean before he gets into his pyjamas.

Try a little togetherness. The rub-a-dub-dub may be more appealing if there's more than one in the tub. Mummy or Daddy make perfect bath buddies (don a bathing suit if you'd rather not bathe in the buff with your toddler). An older sibling or a friend on a playdate makes an ideal bath mate, too (prior parental permission suggested). Or try a washable doll – he can wash his baby while you wash yours.

Hit the showers. If it's the bath that's triggering the rebellion, let your toddler accompany you in the shower instead. Adjusting the water-flow rate to gentle will help make the overhead stream less threatening, as may holding your toddler until he feels confident enough to stand under the shower on his own. A rousing round of "It's raining, it's pouring" can provide a playful note. As with bath water, shower water should be warm, rather than hot, for toddlers.

Keep it short and sweet. Since you're still the one in charge, and because your toddler will need to get clean every once in a while (whether he likes it or not), you may just have to pull rank. A quick in and out of the bath or a fast sponge bath may still prompt protests from your bath balker, but if you keep it short and sweet, and move on to another diversion as soon as the deed is done, you'll end up with a clean toddler no worse for the wear. Keep your cool, too (no taking the bait when your little fish puts up a fight). And remember – this too shall pass.

Hand-Washing Resistance

"Our toddler's hands get unbelievably dirty during a morning of play. But she won't let us wash them before she eats."

No matter what the season, it's what all the toddlers are wearing: blackened knees, filthy forearms, grimy elbows, sticky faces, and dirt-encrusted fingernails.

But though most of the dirt a toddler attracts during a morning's play can stay put until her nighttime bathing, the dirt on her hands should be removed before she eats – particularly since she'll be using them to feed herself. Making sure her hands are scrubbed before every meal won't only keep dirt out of her food (and her mouth) – it'll get her in the healthy, hygienic hand-washing habit.

Easier said than done? Not if you arm yourself with these hand-washing tips:

Put hand washing in her hands. The more control toddlers have over an activity, the less likely they are to resist it. Turn the soap and water over to her, and much of her resistance may go down the drain with the dirt. Don't make a fuss about the splashy mess she'll inevitably make – it can be mopped up afterwards. Do adjust the water temperature for her, though, to avoid burns. (As a safety precaution, keep your home water heater set below 120°F/48°C.) Check her handiwork when she's finished – if her hands don't look much cleaner than when she started, have her try again. Or let her wash your hands while you wash hers.

Make hand washing fun. Because a two-second hand wash won't do the trick (in terms of both dirt and germs), your tot will need a solid 20 seconds of rub-a-dub-dubbing to get clean. Sounds like an eternity (to a toddler) – unless you also make it fun.

It's a Dirty Job

Attention all neat-freak mums and dads: better get ready to lower your cleanliness expectations now that you've got a 1-year-old on your hands (one whose hands are plenty grubby). After all, being dirty comes with the toddler territory. There's sand and soil to sift through, filthy supermarket floors to slide across, food to smear on clothes and body, dust bunnies to collect and play with. Expecting your mini mess-maker to stay clean is like expecting him or her to stay still: neither is in a toddler's job description, and both would keep your little one from exploring and experimenting – two things high on a toddler's must-do list. Plus, the more you gripe about the grime, the more you'll drive those down and dirty ways.

So loosen up. Concentrate only on necessary hygiene: hand washing before eating, after toileting, or when hands have found their way onto something sticky, a nightly bath (see facing page for tips on what to do if your tot tends to reject the bath), and steering your toddler clear of germ breeding grounds like street puddles and animal droppings. Otherwise, let the dirt fly where it may.

Sing "Happy Birthday" or a nursery rhyme while washing up, use a kid's foaming or colourful soap to keep things interesting, or go for naturally scented – coconut or lavender, for instance – to keep things sweet (and don't forget to ask for a whiff after she's finished).

Put hand washing within her reach. One of the most frustrating parts of hand washing for a toddler is the stretch – literally. Providing your toddler with easy access to the bathroom sink (via a step stool) and placing accessories (soap and towel) within reach can help her feel more in control of the process.

Switch to liquid soap. Bar soap is not only slippery and difficult for little fingers to lather, but it collects almost as much dirt as your toddler's hands. So stick with the liquid or foaming kinds of soap.

Wipe it away. When you're away from home, disposable wipes may be the easiest and most sanitary way of giving hands a quick wash, and even a fairly young toddler can use them. Encourage her to make the wipes as "dirty" as she can, so that more of the grime will come off her.

If you do use antibacterial hand gel when you're out and about with your toddler (after a trip to the petting zoo, for instance, or after touching the supermarket trolley handle), keep in mind that while such gels or rinses do a decent job of sanitising the hands, they won't get the dirt off. So use a wipe first to scrub off the grime, and then, if you choose, use a child-safe hand sanitiser (one that's free of alcohol and strong chemicals).

Dry Skin

"My son's skin always seems so dry. What can I do to protect it?"

Many toddlers go through dry skin spells – and some continue to be a little rough around the edges throughout early childhood. Fortunately, there are ways to replenish the moisture that life-on-the-go can steal from tender skin, softening things up in no time:

- Be soap-savvy. If your toddler has very dry, extra-sensitive, or rash-prone skin, choose a cleanser that's fragrance free or even soapless (like Cetaphil).

- Cut back on bath time. Thirty minutes in the bath may seem like a dream for your toddler (so much splashing, so little time!), but too much soaking in water can remove the skin's natural oils along with the dirt. Limiting baths to 10 minutes will allow enough playtime, without paying the price in dry skin.

- Don't rub-a-dub-dub in (or after) the tub. Be gentle when sudsing up and rinsing your toddler's skin – no scrubbing with the flannel. Always pat skin dry instead of rubbing it when your little fish is out of the water.

- Moisturise. Top off every bath (while your little one's skin is still slightly moist) with a generous layer of moisturiser. Reapply as needed, especially when the weather's really cold or your toddler's skin is really parched. The best moisturisers for a toddler's skin contain both water (to replenish moisture) and oil (to seal it in). Extra-sensitive or extra-dry skin will be soothed best by a moisturiser that has few chemical additives and is free of fragrances. Eucerin, Aquaphor, Neutrogena, Cetaphil, Aveeno, and Lubriderm are all top paediatrician and dermatologist picks – though keep in mind the only reaction that matters is your child's skin. Sometimes, even "baby", "hypoallergenic", or "all-natural" products can trigger irritation or a rash – which means it's time to make a moisturiser switch (choose one with a different formulation).

■ Keep those fluids coming. Inadequate fluid intake can lead to dry skin (that moisture comes from the inside out), so make sure your little guy gets his fill. Be especially aware of fluid intake if your toddler has just been weaned and is still working out the mechanics of drinking from a cup, if it's hot out, or if he's been sick.

■ Feed healthy fats. Getting enough of the right kinds of fats can lubricate your little one from the inside out, too. Think avocados, rapeseed, flax, and olive oil, almond or cashew butter (if there's no nut allergy, and spread very thinly). A generally healthy diet also helps promote healthy skin.

■ Avoid overheating in cold weather. When the mercury dips outside, it's always tempting to send the mercury rising inside. But dry, overheated air leads to overdry skin, particularly for toddlers. So keep the temperature inside your home comfortable, but not overly warm. Keep your toddler cosy in tracksuits or jumpers during the day and warm sleepers at night.

Chapped Cheeks

"What can I do about my son's red, chapped cheeks?"

On an average day, a variety of substances (ranging from saliva and mucus to jelly and tomato sauce) manage to find their way onto a toddler's face, where they're promptly smeared from cheek to cheek, causing redness and irritation – especially in winter, when skin is already extra dry. Frequent face washings (to remove these substances) often compound the chafing.

If your toddler's cheeks turn apple red with the first frost and stay that way until the tulips come up, some special attention is needed. To minimise facial chapping:

■ Gently wipe your child's face with warm water immediately after meals to remove any traces of food, then pat dry promptly. If you notice that a particular food or beverage is especially irritating to the skin (common offenders are those that are high in acid, such as citrus fruits and juices, strawberries, and tomatoes or tomato sauce), avoid serving it to your toddler until the chafing has cleared.

■ No rubbing. When washing those chubby cheeks, be extra gentle. And always pat dry. Don't use scratchy cloths or rough paper towels or napkins.

■ Avoid using soap on your toddler's face. When more than water is called for, use a soapless cleanser.

■ Pat his face dry with a soft cloth whenever he's been dribbling (try to catch him before he wipes the dribble all over his cheeks). Gently wipe that snotty nose frequently for the same reason.

■ Soothe chapped skin with a mild moisturiser. Spreading moisturiser on cheeks, chin, and nose before going out in cold weather may also be protective, especially for a teething toddler who is dribbling a lot or a toddler with a runny nose. For tough cases, you may have to opt for an ointment (like Aquaphor), which acts as a barrier while it moisturises.

Eczema

"I noticed a red rash inside my toddler's elbow, and she's scratching it a lot. Could it be an allergic reaction to something, like soap – or could it be eczema?"

Actually, it could be both. Eczema is the blanket name that technically covers the two most common skin conditions in children: atopic dermatitis and contact dermatitis. While both cause rashes – and either could be triggered by an allergic reaction – atopic dermatitis is often chronic, while contact dermatitis usually comes and goes. Initially, they're not easy to tell apart (though the doctor may be able to clue you in). Here's the breakdown on the causes, symptoms, and treatments for both types of eczema:

Atopic dermatitis. When most people (including doctors) talk about "eczema", this is the condition they're typically referring to. Most common in children with a history (or family history) of allergies, hay fever, or asthma, eczema has been aptly described as "an itch that rashes". Once the itch begins, scratching or rubbing the area triggers the rash. In a toddler, the rash usually consists of red small bumps that often weep (or ooze) and crust over when scratched. The rash usually starts on the face and cheeks, spreading to the trunk of the body, the wrists, and body folds (inside groin and elbow creases). This type of eczema is often (though not always) outgrown by age 2 to 3.

What triggers the itch? For most kids, it could be any of the following triggers: dry skin, heat or cold exposure, perspiration, wool and/or synthetic clothing, friction, soaps, detergents, and fabric softeners (though these could trigger contact dermatitis as well; see the next column). Eating certain foods (most often eggs, milk, wheat, peanuts, soy, fish, and shellfish) can also cause a reaction.

Treatment usually includes topical steroid (hydrocortisone) creams or ointments for inflammation and oral antihistamines for itching (especially to help a child sleep). The doctor will prescribe or recommend the medication that's right for your toddler. On the home front, it's important to:

- Clip your toddler's nails to prevent scratching.

- Limit baths to no more than 10 to 15 minutes, and use an extra-mild or soapless cleanser (Dove or Cetaphil, for example) only as needed.

- Limit dips in chlorinated pools and salt water (fresh water is okay).

- Apply plenty of rich hypoallergenic moisturiser after baths, when the skin is damp.

- Minimise exposure to extremes in temperature, indoors and out.

- Use a humidifier as needed to prevent dry air indoors (but don't overdo the humidity, since too much moisture in the air promotes the growth of mould and mildew, common allergy and asthma triggers).

- Dress your child in cotton (rather than wool or synthetics), and avoid scratchy, potentially irritating clothing.

Contact dermatitis. A contact dermatitis rash occurs when skin repeatedly comes in contact with an irritating substance (such as citrus, bubble bath, soaps, detergents, foods, medicines, even a toddler's own saliva or urine – as with nappy rash). The rash, which appears as mild redness and/or small bumps (sometimes with accompanying swelling), is often more localised than atopic dermatitis and usually clears when the irritant is removed (if it doesn't, you may have a case of atopic dermatitis on your hands) and the rash is treated with hydrocortisone creams or ointments. The rash can also crop up when skin comes in contact with an allergen (like nickel jewellery or poppers on clothes, dyes in clothes, plants like poison ivy, or some medications).

Other Skin Rashes

"Our toddler's skin seems so rash prone. Just when his nappy rash seems under control, another rash pops up somewhere else. How can I tell one rash from another and what can I do about them?"

Rashes come and go on toddler skin, but in some toddlers, they seem to come more than they go. Most of the time, a dry patch or a crop of elevated bumps on your tot's skin is nothing more than annoying (especially if it's ruining your toddler's close-ups), and sometimes it's just a reaction to a fragrance or another chemical in a soap or shampoo. But once in a while it's an indication of a skin condition that needs some attention. If your toddler's skin is scaly, itchy, blistered, or oozing, check with the doctor to find out what is causing it and how to treat it. The most common skin rashes in toddlers include:

Ringworm (a.k.a. tinea). This mildly contagious fungal infection (don't worry, no worms are actually involved) shows up as round, red, raised, itchy, and scaly patches that can be as small as a 5-pence piece or can grow up to 2.5 cm or more in diameter. Ringworm can be spread by direct person-to-person contact (one toddler who's been scratching touches another – and bingo) or by sharing towels, brushes and combs, clothes, and anything else that touches skin, as well as through surfaces in warm moist areas (like swimming pools). Your little one can also catch ringworm from a pet

Skin Check

Though the skin is by far the body's largest organ, it doesn't usually get its fair share of attention. While an eye infection or an earache is likely to be treated promptly, a skin condition might not even be noticed – a large percentage of skin, after all, is under wraps most of the time. That's why doctors recommend routine skin examinations that allow parents to become familiar with their children's skin and to be able to note any changes. Make a habit of checking your toddler's skin at bath time, observing any changes in moles or birthmarks, and noting any new marks or lesions you hadn't noticed before. If a mole or birthmark has grown instead of fading, if its colour has changed, if it is itchy, oozing, bleeding, crusting, scaling, or tender to the touch, report your findings to your child's doctor. Also report any sore that takes longer than two weeks to heal or unexplained rashes or other skin symptoms. A before-bath skin check is also a good way to spot mosquito or flea bites when your little one has been outside during summer (see page 443 for insect bites).

(clues that your pet has ringworm and needs treatment: scaly, hairless patches, lots of scratching). Ringworm can turn up anywhere on the body, including the face and scalp (where it can be mistakenly identified as a stubborn case of cradle cap) and can be spread from one part of the body to another by scratching. Since it can be confused with other types of rashes, including eczema and seborrhoea, proper diagnosis is key. Ringworm on the body can be easily treated with an antifungal cream, but on the scalp it may

Screening Out the Sun

Sun may be fun – and it certainly beats rain or snow when you've got to head outside – but it's no picnic for the skin. The sun's ultraviolet A (UVA) rays cause tanning, aging of the skin, and skin cancer, and the ultraviolet B (UVB) rays cause sunburn and skin cancer. That's why all children (even dark-skinned children) need protection from the sun, and those who are most vulnerable to sun damage (children with red or blonde hair and fair skin, those with blue, green, or grey eyes, those with a family history of skin cancer, those with a large number of moles, and those with freckles) need even more. Research shows that serious sunburns during childhood are a more significant factor in the development of adult malignant melanoma (the most serious form of skin cancer) than total lifetime exposure to the sun. To prevent sun damage, take these precautions whenever your toddler steps outside:

Be sunscreen-savvy. When shopping for a sunscreen, start by targeting those that are:

- Labelled "broad-spectrum". This means that a product will screen out both ultraviolet B (UVB) and ultraviolet A (UVA) rays.

- Easy to apply. Creamy products are less drying and stay on the skin longer. But sprays are usually easier to apply – and since a sunscreen can only be effective for your toddler if you manage to get it on him or her, ease of application is a prime consideration.

- Nonirritating. Sunscreens designed for kids usually have more appealing packaging and easier application, but they're not necessarily gentler or less likely to trigger a reaction on tender skin. So it's always a good idea to test your little one for sensitivity to a sunscreen product you're applying for the first time – before you hit the playground or beach. Do this with a patch test: spread or spray a thin layer on a small patch of your toddler's skin. If redness or a rash develops, head back to the shop and choose a product with different ingredients.

- Sporting a high SPF (sun protection factor). The SPF tells you just how much protection a sunscreen product offers. Choose an SPF of at least 30, which theoretically (as long as the sunscreen is applied properly and then reapplied after several hours) allows a user to remain in the sun 30 times longer before burning than would be possible without protection. But since you have no way of knowing exactly how long it takes your little one to burn, or how intense the sun is on a particular day, it's best to be on the safe side. More is more when you're choosing an SPF, so when in doubt, go higher on the SPF scale. Of course, even slathered with sunscreen, an hour or so at a stretch in direct, hot sun is long enough for most toddlers (you definitely don't want to stretch that SPF to its potential protective limits). And don't assume you can safely wait for your toddler's cheeks to start showing some colour before you bring him or her under cover. Pinking of the skin is not generally apparent in the sun. In fact, most sunburns don't reach their peak colour until 6 to 24 hours after sun exposure.

Slather up. Sunscreen is a must-wear whenever your toddler is heading outside. Make applying it as routine as getting dressed and as non-negotiable as sitting in the car seat and you're less likely to face sunscreen resistance in the future.

If it's possible, apply the sunscreen 15 to 30 minutes before going out into the sun, since it takes that long to be thoroughly absorbed into the skin. If you can't manage that, applying it right before going out – or even once you're out – is far better than not applying it at all. Spread the sunscreen generously (err on the side of excess – most people apply far too little) and be careful not to miss any exposed skin – including the back of the neck, the ears, and the feet, three areas often overlooked. When applying to the face, be careful not to get the sunscreen into your toddler's eyes. Since wind and water both thin out protection, reapply every 1 to 2 hours or so if it's windy, if your toddler is sweating a lot, or if he or she has been splashing in a pool or running under a sprinkler. You can reapply it less often – every 2 to 3 hours or so – if you're using a water-resistant product (read the label for recommendations). But keep in mind that even a water-resistant sunscreen can be rubbed off by a lot of towel drying and will need to be reapplied more often under such conditions.

Lips need sun protection, too. Make applying a children's sunscreen lip balm (which should be lickproof) before going out in the sun as routine as applying sunscreen. It will also shield your toddler's lips from wind and cold in the winter, reducing chapping.

Protect year-round. Sunburn's usually associated with summer, but the sun can also burn in the winter – especially when there's snow on the ground. In fact, the sun's rays reflected on the snow can be as intense as those from summer sun. And, although less of the burning UVB reaches the earth in winter, the also-harmful UVA rays remain constant year-round, no matter what the weather. Don't skip the sunscreen when it's hazy out, either, especially if you're on the coast. Much of the sun's ultraviolet light, especially UVA, can penetrate cloud cover.

Schedule outdoor time wisely. When practical, try to limit your child's exposure to the sun – even when he or she is properly protected – during the hours when its rays are at their most intense, between 10 A.M. and 3 P.M. (4 P.M. during the summer months), or when your shadow is shorter than you are.

Play in the shade. Look for playgrounds that are well shaded, and set up play areas in your own garden, if possible, that are in shade all or part of the day.

Beware of glare. On the beach, a beach umbrella can shield you and your toddler from the sun's rays. A beach tent can provide even more protection. But don't stop there. Sunscreen is still a must to help protect skin from the reflected glare of sun on sand. Be mindful, too, of the sun's reflection on snow, concrete, and water (the toddler who's splashing in the pool is more vulnerable to sunburn than the one who's playing beside it).

Cover up. When your toddler is out and about during the hours when the sun is most intense, keep the rays at bay with a pushchair canopy or umbrella, a wide-brimmed hat, as much clothing coverage as is comfortable, shoes and socks (bare feet burn quickly), and sunscreen on exposed parts of the body. Keep in mind, however, that the sun's ultraviolet rays can penetrate sheer and lightly woven, light-coloured fabrics. The typical T-shirt has an SPF of only 7 or 8, which means that toddlers (darker-skinned children included) may need a layer of sunscreen under their thin tees when they are going to spend extended time outdoors. To test a fabric, hold it up to a light; the less light that shows through, the better protection from the sun. If your child takes a medication or has a condition that makes exposure to the sun particularly risky, consider special sun-protective clothes.

require an oral antifungal medication, as well as an antifungal shampoo.

Nappy rash. Stating the obvious, nappy rash is a rash or irritation anywhere in the nappy area. See page 58 for more.

Impetigo. Impetigo is a bacterial infection of the skin that occurs when bacteria, such as streptococci or staphylococci, enter the skin through a break, such as a scratch, bite, or irritation. It can also affect eczema-damaged skin. Either blisters or honeycomb-like crusts form, then weep and ooze yellowish fluid. Impetigo can spread quickly to other areas of the skin, making medical treatment necessary in many cases (topical antibiotics and gentle washing for very mild cases or oral antibiotics for a rash that is more widespread) – the doctor will determine which medication is needed after examining the rash. Keeping skin wounds clean with soap and water, and then applying an antibiotic ointment, prevents impetigo.

Prickly heat. Known mainly as heat rash on the sandpit circuit, prickly heat occurs most commonly in babies, but toddlers, children, and even adults can develop the rash as well. Prickly heat, which results when sweat glands clog up, looks like tiny pink pimples on a reddened area of skin that may blister and then dry up. The rash occurs most often around the neck and shoulders, but it can also appear on the back and face, or anywhere skin rubs against skin or clothing constricts. Since the rash is caused by overheating or overdressing, be sure not to overdress your toddler, and keep indoor spaces comfortably cool.

Sunscreen Struggles

"I know I'm supposed to put sunscreen on my toddler, but that is way easier said than done. She fights it every time."

Toddlers, as you've definitely noticed, fight a whole lot of things that are good for them (say, vegetables) – and even some things that are essential for them (among them car seats, doctor visits, and sunscreen). As always, your best plan of action is distraction. When it's time to slather up, break out a favourite toy for your toddler to clutch or break into a silly (just-for-sunscreen) song. Try some fast talk, too ("Let's get this sunscreen on fast so we can go play in the playground!"), lots of good humour, and a positive, upbeat attitude (approach looking for a battle and you're bound to get one). Being a model of sunscreen sense will also help (apply your sunscreen, then apply your toddler's). As your toddler's comprehension grows, so can an explanation ("Sunscreen keeps the sun from burning our skin"). Make sunscreen (just like the car seat and the doctor visits) a non-negotiable issue – no sunscreen, no go. The more wiggle room you give now (you skip it because you're running late, or because she's having a tantrum), the more struggles you'll get in the future.

Nails

NAIL CARE

For telling clues to a toddler's daily activities, look no further than the fingernails. There you'll find, among other things, mud (from the morning spent digging at the park), Play-Doh (from that playdate), glue (from that collage project), remnants of breakfast, lunch, and dinner, and often, even less savoury substances.

Unless you protect them with gloves (good luck with that plan), there's no way you can keep your toddler's fingernails clean all the time. But since dirty fingernails can harbour germs along with all the collected grime, you should try to:

- Keep them short. The shorter the fingernails, the less they can collect. Short is also best for toenails, which left to grow ungroomed, can curl under and become ingrown. See below for clipping tips.

- Clean them daily. Make nail cleaning part of the regular end-of-the-day routine. Regular hand washing usually does the trick, but if it doesn't, help your child to use a small nail brush in the bath or when washing hands before bedtime. Carefully remove particularly stubborn stuff with a rounded wooden toothpick.

Nail-Trimming Trials

"My toddler's fingernails and toenails get very long and dirty. But she won't let me trim them."

Try to see nail trimming from your toddler's perspective and you'll see why she fights it tooth and . . . nail. First, having parts of her pared off by a clipper or a pair of scissors (even when they're wielded by a friendly parent) is unsettling. A young toddler isn't likely to understand (or remember) that nails don't hurt when they're cut or that they grow back afterward. Second, the process, for safety's sake, requires restraint – something she doesn't like to show, never mind have imposed on her. Not only must she sit still (that most dreaded pose), but she must have her hand and fingers held captive – and motionless – by an adult hand. And third, what's in it for her?

Still, nails need trimming. Long nails can harbour dirt (yuck) and germs (double yuck) even when hands are clean. What's more, a long, sharp nail can cause harm (intentionally or accidentally) through a scratch, pinch, or barefooted kick – and if your little one has an itchy skin rash, like eczema, having the nail power to scratch it can also make the rash worse. Though nail trimming may continue to be a hotly disputed issue for many years to come (until it's replaced by nail nibbling or cuticle picking), these tips may trim some of the resistance – or at least help get the job done:

- Use a blunt instrument. Baby scissors, with their blunt safety tips, or small nail clippers, are good for trimming a toddler's nails. Don't trade these in for pointed nail scissors, at least until your child's old enough to be counted on to hold still.

- Turn the scissors on yourself first. Make a point of trimming your own nails (as well as those of other willing family members) in front of your toddler. Make it look like fun and it's possible she'll want to be next in line for a trim.

- Perform when wet. Warm water soothes toddlers and softens nails, both of which may make nail trimming less of a trial – so try scheduling your toddler's next manicure when she's fresh out of the bath. (Don't try trimming in the water – she'll be too slippery.)

- Play a game. A made-for-nail-trimming version of "This Little Piggy" may be distracting and help replace screams with giggles. Or tell her a story about the "mummy, daddy, and baby" fingers of her hand family while you work ("Baby piggy is going to a party and she wants to look pretty!").

Thinking about tackling that nail trim when your toddler's sleeping? While chances are she'll be far more cooperative when she's snoozing than when she's awake, such sneaky attacks can sometimes backfire – say, if she wakes up mid-trim, especially if she jerks her hand away at the critical moment (leading to an inadvertent nick). If your little one is a rock-solid sleeper (once she's out, she's out), you can give it a try. But if your toddler – like many toddlers – is a restless sleeper, you may not want to try this time-honoured trick at home.

Keep in mind that nibbling a young child's nails off with your teeth is not a good idea. Not only could your nibbles tear the cuticles, but you'll be teaching your toddler that nail-biting is an acceptable habit.

Feet

FOOT CARE

Is your toddler on his or her feet, or soon to be? Either way, it's a sure bet that those tiny tootsies will get quite a workout in the months and years to come. Compared to other parts of your little one's body, though, feet don't need much in the way of care – in fact, less, for the most part, is more. Aside from outfitting them in the right socks and shoes, washing them off every now and again, and entertaining them in the occasional game of "This Little Piggy", your only job as far as your toddler's feet are concerned will be trying to keep track of where they take your toddler (and trying to keep up with them).

Funny Feet

"Sometimes my toddler likes to walk on her tiptoes. And when she does walk flat on her feet, they look, well, like flat feet. Is all of that normal?"

As your toddler grows, changes in those chubby little legs, knees, and feet can keep you on your toes. Among the normal but sometimes peculiar-looking stances you may see your toddler taking are the following:

Toeing-out. Does your toddler walk like a duck, with those piggies pointing out? For new walkers, waddling is normal – and even necessary, allowing them to improve their balance and staying-up power. Gradually, toes will start to straighten out, and by the time most kids are 5 or 6, their feet face forward. A few kids will continue to toe-out, but that's not usually a problem.

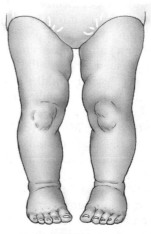

Most toddlers toe-out in the second year, but some walk with their toes in (see above).

Toeing-in (pigeon toes). Is your toddler less duck, more pigeon? Toeing-in early in the second year is usually related to a slight twisting of the tibia (or shin bone), which generally straightens out on its own. But even if it continues into adulthood – as it does in a small percentage of children – it's not considered a problem unless it's extreme. Wouldn't mind a little extra reassurance? Point out the toeing-in at your toddler's next checkup.

Bowlegs. Just about every baby and toddler has a major gap between the knees, though the size of the gap varies (it's definitely going to be more visible in a slimmer tot than a chunkier one). That's because their tibias – the shin bones – are still curved, a leftover reflection of how they spent uterine time: folded up. New walkers also tend to bend their knees to help keep their balance, another reason why their legs appear bowed. With growth, more weight-bearing, more walking, and more steadiness on two feet – usually by the time they toddle into their second birthday party – your toddler's legs will straighten up. Bowing disappears, typically followed by mild knock-knees,

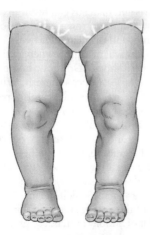

Not to worry – a toddler's legs are normally bowed until some time late in the second year.

> # The Mystery of the Missing Arch
>
> Want to see that seemingly missing arch for yourself? Take a look at your toddler's apparently flat feet dangling from a chair. Without any weight bearing down on those chubby tootsies, you'll most likely spy that hidden arch peeking out.

which often last for a lifetime (it's just more subtle in grown-up legs). In the meantime, make sure your toddler is getting enough vitamin D from milk or from a supplement, since a D deficiency can lead to rickets and permanent bowing. If bowing appears to be worsening after independent walking begins, show the GP so he or she can rule out rickets or a knee problem.

Flat feet. Toddler feet are flat feet – or at least, feet that appear flat. One reason: those tiny feet have bones and joints that are still very flexible, and muscles that are still very underdeveloped. A toddler's own weight pushes the loose joints and the weak muscles towards the ground, making that arch (what arch?) disappear. Toeing-out, which most toddlers do so they can balance better as they walk, puts extra weight on the arch, flattening it still more. Yet another factor is the baby-fat pad that rounds the toddler foot, camouflaging any curve that might be there. By the time your child marches off to school, she is likely to be the proud owner of two well-defined arches. And if for some reason flat-footedness prevails, that's nothing to worry about, either.

Tiptoeing. Many toddlers – and not just for those destined for *The Nutcracker* – enjoy tiptoeing. To a novice walker,

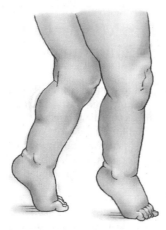

Occasional tiptoeing isn't cause for concern.

tiptoeing is an adventure, a brand-new perspective – and a rest for the rest of the foot. But tots don't stay on their toes forever. Most give up the toe step entirely and switch over to heel first about midway through the second year. If your little one always walks on her toes, though, and/or continues to tiptoe well into the second or third year, mention it to the doctor.

Choosing Shoes

"What are the best shoes for my toddler now that he's on his feet so much?"

The best shoes for a little walker are no shoes at all. But there comes a time and a place in every toddler's life when bare feet or socks won't do – like in a busy shop (where tiny toes can be stepped on) or the playground (where tiny feet can step into something dirty – or worse, onto something that hurts). The next best thing to no shoes (or slip-proof socks) are shoes that are as close to bare feet as possible. Look for:

Just-right fit. Your toddler's feet fit him just right – and so should his shoes. Too big and your toddler may slip, slide, and even trip in them. Too small and they'll pinch and restrict. (See the box on the facing page for shoe-fitting tips).

Lightweight. Toddlers have a hard enough time putting one bare foot in front of another. The weight of a heavy shoe can make this tricky new skill even more challenging. So think lightweight: canvas or soft leather.

Breathable uppers. Walking is a workout for tots. Uppers of plastic or imitation leather keep feet from breathing and trap perspiration. Yet another good reason to choose shoes made from natural, lightweight materials that let air in and moisture out.

Time for New Shoes?

Not like you're ever in any hurry to go shoe shopping with your toddler, but those shoes get outgrown fast. On average, toddlers need a new pair of shoes every three to four months – yet normal growth spurts and plateaus can result in one pair being outgrown after just one month, and the next after five.

How will you know when it's time for new shoes? Do an at-home fit check at least once a month. When there's less than a half thumb's space at the toes, go shopping.

Thinking about saving a few pounds and passing shoes from one child to another? Not the best idea, if you can afford a new pair. A shoe moulds to the shape of the first foot to wear them, which means it may not fit the next foot as well. Fine for a pair of Sunday best, not so great for those daily walkers.

If the Shoe Fits . . .

Trying shoes on a squirming toddler can be a trying experience. But getting the right fit will get your toddler off on the right foot. Here's how:

Start with the right socks. Try shoes on with the same kind of socks your toddler typically wears – and make sure they're the right ones for a new walker. Stretch socks with some cushioning are best, but make sure they fit without restricting the foot, and that they don't bunch up or wrinkle. When socks start leaving marks on the feet, it's time to move up to the next sock size.

Fit both feet. Feet can differ in size. Just because the right shoe fits right, doesn't mean the left will. So be sure both feet get measured, and both shoes get tried on.

Don't fit while your toddler sits. Shoes should be fitted while your toddler is standing with his or her weight on both feet. When checking fit, make sure those tiny toes aren't curled up – a very common habit in little tykes, particularly those who aren't used to wearing shoes. Rubbing your hand along your toddler's calf will help relax leg muscles and uncurl toes.

Check the width. Pinch the side of the shoe at its widest point. If you can grasp a tiny bit of it between your fingers, the width is just right. If you can pinch a good piece of shoe, it's too wide – and if you can't pinch any, it's too narrow. Another sign of a too narrow shoe: you can feel the little toe or the outside bone of the foot when you run your finger along the side of the shoe.

Check the length. Press your thumb down just beyond the tip of the big (or longest) toe. If there's a thumb's width (about a centimetre or two) of room, the length is right. Press down, too, to make sure the toe box has enough height so that toes can be curled and wriggled comfortably.

Check the heel fit. Slide your little finger between your toddler's heel and the back of the shoe. It should fit snugly. If you can't slip your finger in at all, or if it's a tight squeeze, the shoe is too small. If you can move your little finger around freely – or if there are gaps around the ankle – the shoe is too large.

Try before you buy. The best way to tell whether the shoe fits is to see it in action. If your tot's not walking yet, help him or her take a few assisted steps. Be sure toes don't drag and heels don't slide up and down with each step.

Be sure you don't see red. Before you take the shoes to the till, see if they've left any red marks on your toddler's feet. If so, the shoes don't fit.

Don't buy ahead. Considering how fast toddlers outgrow shoes, there's always the impulse to buy shoes "with room to grow". But extra-large shoes, like too small ones, can lead to irritation and blisters, cause unnecessary tumbles, and make walking even more challenging for a newbie.

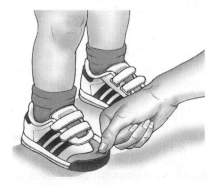

Use your thumb to check for the right fit.

Flexible soles. Feet are flexible, and shoes should be, too. You should be able to bend the toe of the shoe up (about 40 degrees) easily.

Nonslip soles. This time, let your tyres be your guide . . . seriously. A good tyre has good traction to keep a car on the road. Likewise, a good shoe has good traction to keep your toddler on his feet. Nonskid rubber soles, equipped with grooves, will keep your toddler from slipping as he walks and won't be so ground-gripping that it'll be hard for him to lift his feet. When only a dress shoe will do (the kind that has smooth soles), rough the bottoms up with sandpaper or on pavement to improve traction before your toddler toddles off.

Firm, padded heel backs. The backs (or counters) of the shoes should offer firm support – but should also be padded, to prevent rubbing.

No heels. Tempted by heels designed for fashion-forward tots (and their parents)? Resist. Even a slightly raised heel can throw a toddler's posture and balance out of kilter.

Long enough laces. Make sure any laces are long enough to double knot. And then keep them double knotted – otherwise, there's a good chance your toddling tot will trip over undone laces. Velcro is an easy-on option, but keep in mind that it's also easy-off (once your toddler figures out how to undo it, there won't be any keeping shoes on him – and that's not even factoring in the headache you'll get from the sound of ripping Velcro). Or one-two buckle those shoes.

Reasonable price. Shoes should be built to take it, but they don't have to be built to last forever. After all, your toddler will be growing out of them every three months or so. Buying two pairs at a time makes sense, though, since little feet sweat a lot – and switching off will give the shoes a chance to dry out between wearings.

Girl and Boy Parts (a.k.a. Genitals)

VAGINA CARE

Vaginas do a pretty good job of taking care of themselves, but your toddler's will definitely need some help staying healthy. Keeping the vaginal area clean, dry, and irritant-free helps fend off infection. Here's how:

- Change nappies as soon as possible after they become wet or soiled.
- Always wipe your daughter front to back when changing her nappy. Point this out to her, too – so when the time comes for her to tend to this herself, she'll already be familiar with this essential hygiene habit.
- When changing a soft pooey nappy, check around the labia and gently wipe away any stool that may have collected in the crevices. No need to dig around if the area is clean or if you're changing a wet nappy.
- Once she's out of nappies, dress your toddler only in all-cotton underpants to minimise perspiration and maximise ventilation in the area.
- Avoid bubble baths, bath oils, perfumes, harsh soaps, and nappy wipes

that contain alcohol and/or perfumes, any of which may trigger an allergic reaction or irritate or "burn" the vagina. After the bath, it's time for a fresh-water rinse (the water she's been soaking in is a dirt-and-soap cocktail). Rinse her vaginal area with a hand-held shower spray, a cup, or a dripping flannel – and then take her out of the bath so she doesn't sit down again in the dirty water.

- Shampoo your little girl at bath's end so that she won't be sitting in potentially irritating shampoo suds. Have her stand as the water drains, and rinse her hair with a hand-held showerhead or a cup.

If you notice your toddler's vaginal area looking red, or if she seems to be in pain after she pees, it could be a sign of vaginitis – essentially a fancy word for an inflammation of the vagina and/or the vulva. Such inflammation is usually caused by irritation (from bath water, wet nappies, harsh laundry detergents or soap, poor hygiene, and so on). You can treat the irritation with nappy-rash cream or ointment and by making sure to keep the area as dry as possible. The tips above will help prevent a recurrence. If you suspect a urinary tract infection (signs include fever and/or stinging while she's peeing – not after), see page 392.

PENIS CARE

Even though there's extra equipment, a boy's genitals are far easier to care for than a girl's (boys don't have folds and hidden creases like girls do). Here's how:

The circumcised penis. Routine washing with soap and water is the only care a circumcised penis requires.

The uncircumcised penis. No special care is required for the uncircumcised penis, either. Since a toddler's foreskin doesn't usually retract easily, don't try to pull it back. It isn't necessary to clean under it yet anyway. You also don't have to worry about that cheesy-looking material under the foreskin – this is the normal residue of cells that shed as the foreskin and glans begin to separate. These cells gradually work their way out on their own, via the tip of the foreskin, and continue to be shed throughout life. And keep in mind that any adhesion (tissue that keeps the foreskin attached to the penis shaft) will likely loosen by the time your son is 5 years old.

There are a couple of genital-related issues to watch out for in your little boy. First, an undescended testicle, in which one testicle (or less commonly both) has not descended into the scrotum (in other words, it can't be felt in his scrotum) by his first birthday. In this case, it's unlikely it'll come down on its own, so surgery (often laparoscopic) to move the testicle into the scrotum is usually done before he's 15 months old. A retractile testicle (one that comes down into the scrotum occasionally, only to pull back again when exposed to cold temperatures or other stimulation) usually settles permanently into the scrotum closer to puberty, without any treatment.

Another problem to be on the lookout for is urinary flow that's impeded (you'd notice a narrow or dribbly urinary stream and difficulty urinating). This can be caused by a blockage or a narrowing anywhere from the bladder to the opening of the penis, or meatus (this condition is called meatal stenosis). Let the doctor know about any urination issue – he or she will probably want to evaluate your son's stream by watching him pee. Urine should come out in a good strong stream (it should look like it could put out a fire). If it doesn't ever look that way when your little boy pees, it's important to find out why.

The Bottom

BOTTOM CARE

They're cute and sweet as can be – but the same can't be said for what comes out of them. Consequently, toddler bottoms need some cleaning and care to keep them fresh, soft, kissable – and free of nasty nappy rashes. To accomplish this – as well as to treat a simple nappy rash – reduce moisture and exposure to poo (both of which can irritate tender bottoms). Here's the bottom line on bottom care:

- Change your child's nappy as soon as you know it is wet.

- Always pat the bottom dry completely after wiping it and before applying nappy cream or ointment.

- Allow your toddler to wander about the house bare-bottomed when possible and practical – a little air time can help prevent or clear up nappy rash.

- Perfumes and alcohols in soaps, scented baby wipes, and other products that come in contact with your toddler's nether region can irritate his or her skin. Opt for a water-only approach or choose alcohol-free, unscented products if your little one seems particularly prone to rashes.

- Sometimes superabsorbent disposables are so efficient at trapping moisture they lead to more rashes. Try experimenting with different types of disposables to see if that helps prevent nappy rashes.

For nappy rashes that don't clear up after a few days, medication may become necessary, so be sure to put in a call to the GP. For seborrhoeic dermatitis (a deep red rash with yellow scales) and intertrigo (a reddened area where skin touches skin that may ooze white to yellowish gunk), a steroid cream may be necessary; for impetigo (large blisters or crusts that weep, then ooze yellowish fluid, and then crust over), oral antibiotics; and for candida (a fungal or yeast infection that turns the skin bright red and sometimes crops up after a course of antibiotics), a topical antifungal cream or ointment.

Strange Stools

"Now that my son has some teeth, I expected he'd be able to chew up what he eats. But I'm still finding whole pieces of food in his poo."

The contents of your toddler's nappy will continue keeping you guessing for some time to come (is that really a blueberry?). That's because those much-celebrated first few teeth are pretty useless when it comes to chewing. Biting (and looking adorable) is more their business. Until a full set of molars (top and bottom) comes in, a toddler chews with his gums, which means that food doesn't get much of a grinding before it's swallowed. And since a toddler's digestive system is relatively short, what's swallowed passes fairly rapidly through the digestive tract. So it's not surprising that some mouthfuls exit looking more or less the same as when they entered – blueberry in, blueberry out. Among the other interesting titbits you may spy in your child's stool: whole green peas, small chunks of cooked carrot, deep-red slivers of tomato skin, and golden kernels of corn.

As your petite gourmet accumulates a mouthful of molars, he'll be able to chew what he bites off. And as his gastrointestinal transit time slows down, his meals will be more thoroughly digested and his bowel movements less telling (they'll be brown and boring no matter what he eats). In the meantime, be sure that the food you serve is soft enough to be gummed easily (test a new food by trying to mash it in your mouth without using your teeth) and that it's been cut in very small pieces (the smaller the food particles start out, the smaller they end up). If your child, like many toddlers, doesn't seem to bother much with gumming, and prefers the shovel-and-gulp method of eating instead, try encouraging him to chew before he swallows. Take a bite when he does and show him how it's done ("See, I'm mushing up the food in my mouth. Can you do that?").

The New Scoop on Poo

Interestingly, as your toddler takes in more solid food during the second year, he or she will probably poo less. Expect an average of 4 to 20 bowel movements per week, depending on diet, fluid intake, and individual patterns (every digestive system's different).

Is your toddler pooing more – or less – than that? When it comes to healthy bowel movements, consistency is more important than frequency. As long as the stool is soft and easy to pass, your little pooper is popping those stools out just fine. On the other hand, small, hard, and difficult-to-pass poo may signal constipation (see page 388); watery, frequent (as in many times a day), and loose poo may be diarrhoea (see page 390).

The Nappy Wars

"My toddler won't hold still for nappy changes – she fights me the whole time."

Ah, the battle of the bottom. You fight to clean and cover it – she fights to keep you from doing either. She has no patience for lying still, you have no patience for the kicking and rolling around that makes every nappy change a squirming skirmish. Yet, when it's time for a change, it's time for a change. Here's how to quell the nappy revolt:

Check for sore spots. Maybe your little rebel has a nappy rash that hurts when you clean her – so she resists your advances. And maybe her sore bottom feels better when she's bare – so she tries every tactic to stay stripped down. If you think this might be the case with your little one, a little treatment (and a gentle touch) may help. See the facing page.

Come to the table prepared. If you have everything – wipes, ointments, and nappies – at the ready before you scoop her up, changing her can be accomplished 1-2-3, giving her less time to realise what's happening and less time to rebel.

Create a diversion. Pull out a special stash of playthings reserved for nappy changes – the more diverting, the better. Sure, the board book that makes animal sounds drives you to distraction (and drove you to hide it from your toddler last week), but those shrill moos and oinks may distract her, too – long enough so you can get her nappy on without a fight. Ditto a CD of sing-along songs, a talking stuffed animal, a play mobile phone, even the keys you're always trying to keep out of her hands. Or divert with a game of "show me your belly . . . show me your nose . . .", punctuated by some belly raspberries and loud toe kisses. Or appoint your toddler

No More Nappies?

Eager for your little one to give up the nappy and move on to toilet training? It's probably a bit early for that. Most kids don't become fully toilet trained until well after their second birthday – but you can start laying the groundwork for the next stage; see the facing page.

the "nappy helper" and have her hand you supplies (with tops on) as you need them. A little humour can go a long way, too – drape the clean nappy over your head, or pretend to put it on yourself . . . or the dog.

Move the offensive. If the changing table has turned into a battlefield, maybe it's time to retreat to neutral territory. Protected by a towel or waterproof pad, almost any flat surface can be used for changing a nappy. Try the living room floor, a large beanbag chair, the cot, your bed, the bath mat.

Attack vertically. Once a child is toddling on two feet, it's an affront to be forced onto her back. So you may face less rebellion if you change her nappy where she stands – as long as she's standing on a washable surface, of course (don't try this on an unprotected sofa or carpet). Approach the behind from behind. And make sure those diversions are close by as you close in.

Skip the element of surprise. Toddlers don't like surprises. So give a heads-up that it's time for a clean bottom. If your toddler is in the middle of an activity, try to wait until she's finished, or take the toy along to the changing table. And try to keep the mood upbeat. You're less likely to face a fight if you don't anticipate one.

Try a change of command. If Mummy with a nappy signals a struggle to your toddler, it may be time to call up some new troops. Put Daddy on nappy duty, or recruit anyone else who's willing and able.

Take control. If none of the above seem to work, hold your toddler down (or better still, have an ally restrain those swinging feet) and get the job done as quickly as possible. Be matter-of-fact and friendly as you pull your nappy coup – yelling or threatening will only add fuel to your toddler's fury. Remember, it's easier for your tot to fight when someone's fighting back.

Playing with Nappy Contents

"My son has found a fun game: pulling off his dirty nappy and playing with its contents. Needless to say, I'm not enjoying the game."

Toddlers will play with (and sometimes put in their mouths) just about anything they can get their hands on. And if it's squishy, squeezable, spreadable, and forbidden – all the better. Now that your toddler has discovered the delights of nappy-dumping and poo art, it won't be easy to keep his hands out of his stash. Until he loses interest in this pastime (which can take a few days to a few months), you can minimise the problem by:

Limiting access. Your toddler can't get his hands on his faeces if he can't get his hands in his nappies. So secure his nappy tightly (but not so tight that it leaves red marks) and dress him in clothes that limit access, such as dungarees, clothes that button at the crotch (instead of poppers), trousers that are buttoned and difficult to remove, or one-piece outfits. If you get really desperate, put his nappy on backwards so it's harder for him to take off, or use packing or sticky tape to secure the nappy.

Heading him off. Many toddlers keep to a fairly predictable bowel-movement pattern (one moves his bowels after each meal, another just once a day after breakfast, another always wakes up with a mess in his nappy, and so on). If you've figured out your toddler's pooing pattern, try catching him in the act (or immediately after) as often as possible. That way you can get to his nappy before he does.

Providing a substitute. Squishing, squeezing, and spreading are irresistible tactile experiences for toddlers. Supply your toddler with plenty of alternative opportunities for that kind of play, and he may not feel as compelled to look for them in his nappy. Give him squishy, squeezy toys (make sure they're age-appropriate and safe), and opportunities for finger painting, sand play (especially satisfying when water is mixed with the sand), and playing with Play-Doh. (Most of these activities will require careful adult supervision.)

Remaining unfazed. Chances are excellent that, in spite of all your efforts to discourage or distract, your toddler will still find the will and a way to pursue his nappy probing. And chances are even better that the more attention (either negative or positive) you pay to his dirty little game, the more eager he'll be to keep playing it. So keep both the smiles and the scowls off your face, and don't make a stink about the stink (disparaging his bowel movements may lead to future potty problems). Instead, calmly but firmly make it perfectly clear that the behaviour is unacceptable ("Don't touch the poo. It's dirty").

Telling him where to put it. Teachable moments are everywhere when you have a toddler – even on those poo-smeared hands. While his faeces fascination isn't a sign that he's ready to start using the potty, it is an ideal opportunity to introduce the toilet to your toddler – and to show him where poo ultimately belongs. Take him into the bathroom, empty what remains of the contents of his nappy into the toilet, and explain, "Poo goes in the potty." You can even let him flush, if he seems interested, and if the noise doesn't frighten him. Then finish cleaning up in the bathroom – including, of course, a thorough hand washing (along with another reminder: "We always wash our hands when we touch poo, because poo is dirty").

Offer a snack if he goes for a sample. Did your toddler go in for a lick? Again, don't freak. Matter-of-factly say, "Poo isn't for eating. Food is for eating. Let's clean up and then have a snack."

ALL ABOUT:
Thinking About Toilet Training

When is the right time for toddlers to ditch those nappies and take a seat on the potty? Actually, there is no right time. Like all developmental achievements, children pick up potty skills at their own speed, and when it happens has no correlation with other areas of development (like walking, talking, or teething). On average, most toddlers master toileting between the ages of 2 and 3½. The average for girls is 35 months, the average for boys is 39 months, with peeing usually ahead of pooing for both genders.

Studies show that there's no inherent advantage to starting toilet learning early. In fact, it typically takes longer to completely train an under-2-year-old than to wait until the beginning of the third year to get the potty party started. That said, there's no reason to postpone the potty programme if your toddler seems eager and ready to roll – and, in fact, there's no better reason to get started. Since cooperation is key in toilet training (this is definitely one agenda you can't force), you're bound to get better results when your little one's on board, both developmentally and emotionally. Most toddlers show signs of readiness between 20 and 30 months, though some children will hop on board earlier and others later.

In other unscientific words (because potty training definitely isn't a precise science), kids are ready when they're ready. That's why it's important to let your child set the potty pace – if the timing isn't right, even the best toilet-training tactics won't get the job done.

POTTY READY SIGNS

Here are some signs of potty readiness:

- You're changing fewer wet nappies. Until the age of about 20 months, kids pee so frequently that expecting them to control their bladders is probably unrealistic. But a toddler who stays dry for an hour or two at a stretch – and occasionally awakes without wetness – may be physically ready to take the next step.

- Your toddler starts giving a BM blow-by-blow. Some children happily

---

MILESTONE

Potty Readiness

Ready to give up nappy changes, but not sure if your toddler's ready for the big change? Here's the toilet timeline for most 1- to 2-year-olds:

12 to 15 months. Most children early in the second year aren't showing any signs of toilet readiness (though a small minority may be ready earlier than others). By age 15 months, some children will start showing signs that they can "feel it coming".

15 to 18 months. As your toddler's language skills start to improve, he or she may start using potty words to describe what's going on in the nappy area. Your little one may also

enjoy watching bigger ones (you, your spouse, an older sibling, cousin, or friend) use the toilet. Since observing the process in progress can demystify it, consider an open-door policy, if you're comfortable with one.

18 to 24 months. As the second birthday approaches, potty readiness signs will probably become more apparent. Your toddler may enjoy sitting on a special little kid potty (with nappy on), reading toilet books, or even pretending a doll is using the potty. It may be time to start thinking about toilet learning, but watch for those signs before you move ahead.

But Are *You* Ready?

Maybe you're giddy at the thought of giving up nappy changes – and those midnight nappy runs. You're already mentally spending (or banking) the money you'd save on nappies each month. You're imagining all the space you'll have in your little one's room without those piles of nappy boxes and once you move out that changing table or convert it into a dresser. And who's going to miss the Nappy Genie?

Or maybe you're dreading the potty process like nobody's business. You're worried that you're too busy right now to play potty police. Or that the holidays are coming up, and you don't want to be wiping up pools of pee while entertaining a houseful of guests. Or you're just worried about your new living room rug.

In deciding when to take the potty plunge, your toddler's readiness is definitely a top priority – but your readiness counts, too, as do circumstances at home and at work. Potty training takes eagerness, willingness, and cooperation from your toddler, but it also takes time, attention, commitment, consistency, and loads of patience (not to mention, many loads of laundry) from you. Tackling the project when you're inundated at work or overwhelmed by other stresses (the child minder quit, the dog's sick, the dryer's on the blink) may be asking for trouble. Ditto, you may want to consider postponing potty happiness if there's about to be a major change or disruption in your child's life (like a holiday or a parent leaving on a business trip).

announce when a bowel movement is about to make an exit ("Me poo!"). Others communicate through less verbal means – by retreating to a corner, for instance, or producing a preemptive grunt. Either way, your little one's aware that a poo's about to pop – and is letting you know.

- Your toddler dislikes those dirty nappies. Is your little one eager to escape a nappy as soon as it's wet or soiled? That could be another signal of readiness to ditch the nappies.

- Your toddler can undress for potty success. When nature calls, the potty won't be of much use unless your child can quickly yank down his or her trousers and pull-ups or underwear.

- Your toddler can talk the potty talk. Whether you prefer child-friendly jargon like "poo" and "pee" or technical terminology like "defecate" and "urinate", it's important that your child understands and can use the family's words for bathroom functions and any associated body parts. Communication is key to potty success.

POTTY ABLE SIGNS

Keep in mind that even if all signs point to your toddler being "ready," there's still the "able" component to consider. Key to potty proficiency is being capable of performing a challenging 10-step potty process:

1. Feel it coming

2. Hold it in

3. Get to the potty

4. Pull down pants

5. Sit on the potty

6. Push

7. Wipe (with help)

8. Get off the potty

9. Pull up pants

10. Flush (though this step isn't a deal breaker)

In other words, even if all the readiness signs are there, it doesn't mean your toddler is going to take to toileting in no time at all. Your little one can be "ready" to start the process for months before he or she has what it takes to perform it completely without your assistance. Take your cues from the expert – your toddler.

POTTY PREP

The second year may be too soon for most toddlers to embark on a full-fledged potty training mission, but it's also never too early to start laying the groundwork. While you shouldn't push a tot who clearly isn't interested or ready to try a toilet (it could backfire – and the mission could end up taking a whole lot longer than it has to), if your toddler is definitely showing signs of readiness, you can begin setting the stage for some practice runs. Here's how:

Gear up. Choose either a child-size potty (look for a model that's durable and won't tip over when your child jumps up to check progress) or a potty seat that simply attaches to the grown-up toilet. Then remind your toddler what the potty is for: "Whenever you feel ready, you can use this potty instead of a nappy to pee and poo in." Buy some fun underwear, too, and point to it occasionally: "One day, you can wear pants, like Mummy and Daddy do!"

See it, suggest it. When you notice that your little one is about to poo or pee (most tots show obvious signs that a poo is coming, while around half indicate they're about to pee), suggest to your toddler that he or she do it on the potty instead of in the nappy. If the answer is a resounding "no!", leave it alone.

Give a demo. Of course, you could explain to your child how to squat, push, wipe, and flush, but it's much more effective – not to mention efficient – to simply bring your potty pupil to the bathroom and demonstrate. Not all parents are comfortable doing their business with an audience, though, so don't feel bad about skipping this step if it's not quite your speed. Of course, the demonstration will be most helpful if the parent who has the same plumbing as your toddler performs it.

Play up the potty positives. Well before your first nappy-free trial run, highlight the perks of using the potty. You might say, "Wearing pants is fun!" or "Pretty soon you can flush, just like Mummy and Daddy!" But don't knock nappies or call your child's old habits babyish – or the contents of a nappy smelly. That could provoke the kind of trademark negativity that's likely to lead to real resistance ("You want to see baby . . . I'll show you baby!").

Read all about it. Seek out a potty-training book geared to toddlers and read it together. (Check out *What to Expect When You Use the Potty*, *The Pop-Up Potty Book* or *Have You Seen My Potty?*) But don't feel you need to hammer home a lesson or compare your toddler to the characters. Just hearing about other children using the potty and seeing them do it will help your little one feel more comfortable when making the leap onto the seat.

Toilet-Training Trends

There's a reason why nappies are getting bigger and bigger: the children wearing them are getting older and older. The average age for ditching nappies has definitely crept steadily up over the years, now hovering at just over 3. And studies seem to back up a somewhat later starting date for Project Potty, showing that while it's definitely possible to train very young children (under 18 months), it typically takes far longer than it does for those 24 months and up. That's because toddlers under 2 aren't typically ready to master toileting.

Still, you may have heard about a toilet-training trend called "elimination communication", designed for very early learners (infancy and up) and the parents eager to train them. Maybe you've even spotted one of those apparent potty prodigies sporting a nappy-free profile at the playground and wondered: how does it work? Essentially, parents put their little ones on the potty according to a schedule or as soon as they notice the signs of elimination in progress. Whether it's the parents or the children who are trained is debatable, but when it works, it allows nappies to be ditched early in the second year or even late in the first. Regardless, it's definitely labour intensive (for parents), requiring a very flexible schedule and very quick reflexes.

Up for the challenge of super-early training? Go for it if you want – just be prepared to spend lots of time on the project. Not in any hurry? That's fine, too – just wait until you're both ready. One thing's for sure: your toddler will learn how to use the potty eventually. Potty promise!

Bridge the gap between nappies and the potty. If possible, start changing your toddler's nappies in the room where the potty is stashed (probably the bathroom) – this subtly reinforces the connection between the two. After a BM deposit in the nappy, bring it to the big toilet so your tyke can watch you flush the poo (or you can flush it together). You can even add a "bye-bye, poo" ritual, which many toddlers enjoy. If your child is frightened of the flushing sound, just dump together and flush later.

Let your child be the teacher. Buy or borrow a special doll that wets and encourage your child to help the doll use the potty. This can boost understanding of the process, provide practice, and give your toilet learner a greater sense of control over a pretty daunting process.

Provide easy access. Get in the habit of dressing your toddler in easy-on, easy-off bottoms (trousers that pull up and down without any fiddling – no dungarees or tricky buttons), and then practise the all-important pull-down manoeuvre. Ask your toddler to pull down his or her trousers before nappy changes and then pull them back up after. You can even have a contest: "Let's see if you can pull down your trousers before I count to three!" or "Let's see who can pull trousers down faster!" Remember, there will be no time to spare when nature calls your potty newbie, so the more practice, the better.

Prevent potty overload. If all the potty talk starts rubbing your toddler the wrong way, boredom starts to set in, or it becomes clear that the time isn't right after all – give it a rest for a while. Pushing the potty – whether you've started the training process or you're just gearing up for it – rarely works.

READY . . . SET . . . GO POTTY

All potty systems are go? Your toddler's ready, you're ready, the new potty or potty seat's at the ready? While there are plenty of approaches to potty learning – from the super-scheduled to the really relaxed – there are five basic steps to potty proficiency:

1. Switch your toddler into pull-ups or training pants – or take the plunge to regular pants (you'll want a mop handy if you do). While pull-ups will make the process less messy (you won't be cleaning up pools of pee like you would with training pants or underwear), it'll also make it last longer. Like nappies, pull-ups whisk moisture away from your tot's bottom, making him or her less likely to notice (or be bothered by) wetness. It also strips away some of the motivation for getting to the potty on time, though some pull-ups have child-friendly features, like colour or temperature changes, that alert little ones to wetness – and that can pump up interest considerably. Switching from nappies directly to cotton training pants or even regular boys' or girls' underwear will definitely be messy (accidents will happen), but will likely shorten the training process for a potty-ready toddler. Another incentive with big-boy or -girl underwear: they're for a big boy or girl – something that most every toddler aspires to be. Want the best of both worlds? Use a combination of pull-ups (for times when an accident would be extra-inconvenient) and cotton underwear (for at-home training sessions).

2. Remind your toddler throughout the day to go to the potty when he or she has to poo or pee: "Don't forget, Max. If you have to pee, do it in the big boy potty." But don't stop at just verbal reminders. Take your toddler to the bathroom at regular intervals and sit him or her on the toilet (you never know . . . something might come out). You can even encourage the flow of urine with a trickle of water: turn on the bathroom tap while your toddler sits on the potty (it's an old trick but a good one). And watch for those cues (grunting, squirming, going off to a corner); if you pay attention, you'll know just when to whisk your little one right to the potty. Even if you're too late and your tot's already done the deed, try having him or her sit on the potty anyway to reinforce the connection. And, of course, if your tot poos at predictable times (such as right after he wakes up in the morning, or right after she eats her lunch), be sure to make a break for the bathroom at those times, too.

3. Boost your toddler's awareness of body signals by allowing your little one to scamper about (in a private garden or a room with a washable floor) with his or her bottom bared. It's hard to ignore the urine when there's no nappy to hold it in. Keep the potty close by so your child can act on those body signals (or that trickling-down-the-leg pee) quickly.

4. Bring on the praise – and the stickers. Be a big potty booster, cheering on your toddler every step of the way, even when those efforts don't always bring success. Playing up the "big girl" angle can be especially motivating ("You made a pee-pee on the potty, just like Mummy. . . . what a big girl you are!"), but avoid making baby references when your toddler's attempts fail ("Only babies pee in their pants!"). Positive reinforcement (especially in the form of special rewards) can help spur on your little potty pooper. Each time he or she produces in the toilet, reward your toddler with a sticker, a big hug, a star on a toilet chart, and so on. Skip big-ticket rewards (your toddler will come to expect them) and food rewards (never a good precedent to set).

5. Let your toddler set the pace. Keep it casual when reminding your tot about using the potty – nagging will only provoke resistance. Ditto, when it comes to forcing. Never make your toddler sit or stay on the potty if he or she is ready to get up – even if you know there's a poo about to happen. Squabbling over pottying is sure to prolong the process. If you meet with total defiance, it's best to throw in the towel (and the toilet paper) for a while.

Nothing happening? Or has your potty student taken a turn for the reluctant, or even the rebellious? Maybe you pushed a little too hard. Maybe your tot's not as ready as you thought. Either way, don't worry about false starts. Just bring back the nappies, back off from the potty, and wait till everyone's had a break and the time's just right.

CHAPTER 3

Your Toddler On the Go

E VEN IF YOUR LITTLE EXPLORER isn't yet on two feet – and especially if running and climbing have already left walking in the dust – there's no doubt about it: your toddler is living life in the fast lane, and sometimes . . . right on the edge. And it all happens in the blink of an eye (but don't blink – otherwise your toddler will be halfway down the street without you). Soon after those first steps, it's a hop, skip, and a jump to more advanced motor skills like running, climbing, and kicking. This rapid mastery of large motor skills will quickly leave you realising that the days of staying a comfortable step ahead of your little one are gone – and that you'll now be racing just to keep up. Sure, it'll take plenty of practice for your toddler to coordinate the many movements he or she will need to perform some of those advanced skills (hey, this stuff isn't as simple as it looks!), but your encouragement will make the moving move along faster than you expect.

What You May Be Wondering About

Walking

"When will my 13-month-old son start to walk?"

While few moments are as cute (or as recordable) as your little one's first wobbly steps (unless of course you count that first smile, that first clap, that first crawl . . .), not all tots are ready for their video moment the moment they turn a year old. But just because your toddler isn't yet performing great feats on two feet doesn't mean he isn't in the running for on-time walking. Of

Getting Up and Going

Is your toddler still on all fours? Or has your mini-marathoner already broken into a sprint? Is your barely 1-year-old a master mountaineer (at least when it comes to flights of stairs and piles of cushions)? Or is your almost 2-year-old still taking every step like it's Mount Everest? Toddlers are all over the developmental map when it comes to those large motor skills (walking, running, climbing), but most fall into the following age-by-age categories:

12 to 15 months. Some 12-month-olds are already walking on their own, and a few have even been at it for months. Others are just beginning to pull themselves up to standing early in the second year, and still others may have been on two feet for many months, but still haven't gotten up the nerve to take a first unassisted step. By 15 months, a sizeable majority of toddlers who aren't yet walking solo will be cruising – taking a few cautious steps while clutching the sides of furniture, or holding your helping hands or the handle of a push toy.

15 to 18 months. By 15 months, the early walkers are probably already proficient at toddling, though their stance and gait may still be more wide-legged than graceful (they're called toddlers for a reason). Newbie walkers who are just now getting the hang of balancing on two feet will still be a little shaky, with first steps that tend to be tentative and wobbly. But as their legs become more muscular, their walk will become more steady and firm, allowing little ones to explore with more freedom than ever before. By this time, most tots (even those who aren't yet comfortable on their feet) enjoy push toys, which offer something to lean on while they take their practice laps. Once they're confident in their walking skills, they'll be able to drag a pull toy behind them.

18 to 24 months. By the second half of the second year, the majority of tots have mastered the art of the squat (yoga anyone?). Most later walkers have also caught up to the early movers and shakers and have graduated to upward mobility: climbing (up and down stairs, out of the high chair, onto the kitchen counter) – there's really nothing some toddlers won't attempt to scale, so don't forget to toddler-proof your home; see page 405). Running isn't far behind (though for some tenacious tots, running is already the name of the game), so you'd better lace up your own trainers. It'll be hard to keep up!

Be on the lookout: If by 12 months your child is not trying to stand, still seems uninterested in cruising by 15 months, or hasn't stepped out on his or her own by the last few months of the second year, talk to your GP for reassurance. Your little one's probably just busy focusing on other skills, but in some cases, there may be a physical or developmental delay or muscle weakness that could benefit from physical therapy or do-at-home exercises.

course, some precocious little ones master upright mobility before their first birthday, but others don't take a single step until 15 months, and still others don't start putting one foot in front of the other on their own until as late as 18 months.

That very wide walking range of normal is just that – wide and normal. Even if your sweetie ends up taking his sweet time stepping out on his own, he's likely to catch up quickly. Many slowpoke walkers break into a run just weeks after they've started to walk.

When your little one starts taking those first steps can be related to a number of factors: his genetic wiring (if either parent walked late, he may, too), his temperament (a high-energy toddler may walk earlier than a mellow one), his build (a lean baby will likely strut his stuff sooner than a Buddha-baby), and his confidence level (cautious kids may want to wait until they're steadier on two feet, while daredevils are often raring to go, taking tumbles in stride). The good news about the timetable for walking is that there's no timetable at all. Whatever age your toddler starts toddling, whether at 9 months or 16 months, it's no reflection on his developmental potential.

Your toddler will start toddling when he's ready. Meantime, lend a helping hand (and a couple of clapping hands to cheer on his efforts), but rather than focusing on the finish line, embrace the journey (and the bumps, falls, baby steps, and false starts along the way). It's a journey that will make his victory lap – when it finally comes – seem that much sweeter.

Encouraging Walking

"Is there anything I can do to encourage my daughter to walk? She's already 15 months old but seems plenty happy to sit in one spot or just crawl when she wants to get somewhere."

Tired of just sitting there watching your child just sitting there? Don't sweat those first steps, or try to rush them (if she's not ready to step out on her own, no amount of parental prodding will motivate her to reach that milestone faster – and, in fact, too much pressure can slow her down plenty). Just give your little one lots of space and opportunity to practise her prewalking skills, offer lots of encouragement and

positive reinforcement (think gung-ho cheerleader, not drill sergeant), and provide conditions that won't trip her up when she makes those tentative attempts at walking.

Start with a small shopping trolley, pint-size lawn mower, or other stable push toy that can give your toddler the supportive cruise control she needs as she works those legs, refines her balance, and boosts her confidence. Look for push toys with a bar or handle she can lean on and big wheels and weighting that make it harder for the toy to tip over, which could take her confidence down with it. Encourage her to push the toy to reach the reward across the room: you – with a big smile on your face, your arms wide open and poised for a hug.

If your not-yet-toddling toddler still doesn't seem to want to get up and go, also consider what she's wearing. Slippery socks and bulky clothes may keep a new walker grounded, so no matter the season, keep her outfits streamlined when she's in trekker training mode – steer clear of tight or stiff clothes that could constrict movement, and avoid loose and flowing clothes that could tangle her up. Make sure her shoes are made for walking (see page 54), and while you're at it, keep your

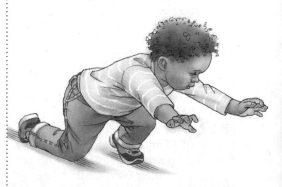

A new walker will take lots of spills and falls.

Walking to Different Beats

Have your twins been running (and crawling, and cruising, and walking) on just about the same developmental schedule since day one? Or does one always seem to be leaving the other in the developmental dust? Or do they seem to switch off making milestones first? The truth is, all children develop at the rate that's right for them – a rate that twins may share a little, a lot, or not at all. After all, despite rooming together in the womb and being born on the same day, twins (and other multiples) are very much their own little people. They have their own personalities, their own interests, their own abilities, and their own developmental blueprint for all skills, including those gross motor ones. While developmental patterns may be quite similar in identical twins (yes, sometimes even nearly identical – they take their stand for the first time on the same day, take their first steps on the same day), they often aren't in fraternal twins, who are genetically no more alike than any two siblings (though the achievements of one may motivate the other). As long as both your little ones are reaching most milestones within the very wide range of normal (with adjusted age factored in, if they were born prematurely), their development can be considered on target – even if they're not developing the same skills at the very same time.

Have a habit of comparing your twins when it comes to development? Resisting comparing any child to another child (whether it's a sibling or another tot at nursery) is always easier said than done – but it can be especially challenging for you, since you're watching the differences between your toddlers play out in front of your eyes every day. Still – and you probably already know this, at least deep inside: it's not fair to compare. So try to treat each twin like an individual when celebrating his or her amazing achievements – whether or not those skills match up pace-wise. And remember, few toddlers develop at the same rate across the developmental boards. Maybe your not-yet-walking tot is cruising ahead in verbal development, or busy focusing on perfecting fine motor skills ("Look, I can eat with a fork!") instead of concentrating on putting one foot in front of the other ("I'll leave that for later"). Just don't forget to applaud as loudly for the second set of first steps as you did for the first.

If you notice that one or both of your twins is consistently missing milestones or seems to be suddenly slipping significantly in development – or if you have a gut feeling that something isn't right – check in with the doctor.

---

daughter's tootsies bare as much as you can for a closer encounter with the floor (bare feet offer optimum traction and flexibility, helping her develop balance and coordination). Next best to barefeet are socks with rubberised treads on the bottom.

One last bit of advice: ban the baby walker (it can slow motor development and worse, can tip over or roll down the stairs, causing injuries) and put away the activity centre (while it doesn't carry rough-and-tumble risks, it doesn't boost skills, and can even cause lags).

Delayed Walking

"Our 18-month-old son is the only child in his playgroup not walking on his own. Should we be concerned?"

Most children are stepping out on their own by 18 months, but occasionally a toddler refuses to toddle until later. Sometimes fear (because of a previous nasty fall) keeps a toddler from letting go and taking off. Sometimes it's proficiency as a crawler (he knows he can get around more quickly on hands and knees than on feet). Sometimes a gross-motor developmental timetable that's on the slow side of normal is responsible. And sometimes walking is delayed by a problem that needs medical attention.

Your first step in finding out why your son hasn't yet taken his first solo steps is to consult his doctor. You'll probably get the reassurance you're looking for. If a problem is discovered, the news is still good: early physical therapy can help your toddler catch up.

Going Back to Crawling

"Our daughter started walking a week ago, but has suddenly gone back to crawling. Is something wrong?"

There's no better way to describe the feat of walking than as a one-step-forward, one-step-back process. After all, you can't expect your toddler to master the art of walking one day and then never plop back down again for a quick crawl (especially since crawling will get her from point A to point B a lot faster than walking will these days). It's only natural for your little one to switch off between her newfound skill (walking) and her previous – and possibly favoured – mode of getting around (crawling).

A return to crawling can also be due to these factors:

- Frustration. It takes patience – an attribute most toddlers have in short supply – to perfect walking. Frustration over frequent falls, slow speed, or an inability to turn a corner without bumping into it may prompt your toddler to take to her knees again until her legs and feet have worked out their kinks.

- A nasty fall. Taking a traumatic tumble can cause a cautious toddler to think twice about getting back on her feet again. Until she recovers her nerve, crawling may provide the most comforting form of mobility.

- A new accomplishment. Often, a still-wobbly skill, such as walking, will be temporarily dropped while a toddler focuses her full attention on honing another, such as talking.

- An upcoming cold or other minor illness. For a few days before the symptoms of a cold, flu, or other virus become apparent – and, of course, during an infection – children often suffer from a run-down feeling that keeps them from running around. In this case, walking, which is still a challenge, might well be dropped in favour of the more familiar and less stressful crawling. Teething can have the same effect.

- A bad day. Everybody has them – and some toddlers have them quite often. Grumpiness and fatigue can temporarily sap a toddler's mojo and dampen her enthusiasm for challenging activities, including walking.

Of course, if your toddler is unusually irritable, or seems to be limping or unable to stand upright, check with her doctor to make sure there is no physical problem, such as an injury or illness.

Also check with the doctor if your child has been walking for a few months already and all of a sudden no longer seems capable of doing it.

Coordination . . . or Lack of It

"My son is always bumping into things – or falling down. Could it be his coordination? His eyesight?"

One-year-olds, collisions, and falls go hand in hand – and often, head over heels. There are several good reasons why your toddler is an accident (and an accidental fall) waiting to happen, all of them completely age-appropriate:

He's a new walker. Walking looks easy, doesn't it? Well, not so much when you're first starting out on two feet, not to mention trying to put one foot in front of the other for the first time. It'll take plenty of time and experience before he's steady as he goes – and before he can avoid head-ons with the wall . . . or always being the fall guy.

He's short on balance and coordination. Both of these skills take practice to perfect, especially when you're trying to put them together. Ever tried to learn how to snowboard or surf or water ski as an adult? Then you have an inkling of what your toddling tot is up against. And why he often walks into walls, tables, or people – and has a hard time staying on his feet (and off his fortunately well-padded bottom).

He doesn't look where he's going. Understandably preoccupied with the challenging mechanics of walking, your little guy often focuses on his feet instead of where they're taking him. Or he fixes his attention on the person or object he's trying to reach – Daddy, a favourite stuffed giraffe, the

remote control he just spied on the sofa – instead of the lorry he's about to trip over, or the coffee table he's about to barrel into. Even if he does glimpse a roadblock or stumbling block at the last minute, he may not be able to veer around it or stop short of it, especially if he's picked up some speed. Figuring out how to step on the brakes comes later.

He has a limited attention span. This may be stating the obvious, but a toddler is easily distracted. He's on his way to the toy car garage when he sees his stuffed dog – and trips trying to change direction. He's toddling over to the kitchen when the doorbell rings. He turns and looks – and promptly takes a tumble.

His sight is far from perfect. Another reason your toddler's such a flopper (and apparent klutz): he's longsighted. A 1-year-old's eyesight has come a long way since those fuzzier baby days, but he still has limited depth perception, which makes judging distances tricky, even if you could rely on him to look where he's going. By age 2, vision improves to about 20/60; by age 3 to

---

Born Early?

Wondering how your premature baby will stack up development-wise to his or her peers now that they're all toddlers? While it's true premature babies may reach milestones a little later (especially during the first year), the developmental gap typically narrows and disappears entirely by the second birthday. Until then, use your toddler's "adjusted" age when calculating all milestones.

Taking the Ouch Out of Falls

Falling for your little one . . . well, that's the easy part. The harder part is trying to prevent your toddler from taking as many of those tumbles as you can, and to protect against injury when you can't. Here's how:

- Factor in flooring. Of course, wall-to-wall carpeting can be a stain-magnet when there's a toddler in the house, but it's also the most forgiving surface for a new walker, cutting down on slip-ups and softening the falls that do happen. Rugs, on the other hand, are notorious for tripping up even the most seasoned walker (sound familiar?). If you do have rugs, make sure they lie flat on a nonslip pad. If you have slate, tile, stone, brick, wood, or otherwise slippery or extra-hard floors, and don't feel like remodelling, you'll just have to be extra vigilant until your toddler's steady on his or her feet (see the tips that follow).

- Let your toddler go barefoot when possible. Those adorable tootsies help your toddler put his or her best foot forward, providing more traction and comfort, the most padding, and the most flexibility. When bare's not an option, socks are next best. Select socks that fit well, can be trusted to stay on, and most important of all, are slip-proof. When only shoes will do, choose those that most closely mimic nature's design (comfortable, flexible, well-fitting, and with good traction). See page 54 for more on toddler shoes.

- Keep drawers and doors closed. That goes for dressers, kitchen doors and drawers, room doors, appliance doors – anything your toddler might collide with or trip over. You'll save yourself some bruises, too (how many times have you banged your shin into the open dishwasher door this week?).

about 20/40. But it's not until roughly school age that normal 20/20 vision can be in the cards (that is, unless he needs glasses).

A lack of reason. Right now, he's on auto-pilot. He's (sort of) mastered the physical skill of walking, but not the reasoning skills that will keep him from walking into trouble. With time, he'll be able to coordinate not only his feet, but that vital communication between his feet and his brain ("Warning . . . toy car ahead!").

Oops, he did it again . . . and again? Fortunately, coordination, balance, attention span, and vision sharpen with time – as will his ability to navigate his world more safely and steadily (though don't expect him to win any coordination contests until about age 8 or 9). Until then, you can protect him from some of life's little bumps and falls by making his world safer (see box above).

Climbing

"My 18-month-old loves to climb on everything and anything. Should I try to stop her?"

What goes up and doesn't like to come down? Most toddlers – every chance they get. Once they've

- Look out for electrical cords that your little explorer could trip over. Two more reasons to keep cords inaccessible or tacked down: they can pose a strangulation hazard, as well as pull down heavy objects – like computers or lamps – onto your toddler.

- Screen each room for flimsy furniture your toddler could tip over, and temporarily move those pieces to areas your toddler can't get to. Remember, your little one is far from steady, so any furniture that might be clutched on to for support should be reliably stable.

- Keep stairs safely blocked off so your toddler isn't tempted to practise climbing skills on his or her own, or worse, trip and tumble down a flight (see page 407).

- Outfit your toddler with the day's adventures in mind. Long trousers will cushion blows to those dimpled little knees, but if trousers are too long – or falling down – they can trip your toddler up.

- Check out all of the toddler-proofing tips starting on page 405.

Done everything you can to protect your toddler? Now, relax. Toddlers are built to take it. Those little bodies are made with not only cuteness but practicality in mind: close to the ground, well-cushioned with baby fat, and usually in nappies (for extra cushioning). Plus, their skulls are still somewhat flexible (that soft spot won't close up completely until 18 months), which means that a toddler can generally handle minor bumps to the head with nothing more than a few tears. Keep a close watch as you enjoy those exploits on two feet, but avoid overprotecting – or overreacting when your toddler takes a minor tumble.

mastered life on the ground, they're usually eager to explore their world vertically – scaling chairs, beds, and tables; climbing stairs; and clambering onto anything that will enable them to reach higher and higher heights. The particularly intrepid might even learn to stack objects to reach entirely new levels ("Hmmm . . . if I put my stool on top of the couch, I can reach that lamp!").

Your toddler's monkey-like tendencies may drive you bananas – and "get down from there!" may have already replaced "don't touch that!" as your most frequently screeched phrase (though come to think of it, you may be using them both in quick succession). But there's no need to completely squelch your little climbing-crazy tot's desire for upward mobility. After all, climbing is another way she can explore her environment, experiencing it from totally different vantage points – which can be exhilarating when you're 0.6 m tall. It's also a vital skill to practise and perfect – after all, even if she never does any mountaineering, she'll still have to climb a flight of stairs every now and then. Plus, climbing allows her confidence to soar, literally, along with her coordination, her spirit of independence, and her drive to take on and conquer life's challenges.

Still, your toddler can climb into a heap of trouble if you're not careful – and watching her like a hawk. To keep

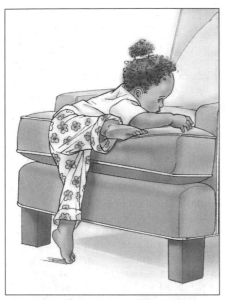

Up, up, and away – most toddlers are vertically motivated and resourceful when it comes to getting to the top.

her safe while she indulges her vertical urges:

- Provide safe outlets. Let her climb to her heart's content on a small plastic slide or climbing frame, and buy a sturdy children's step stool so she can access out-of-reach toys or books without resorting to makeshift (and very tip-prone) climbing structures – or trying to scale a bookcase one shelf at a time. Outdoor playgrounds (or indoor ones for when the weather's less than perfect) that allow your champion climber to practise her skills (and that have soft surfaces underneath to tumble onto) can channel her acrobatic energy to more appropriate frontiers than the dining room table.

- Provide a safe environment. If you haven't already, it's time to assess your home's safety from a climber's perspective. Put away rickety chairs, bookcases, or side tables, and securely

anchor wall units, dressers, and large bookcases to the wall (even those you think are too heavy to topple over). Never leave stepladders or stools out and unattended, or leave a chair too close to a counter or table, and don't invite your child to climb (and maybe fall) by placing tempting objects (like a remote) in view on a high surface. When gating off stairways, place the bottom gate three steps up so that your climber gets practice attempting that irresistible ascent, but won't get hurt if she does take a tumble. And speaking of tumbles, remember to cushion the base of favourite climbing mountains (your bed, the sofa) so falls don't turn into crash landings. See page 405 for more on childproofing.

- Provide safe limits and supervision. Be clear and consistent about what your little adventurer is allowed to climb on and what she's not. And remember that no amount of childproofing can substitute for constant supervision. Watch her inside and outside – and no matter where she's climbing or what she's climbing on, stay nearby in case she takes an unexpected tumble.

Climbing Out of Cot

"Our son is very tall for his age and an exceptional climber. We're afraid he'll try to climb from his cot in the middle of the night. What should we do to prevent this?"

If your tall tot has reached the 89-cm mark (the height usually required for a successful escape from the cot) or is quickly inching towards it, he may try to make a break for it any time now. Ditto for the particularly proficient climber, no matter what his height. But since scaling the cot's railing can result not only in freedom for the escapee but a big bump on his head (or worse), you're wise to start thinking about protective measures now. Here are some basics:

- Be sure that the cot mattress is at the lowest setting.

- Continue to leave large stuffed animals, pillows, and cushy duvets out of the cot, not for the old reasons, but for a new one: toddlers can use these as a step up to sweet freedom – and a bad fall.

- Pad the escape route with something (sofa cushions or an old quilt, for example) that will soften the landing should your toddler make it over the side.

If your toddler does manage an escape, or if you catch him in the act of attempting one, tell him calmly and firmly that climbing out of the cot is dangerous ("You could fall and get a nasty bang") and that it's not allowed. If that doesn't discourage further cot breaks, you can consider making the move to a bed. While experts recommend transitioning to a bed at about age 2½ or 3 – most kids are safer in the confines of a cot than out of it – a child who repeatedly climbs out of the cot, despite your repeated reminders to stay put, may be a good candidate for earlier graduation. But don't rush the move to the bed, especially if your tot climbs out only once or twice (he may just be testing his ability and then move on to the next skill, especially if he takes a fall). And if all's quiet on the cot front, there's definitely no need to make a change – no matter how tall or agile your toddler is.

Very Active Toddler

"Our daughter never stops moving, from the time she wakes up in the morning until she finally falls asleep at night. I know toddlers are supposed to be active, but *this* active?"

If there's a law of toddler physics, it's that little bodies in motion stay in motion. From the time they start jumping up and down for their early dawn cot release to the moment they finally lay their tired-out heads back down at night, toddlers are perpetual motion machines. Their energy seems endless and, for the parents struggling to keep up with them, exhausting.

In other words, your toddler's pace is age-appropriate. That said, some toddlers are definitely more active than others, ranking at the high end of the high-energy spectrum – and it sounds like your daughter's among that lively group. While you'll be living in the fast lane with your toddler for some time to come, there are some tricks you can try to slow her down, at least a little, at least once in a while:

- Stick to routines. Keep meals, snacks, naps, outings, and playtime on a regular schedule each day to bring some order to your toddler's otherwise frenetic life. See page 180 for more on routines.

- Relax with her. Your active toddler won't stand for sitting still? Gradually, with a little parental perseverance – and enough enticing activities – you may be able to convince her to take periodic (if fleeting) breaks from the action. Make downtime fun. Read a book, do a puzzle, build a castle out of bricks, play finger games, try some scribbling, or pound some Play-Doh. Or make a game out of doing nothing – you can call it the "quiet game". Say "Let's see if we can sit quietly until the buzzer rings" or "until the song is over". Or better still, challenge her: "Let's see who can stay still longer."

Let's Play Ball

It's no toss-up . . . toddlers love balls. And while your budding bowler may not be ready to pitch a strikeout yet (and catching is pretty iffy), there's a lot to gain from playing catch. Not only will a ball game boost your toddler's gross motor development, but it'll fine-tune hand–eye coordination and body coordination in general. So provide your toddler with a variety of balls to toss around and catch, from soft cotton-covered balls to light plastic balls, from big bouncy balls (if it's a blow-up kind, keep the ball slightly underinflated to make it easier for your little one to "catch") to beanbags. Add a bucket or basket to the mix when your tot is old enough to aim, shoot, score. Here's what to expect on the field:

12 to 15 months. Your toddler is starting to have a ball – first by rolling that curious round thing you've handed him or her (show your child how to spread his or her legs so the ball will roll into an easy-to-capture spot), and then by attempting to throw it – or more likely, dropping the ball and watching in delight as it moves across the floor.

15 to 18 months. Your little slugger is working on those throwing skills by practising projecting the ball away from his or her little body and hurling it towards someone (or something) else. Bouncing the ball (really, throwing it towards the floor and watching it bounce back up) is also a skill that your toddler will get a kick out of.

18 to 24 months. Speaking of kicking, as your little bowler ambles towards the second birthday, a new skill – kicking a ball – starts to emerge. That first football kick may be more involuntary than intentional (foot contacts ball, ball moves . . . cool). But once cause and effect become clear, your baby Beckham will aim for more deliberate foot–ball contact. Goal!

Be on the lookout: Watch for these emerging skills, and if you notice your child lagging behind in any skill (such as your 20-plus-month-old never attempting to kick a ball, for instance), mention it to the GP.

- Catch her being calm. Okay, it won't be often, and it won't be for long – but try to notice any time your toddler is calm or playing quietly and praise her for the effort, even if the quiet time was brief.

- Channel that endless energy into constructive activities (see box, page 80).

- Minimise frustration. Sometimes, frustration leads to bursts of very active behaviour. To head off that kind of hyped-up activity, help your toddler work through the many challenges she faces in a day (trying to get those bricks to stop falling down, trying to tell you what she wants for lunch, trying to match the circle you made with a crayon).

- Make sure she's getting enough sleep. Sometimes, an overactive toddler is actually an overtired toddler. If she's stopped one or both of her naps, make sure she's getting enough sleep at night. Or try reinstituting naptime or an enforced "rest time" if she seems to need it. And spend plenty of time winding her down before you expect her to brake for bed or a nap. See Chapter 5 for more on sleep issues.

- Watch what she eats. Some, though not all, toddlers seem to get extra energetic from extra amounts of certain foods (such as those that contain too much sugar, and/or artificial colours and flavours). If you notice a spike in activity level after an overloaded sugar-fest or a red-dye #2 frenzy, see if cutting them out of her diet helps her slow down. And of course, keep your little live wire away from caffeine in all its forms (including too much chocolate).

In time, as your toddler gains a little more self-control and a little more attention span, her activity level will likely come down a notch or two. That doesn't mean she won't continue to be very active – and being active definitely beats being sedentary, at least from a health perspective – just that she won't spend the whole day on the run. While you're waiting for that breather, be accepting of your bouncing (off the walls) baby girl. Remember, she's just doing what comes naturally to toddlers in general, and to her in particular. Keep your expectations of her realistic (for instance, don't expect her to sit still for long dinners, and make sure she gets plenty of running around during breaks on a car journey). Also, keep your guard up: active toddlers can get into a whole lot of trouble in a hurry, inside or outside the home.

Looking for some good news as you race from room to room with your little marathon girl? Researchers have found that toddlers who are very active, stimulation seeking, and curious tend to score higher on IQ tests and have above-average reading skills in primary school – once they manage to sit down with a book, that is.

Less Active Toddler

"I thought toddlers were supposed to be active, but mine just sits and plays quietly, while everyone else his age is running, jumping, and climbing."

Toddlers, like humans of all ages, come in all kinds of personality packages. Though as a group they've earned their high-energy reputation, there are plenty – like your mellow fellow – whose temperament is more laid-back. While most tots follow the Duracell Bunny model – and some definitely outrun it – others are content to sit and watch the world whirl by.

By all means, try to coax – but don't pressure – your toddler into more active pursuits. Play lively music and invite him to dance along with you. Try to get him interested in rolling a ball, or pulling a trolley, or joining you in a jumping game. But don't push the athletic agenda, which might only make him more activity averse. Take him to the playground more often, but if he'd rather stand and watch the other kids going down the slide than attempt it himself, let him. Go for a romp in the park, but if he'd rather stop and study a rock than toddle along the path, that's fine, too.

Celebrate the unique little person your toddler is (and the fact that you don't always have to be running after him). Compliment him on his drawings, on how carefully he stacked those three bricks, on his choice of books. Take advantage of the fact that he'll sit still for a story, unlike his on-the-run peers. And whenever he joins the movers and shakers or does a little moving or shaking on his own, cheer him on.

If your toddler regularly resists all activity, check with his doctor to be sure there isn't a physical trigger for his unphysical nature.

ALL ABOUT:
Getting Physical

You might be wondering why anyone would actually need to encourage a toddler to be active. Aren't tots active enough? Don't you get exhausted just looking at yours go, go, go – never mind trying to keep up with him or her? No one needs to tell you that most toddlers are naturally bundles of energy, perpetually in motion, no windup necessary. Even the most mellow have energy to burn – they just do it without bouncing off the walls. All that physical activity – the crawling, the cruising, the toddling, the climbing, the throwing, the running – is definitely age-appropriate for your toddler, but there's more to it than that . . . a lot more. Toddlers who stay active:

Sleep better. Here's a perk of toddler activity that's sure to perk you up: kids who are active during the day conk out more easily at night (they're tired out from all that activity) and have deeper, more restful sleep than children who tend to sit much of the day (cooped up in a car seat or a pushchair, or in front of the TV). Just make sure that your little one starts to wind down as the day winds up. Too much activity too close to bedtime can rev your toddler's engine just when it should be settling down, and that could actually prevent a good night's sleep.

Are happier. Physical activity boosts mood by stimulating chemicals in the brain that leave your toddler more cheerful and, paradoxically, more relaxed (and a happier and more relaxed child translates to a happier and more relaxed parent).

Outlets for High-Energy Toddlers

All toddlers need to blow off steam once in a while – and some need to blow off more steam more often. Whether your tot's especially active by nature (even by toddler standards), or just having a particularly frustrating day (every toddler has plenty of those), providing acceptable outlets to blow off that extra steam can prevent those much-dreaded blowups. Encourage your toddler to try these activities when he or she is reaching a boiling point:

- "Drumming" on pots
- Hammering on a workbench
- Pounding on Play-Doh
- Splashing in the bath or toddler pool
- Pulling weeds in the garden (only for toddlers who won't be tempted to taste)
- Pillow fights (in a safe space)
- Punching a punching bag or a pillow

Once your child has calmed down, try to figure out whether there was a trigger setting off the wilder-than-normal behaviour (he became overly frustrated, she didn't nap, an entire chocolate cupcake was consumed) and see if you can find a way to circumvent it in the future, preventing a repeat.

Burn up energy in more positive ways. All that excess toddler energy has to burn off somehow. A toddler who's physically active has opportunities to burn more of it off in constructive ways (rolling a ball, dancing to music, scooting along on a riding toy, chasing butterflies in the park) instead of in not-so-constructive ways (let's say, tantrums). Being active helps a toddler work out frustrations, too – something every little one has lots of. And it's frustrations, of course, that trigger so much of the behaviour you find so frustrating (let's say, tantrums).

Are healthier. Being physically active has long been linked to a more robust immune system in adults, and the same appears to hold true for little ones. Which means all that running around could actually cut down on your toddler's runny noses.

Have better appetites. Sure, it's hard to get your on-the-go toddler to break for a meal. But an active lifestyle actually does promote a healthier appetite. After all, the more active your tot is, the more fuel that busy engine will need to keep going . . . and going . . . and going.

Are less likely to become overweight. Since exercise helps control body fat, children who are active in the toddler and preschool years aren't only at a lower risk of childhood obesity, but are less likely to be overweight down the road. A leaner body, in turn, lowers the risk for developing type 2 diabetes, high blood pressure, high cholesterol levels, and even many cancers – giving your little one a healthy start to a healthier future.

Are more likely to become active adults. Habits have a way of sticking around, and the earlier they're formed, the more likely they are to stick for life. That goes for good habits (healthy eating, regular exercise) and bad ones

(fast-food allegiance, couch-potato proclivity). Yet another compelling case for making physical activity a habit for your toddler now.

Convinced about the benefits of building lots of physical activity into your toddler's routine, but not sure how far you'll have to go (or how much time or money you'll have to invest)? Actually, since toddlers appreciate the simple things in life, it'll be practically effortless. In other words, signing up for those toddler tumbling classes or daily trips to the playground – while fun – won't be necessary. Instead, just:

- Turn off the TV. Television-watching tots – like television-watching adults – rarely get the physical activity they need. In fact, there's no activity that burns less energy than watching TV – even sitting around doing absolutely nothing burns more.

- Limit time spent cooped up. True, a toddler-on-the-go needs a whole lot of supervision – and that supervision can sometimes be inconvenient (as when you're rushing to get through the supermarket, dashing to the post box, running errands in town). But a toddler constantly cooped up in a pushchair, a shopping trolley, or a carrier doesn't get the chance to flex those little muscles. Another benefit of leaving the pushchair at home at least some of the time? You'll be getting your exercise, too, chasing after your go-getter.

- Get physical together. There's no better way to encourage your toddler to be physically active than to get active yourself. Whether it's a morning walk or an afternoon dance party, a yoga session on the living room floor or a beach ball roll in the back garden, getting physical together will keep you healthier together.

In the Swim

Your toddler loves to splash water, can't get enough bath time, squeals in delight at the sight of a swimming pool, and tries on those beloved arm bands every chance he or she gets. All signs that it's time to sign up your water baby for swim classes, right? Maybe.

There is some evidence that suggests that children over age 1 (read: not infants) may be less likely to drown if they've had formal swimming lessons. Of course, standard swim strokes like the crawl are typically beyond their developmental reach, but even 1-year-olds can be taught a few basic moves (like the doggy paddle). Formal swimming lessons definitely aren't a must-do this early on – and they aren't for every toddler, either. But if you're inclined to have your little one take the plunge, there's no reason to postpone getting in the swim of things (or at least, the swim-readiness of things). Keep in mind, however, that there's no one age that fits all when it comes to swimming classes. Some tots are ready for lessons earlier, some later.

How will you know if it's the right time to get your fish into the water? Ask yourself: is my child exposed to water and its potential dangers often (for example, do you have a pool at home, live near the beach, take holidays by the sea or at resorts with pools)? Is he or she developmentally ready to take a formal class (i.e., able to

understand and follow instructions)? Physically ready (Will he be able to kick? Will she be able to paddle her arms? Do it in a coordinated way?)? Emotionally ready (a child who's fearful of the water may need to wade into swimming gradually)? If all swim systems seem to be a go, go right ahead and sign up your 1-year-old for a swim-readiness class (full-on "drown-proof" swimming classes are still not appropriate for a young toddler, so steer clear of those). Your child's not ready, or maybe you're not? It's fine to wait until the time's right.

The most important lessons about swimming classes: they don't protect toddlers from drowning and they're never a substitute for adult supervision in the water. Neither are floats, arm bands, or rubber rings (they're fine if you're in the pool, right next to your tot at all times, but can't be counted on to keep your toddler safe). It is recommended that you practise "touch supervision" in the pool – being close enough to reach out and touch your child at all times. Be sure, too, to keep underwater submersions brief and watch carefully to make sure your toddler isn't swallowing a lot of water (something young children are prone to doing, and which can be harmful).

For more on safety in and around the water, see page 430.

■ Take it outside. A little fresh air actually kicks up the benefits of physical activity – especially when it comes to better sleep and mood. Exposure to daylight also pumps up the exercise perks. So as long as the weather cooperates, try to give your toddler at least some of that daily run-around outdoors.

■ Keep it fun and simple. Try any of these energy-expending activities, all toddler favourites:

□ Dancing to lively music

□ Tumbling and rolling (on a large mat or carpet, away from sharp corners and other hazards)

- Jumping into a beanbag chair
- Kiddie aerobics (lead your toddler in just-for-fun toe touches, head-shoulder-knees-and-toes touches, and star jumps)
- Beanbag tossing (in an area where no lamps or fragile items can be knocked over)
- Lively circle games and action songs, such as "Hokey Cokey", "Ring a Ring o' Roses", "If You're Happy and You Know It"
- Action games: Hide-and-Seek; Follow the Leader; Catch Me If You Can; Simon Says; Red Light, Green Light
- Pushing a push toy, pulling a trolley, or riding on a tricycle
- Practising climbing stairs (supervised)
- Free play: running, jumping, climbing, rolling, hopping
- Playground play: swings, slide, climbing frame, seesaw
- Ball rolling, bouncing, throwing, kicking
- Bubble catching

Ways to Unwind

Sometimes, a bundle of energy can become so overwound that constructive channelling (or getting ready for a nap or bed) is no longer possible. When this happens, it's best to begin the unwinding process promptly. Try relaxing your toddler with any of these soothing activities:

- Hugging, cuddling, or massage (accompanied by a gentle "shhhhh")
- Soft music, with or without lyrics
- Reading a relaxing story
- A warm bath
- Playing simple puzzles (but only if your toddler doesn't tend to be frustrated by them)
- Doodling, painting with a brush or fingers, drawing with crayons or chalk
- Play-Doh play
- Water play
- Watching fish in a fish tank
- Lying down on the grass and looking at the clouds
- Stroking a stuffed animal

CHAPTER 4

Feeding

WHAT'S YOUR BIGGEST TODDLER FEEDING CHALLENGE? Pokiness? Pickiness? An allegiance to beige foods – preferably those that don't comingle – or a suspicion of anything (naturally) green? New texture intolerance? A sweet tooth, or a fried fetish? All of the above? If so, that's not surprising. Even babies who used to open up wide for whatever was spooned their way often start taking the path of most mealtime resistance (resistance, that is, to anything their parents want them to eat) once they've entered their second year. Should you wave the white napkin of surrender, and give up on the idea that your toddler will ever eat a varied, balanced, healthy diet (or even one out of three)? Absolutely not – and here's why. As finicky as your toddler's eating habits may seem now, they're actually more malleable than they'll probably ever be again (not to mention, your 1-year-old can't reach the ice cream stash yet or drive to Burger King). Offer up healthy foods now, and your little one will be more likely to reach for them later. Advocate eating for the right reasons (hunger, instead of boredom, for instance) and in the right setting (at the table, not on the sofa in front of the TV), and you're more likely to raise a child who eats right. Serve up surprises along with those standards (a side of curried cauliflower with that pasta and cheese, a slice of ripe mango with those fish fingers), and you may be surprised to see your toddler's tastes expand beyond the bland and blander (or the sweet and sweeter, or the salty and saltier).

The Second Year Diet

Your toddler's eating habits are a work in progress (though sometimes, it may be hard to see the progress – especially after the second cereal-only week in a row). They're busy forming, but they're far from formed. Which means you've got the opportunity of a lifetime to help your toddler form a lifetime of healthy eating habits, ones that can actually help shape a longer, healthier life (new science keeps backing up the old adage: you are what you eat). And there's no better time to start instilling those habits than now.

INTRODUCING . . . HEALTHY HABITS

To get your little one's eating habits off to the healthiest start possible, start with these healthy feeding basics:

Bites count (but don't have to be counted). Given that tiny tummy, that tender appetite, and probably limited tastes, there are just so many bites your toddler can take. In fact, toddlers run on surprisingly few bites a day – and that's completely normal. That's why it's smart to focus – as much as you possibly can – on quality, not quantity. Serve your little one foods that pack nutrients into every bite, however small or few the bites may end up being: whole grain bread instead of white, whole wheat cereal instead of pastries, baked sweet potato wedges instead of chips. Try to limit the number of bites wasted on foods that don't give back nutrition-wise (a.k.a. junk food).

You pick, your toddler chooses. Let's face it. If toddlers were in charge (especially older ones), all meals would feature icing, and broccoli would never find its way into the shopping trolley. Fortunately, they're not in charge – or at least they shouldn't be. Don't forget – though it's easy to when your little one screams for ice cream or clamours for cupcakes – who's actually running

Additives Add Up

Does your little one love that neon-rainbow cereal? Those brightly coloured ice cream sprinkles? Anything that leaves his or her tongue blue? You might want to reconsider making such artificially coloured foods (and other foods with certain types of additives) part of your little one's diet. Why? First, while the cumulative effects from artificial additives on future general health aren't fully known yet, those additives are certain to accumulate faster and with more potential for harm in a body that's so little and still growing. Second, there's some research that suggests that certain children may be extra-sensitive to artificial colouring, dyes, and preservatives in processed food, possibly leading to behavioural issues and attention problems. The final reason, though, may be all you need to know: most of the foods that these kinds of artificial additives are added to aren't good for your toddler, anyway. They're likely to contain lots of other less healthy ingredients, including too much sugar, too much sodium, and too much fat.

Keeping additives off the menu is easy to do if you limit the amount of processed foods you serve up (choose fresh, unprocessed or minimally processed, whole foods as often as you can); read labels carefully; avoid buying foods that contain artificial colours (like red E124, blue E133, yellow E160$_6$) and look instead for foods that use natural food colouring (such as annatto extract, beta-carotene, beetroot, fruit or vegetable juice, paprika, saffron, or turmeric); and pass up artificially flavoured drinks and milks (did you know that some strawberry milk doesn't have a single strawberry in it?).

the food department: you. As the adult, you get to pick which foods make it home, and which foods don't. You also get to pick when foods are appropriate (steamed carrots and hummus before dinner) and when they're not (biscuits for breakfast). After you've picked, it's fine for your toddler to choose from the selection of healthy foods you've provided (and remember, it'll be a lot easier to say "no" to chocolate marsh-mallow cereal when there isn't any in the cabinet).

Appetite rules. Toddler eating pat-terns . . . well, let's just say that there's no predicting them. One day, your toddler ploughs through two bowls of cereal, a banana, and a yogurt for breakfast, turns down a snack, and manages barely a nib-ble at lunch and dinner. The next day, breakfast is a bust, lunch is lacklustre, but a pile of pasta and cheese is demol-ished at supper. The third day, snacks attack, while meals take a low profile.

The best strategy for you, the feeder? Go with the appetite flow. Serve up a predictable schedule of three meals, supplemented by well-timed snacks, and let your toddler's appetite dictate how much (or how little) is eaten at each. No pressure to eat more, no recriminations for eating less, no prob-lem over leftovers or mainly skipped meals. Remember, healthy kids eat as much as they need. Take a look at the big picture – your toddler's diet over a week, for instance – and you'll prob-ably see that all those ups and downs in appetite balance out.

Snacks are essential. A toddler's teeny tank fills up quickly, which means it needs frequent refills, too. That's where snacks come in. For little ones, snacks provide a steady supply of much-needed fuel for that on-the-go lifestyle, while covering any nutritional gaps barely touched meals leave behind.

As long as they're healthy (think of them as mini-meals – scaled down, but still nutritiously substantial versions of those three squares), they're just another opportunity for your little one to eat well.

Liquids drown solids. As recent gradu-ates of liquid-only diets, it's not surpris-ing that most toddlers are big fans of fluids. The problem is, when the fluid of choice is filling (as in juice) and the method of beverage delivery is easy-to-use and readily available (as in the bot-tle or the beaker), a toddler's appetite for solids can be drowned by too many liquids. To encourage healthy eating, discourage excess drinking. Limit milk intake to 500 ml a day, juice to no more than 100–200 ml.

Carbohydrates are a complex issue. Bagels, bread, crackers, spaghetti, cereal – even the most finicky toddler usually enjoys at least one member of the carbohydrate family, and some seem to be carb-only consumers. But since all carbs are not created equal, nutrition-ally speaking, it pays to be picky – and to pick mainly complex carbs when feeding your toddler. Complex carbs provide a wide range of the naturally occurring nutrients, nutrients that are stripped away during the refining process (the process that makes whole grains white) – and nutrients that fuel your little one's growth and develop-ment. Whole grains and other complex carbs (see page 91 for examples) are also digested more slowly than refined ones are, which means that they'll pro-vide a more steady supply of the energy your toddler needs – while helping pre-vent those blood sugar crashes that can send a little one's sunny mood south in a hurry. What's more, a diet that favours complex carbs over refined ones – espe-cially if it's started early in life, when those taste buds are being formed – is

Mix It Up

One-year-olds aren't generally known for their daring at the dinner table (unless you count standing up in the high chair). For many toddlers, dietary variety might mean switching between jam sandwiches cut into triangles and jam sandwiches cut into squares.

Still, a diet that mixes it up offers the best nutrition – after all, the same-old-same-old foods mean the same-old-same-old nutrients. Variety also keeps mealtime monotony from setting in, while expanding a toddler's dietary repertoire (at least, potentially . . . eventually).

So dare to think outside the lunch box and the breakfast bowl:

- Alternate oat hoops with wheat flakes; porridge with Weetabix.
- Top cereal with bananas one day, strawberries the next.
- Mash winter squash, then celeriac, then edamame.
- Get crazy with quinoa, then lentils, then halved black beans, then halved chickpeas.
- Spread sandwich fillings on pitta or roll them up in whole wheat tortilla wraps.

- Serve Cheddar cheese cubes, string cheese sticks, or Swiss cheese slices.
- Create salmon burgers, burritos, or teriyaki.
- Cook your own baked chicken fingers, chicken parmigiana, or chicken quesadillas.
- Take on tofu in a stir-fry, or a lasagna, or in crunchy nugget form.
- Make meatballs from minced turkey or lamb, not just beef.
- Dice ripe papaya and mangoes, as well as apples and pears.
- Pour apricot juice at one meal, vegetable juice at another.
- Toss peas into the cheesy pasta, then cauliflower.
- Offer your little dipper a variety of dips – cheese sauce, tomato sauce, yogurt, guacamole, tartare, apple purée, mustard. Experiment with spices, too – a hint of ginger or curry, a little garlic (how do you know for sure your picky eater won't eat pesto?).

Think your toddler won't buy into variety? While food ruts are definitely age-appropriate, they're not inevitable. Mix it up, and you may be surprised.

---

less likely to lead to obesity and type 2 diabetes. That's because complex carbs regulate blood sugar best, limiting the amount of circulating sugar that can be converted to fat.

Healthy foods come in colourful packages. So, your little one may not know red from blue, or green from orange yet. But here's something you should know about colour: it can clue you in to nutrition. When a food comes by a vibrant colour naturally (red raspberries, not berry-flavoured fruit snacks), it's a sure sign that it's packed with nutrients your fast-growing toddler needs. Think of all the natural colours of the rainbow when you shop: red tomatoes and strawberries; orange carrots, sweet potatoes, and melon; blue blueberries (and if you can find them, other blue produce, like blue potatoes); yellow sweetcorn and mangoes; green kiwis and broccoli. And the colour connection isn't exclusive to the produce aisle. Whether you're picking out bread, rice, or cereal, you'll make a healthier choice if you look for deeper colours (white bread, rice, cereal, and pasta pale in nutritive value next to the darker, whole-grain varieties).

Sugar's not so sweet. Of course, little ones are sweet on sugar – usually from that very first lick of icing or crumb of cake. But here's the news on sugar, in case you haven't heard: it's full of calories, but empty of nutrients. Foods high in sugar are fine for a once-in-a-while treat, but not-so-fine as a steady diet. Since they're a waste of precious tummy space (space that's limited in a toddler), filling up on sugary treats means your little one won't have room – or appetite – left for healthy foods that offer something to grow on. Worse still, sugary foods are linked to tooth decay (even in those cute little baby teeth) and obesity (in childhood and beyond), and even to other health problems in the future (like heart disease). Plus, once little ones get a taste for the sweet life, it's hard to get them unhooked (that sugar craving can be tough to kick, as you may know from personal experience). The best sugar strategy? Limit the amount your toddler eats right from the start. Help nurture a taste for foods that are sweet, but not sugar-sweetened (like fruit, sweet potatoes, carrots) and for foods that introduce other tastes altogether (the tanginess of yogurt, the garlicky goodness of hummus, the creaminess of avocado, the spiciness of salsa).

Salt's hard to lick. If there's one ingredient as common in the UK diet as sugar, it's salt – in copious quantities. Scan nutrition labels on packaged foods (it's listed as "sodium") and you'll uncover it in obvious places (those salty-tasting crisps) and in not-so-obvious places (that sweet-tasting cereal). Too much salt, like too much sugar, is a recipe for future health problems. A high-sodium diet is linked to high blood pressure (which is in turn linked to heart disease) and obesity (because salty foods are often also fattening foods). And like a taste for sugar, a taste for salt is hard to lick once it's acquired (which may be why you can't imagine life unsalted) – another compelling reason to limit the salt your toddler consumes now. Consider this: most kids eat about twice the sodium they should.

The best foods remember where they came from. The closer foods stick to their roots, the more natural goodness – and naturally occurring nutrients – they can offer your toddler. That's why whole wheat bread beats white bread; fresh fruit juice trumps "fruit squash"; real cheese triumphs over the processed kind; an artificially flavoured (and coloured) blueberry yogurt can't stand up to one that's blended with real blueberries. So, whenever you can, choose foods with that fresh-from-the-farm pedigree: fresh (or fresh-frozen) fruits and vegetables, unrefined breads and cereals, unprocessed meat. Prepare those healthy foods in the healthiest way possible, too (steam or roast veggies to preserve vitamins and nutrients, bake chicken instead of frying).

Healthy eating habits begin at home. Where did you form your eating habits? Of course, there were friends' houses involved (especially once you got to sleepover age), school lunches, ice cream vans, cinema snack bars, possibly school cafeterias. But chances are, when you break it down, most of what you learned about eating you learned at home. So make your home a place where healthy eating lives – and a lifetime of healthy eating habits start. Don't forget what's in it for you, either. A family that eats healthy together stays healthy together.

THE SECOND YEAR DAILY DOZEN

Ever tried to keep track of your toddler's food intake (so, let's see: that's 2½ bites of eggy bread, 3 blueberries, and a spoonful of yogurt . . . half a cheese stick and a banana slice . . . six spoonfuls of Cheerios, counting the ones that ended up crushed into the car seat . . . the majority of a meatball, 10 pasta shapes, and a squeeze of tomato sauce, most of it used as face paint)? It definitely isn't easy – and fortunately, it definitely isn't necessary.

So put away the scorecards, the calculators, the measuring spoons and jugs – and stop struggling to add up those nibbles, licks, crumbs, and scraps (which add up faster than you'd think, anyway). The Second Year Daily Dozen outlined below aren't dietary guidelines to stick to strictly, but a general guide to the types of foods (and food groups) your toddler should be sampling. Instead of trying to keep that running tab of food intake or serving up pressure (in the form of bribes, pleas, or punishment) in an attempt to meet daily quotas, aim to offer a variety of healthy foods for your little one to eat – or not eat – based on appetite. Keep in mind, too, that toddlers need to eat a lot less than their parents usually think – which means those tiny appetites are typically right on target.

Calories. It is recommended that toddlers get about 1,000 calories per day. But now that you know that, forget it. You don't have to count calories to tell if your toddler is getting enough – or

Drink Your Vitamins?

They're sweet. They're sippable. They come in the kid-friendliest flavours. And they're packed with all of the nutrients a toddler could possibly need, from protein to calcium to DHA. But should you pick a liquid nutritional drink to supplement your toddler's picky eating habits? Probably not, for multiple reasons. First, most are loaded with sugar and contain both artificial flavours and artificial colours. Second, they're super-filling and go down easily, leaving a tiny tummy with precious little room for solids. And most important: they're no substitute for real food – the real food your toddler should be getting a taste for (and experience eating) now. Though they may fill in some nutritional gaps, they'll also open up more (even those with added fibre are no competition for a slice of whole wheat bread). Plus, offering these drinks could set up a cycle of even pickier eating habits (as in, only chocolate-, strawberry-, and vanilla-flavoured need apply). Remember, the vast majority of toddlers – presented with whole, healthy foods – will eat all they need to grow . . . no sweet supplements necessary. Still concerned that your toddler doesn't eat enough? Check with the doctor.

too many. Instead, simply keep track of his or her weight at checkup times. If it's staying on approximately the same curve – allowing for a jump or dip as a thin toddler fills out or a chubby one slims down – caloric intake is on target. Remember, too, that healthy toddlers (ones who aren't pressured to eat more

Don't Get Your Toddler Juiced

It's brimming with vitamin C (and, increasingly, other added nutrients, like calcium), thirst-quenching, and a big-time favourite among the beaker set. But too much juice – and it's easy for your little one to get too much – can actually lead to a whole host of health problems, from obesity (from too many empty calories) to malnutrition (from too many empty calories taking the place of nutritious ones) to chronic diarrhoea. So always dilute juice at least half and half with water, and limit the total tally of juice your toddler drinks to no more than 100–200 ml a day. (Your tot's not a juice lover? No need to serve any.) Also, read labels to make sure what you're pouring is 100 per cent fruit juice, not a "fruit drink".

or eat less) are pretty good at self-regulating their caloric intake. They'll eat as much as they need in order to grow.

Protein. Little bodies need protein to grow big – but in surprisingly small amounts. In fact, two 250 ml glasses of milk provide just about all the protein a toddler needs in a day (approximately 16 grammes). Anything else – that spoonful of yogurt, that half a fish finger, those three bites of cheese – is just gravy. That said, it's a good idea to start your tot on a wide variety of protein foods, not only for the nutritional perks (different types of protein foods offer up different nutrients), but for the taste experience. Mix it up as much as you can: dairy products (besides milk, look to yogurt and cheese, including ricotta and cottage cheese), eggs, fish, chicken

and turkey, lean meat, beans, edamame, tofu, and whole grains (especially the protein-packed quinoa). Peanut butter and other nut butters (like almond butter) count, too, but be sure to use creamy (not crunchy), spread thinly, and avoid altogether if there are allergy concerns.

Calcium. Your always-busy toddler is busy behind the scenes, too – busy building strong and healthy bones, muscles, and teeth. Essential to that construction project: calcium, and plenty of it. In the second year, your child will need about 500 milligrammes of calcium per day – no challenge if you have a milk-lover on your hands (there's 300 milligrammes of calcium in every 250 ml of the white stuff), and actually not even much of a challenge if you don't. Other dairy products, such as yogurt and cheese, can also help your toddler bone up on calcium (if you're counting, yogurt cashes in as much calcium as milk, cup for cup; about 25 g of cheese does the same). Nondairy sources can contribute, too – including calcium-fortified juice, tofu and many soy products, and some dark green veggies (admittedly a long shot for little ones, but you never know).

Vitamin C foods. This vital vitamin boosts the immune system, helps heal those scrapes and bruises, and strengthens muscles and blood vessels, putting it high on your toddler's must-have list. Since the body can't store vitamin C, you'll have to serve up a fresh supply daily (yesterday's berry fest can't be applied today). Happily, most little ones don't need any coaxing when it comes to vitamin C. This multitasking vitamin can be found in a multitude of toddler-pleasing fruits and veggies, among them citrus fruits (including the standard orange juice), berries, melon, mango, kiwi, broccoli, leafy greens, bell peppers, tomatoes, tomato juice and tomato sauce, and sweet potato. Just one or two servings will C your toddler through the day.

Green leafy and yellow vegetables and yellow fruits. These vitamin A-listers boast a long list of body-building benefits (they're important for vision, bone and tooth development, immune system maintenance, healthy skin and hair, and much more). Even if green's not your toddler's colour (broccoli, cooked greens), he or she will find plenty on the yellow/orange A-list to pick from: apricots, cantaloupe, mango, papaya, yellow peach, carrot, winter squash, sweet potato, pumpkin, tomato and tomato sauce, red bell pepper. Aim for one to two servings per day (keeping in mind that many vitamin A-rich foods are also packing C – there's no need to double up).

Other fruits and vegetables. Round out your tot's nutritional profile with one or two servings of these other fruits and veggies, which pack vitamins, minerals, antioxidants, and fibre: apple, pear, banana, cherries, berries, grapes (cut in half), pineapple, cooked raisins, avocado, green beans, beetroot, aubergine, turnip, mushrooms, courgette, okra, green peas, sweetcorn.

Whole grains and other complex carbohydrates. Most toddlers are carb cravers, but not all carbs make the nutritional cut. Skip the simple carbs (white bread, white rice, and refined cereals lack naturally occurring nutrients and fibre your little one needs) and go for the whole grain. Aim for about 4 to 6 toddler servings a day (sounds like a lot? A single slice of whole-grain bread offers up 4 toddler servings). Choose from whole-grain bread, pitta, bagels, tortillas and wraps, muffins, and crackers; brown rice, quinoa, barley, and

---

It's Milk Time

Now that the second year has arrived, it's time to turn in the formula and make the switch to milk (in case you're wondering, there is absolutely no reason to "graduate" to toddler-type formulas instead). Most toddlers happily lap up cow's milk as soon as it's introduced, but an occasional formula-fond child snubs this beverage-come-lately. One way to make the transition easier for those finicky tots is to start by diluting their formula with a little cow's milk. Gradually, over a period of a few weeks, decrease the proportion of formula until your child's drinking milk and nothing but. If your toddler has been formula-free until now, and you plan to continue breastfeeding, you might want to consider introducing milk anyway – not only for the experience but also because it contains more vitamin D than breast milk does – and that's something a growing body definitely needs in adequate supply. Besides, there's nothing like milk poured over cereal, or into smoothies – or, of course, as a dunk for biscuits and muffins.

What type of milk should you pull off the dairy case? Most likely whole, because 1-year-olds need extra fat to boost brain development (but check with the doctor).

---

bulgur; whole wheat pasta; whole-grain cereal, pancakes, and waffles; lentils, chickpeas, pinto, kidney, haricot, or other beans. Keep in mind that wheat isn't the only grain that comes whole – look, too, for whole corn, whole oats, whole rye, whole barley, and more. How do you know you're getting those grains whole? Check out the ingredients list – it has to specify "whole" to be whole.

Iron-rich foods. A lot of little ones don't get enough iron, especially once they've moved on from enriched baby cereal and formula. Since this mineral is needed to manufacture red blood cells – and red blood cells are needed to deliver oxygen to every part of the body – it's important to keep an eye on your toddler's iron intake (shortfalls can lead to iron-deficiency anemia). Pump up your tot's diet with good sources of iron, including lean beef, pork, poultry, salmon, eggs, beans, tofu, prunes, cooked raisins, leafy greens, porridge, and whole-grain breads, pasta, and cereals. Not sure about your tot's intake? Check with the doctor.

High-fat foods. No need to be fat-phobic when it comes to your toddler (even if you're wisely trying to prevent obesity later in life) – just fat-selective. The right amount of the right kind of fat is vital to the development of your toddler's fast-growing brain and quickly-developing nervous system. Sticking with whole milk until your toddler turns 2 (unless the doctor has advised otherwise) will provide much of that needed fat. When adding other fats, think heart healthy (arteries start clogging early in this fast-food-fed nation): olive and rapeseed oil, avocados, smooth, thinly spread nut butter (if there's no allergy risk). Stay away from saturated fats (most often found in fast food, junk food, and processed food), particularly trans fats.

Fluids. Your toddler needs no more than 4 to 6 cups of fluid a day (around 500 ml milk, 100–200 ml of juice, and 500–700 ml of water will do the trick) – but no need to count millilitres (and what with all those spills and leftovers, it's tough to keep track). Since it's a matter of fluid in, fluid out, just keep an eye on those nappies: a toddler who's getting enough fluid will produce plenty of clear urine; one who isn't will have dark, scant urine. You'll need to step up fluid intake to prevent dehydration in hot weather, and also when your little one is down with a cold or fever, has diarrhoea, or is vomiting. Water is the most obvious source of fluids – and a great one for your toddler to get a taste (or, non-taste) for – but keep in mind that there's water, water everywhere, including in fruits and veggies (they're mostly water), milk, soup, and juice.

Omega-3 fatty acids. Part of the family of essential fatty acids, omega-3s (such as DHA, EPA, and ALA) should be an essential part of your family's – and your toddler's – diet. That's because omega-3s are vital for your tot's normal growth and development, are beneficial for his or her vision and healthy brain development, can help stabilise mood and behaviour, and are heart healthy. You'll find omega-3 fatty acids in plant foods like walnuts, flaxseeds (grind them up and hide them in your tot's porridge), tofu, edamame, and rapeseed oil, and also in fatty fish, especially salmon. If you're still breastfeeding, remember that breastmilk is a great source of omega-3s. You'll also find it in DHA-enriched foods like yogurt, cereal, eggs, nut butters, and even ice cream.

Vitamin supplements. What happens when breakfast (porridge with pears) ends up on the floor, lunch (yogurt and cut-up fruit) ends up mashed in your tot's hair, and dinner (a well-balanced meal of cheesy pasta with hidden salmon flakes and mashed cauliflower) never leaves the plate? You end up with a toddler who's missed out on his or her share of daily nutrients. It's typical, as toddlers are notoriously eccentric and erratic when it comes to eating, and nothing to be concerned about. Your child will probably make up the shortfall another day or tap into his or her

Serving Size Matters

Does your toddler barely make a dent in the piles of food you offer up each day? Perhaps it's because you're offering far too much. Most parents do – because most parents think their tots need a lot more food than they actually do. The problem with overserving toddlers isn't just the potential for waste – it's the potential for waist. Pushing too much food can lead to eating too much food (especially if kids start buying into the "eat what's put in front of you" mindset), which can quickly lead to overweight. And talk about out-of-proportion portions: many children (and adults) routinely eat double and triple the recommended serving sizes. There's definitely no need to measure out your toddler's portions precisely (or even at all) – the best strategy is always to let little ones eat to their appetite. But to avoid overwhelming that appetite with heaping servings, it helps to have a little portion perspective. Check out the approximate recommended serving sizes for tots – you'll notice that they run about one-quarter the size of a recommended adult serving size:

- Fresh fruit: ¼ cup
- Cooked fruit: 2 tablespoons
- Cooked vegetables: 1 to 2 tablespoons
- Meat, fish, or poultry: 25 g
- Bread: ¼ slice
- Crackers: 2 small
- Cold cereal: 35 g
- Porridge: 2 tablespoons
- Cooked pasta, rice, or other grain: 2 tablespoons
- Beans: 2 tablespoons
- Cottage cheese: 25 g
- Egg: ½
- Yogurt: ¼ cup
- Cheese: 10 g, or about 2 tablespoons grated

So before you worry that your toddler's not eating enough, remember how little enough really is. In fact, serve up just the right amount of food, and you'll probably realise your toddler is eating just the right amount.

---

stores from the healthy eating he or she did yesterday or last week. But there are some nutrients (vitamin C comes to mind) that can't be stored and that need to be replenished daily, and others (like vitamin D) that are in short supply in food. Add to that the standard-issue parental worry that can leave nagging doubts in your head about whether your little one's nutritional intake is up to snuff. Enter a vitamin supplement – a kind of nutritional insurance that can put your mind at ease. But since giving a daily vitamin to toddlers is not an official recommendation (there is no official position on the subject), it's up to you, along with the doctor, to decide whether or not to invest in that insurance. If you do opt to add a vitamin supplement to your toddler's diet (ask your GP for a brand recommendation), use a liquid preparation until your toddler's molars are in, then switch to chewables when your child can be depended upon to chew a tablet thoroughly. Store them well out of your toddler's reach, and never refer to them as "sweets". Their colours and shapes, aroma and taste can be extremely enticing, which is good, since it makes them attractive and palatable to children, and bad, since it can make them too tempting. Most of all, remember that vitamin supplements should never be viewed as a replacement for nutritious foods. The body absorbs nutrients from foods much more effectively than it absorbs nutrients from supplements. So if you constantly find yourself relying on a multivitamin to counteract the chips your child clamours for or to make up for the fact that produce always seems to be passed up, you probably should rethink your strategy.

What You May Be Wondering About

When to Wean from the Breast

"I'm still breastfeeding my daughter, and neither one of us is ready to give it up. Is there any reason to wean?"

Actually, if you're still both on board with the breast, there's absolutely no reason to jump ship. In fact, the World Health Organisation has an official policy to that effect: breastfeeding should continue, ideally, for at least 6 months – and then continuing with other foods up to 2 years. For some breastfeeding teams, a year (or even less) is enough, while others are still going strong through the second year and beyond.

So wean when the time's right for both of you (if the time is right for her but not for you, see the next question). Just keep an eye – as you keep up those cuddly breastfeeding sessions – on solids intake (once that first birthday is celebrated, a busy toddler needs more protein, vitamins, and other nutrients than breast milk alone can provide) and appetite (toddlers who drink too much from breast or bottle can drown their appetite, so if your little one seldom seems hungry for solids, breastfeed after meals instead of before). Supplementing with cow's milk may also be a smart move – even as you continue to breastfeed – since it offers up essential vitamin D. Also, try to brush your toddler's teeth after nighttime breastfeeds and consider nipping middle-of-the-night feeds altogether (some dentists link these to baby-bottle mouth, though it's clearly less common among breastfeeding toddlers than those who sip from a bottle or a beaker).

"My son seems ready to stop breastfeeding – he struggles and pushes away from my breast when I try. But I'm so not ready."

Breastfeeding can be one of life's most satisfying experiences, but it definitely takes two willing participants. Before you decide your toddler is no longer willing, though, you may want to take a closer look. Sometimes, a baby or toddler will go on a temporary breastfeeding strike because of a stuffy nose, an achy ear, a painful bout of teething. If it's clear, however, that he's had enough of this good thing – if he seems just as happy (or happier) with a cup of milk, a meal, and his freedom from laptop feedings – it's time to move on, Mum. So follow his lead, as understandably hard as it may be for you to make the break. If you can convince him to

How to Wean: From the Breast

Is weaning from the breast around the corner? You might want to take that turn slowly. Weaning gradually – instead of suddenly slamming the brakes on breastfeeding – is usually best for both breastfeeding team members, allowing you, your body, and your toddler enough time to adjust before this special era comes to a close. Extra helpings of one-on-one time can fill in the emotional and physical gaps for both of you while you ease out of breastfeeding. (Many of the same tips that help bottle weaners can also help a breast weaner; see page 96.)

Weaning now may be pretty easy (if both of you are ready to quit the breast) or quite the challenge (if one or both of you are still strongly attached to it). Either way, a multistep programme helps get the job done:

- Step 1: Get that cup going, if you haven't started yet (see page 99), so you have something to wean to besides the bottle (which should ideally be kicked at about a year).

- Step 2: Time it right. There's no predictably perfect time, since nothing's predictable or perfect when it comes to life with a toddler. But if you can, try not to start your weaning campaign when there are other stresses, changes, or adjustments going on. Wait until all is (relatively) quiet on the toddler front.

- Step 3: Fill with food first. At those usual daytime feedings, don't offer the breast first. Instead, try to pre-empt with a snack or meal and a cup of milk, along with some cuddle time. At the very least, the appetite edge will be off, and your toddler will take less breast milk when you do serve it up. Decreased demand will result in decreased supply – which will in turn make your breasts a whole lot more comfortable as you wean.

- Step 4: Shake up the bedtime routine. The idea is to keep your toddler from falling asleep on the breast, so that a breast-free bedtime won't be an impossible dream. If you've always saved breast for last, wedge breastfeeding somewhere else in the ritual instead, such as after bath, pyjamas, and bedtime snack but before other relaxing activities (like story and cuddles) and definitely before toothbrushing.

- Step 5: Start cutting back. First to go should be the feedings your toddler can take or leave – most likely those midday ones. Over a couple of weeks, cut back to just two feedings a day, then one (bedtime's usually last to go). As you cut feedings, keep your toddler's schedule busy and blood sugar up with activities and regular, healthy snacks and drinks of milk. Heap on the affection and attention, but try to avoid anything that involves close proximity to your breasts (and it's definitely not the time to go bra-less or low-cut). And speaking of which, if engorgement becomes an issue, express just a small amount of milk to relieve the pressure, without encouraging production.

- Step 6: Drop the last feeding. When you're ready to go all the way, say bye-bye to the last feeding (though if you're both still invested in the breast, you can opt to hang on to that bedtime feed until the milk runs out or interest wanes on either side or both). To make that emotionally charged milestone easier for both of you to pass, try to stay out of the picture for a night or two. With Daddy or a favourite baby-sitter in charge of bedtime, go shopping, to the cinema, or out to dinner with friends, or if you don't feel like getting out of the house, at least keep out of sight (and sniff) at home.

How to Wean: From the Bottle

Is it time to say "bye-bye, bottle"? Choose the technique that best fits you and your toddler (no one technique fits all) and get ready to wean. Just make sure that everyone else in your little one's life, such as childcare providers, is in the loop with the plan.

Quick withdrawal. If your toddler is relatively easygoing, doesn't panic in the face of change, makes transitions smoothly, isn't especially hooked on the bottle, and has a good working relationship with the cup, you may be able to wean cold turkey. (These tips can also be useful, in a modified form, with "gradual withdrawal"; see below):

- Pencil in a start day that's just right, one with no (other) dramas going on and with lots of time to devote to Project Wean. But keep your eraser handy. If your toddler wakes up on the wrong side of the bed on that selected morning (or you do), or if something has come up unexpectedly that suddenly demands your attention (like the contents of a clogged toilet or your toddler's tummy), put weaning on hold.

- Hype it up. Generate weaning-day excitement: "You're a big boy (or girl) today! Just like Mummy and Daddy! Just like cousin Alex! Hooray!" Explain that just like all big boys and girls, your toddler can now drink from a cup, instead of a bottle. Toast the occasion with sips of morning milk, and don't forget to say "Cheers!"

- Shop it up. If your toddler is into new possessions (and most toddlers are), mark this special day with a trip to the shops for a brand-new "big boy or girl cup".

- Have a bye-bye ceremony. There are several options for kissing the bottle good-bye. You could have your toddler toss it in the recycle bin. Or put it in a gift box for "babies who need a bottle". Or leave it for the "bottle fairy" in exchange for a little token of her appreciation (some stickers, a book, a toy). Or have your little weaner use it to feed teddy bears or dolls. If, however, you sense the less time spent dwelling on the bottle, the better, just stash it yourself without any fanfare.

- Stay busy, busy, busy. Plan to keep your toddler occupied with favourite activities – finger painting, a trip to the playground, a visit with Grandpa (or other favourite people who don't drink from baby bottles). If possible, stay out of stressful locales (did someone say supermarket?). Don't skip naps or regular meals while staying busy – giving up the bottle can be grumpy-making enough without adding in fatigue and low blood sugar.

continue just long enough to make the break less painful for your breasts, try to wean gradually. If not, just add that to the long – but well worthwhile – list of sacrifices you'll be making over your mummy career.

Either way, try not to take his rejection of your breast as a rejection of you – it isn't. It's a rejection of dependence – and that's a normal developmental step some kids take sooner, some take later, but all take

- Be patient, patient, patient. Depending on how strong the bond between your toddler and the bottle, you can expect tough times during weaning day, and possibly the days ahead. Extra cuddling, extra comfort, and extra patience will see you both through. At night, an extra-relaxing bedtime ritual (soft music, low lighting, a soothing snack, a whole lot of lap time) can fill the gap left by that abandoned bottle. If the "big boy or girl" theme is fizzling, let it go for now. Your toddler may need a little babying and other comfort habits (thumb sucking, blanket clutching) during this tricky transition.

- Be flexible. If it turns out that a one-day turnaround, or two, or three, isn't emotionally or physically possible for either or both of you, extend the programme to gradual withdrawal. Or offer a bottle with water only for now.

Gradual withdrawal. Is your toddler not cut out for cold turkey – or maybe it's you who'd rather take things slow? Try a slower, multistep approach instead. All the tips from "quick withdrawal" can help when you're weaning gradually too.

- Step 1: Set bottle limits. Allow the bottle only while your child is sitting on your lap, or in a certain chair – and no wandering off clutching it. Calmly but firmly end bottle sessions when your toddler's had enough sitting.

- Step 2: Get in the cup habit. Before usual bottle times – and definitely before any whining for the bottle begins – offer a cup of milk and a snack or meal. Hopefully, a full tummy and quenched thirst, along with some attention and distraction, will keep the bottle cravings from kicking in. If not, maybe your toddler will take less from the bottle than usual, and cravings will gradually ease.

- Step 3: Start cutting back. Over a couple of weeks, systematically cut down on the number of bottles you give. Drop the one your child shows the least interest in first, and the most beloved bottle last. You can also start decreasing the amount of milk or juice you put in each bottle, and filling up the cup instead. Or switch to water-only bottles – better for your toddler's teeth, less appealing to your toddler (talk about win–win). A somewhat sneakier, sometimes effective strategy: substitute a teat with a tiny hole. Your toddler may be less excited about working harder for that drink.

- Step 4: Cut it out. When you've worked it down to one bottle, and the time seems right (or as right as it's ever going to get), say bye-bye bottle, with or without a ceremony – but with loads and loads of positive reinforcement. Keep the extra comfort and distraction coming as long as your toddler (big boy or girl!) needs it.

eventually. It's also probably a rejection of being stuck in your lap for hours a day when he'd rather be on the go.

Best to get your cuddles when you can, most likely on his terms from now on. Make your lap available, but not required seating. And remember, there are plenty of other ways to stay close with your toddler, now and later, that won't threaten his newfound autonomy.

When to Wean from the Bottle

"I know I'm supposed to start weaning my son from the bottle now that he's a year old, but I can't imagine he's ready."

Timing may not be everything when it comes to weaning – but it's a lot. And if there ever was an ideal time to wean your toddler from the bottle, you're looking at it now, for all sorts of reasons, including:

- You've got flexibility. Okay, it's relative. Your toddler's not the putty in your hands he was six months ago. But he's also not the independence-fighting insurgent he's scheduled to become six months or a year from now. Once he really gets the hang of kicking and screaming (peaceful protests aren't so much a toddler's thing), getting your little one to cooperate in just putting his shoes on – never mind in major lifestyle changes, like giving up the bottle – may become a much bigger challenge.

- You've got milk. Those formula days are over, and there's a new beverage in town. What better time to retire that old beverage conveyer, the bottle?

- You've got solids. Back in those baby-bottle days, your little one got fed by drinking (breast milk or formula or both). But solids are the new liquid for toddlers – and they've taken on much more nutritional significance. Bottle drinkers tend to take in too many calories from milk and juice, leaving them little appetite for the solid food they need to help them grow and help them gain eating experience. Those who manage to find room for the solid calories on top of the liquid ones can end up gaining too much weight. More good reasons to make the break from the bottle now.

- You've got teeth to consider. So-called "baby-bottle mouth" (bottle-induced tooth decay) can affect any child with teeth, but the more teeth, the greater the potential for those serious dental problems. The issue isn't just the fluid in the bottle (unless that fluid is water), but the mechanism of bottle-feeding. Instead of sipping and swallowing – as a child does with a regular cup – a bottle (and to a certain extent a beaker) allows liquids to pool in the mouth before they're swallowed. Unless they're brushed away, the sugars in the liquids (lactose in milk and fructose in juice) are broken down by bacteria in the mouth. During the process an acid is formed, which feasts on protective tooth enamel, causing decay.

- And health issues, too. Toddlers who keep nipping from a bottle, especially when they're lying flat on their backs, run a higher risk of ear infection.

- You've got support. Healthcare professionals recommend weaning children from the bottle at 12 months.

That pile of reasons for weaning now, however, may not stack up against other considerations you're facing – like a big change or stress in your child's life (a new home, a new child minder) or in yours (a new job or a job search, a sick parent, financial issues). The time that's right for you and your toddler is always the best time. No matter when in the second year you get around to weaning, amen to the expression "Better late than never"!

Cup Conflict

"I know it's time to get my toddler on a cup, but whenever I hand her one, she pushes it away and points to her bottle – and I give up, again."

Having trouble getting your little one to join the cup club? That's probably because membership wasn't her idea. A toddler usually has no problem trying new things – that is, as long as the new things aren't offered up by others (namely, parents). Grabbing a handful of green grass and shoving it into her mouth? Fine. Having a spoonful of green broccoli waved her way? Not so fine. Going for Dad's cup of coffee when he's not looking? Just the ticket. Having Dad hand her a cup of her own, and encouraging a sip? Not a chance.

Of course, you know your toddler will take a cup eventually. The trick will be getting her to sign up for the cup club sooner than later, so she can leave bottles to the babies. Here's how:

- Stop passing the cup. For a few days, don't even bring up the cup. This will allow for a fresh start to what's become a stale campaign. Stash the cups you've been trying to foist on her out of sight, so you don't resurrect any conflicts.

- But pass the glass. If she makes a grab for your juice glass or your water bottle, by all means let her have a supervised sip. Just because she doesn't want to drink what Dad puts in front of her doesn't mean she doesn't want to be just like Dad. Some children like to bypass the baby stuff and move right on to adult drinking equipment (anything breakable or spillable will need adult supervision).

- Go shopping . . . together. It goes without saying that taking your toddler to the shops is something you do only when you need to. Well, you need to. Letting her pick out a new cup or two will help give her that sense of control she craves. Show her two at a time, and allow her to select her favourites (if you can, get a couple of different styles, maybe one with handles, one without, one with a straw, one that has a spout) – and don't underestimate the power of cute characters or magical gimmicks, like cups that change colours.

Straw Power

You probably associate them with the unhealthier side of eating (want chips with that?), but straws are actually good for your toddler – and definitely a whole lot better than a beaker or bottle – for a couple of impressive reasons. First of all, sucking from a straw requires complex movements by the jaw and mouth muscles, giving them the workout they need to develop well (and, ultimately, to coordinate to form a variety of sounds and to string those sounds into words and sentences).

Second, instead of encouraging liquids to pool in the mouth, where they can lead to tooth decay (especially if there's sugar in the liquids, even milk sugar), straws send liquids on the fast track to being swallowed, so teeth are largely bypassed and protected. Not to mention, they're fun for toddlers to use – especially when they're bendy or colour-changing.

Beaker Know-How

What's not to love about beakers? They're virtually indestructible, practically spill-proof, and totally portable. Unlike other cups and glasses, they can be used on the go. And best of all, they allow beginners to sip on their own.

While parents and children may find them easy to love, however, some experts aren't quite so keen on beakers. Call it media buzz, scientific buzz kill, or a little of both, but research making the rounds has shown several potential pitfalls to beaker use. One: tooth decay. Because most beakers, like bottles, release liquids slowly, there's more time for them to pool in the mouth – not a problem if water's being sipped, but a recipe for cavities if the cup is filled with milk or juice. Brushing after drinking is one solution to this problem, albeit not very realistic when toddlers do round-the-clock sipping.

Then there's the germ factor. When beakers – like bottles – become a child's constant companion, they also become safe havens for bacteria. The longer they're dragged from activity to activity – or emptied and then filled again without washing – the more bacteria they breed. And if that's not enough to make you queasy, consider how many times toddlers ditch a beaker in a pile of toys, then retrieve it (and sip from it) three days later.

Another health concern: when the beaker (like the bottle) is filled with juice, chronic sippers can develop chronic diarrhoea. Or drown their appetite for solids. Or get too chubby, from all those easily chugged juice calories.

And there's more. Researchers have suggested that exclusive beaker use may possibly slow speech development, since drinking with a spout doesn't give mouth muscles the workout they need. Any slowdown would be temporary – still, it's food (or drink) for thought.

On the plus side . . . well, you already know the plus side of beakers.

- Have a cup playdate. Getting to know the cup may help her get to love it, or at least, try sipping from it. Show her how she can use it to feed her dolls or serve you "tea". Seeing you sip from it, by the way, may ignite a typically territorial reaction in your toddler – before you know it, she may be clamouring to drink from "my cup"!

- Make it available, not an issue. Remember, she's more likely to sip from the cup if it's her idea than if it's yours. So instead of trying to coerce or cajole a sip before the breast or bottle (good luck with that plan), casually make it available at meals.

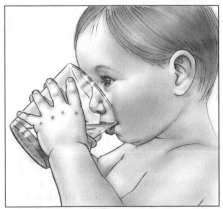

Drinking without dribbling will take lots of practice. Nappy-only practice sessions minimise mess.

They're a terrific transition from breast or bottle to traditional cups. They minimise mess, maximise convenience. But they're not the only choice. Toddler cups with straws are also a good option in this transition stage – without the downsides of traditional beakers (see box, page 99). Still, if you'd like to go the beaker route, here's how to get the pluses without too many minuses:

Compare and contrast sips. Some beakers claim to be better for dental and mouth development than others. Check the current field out before you buy (and look for cups that are BPA-free; see page 130).

Switch sips. Instead of starting and sticking with a beaker, try teaching your toddler the fine art of sipping from a spoutless cup from the start, too. Opt to alternate if your little one is amenable. Or, let your toddler master a straw.

Set some beaker limits. Make a beaker-with-meals-and-snacks-only rule. That will cut down on tooth enamel wear and tear, prevent juice overdosing and bacteria cocktails, and keep beaker use from slipping into beaker abuse. Or, limit on-the-go beaker use to water.

Remember the point of sipping. The breast and bottle – those were (or are) for feeding your toddler *and* providing sucking comfort. The point of the beaker (or any cup) is to provide your toddler with fluids. If you're using the beaker to calm your toddler down during stressful moments, or keep boredom from setting in during trips to the shops or while riding in the car or pushchair, or to keep those little hands busy and that little mouth occupied . . . then you're overusing it. Does your toddler crave the comfort of clutching the beaker? That's totally fine – as long as it's filled with water, and washed frequently.

Know when to quit the beaker. Once your child can handle a glass or regular cup without too much spilling, ditch the beaker.

The less attention you pay to the cup, the more likely she is to pick it up and surprise you with a sip.

- Pull a switch. You've been filling it up with milk? Switch to watered-down juice. Or try something completely different – something she likely never encountered in a bottle – like a sipable fruit-and-milk smoothie.

- Let the weaning begin. The immediate objective is trying the cup, but don't lose sight of the ultimate goal: Giving up the bottle. Just don't let your toddler in on your plan. As she starts getting on friendlier terms with the cup, gradually cut back on the fluids she's taking from the bottle (just keep an eye on her fluid intake, to make sure she's getting enough). Whatever you do, try not to associate joining the cup club with revoking her membership in the bottle club. Otherwise, she'll reject the former and cling to the latter.

- Cover all bases. Drinking from a cup will be a messy business until your toddler becomes a pro (unless you're using a spill-proof cup – and for experience's sake, you shouldn't always do so). Prepare for messes, but keep your cool when they happen . . . and they will.

Belated Bottle Weaning

"I just never got around to weaning my daughter from the bottle. Since she seemed so happy with it, I kept putting it off. Now that she's almost 2 and is so stubborn about everything, I don't know how I'll ever get her off it."

Weaning from a bottle at any age can be challenging, and weaning at the infamously inflexible age of 2, as you've guessed, considerably more so. But with a lot of patience and determination, a little friendly persuasion, and a minimum of pressure, it can be accomplished. Here's how:

▪ Try the weaning tips on page 96. They can work just as well for an older toddler as a younger one.

▪ Bottle water. A water-only policy will almost certainly make the bottle less appealing. It'll also protect her teeth while she's kicking the bottle habit.

▪ Hand over the choice. If there's one thing you've learned about your toddler over the past year, it's that she's a control freak – most toddlers are. So instead of forcing the issue (you know where that's going to get you), put the choice in her hands next time she asks for a bottle . . . literally. Offer up a bottle of water in one hand, a cup of her favourite beverage in the other, and let her choose. After she realises she can't hold both at the same time (she'll probably try that first), she may decide that having her favourite drink beats having her favourite container. Even if she doesn't take the cup the first time, or the second, keep on trying – eventually, she's likely to reach for it. Of course, the success of this strategy – like most strategies involving your toddler – depends on you not caving. Stand firm on water-only in the bottle, even if she whines to have her choice refilled with milk or juice.

▪ Offer incentives. Here's the good part about belated bottle weaning – your older, wiser toddler can now understand the concept of a rewards programme (I-do-this, I-get-that). Incentives work well, especially for one-time developmental achievements (though they can clearly be overused – as in, you start using them every time you want your toddler to comply with anything). Let your toddler know that there's something special in store for her if she gives up her bottle: a new book, stickers, a toy, a trip to the zoo – nothing over the top, but just enough to convince her that quitting is worth her while.

▪ Play up the perks. She knows the benefits of sticking with her bottle. Now it's time to try selling the benefits of giving it up – namely, being a big girl, and all the privileges that go along with that status. Entice her with a few big-girl perks: sitting in a grown-up chair instead of a high chair for meals, using a big-girl spoon instead of her baby spoon, and so on.

▪ Use the tooth defence. Explain that drinking from a bottle can give her teeth sore bits, and that drinking from a cup will make her teeth strong, happy, and healthy.

▪ Call the authorities. Your little one may be just about big enough to be impressed (possibly even influenced) by the powers that be, at least the nonparental powers that be. That definitely goes for doctors and dentists. So make an appointment with the doctor or dentist and have them explain why drinking from a bottle can hurt her teeth.

- Cheer her on. Breaking a habit is hard to do – as you probably know from your own experience. What makes it harder? Anything that steps up stress (like pressure from your parents – which, of course, also steps up rebellion). What makes it easier? Lots and lots of positive reinforcement. So, keep pressure to a minimum (and definitely don't threaten or belittle your little one because she's having a tough time giving up the bottle), and offer her the support, understanding, and extra attention she may need while she weans. Once she's reached this major milestone, provide both the reward she's earned and the cheers she deserves.

Milk Rejection

"We've been trying to switch our son over to cow's milk, but he won't touch it. I'm afraid he won't get enough calcium without it."

Milk may be the most popular source of calcium in a healthy diet – especially among the playground pack – but it's certainly not the only one. A 250 ml glass of milk contains about 300 milligrammes of calcium, but so does about 25 g of cheese or 25 ml of yogurt (opt for whole-milk dairy products to ensure adequate fat intake, unless the doctor has recommended otherwise). Calcium-fortified juices count, too – though since juice intake should be limited, you won't be able to fill your tot's calcium requirements on juice alone.

Sometimes, it's just a matter of time before a tot develops a taste for milk – so definitely don't give up, and absolutely keep offering (but not pushing) sips. If you haven't already, you can try mixing milk half and half with familiar

Milk Measures

Once your toddler's weaned and you no longer have those bottle calibrations to count on, how do you do the milk maths? Here's one way to keep tabs on intake – and to make sure your little one gets the 500 ml per day he or she needs. Measure that 500 ml of milk into a covered jug each morning, keeping it in the fridge and reserving it for your toddler's needs. Pour just a little at a time, to cut down on leftovers that'll mess up the tally. At the end of the day, you'll have a pretty good idea of how much milk is actually being drunk. If there's consistently milk left in the jug, be sure your toddler's getting enough calcium and vitamin D from other sources.

formula or breastmilk, gradually transitioning to all milk as your little one becomes accustomed to the new flavour. Or sneak milk into fruit smoothies, soup, and cereal (make hot cereal with milk instead of water).

While you're smart to keep an eye on your little one's calcium intake, there's another vital bone-boosting nutrient he might be missing if he's not a milk drinker: vitamin D. Check in with his doctor to see if a supplement's a good idea to fill in any gaps.

Milk Allergy

"I just weaned my toddler from the breast to cow's milk, and all of a sudden she's having some symptoms – a little diarrhoea, a little runny nose, some wheezing – that make me wonder if she could have a cow's milk allergy."

Milk and toddlers usually go together like . . . well, like milk and biscuits. But it's not always a match made in high-chair heaven. For 2 per cent of little ones, a milk allergy stands between them and childhood's favourite biscuit chaser. The symptoms include some that your toddler has shown (diarrhoea, wheezing, a runny nose), as well as an uncomfortable host of others she hopefully escaped (such as eczema, constipation, irritability, poor appetite, and fatigue). They usually kick in as soon as milk is served up (in the first year if cow's milk formula was given, or once a breastfed or soy milk formula-fed 12-month-old takes that first sip of whole milk). To find out for sure whether your toddler is among that milk-allergic minority, check with the doctor for an official diagnosis.

Happily, milk allergies are often short-lived – and most kids can move on to milk by the end of the third year, just in time for those classic after-preschool snacks. Until then, she'll probably have to stick with the less conventional – but nearly as nutritious – soy milk, that is, if she doesn't turn out to have a soy allergy, too (almond milk and coconut milk, in case you're wondering, are not nutritionally equivalent to cow's milk, and goat's milk is likely to trigger an allergic reaction, too). Cow's milk cheese, yogurt, ice cream, and other dairy products will also have to stay off the menu until she's outgrown the allergy, though there are soy equivalents

of all of these, too. Meanwhile, discuss with the doctor how she can make up for the nutrients she's missing in milk, most notably calcium and vitamin D. Check in with the doctor, too, about her fat and protein intake, since most tots get a hefty share of these nutrients from whole milk.

Appetite Slump

"Our daughter was the world's best eater when she was a baby. But now she barely eats anything. What's going on?"

Is your 1-year-old clamping shut instead of opening wide? That's not surprising, and it isn't unusual, either. Here's why:

- An identity crisis – the crisis being, she's just realised she has an identity. It's no coincidence that toddlers start to put their foot down (at mealtime, bedtime, really any time) just about the same time they start standing on two feet. Derailing that "choo choo train" delivery of cereal that's trying to access the "tunnel" is one of many ways she'll be establishing her autonomy – and she's right on schedule.

- A normal weight slowdown. My, how your little one has grown in the first year – more than tripling her birth weight by the time you served up her first birthday cake. Problem is, if she kept growing at such a rapid rate, she'd weigh as much as a 10-year-old when she turned 2. Fortunately, her body opts to put the brakes on her appetite instead, slowing down weight gain before it reaches Humpty Dumpty proportions.

- Life on the run. Who has time to pencil a meal into a schedule as busy as your toddler's? There's walking to practise, climbs to attempt, trouble

---

Food Allergies

Wondering if your toddler has a food allergy? And if he or she does, what to do about it? See page 392 for all the details.

Self-Feeding

Your days of spoon-feeding your little one are over – or they should be soon – so get ready to pass the spoon (and fork) to a new generation. Letting your tot self-feed may not be the neatest endeavour, but it's a crucial developmental step, and it doesn't happen overnight. Here's what you can expect as your toddler journeys along the road towards independent eating:

12 to 15 months. By now your 1-year-old is likely a pro at using fingers to pick up foods and shovel them into his or her mouth – and finger foods are uniquely suited to toddlers, so keep serving them. Early in the second year (if not before), your toddler will start showing interest in using a spoon – an interest you should definitely nurture. But with those still developing fine motor skills – and eye–hand coordination – proficiency may not keep pace with that interest just yet. Since practice will eventually make perfect, give your tot plenty of opportunity to wield that spoon. As for cups, by now your little one should be pretty handy holding a cup, at least with two hands. Beakers are easier to handle, not to mention less messy, but alternate beakers with regular cups and cups with built-in straws. Adding a straw to a regular cup can make it more fun to drink from.

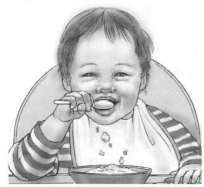

Self-feeding is messy feeding.

15 to 18 months. By 15 to 18 months, most toddlers have made the connection between spoon (or fork), bowl (or plate), and mouth. But actually making smooth connections, well, that's another story. There's the challenge of scooping the food onto the utensil, lifting it towards the mouth without inadvertently flipping it over and dumping its contents on the floor, manoeuvring the food into the mouth, and then repeating. It's a messy job, for sure, but one your tot will have to do . . . again and again and again until it's seamless (and don't expect anything approximating that until age 4 at least).

18 to 24 months. By the second half of the second year, it'll be hard to pry the spoon or fork out of your toddler's hands – not that you should try. "Me do it!" will be a familiar battle cry – especially when it comes to self-feeding (though you'll hear it in just about every context). You can't expect neat eating yet, but you can expect better compliance when it comes to the rules (as in, if you throw your pasta on the floor, lunch is over). A normal cup should appear regularly at meals – in fact, it's a good idea to start transitioning completely from the beaker soon. Straws continue to be a toddler favourite, and that's fine, since using a straw gives those mouth muscles an important workout while protecting teeth from decay.

Be on the lookout: If your toddler isn't self-feeding finger foods by 15 months or attempting to use a spoon by the middle of the second year, mention it to the doctor. Also let your doctor know if your child always gags when eating, has a hard time chewing, or shows a strong preference for puréed foods after 15 months.

to get into. Plus, eating is something that's done sitting down, at least when parents have their way – a real downer for someone who's just learned to stand up.

- An improved memory. A baby feeds like there's no tomorrow – or no next feeding. But a toddler is able to reason, "They feed me several times a day around here. If I don't eat now, I can eat later." If she's otherwise occupied (and when isn't she?), she may see no need to break for a meal.

In other words, your little hunger striker is just being a textbook toddler – taking her developmental cues from Mother Nature (and not her own mother, or father). If that doesn't reassure you enough, consider this: study after study has shown that healthy toddlers who aren't pushed or prodded to eat consume all the food they need to grow on. What's more, they're less likely to develop eating issues or weight issues later on.

Still not quite convinced that your toddler's appetite slump is normal? Here's something else you should know. Toddlers need to eat a lot less than their parents usually think. Case in point: a toddler-appropriate serving of sweet potato? Only about two to three 2.5-cm cubes (see box, page 93). So get in the habit of thinking spoonfuls, not platefuls. Too much food on a plate can easily overwhelm a petite appetite. If she's hungry at meal's end, she can ask for seconds.

Need even more reassurance? Check with the doctor, especially if symptoms of illness are accompanying an appetite slowdown.

Is your toddler picky, picky, picky too? See page 109 for tips on finessing the finicky eater.

Up-and-Down Appetite

"One day my son will eat nonstop, the next day he'll eat next to nothing. Is that normal?"

Left to his own appetite – and it's best if he is, as long as he's thriving – the typical toddler's food intake will vary from meal to meal, day to day, week to week, month to month. Maybe he'll consistently eat one big meal a day and pick at the others. Maybe he'll graze his way through every meal. Or nibble one day, gobble another. His appetite may speed up when he's going through a growth spurt, or slow down when he's teething or otherwise out-of-sorts. Scrutinise each meal, or even each day's worth of meals, and you're bound to see a lopsided nutritional equation. Check out the big eating picture (instead of the leftovers on his plate last night), and you'll almost certainly see that his food intake balances out over time.

So instead of trying to micromanage your toddler's eating habits (you'll meet with limited success), try letting him be the master of his own appetite. Offer small portions of healthy food at regular intervals, and let him decide if he's hungry and when he's full – no matter how much he's eaten, or not eaten, whether he's ploughed through a third portion or hasn't made it halfway through the first. There are two bonuses to this approach. First, you won't be driving yourself (or your toddler) mad at mealtimes by counting uneaten peas or prodding for "one more bite". Second, and most important, you'll be raising a child (and eventually, an adult) who has healthy attitudes towards eating ("I eat when I'm hungry, I stop when I'm full").

Messy Eating

"I wasn't exactly expecting neat eating at this age. But my toddler throws and smears more food than he actually eats."

For toddlers, enjoying food means smearing it, tossing it, mashing it, and squishing it (the tot equivalent to a wine taster's sniffing and swishing ... and come to think of it, both involve spitting, too). Sure, you don't want to spoil your toddler's food fun – and yes, you've heard that toddlers learn about their environments through tactile experimentation and feeling the food between their fingers – but must you wave the white paper towel of surrender in the name of your toddler's good time at the table? Let the food fly – and spill, and crust – where it may? Well, not exactly. You can try these mess-minimising mealtime tactics:

- Rationing. Serve up a mess of food to your toddler, and he's sure to serve up a mess to you. Instead, place just a few bites in front of your child at a time. Add a few more as those are consumed, if they're consumed.

- Occupation. To keep those chubby hands busy, give your toddler props. Literally. Hand over the spoon, if you haven't already. Not only will your toddler love running the eating show, the challenge of bringing food to his mouth with this novel gadget may also distract him from overturning the cereal bowl onto the cat's head. A little high-chair chat may divert, too, while passing on valuable social skills. If conversation doesn't work, substitute an acceptable game for the objectionable one: "You take a bite of your cheese and then I'll take a bite of mine."

- Suction. Forget sliced bread (it's only going to land on the jam side when it's tossed to the floor) – there is no better invention, at least as far as parents of little ones are concerned, than a bowl that attaches to a table or high-chair tray with suction. It can't promise no fuss or no muss – but it can promise no bowl of pasta flung across the kitchen like a Frisbee.

- Stick-to-it-ness. Try to serve foods that don't just stick to his ribs, but to the bowl, plate, and spoon. Mashed potatoes, sweet potatoes, cottage cheese, chunky fruit purée, slightly mashed bananas, porridge, or egg mayonnaise.

- Protection. Besides the obvious – paper towels or dish towels and wipes (and lots of them) – you can cut down on cleaning by spreading plastic or newspaper under the high chair and seating your toddler as far from nonwashable furniture as possible. Preferred mealtime dress code: an over-the-shoulder bib or nappy only.

- Reinforcement. When your little mess-maker makes a little less mess at mealtime, reward him with a reinforcing round of applause. On the flip side, when he flips the scrambled egg over the side of the table or pours milk down his T-shirt, skip the eye roll or exasperated groan. The more attention paid to mess-making, the more mess he'll make.

- A three-chances policy. Or two chances, or four, or whatever you feel you can stick to. Let your toddler know – calmly, firmly – that when the mess leads to mealtime mayhem, the meal will be stopped. After the requisite number of "No playing with your food" warnings, follow through – and take the meal away.

Self-Feeding Sloppiness

"I know I'm supposed to let my daughter feed herself. But I really hate the mess she makes, so I always end up taking the spoon from her."

If a toddler with a spoon can be considered armed and dangerous, this could be your year of living dangerously. Disarming her – and wielding the spoon yourself – will definitely cut down on the mess, but it'll also cut down on the opportunities she has to self-feed (something she'll have to learn eventually anyway, unless you plan on following her around with a fork and knife for the next 20 years). Feeding herself feeds her independence, social skills, and healthy attitudes about food (she won't ever force herself to eat when she's not hungry, but you might).

No, she won't be giving Miss Manners a run for her table etiquette any time soon. And you'll still need to continue the search for the most absorbent paper towels and the best dish cloths that supermarkets have to offer. But there's no better way to instil a future of good eating habits than by putting up with some messy ones now. Toddler, feed thyself.

Food Spitting

"My toddler has started spitting his food. It's cute, but annoying – and messy. And the problem is, I can't help laughing."

Nothing brings out the joker in a toddler like an audience – and nothing brings out the porridge, puréed carrots, and yogurt like one, either. At 6 and 7 months of age, your little guy probably started making raspberry sounds (and may even have picked them up from you, when you blew juicy raspberries on his adorable belly after the bath). Innocent enough, at first. But it wasn't long before he realised that a raspberry sound combined with squishy or liquidy food creates the ultimate sight-and-sound show. This realisation, of course, is reinforced every time you react, whether by giggling, jumping a metre in the air (as a mouthful of soggy cereal goes splat onto your freshly blow-dried hair or dry-cleaned suit), or even going ballistic (negative attention, every toddler knows, is better than no attention at all). Clearly, it's time for some stage managing:

Give him new props. Certain foods, he's probably learned, spit better than others. So beat him at his own game. When possible, substitute slivers of soft melon or a cube of well-cooked sweet potato over strained fruits and veggies. Think easy to gum, but not easy to spit: cubes of soft eggy bread, pasta shapes, titbits of cheese, fish fingers. Serve the gooey stuff – like yogurt – as a dip, instead of as the headliner.

Don't let him blow you away. This is the hard part, but try not to flinch . . . or chuckle . . . or smirk . . . or blow a gasket when he spits food your way, or any way. No reaction, no satisfaction. If he's not getting the attention he's looking for, he'll get bored by his own tricks.

Bring down the curtain. He needs to know that if he keeps spitting or blowing, he's blown it. With a poker-straight face, give him a simple, firm warning, "No spitting food. We eat food." If the spitting continues, repeat, "No spitting," and add, "If you spit food, I am going to take the food away." The third time he blows raspberries (but be consistent, whether it's two, or three, or four warnings), remove the meal promptly. Even if he doesn't understand at first, he'll make the connection – and get the message – soon.

Food Fetishes

"Help! My son won't eat any food that's touching another kind of food."

Of course he won't. He's a toddler – and most toddlers have plenty of faddy food fixations. For this particular fetish, keep your purist happy by dividing to conquer. Use a divided dish and fill each compartment with a different food. Or serve each food in its own separate bowl. And don't worry that you're catering to your toddler's compulsion. If you matter-of-factly comply, this very common fetish will eventually run its quirky course. On the other hand, if you scold, dish up snarky comments, or roll your eyes, it may very well get worse.

"My toddler has a fit if the cracker or biscuit I give her has a piece broken off. What's her problem?"

Most toddlers like things just so – consistently just so. A predictably intact biscuit brings a little one comfort, the same kind of comfort that comes from knowing that cereal will always come in the blue bowl every morning, and that she'll always be wrapped in the bunny towel after every bath. Sounds a little compulsive, but it's just one more of the many ways that a toddler tries to control her environment.

When the age of reason dawns (probably some time after her third birthday), your child will begin to accept the way the cookie crumbles – and that broken biscuits taste exactly like unbroken ones. In the meantime, humour her when you can (if you have an unbroken biscuit on hand), and offer a sympathetic reality check when you don't ("See, all the biscuits in the box are broken – let's just pick the one you like most"). And when she breaks her own biscuit, think of that as a teachable moment (actions have consequences – she's broken her biscuit, she lives with it . . . or eats it).

The Fussy Eater

"My daughter is such a picky eater. She'll never try anything new, just the same-old-same-old – and sometimes she won't even eat that. I'm so frustrated!"

Picky, picky, picky? Most toddlers are. Some are predictably picky (only Weetabix, banana slices, and pasta-no-sauce need apply). Others, selectively so (one day, cauliflower makes the cut, the next day, it's snubbed). Control ("I'm

---

Try, Try Again

You've proposed papaya – no go. Served up spinach – uh-uh. Tried to tempt with tuna fish – not in a million years. Tired of rejection, and ready to give up on offering your toddler new foods (after all, what's the point)? Not so fast. Studies show it can take up to 15 tries for a child to get used to a new food, never mind like it. Bottom line: be patient with your tot's slow-to-adjust palate, which takes time to warm up to new tastes and textures. If at first a food gets rejected, just try, try again.

Also don't assume – as many parents do – that your little chicken nugget nut or toast freak definitely won't like a food because it's spicy, saucy, or not beige. Offer a taste of your tomato salad, a bite of your beef chilli, a sip of your lentil soup. Sometimes, seriously finicky toddlers decide to latch on to a completely unexpected taste (which may mean you'll have to keep that green chilli coming!).

the boss of me, you're not") certainly factors into fussiness, as it does into most stereotypical toddler behaviours. So does the need for comforting consistency, without any unsettling surprises (like discovering blueberries in the Weetabix instead of the accustomed banana). But there's another reason why some little ones won't venture out of the familiarly bland, and it's a product of physiology, not psychology: their taste buds are hypersensitive to new flavours, especially strong ones. So when your toddler turns up her button nose at broccoli, it may actually be because it tastes really bad to her. New textures may also be literally hard to swallow.

So what's the parent of a fussy eater to do? Continue pushing and prodding a varied-diet agenda? Or give in to her menu of monotony (and sometimes, not even that)? Actually, neither. Instead:

Start small. Sometimes size matters. A mountain of food (no matter what food) can overwhelm a little eater – causing her to give up before she's started. Keeping first portions small (see the box on page 93) will make them easier to negotiate. You can always offer seconds if the first little pile is polished off.

Serve up a side dish of new. Of course she's having the usual, and that's fine. But that doesn't mean you can't offer up a side dish of something new and unexpected (on a separate plate, so it doesn't mess with the pasta): a slice of avocado, a spoonful of tomato sauce, a cube of mango. Or bridge the gap between the familiar and the unfamiliar – drizzle some of her standard cheese sauce on a floret of steamed broccoli or cauliflower, a small meatball, or a few flakes of fish (on a separate plate, so there's no mingling with her precious pasta).

Try family style. Eating as a family comes with lots of benefits, long and

Banishing Beige Boredom

Is your tot on the beige food plan (the plan being: all beige food, all the time)? It's probably a little one's intuitive way of avoiding foods with strong flavours (if you think about it, beige is usually bland). A variety of colour does offer the best variety of nutrients, but you'd be surprised how far beige can take your toddler nutritionally – that is, if it's carefully selected. Wholesome bananas are beige. Whole wheat bread and whole grain cereal (especially porridge) are obvious beige standouts, as are whole wheat pasta, brown rice, quinoa (it's a protein-packed grain that's fun to eat), and mashed white beans or chickpeas. Cauliflower is sort of beige (toss it in a white Cheddar sauce), as are hummus (a chickpea dip that toddlers often lap up), tahini (a sesame dip), and tofu. You can roll tofu in toasted whole wheat bread crumbs and bake it like chicken fingers – which can also be made, by the way, with a coating of healthy whole wheat crumbs (as can fish fingers).

Continue offering brightly coloured side dishes (add a blueberry smile on that beige toast), but don't push the rainbow agenda. Left to run their course, beige fads typically don't last very long.

short term. But here's one you might not have thought of: family-style eating may encourage your picky toddler to eat more adventurously (as in, "I'll have what she's having"). Pass around a bowl of pasta with veggies and pesto or a plate of teriyaki salmon and brown rice, and you may be surprised to see your tot reach for a taste. When you can't sit

Ordering Trouble?

Feel like you've been running a restaurant in your kitchen, taking orders from your toddler around the clock ("boiled egg, crust trimmed, sliced apple!")? There's definitely something to be said for accommodating your toddler's picky palate – after all, toddlers are picky for a variety of legitimate reasons, from their tender taste buds to their craving for comforting consistency and control, and besides, nobody forces you to eat foods you don't like.

Still, there's a fine line between being accommodating and being taken advantage of, between letting your toddler have some control over the menu and allowing a kitchen coup. To avoid problems in your kitchen:

- One order per customer, per meal. Your toddler has requested eggy bread, you've prepared and served it, and now he or she decides to change the order to cereal? No – eggy bread is ordered, eggy bread is eaten. Otherwise you'll find yourself caught in a revolving kitchen door, and your toddler will learn nothing about sticking with a decision.

- You set the menu. Offer two, or at most three, healthy choices at meals and let your toddler choose between them. Endless options are overwhelming to toddlers, and offering free choice in the kitchen is asking for trouble (and an order of biscuits for breakfast, and ice cream for dinner – or an order of pasta and cheese when you've run out of pasta).

- All meals come with a side dish of what everyone else is having. The house rules: your toddler can have a preferred meal but served with a little bit of what the rest of the table are having.

Rather not cater to your fussy toddler's picky tastes at all? Some parents decide that offering choices isn't for them, and opt to stick with the time-honoured eat-what's-put-in-front-of-you approach. Others decide that having a toddler who eats adventurously is essential (though they may discover that their tykes just won't favour curry or savour coriander no matter what their culinary DNA). The last word, as always: do what works best for your family.

down together for a full meal, try to have a healthy snack while your little one digs in – and don't forget to share.

Hire a junior chef. Older toddlers love to pitch in, and studies show that children who help at mealtimes are more enthusiastic about trying the fruits (and veggies) of their labour. Start at the supermarket, by letting your picky tot pick between pasta shapes, choose a tomato, plop green beans into a bag. And then it's on to the kitchen – yes, the kitchen. While your first instinct may be to shoo your toddler from the kitchen

(the stove's too hot, the knives are sharp, and you just want a little peace when cooking), inviting her to "help" you instead can be just the (meal) ticket for a picky eater. So let your toddler sprinkle cheese onto the pasta, stir the cake mix, toss the blueberries into the porridge, or pat the salad dry. Her role as junior chef may not open up a world of eating experiences right away, but chances are she'll be more willing to try something she helped make.

Take no captives. Sometimes it's not the meal itself that a toddler finds objectionable, but the confinement (in a high chair, for instance). See page 117 for less-confining seating options. Allow the freedom of self-feeding, too, for best eating results.

Make the name part of the game. Just as you'd be more tempted to order "a mélange of baby spring greens tossed in a mustard vinaigrette" than a "house salad", your toddler may be more tempted to eat egg mayonnaise if it's called "egg sand" and scooped up with "spade" crackers, a peanut-butter-and-banana sandwich if it's called a "pb&b," a fried egg if it's sunk into the centre of a piece of toast and called "egg in a hole", a miniature meat loaf if it's called a "meat cake". For other strategies for making food fun, see box, page 114.

Leave pressure off the menu. Leave the pushing, prodding, coaxing, bribing, and cajoling – stop even those time-honoured "here-comes-the-choo-choo-into-the-tunnel" games. Let your little one eat as much, or as little, as she's hungry for – and when she's had enough, let her stop. Letting her appetite call the shots will help her develop healthy attitudes about eating, instead of setting the table for future food issues. Plus, when was the last time putting pressure on your toddler convinced her to do something she didn't want to do?

Let the picky pick, to a point. As long as there are only healthy options to choose from, let your picky eater at it. Encourage her to eat outside the box (of frozen fish fingers) and to try what everybody else is having, but don't insist. On the other hand, make her stick with what she picks (you don't want to fall into the restaurant chef trap – if it's pasta and cheese she's selected, it's pasta and cheese she eats). And when picking's just not possible – you're at a friend's house, and it's omelettes for

brunch – end of story. Let her know: "You can have the omelette and some bread, or you can leave the table and go play." After all, in the real world, you don't always get to pick.

Let the poky poke, to a point. Many toddlers are slow eaters, particularly once they've started feeding themselves. Each pea must be popped in the mouth individually, strands of spaghetti sucked up one at a time. So give your toddler all the time she needs to complete the meal, even if it means starting breakfast 10 minutes sooner so you can get to nursery on time. When eating dissolves into playing, however (the peas are being plopped into the orange juice instead of popped into the mouth, the spaghetti strands are being strung from the high chair like garlands), end the meal promptly. Limiting distractions will help keep your toddler on task, so turn off the TV at mealtime, and if she wants to bring a toy to the table, let her know it'll have to watch her eat.

Feed when hunger strikes. It may sound obvious, but kids who aren't hungry at mealtime don't eat well. Some toddlers get out of bed in the morning ravenous, ready to dive into their bowl of cereal; others need some time to wake up and work up an appetite. Some can wait for a late family dinner hour; others have long lost their appetites by the time everyone's home and ready to eat. Try to tune in to your toddler's individual hunger pattern, then set mealtimes a little before each hunger period. And once you've set the mealtimes, try to stick with them; for most toddlers, regular and predictable mealtimes, with food served in the same place at the same time, works best. Another obvious appetite saboteur: too many snacks, or snacks that are too filling or served up too close to a meal. Ditto too many filling drinks.

Vegetable Snubbing

"My toddler won't eat anything that resembles a vegetable, especially if it's green. I know that's age-appropriate, but how's he supposed to get the nutrients he needs?"

It's not easy being green – especially if that something green is sitting on a toddler's plate. It'll be pushed to the side, hurled across the room, or fed to the dog . . . but eaten? Not likely. That childhood cliché holds true for most little ones, at least during the picky second year. And it's not surprising. Many green vegetables have strong flavours that can easily offend timid taste buds. Some have challenging textures or smells. Some, all three. Fortunately, not all veggies are green, and none of them has cornered the market on a particular nutrient. Here's how to get your toddler to eat his vegetables, or at least the nutritional equivalent of them:

Be a little sneaky (but not too sneaky). Vegetables don't have to be recognisable to be nutritious, and it's fine to sneak some into the foods your little one loves. Add chopped or puréed vegetables or tiny peas to the macaroni and cheese (cauliflower is especially hard to spot in an otherwise white dish). Toss little bits of cooked broccoli or red pepper into the spaghetti sauce. Stir a small amount of grated carrot into scrambled egg, meatloaf, or burgers. Bake some pumpkin bread. Pour some vegetable juice (some kids love the taste). But don't get in the habit of trying to disguise all the vegetables you serve – or try to serve – your toddler. First, because all that sneaking around will have to stop somewhere: do you really want

---

Gratifying a Snack Attack

Tiny tummies need frequent, small refills. Besides the obvious snacks (multigrain hoops by the cupful, and crackers by the bagful), try these wholesome nibbles:

- Carrot mini-muffins
- Cheese (sticks, cubes, slices, or coarsely grated)
- Shelled halved edamame or chickpeas
- Fresh fruit (small chunks or thin slices of peeled apple or pear, apricots, bananas, kiwi, peaches, nectarines, mango, melon, and so on) with a yogurt dip
- Dried fruit (no-sugar-added varieties), bite-size
- Small banana chunks

- Hummus, tahini, or salsa dip with crackers, pitta, or soft-cooked veggies
- Peanut butter (if allergy isn't an issue) spread thinly on half a whole grain mini bagel or on thin slices of peeled apple
- Microwave-cooked apple, peach, or pear slices sprinkled with cinnamon, topped with yogurt
- A small cup of soup
- Baked sweet potato wedges
- A turkey–cheese roll
- Egg mayonnaise, eaten with crackers or cooked veggies
- Mini-pizza (tomato sauce and cheese melted on bread)

Fun with Food

For toddlers, eating can be a drag – especially when they have to eat while sitting at the table. Add a little fun to food, though, and it's a completely different story. Here's how:

Shape up. Cut sandwiches, bread for eggy bread, even chicken fillets (pounded flat) into intriguing fillets – circles, diamonds, triangles, animals, hearts, stars – with a knife or a biscuit cutter. Spread thin pancakes, bread (flatten slightly first), or whole-grain flour tortillas with jam, peanut butter, cream cheese, tuna mayonnaise, or another favourite filling, and roll them up. You can serve the roll-ups whole, or slice them into wheels. Pour pancake batter to form faces, letters, teddy bears, and hearts, or shape already-cooked pancakes with biscuit cutters; decorate with chopped cooked raisins, banana slices, blueberries, or other fruits (fresh or freeze-dried). Seek out interesting shapes when buying pasta: wagon wheels, shells, twists, and alphabet letters (for fun and learning).

Sculpt a dish. Let loose the artist in you – and in your toddler – as the two of you create masterpieces good enough to eat: a cheese cube "brick" tower; a landscape of cooked broccoli and cauliflower "trees" dusted with grated cheese "snow"; a newfangled "ants on a log" (¼ of a banana slightly hollowed out, then filled with yogurt, and dotted with halved blueberries); a skyscape (mashed potato clouds, with green pea rain or a slice of baked sweet potato sun).

to be performing disappearing vegetable acts when your child's at junior school? Second, because it's not going to be effective forever (it won't be long before your little one cottons on to vegetable deception). But most important, because the ultimate goal should be a child who chooses to eat well – who reaches willingly (maybe even happily) for that stalk of broccoli, that asparagus spear, that mushroom slice – not one who's tricked into eating well.

Vary those veggies. So you keep offering up broccoli, and you keep getting turned down. Don't give up – you never know when you'll hit broccoli bingo – but do offer up vegetable variety: chunks of soft-cooked butternut squash, beetroot, cauliflower, Brussels sprouts, parsnips, bell peppers (in red, yellow, orange). And never assume that because your toddler has rejected one veggie he'll turn down another. Here's another assumption you should never make: that he won't like a veggie or other food just because you don't.

Sauce them up. Just because your toddler doesn't like veggies plain, it doesn't mean he won't like them with sauce. Try cauliflower in a mild coconut curry sauce. Broccoli in a stir-fry. Feature veggies in stews and soups (minestrone is a toddler favourite, but you can also add extra grated carrot to chicken noodle). Dipping, because it's interactive, elevates veggies of all kinds to fun finger food. And for those pint-size cheese lovers, melting a little grated cheese on any veggie can turn it into a tempting treat.

Eat your vegetables. Toddlers model all kinds of behaviours, including those they spy at the dinner table. If you dive enthusiastically into that bowl of green beans and carrots or take seconds on the salad, your little one's more likely to.

Think mini. Bite-size is just the right size for little fists, mouths, and appetites. Cut sandwiches or eggy bread into tiny squares, chicken fillets into nuggets or "fingers"; make mini pancakes; serve soft-cooked carrot "pennies"; use mini cake tins to bake tiny cupcakes, miniature meat loaves, single-serving carrot cakes. Look for baby carrots, tomatoes, courgettes, squash, sweetcorn, beetroot, and other mini-vegetables, and serve steamed or stir-fried until soft.

Sauce and dip. Some toddlers prefer their food plain, others like everything sauced or dipped (dipping is a particular favourite, because it's so interactive – a process fully under their control). Many latch on to one particular sauce or dip (tomato sauce, ketchup, cheese sauce, apple purée, yogurt dip, hummus, chilli sauce), and want everything they eat coated with it. Play along, even if the combinations seem a little peculiar (as in apple purée on chicken, tomato sauce on mashed potatoes, toast with cheese sauce, or toast dunked in yogurt).

Grate great food. Serve a mound (you can call it a "mountain" or a "hill") of finely grated carrot. Combine grated carrot, cabbage, and apple with a vanilla yogurt dressing for a tasty, nutritious coleslaw. A pile of grated cheese makes a fun snack, especially served next to a pile of grated apple.

Don't have the time, patience, or artistic inclination for preparing fun food? Or, do you feel strongly that food should be served up as is, no bells or whistles necessary? Your kitchen, your choice. Chances are, a hungry toddler will be happy having it your way.

Grow your own. There's no better way to get a little one interested in vegetables than to grow some together (talk about ownership!). Next best, visit those who do grow their own, at the farmer's market or a local grocer's. Out of season, or out of area? Visit the vegetable aisle, and enlist your toddler in veggie selection, and later on, in preparing them.

Switch colours. Your toddler still isn't going for the green? It's by no means required eating. In fact, the very same nutrients found in green vegetables can also be found in those more toddler-friendly colours, orange and yellow (think carrots, sweet potatoes, butternut squash). What's more, fruit covers all those nutritional bases just as well as any vegetable, especially fruit that's vibrant in colour (mango, papaya, cantaloupe, apricots, peaches, and berries). Add fruit to yogurt, to cereal, to smoothies – it's also yummy to dip with.

Favourite Food Rejection

"All of a sudden, my daughter has started rejecting her favourite dishes. What's wrong?"

Is yesterday's favourite food suddenly on today's blacklist? That's a toddler for you. Just when you think you've finally found a food you can count on your toddler eating, she stops eating it.

Sometimes it's just trademark negativity or an effort to gain control ("You can't make me eat my favourite food!"), sometimes it's a whim, sometimes it's a bout of teething or an oncoming cold, and sometimes it's just boredom that turns a toddler off an old favourite food. Whatever the reason for rejection, keep these dos and don'ts in mind:

Don't stress. Your toddler won't starve – she'll just eat something else.

Healthy toddlers who aren't pushed to eat always eat what they need. And making a big deal about the rejection only reinforces what she probably already senses: that the best way to push your buttons is to push away what's put in front of her. Instead, keep your cool when she suddenly spurns her beloved toast.

Do give it a break. Matter-of-factly take the rejected food away, and don't serve it up – or bring it up – for at least a week, unless it's asked for. In the meantime, offer nutritionally similar foods – if it's frozen waffles that have got the cold shoulder, serve pancakes. If it's yogurt, try cottage cheese. If it's apples, go bananas. Even toddlers get bored with the same old foods, after all.

Do bring it back with a twist. When you return the rejected food to the menu, serve it with a different spin. Cereal for lunch instead of for breakfast. Butter and Marmite toast rolled up and cut into wheels instead of standard squares (or for something completely different, try using a whole wheat tortilla in place of the expected bread – or banana instead of jam). Melon scooped into tiny balls instead of chunked. Chicken topped with tomato sauce and cheese instead of cut up into nuggets. Melted cheese made with mozzarella instead of Cheddar (and maybe served with a salsa dip).

Don't miss an opportunity. If you think about it, rejection of a favourite food is the perfect chance to offer up some new foods. So take the opportunity to add an item or two to your little one's repertoire.

Do try it yourself. Toddlers are notoriously possessive. Helping yourself to that rejected yogurt or bowl of cereal may inspire your toddler to dig in.

Don't write off rejected foods. What's off the menu today may be back on tomorrow, so don't give up (yet) on the six boxes of ricecakes you've stockpiled in the cupboard. In fact, if the favourite food strike is being triggered by teething discomfort or a soon-to-appear cold, it may be back in favour once your little one's back to her usual self.

Restless Mealtimes

"Our son won't sit still for a meal. He tries to stand up, squirm, and twist in his high chair – and he usually wants to come out before he's eaten very much."

In his baby days, your little guy did much of his exploring via his mouth – making eating an exciting experience. As a toddler, he prefers to explore on foot – making eating an exasperating waste of time, at least from where he sits (and twists, and squirms). And yet, food breaks are necessary to fuel his other activities. To help him refuel in spite of himself:

- Consider a new seating arrangement. Toddlers aren't big fans of confinement. It's possible that a seat at your table in a booster or clip-on chair, or at his own child-size table, might make your little one feel less cooped up and more cooperative at mealtimes.

- Stop feeding him. Letting him self-feed will definitely keep him occupied longer, particularly if he has new challenges before him (a cup with a straw, a spoon, a sauce for dipping food into).

- Keep him company. Even if you're not eating a meal at the same time, have a seat next to your toddler while he eats. No need to provide dinner theatre entertainment, but a little conversation may keep him from becoming bored too fast (just don't talk about how little he's eating or how much he's fidgeting).

- Avoid on-the-go eating. Make even snacking a seated activity. If your little diner gets to graze while he plays, he won't see the point of ever sitting down to eat.

- Sit yourself. Your toddler watches every move you make – and picks up habits accordingly. If you're always eating on the run (or straight out of the fridge, or standing at the counter), you're teaching your toddler to do the same. Yet another reason to regularly put family meals on the agenda, and to seat yourself even for those quick bites.

- Have toddler-size expectations. There's a limit to how long your toddler will sit, and you'll know he's reached that limit when he starts doing more fidgeting than eating. Release him without a fuss, even if he hasn't eaten much. Later there'll be another meal (or snack) where that one came from – that is, as long as he sits down for it.

Mealtime Entertainment

"Recently, mealtimes have become disasters. Our daughter won't eat anything without being entertained – and sometimes my husband and I feel like a circus act. What can we do?"

Stop sending in the clowns – and quickly. A toddler who is coaxed into eating by parental song and dance, stand-up comedy routines, magic tricks, and other (desperate) acts soon comes to expect equal servings of entertainment with her food. And guess what happens when it isn't served up?

Your goal isn't to get your toddler to eat, but to let her eat as little or as much as she's hungry for. Using entertainment to keep her in her seat at the table, if only for a few extra bites, undermines the natural function of her appetite, a process that's vital to self-regulating her food consumption. To develop healthy attitudes towards food, she should associate eating with being hungry ("My tummy's growling, so it must be time for me to eat"), not with being amused ("Daddy's standing on his head again, so it must be time for me to eat").

Of course, pulling the mealtime performance plug isn't likely to go over well at first. But resist the temptation to don your tap shoes and funny hats for one last show. Stay calm, nonchalant – as if her eating, or not eating, doesn't matter to you in the least (which it shouldn't, as long as her growth's on target). She'll eat when she's hungry, even if the show doesn't go on. And speaking of shows, avoid the mealtime TV trap. While watching TV may prolong the meal, it also promotes the unhealthy habit of zoned-out eating.

For a better form of mealtime entertainment – one that provides her with valuable social experience while making her meals more interesting – sit down for a conversation with your toddler while she eats.

Switching Out of a High Chair

"When do we switch our little man from a high chair to a booster seat?"

The best seat in the house for a toddler depends on the toddler who's sitting in it. Some little ones are perfectly happy in their high chairs until they physically grow out of them, but the wriggling and whining of other high-chair captives makes it clear that they're ready – and eager – to be relocated as soon as possible.

If your child does more fidgeting than eating in his high chair, it's time for a place at the table – in a booster seat

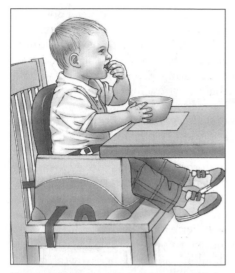

Most toddlers are ready to move out of their high chairs and into a less confining booster some time in the middle of the second year.

or hook-on chair, that is. Even if he's content with his solo eating arrangement, bringing him to the table helps him hone his social skills and pick up (eventually) some polite eating habits.

Once you transition, make sure the booster's always attached securely to the chair, and that your strapping tot is always strapped in. Hook-on chairs should never have a chair under them – otherwise a toddler can easily push off against it, dislodge his seat, and go flying. One other toddler-proofing tip: be sure the table isn't one big booby trap, especially now that he's joining the adults. Keep the surfaces he can reach (you may be surprised at how far those monkey arms extend) free of breakable, spillable, and dangerous items: knives, pointy forks, glass vases, and foods that pose a potential choking hazard.

Another seating arrangement that many toddlers love: a child-size table and chair, which also comes in handy for drawing and other art projects. Just keep in mind that your party-of-one will also need the social practice he'll get

sitting down with you and the rest of the family at the big table.

A Vegetarian or Vegan Diet

"We'd like to raise our toddler as a vegetarian, like us. Are there any nutritional requirements he won't be able to meet on a vegetarian diet?"

If you think about it, many toddlers are voluntary vegetarians, or nearly so – after all, they're more likely to be big consumers of carbs than of meat, chicken, and fish. Happily, vegetarian kids and vegan kids can be just as healthy as meat-eaters. Whether it's a family's philosophical commitment that's keeping meat off the menu or a passing food phase, there's no need to worry that your child will go hungry or miss out on key nutrients. Just remember to:

Keep track of protein. Toddlers who eat dairy products and eggs can easily fulfil their daily requirement for protein (often by lunchtime). But vegan toddlers, who eat no animal products at all, can fall short in this category, which is essential to growing, something toddlers are supposed to be busy doing. To fill in the gap, offer up protein-rich complex carbs, such as quinoa and high-protein pasta (most whole grains are actually pretty protein-packed) and all things soy (soy milk, soy cheese, tofu, edamame, along with carefully selected meat replacements, such as soy veggie burgers and soy "chicken" nuggets, though watch out for those that are high in sodium). And don't forget beans – a great source of protein, not to mention other key nutrients. Thinly spread creamy nut and seed butters (if there's no allergy) can also contribute small amounts of protein.

Be savvy about B_{12}. Vitamin B_{12} is right up there on the necessary nutrient list – important for normal growth and development. And while meat is an exceptional source of B_{12}, all animal foods provide a fair share. So if your toddler is a lover of dairy products and eggs, he's all set as far as B_{12} is concerned. If all animal products are off the table, make a point of including some B_{12}-fortified foods in your tot's diet. Many cereals are fortified with B_{12}, and you'll also find it in enriched soy milk (check the labels). Ask the GP if adding a B_{12} supplement might be a good idea, too (not all toddler multivitamins contain B_{12}).

Pump up iron with C. With all the produce and grains that vegetarian children eat, they typically get lots of iron. The only problem is that plant-based iron (called non-heme iron) is not as easily absorbed by the body as iron that comes from animal sources (heme iron). To make sure your toddler makes the most of the plant-based iron he's eating, serve a vitamin C-rich food (which boosts iron absorption) at every meal: some kiwi with that whole-grain toast, strawberries on that porridge, tomato sauce on that pasta.

Pour on the calcium. For those milk-drinking (and yogurt-and-cheese-eating) toddlers, getting their fill of bone building calcium is easy. Vegan toddlers can cash in on the calcium in fortified soy milk (but do check the label – not all soy milks contain calcium), and some other soy products, as well as fortified juice.

Be doubly sure about D. Vitamin D is essential for good bone growth, and a D deficiency in young children is linked to the development of rickets. If you've got a milk drinker, you've got vitamin D sorted. But getting enough vitamin D into a vegan tot can be a challenge unless you're serving soy milk that's vitamin D-fortified. To make sure that your vegan toddler is getting enough of this vital nutrient, check in with the GP

to see if a vitamin D supplement should be on the menu.

Don't forgo the fat. In the second year, toddlers still need plenty of healthy fat for brain development, and most get what they need from whole milk and whole milk dairy products. A vegan tot doesn't get that fat boost from soy milk, since it's naturally lower in fat than whole cow's milk. Even if you serve full-fat soy milk (which you should, since reduced fat or nonfat varieties contain even less fat), your toddler may not get enough of the fat he needs. Enter other healthy sources of dietary fat, like avocados, rapeseed and flaxseed oil, and ground seeds or nuts (if allergy's not a problem) – some of which are also good sources of omega-3 fatty acids, an important addition to your little vegan's diet.

Make more bites count. Since vegan toddlers need to eat even more plant-based foods to make up for the meat they're skipping (it takes nearly 150 g of beans and rice to equal the protein in a few bites of chicken), finding enough room in their tiny tummies can be challenging. That's why filling up that precious stomach space with junk food is an especially bad idea for little vegans, and offering healthy between-meal snacks is a particularly good one.

Eating Out with a Toddler

"We'd like to eat out more, but our toddler's not the best eater around – and she doesn't exactly have perfect table manners. So we've mostly been staying home."

Have reservations about eating out with your toddler? Don't. Eating out is valuable social practice for toddlers (and who wants to cook every night, anyway?). But before you secure a table for three – or two-plus-a-booster – consider the following:

Cuisine. You may savour scampi, but your toddler's tastes probably lean more towards pasta (hold the cheese and the green stuff) and chicken fingers (sauce on the side). In the interest of a peaceful meal, let your toddler's palate help guide your selection of a restaurant. A children's menu is a plus, but most restaurants will create a toddler-friendly meal upon request. That said, sometimes a change of place convinces a toddler to try a change of taste – she may be inspired to sample a stir-fry at a Chinese restaurant that she'd never sample at the kitchen table (and if not, there's always rice and small chunks of pineapple). So, once in a while, think about taking a leap of faith with your toddler into an unfamiliar culinary territory – you may be surprised at what she opens up to.

Amenities. Call ahead to make sure there's an ample supply of toddler seating (high chairs, booster seats) available – if not, bring your own. Restaurants that provide crayons and paper tablecovers or place mats get extra points. If the restaurant you're going to doesn't offer these perks, don't leave home empty-handed – you'll need kiddy entertainment galore. Pack a bag full of books, crayons, paper, or a few small and quiet toys. Toting a few crackers, a little dry cereal, or a cheese cube or two isn't a bad idea as backup (especially if the food takes a while to arrive), but try not to oversnack your toddler before the meal starts – or there goes any incentive to sit still. And don't forget a beaker, to avoid embarrassing spills.

Attitude. How will the restaurant react to a pint-size patron? When in doubt, ask straight out: "Are toddlers welcome in the restaurant?" The response will tell you what you need to know, even if not in so many words.

Noise level. A high noise level may be a conversation buster, but it also can drown out toddler whining and fork banging. Lively music is a good diversion for your toddler – and a good cover-up for those noisy antics (what the next table can't hear can't irritate them).

Dining time. When possible, arrive before the mealtime rush, when the restaurant isn't crowded and the staff isn't frazzled . . . yet.

Waiting time. Don't leave the wait up to fate. When you can, select a restaurant that takes reservations or that you can count on having free tables. If there's a wait, let your toddler burn off some energy outside (under your watchful eye). Toddlers don't usually do well when they have to sit and wait for a table and then have to sit and wait for dinner – and then have to sit and wait while everyone finishes eating.

Seating. Try to reserve the perfect table. Both you and the restaurant will appreciate it if you're seated in an out-of-the-way area (far enough from other diners that your toddler's screeching won't annoy them too much – and far enough from the kitchen door or the waiting station that there won't be a catastrophic collision if your toddler suddenly bolts from the booster). A window is a nice plus, especially if there are cars and passing people to distract your little one, and you might also want to consider a table close to an exit – in case your toddler needs a break from a long meal.

Once you've arrived at the restaurant:

Go for speed. There's nothing like a leisurely dinner – if you've left junior home with a babysitter. But if she's sitting between the two of you, pounding

Choking Risks

Good-bye baby purée, hello grown-up textures. With a rapidly increasing complement of teeth, most toddlers are ready to enter a whole new world of eating experiences. Yet even with their ever-widening culinary horizons, there are still certain foods that must remain off-limits to toddlers because they can cause choking.

Though anyone of any age can choke on food, several factors may combine to make toddlers and pre-schoolers more vulnerable to a choking incident. Even once they have a full set of teeth (usually by the middle of the third year), their chewing and swallowing skills aren't well developed. They tend to bite off more than they can chew or swallow, to overstuff their little mouths for fun or out of impatience, to gulp food so they can get a meal over with and get back to play, and given the chance (which they shouldn't be), they're quick to eat on the run – and to eat while running.

To minimise choking risks, keep the following foods off-limits to your toddler (with the exceptions noted):

- Nuts and seeds, unless ground

- Hard sweets, marshmallows, toffee, and other sticky sweets or fruit snacks, chewing gum

- Sausages (slice them lengthwise before cutting crosswise to reduce risk)

- Chunks of meat

- Grapes (unless peeled, seeded if necessary, and halved)

- Raw cherries (unless peeled, pitted, and halved or quartered)

- Raw celery

- Whole raw carrots (thin slivers are fine for those with all their teeth, and finely grated is okay for those who are still gumming)

- Peanut butter or any other nut butter by the spoonful or fingerful (it's okay spread thinly on bread or fruit, but should never be eaten by the mouthful at any age)

- Popcorn

- Dried fruit (unless it's cooked and chopped). Bite-size freeze-dried fruit is safer, as long as it readily melts in the mouth without chewing (check a piece in your mouth first).

No matter what your toddler is eating, you can reduce the risk of choking even further by:

- Feeding your toddler in a sitting position only. Eating on the run, or while walking, playing, lying down, or semi-reclining presents a choking risk.

- Discouraging your toddler from overstuffing his or her mouth by offering small amounts of food at a time.

- Encouraging your toddler to swallow before talking or laughing (this will be easier to enforce if it's an across-the-table policy).

- Being especially careful about snacks in the car. A sudden stop can send a too-large piece of food down a toddler's windpipe.

the table for food, climbing over the back of the chair, and clanging the silverware, speed is of the essence. Your goal should be to get in, get fed, and get out as expeditiously as possible. Eating at restaurants that specialise in speedy service will help (but best not to overdo visits to fast-food eateries that specialise in high-fat cuisine). Some that offer take-away (pizza restaurants, for instance) will accept a call ahead to place your order, then serve you when you arrive. When that's not a possibility, ordering promptly and all at once saves time (if you start with drinks, you're in it for another 10 minutes, easy). Checking out the menu online before you go – so you're all ready to order as soon as you sit – can also save waiting time. Thinking about ordering your toddler's food first so she'll get to eat sooner? Sounds like a plan, until you consider that she'll be finished eating – and long finished sitting – before you've even been served. Unless your toddler is a really slow eater (the kind who can keep nibbling and nibbling), ask that everyone's food be brought as soon as possible. And that salad you were going to start with? Instead of ordering it as a first course, order it on the side of your main meal. Another way to put time on your side: order dishes that are ready quickly (ask the waiter which ones are).

Clear the area. Move everything breakable, bangable, and spillable out of your toddler's reach, not to mention all sharp objects (knives and forks), and flowers fake and real (you don't want her nibbling on the centrepiece).

Think small and familiar. If you can, order up something tried, true, and toddler-friendly (she can take her taste tests from your plate). Too much food will overwhelm her, so ask for an extra plate to scoop spoonfuls onto, and go for a half portion if there's no child size available.

Nothing looks familiar on the main meal side? Combine side dishes into a meal (some baked potato, cooked carrots and peas, rice, a slice of cheese). If your toddler is a purist, warn the server to leave off the garnish – that artistic sprinkle of parsley or chives could spell rejection and a return trip to the kitchen.

Set limits. Okay, it's not fair to expect a toddler to sit through a restaurant meal as the model of decorum. But it's not fair to subject fellow diners to an hour of toddlers-gone-wild, either. Consider, after all, that the people at the next table may be paying good money to a babysitter so they can relax without their own offspring for an evening. Enforce a few simple rules of civility (no banging, no clanking of silverware, no screaming), and definitely go out of your way to keep your toddler relatively quiet and content during the meal – though if she becomes so disruptive that other diners are giving you the evil eye, it's high time to march her out of there for a while. If there are two adults, one can supervise a toddler outside for a few minutes while the other enjoys a little solo dining, but don't take your junior diner home before the meal is finished, or she'll get the idea that she can change your dinner plans just by acting up. Another restaurant rule: no leaving the table unescorted. Children wandering alone around a restaurant can walk into someone carrying a tray of hot food or drinks and cause a serious accident – not to mention get hurt themselves.

Tip well. The special requests, the pasta ground into the carpet, the tomato sauce splattered across the table, the drinks upturned, and the plates tipped over – a few good reasons why anyone who waits on a toddler deserves a little something extra for his or her efforts. Be especially generous if you plan to return to the restaurant.

ALL ABOUT:
Food Safety

Lots of whole grains? Tick. Fresh fruit? Tick. A variety of veggies? Tick. Omega-3-packed fish? Tick. Bacteria, pesticides, and other assorted chemicals? You might want to make sure.

Feeding your toddler well isn't just about feeding healthy foods (or trying to work out how to get your toddler to eat them). It's about making sure the food you buy, prepare, and serve your little one is as safe as it can be. Happily, with just a few precautions and a lot of common sense, you'll be all set when it comes to food safety.

SAFE PRODUCE

Fruits and vegetables have earned their reputation for being healthy – especially for fast-growing toddlers. And although vegetables typically get mixed reviews from the booster seat crowd, what toddler doesn't enjoy a nice juicy chunk of melon or mango? A sweet slice of apple or pear? A blueberry-banana smile on their cereal? Just remember, as you pick the fruit bowl clean for your little fruit fan, that all fruit is healthy, but not all fruit is safe – at least, not right off the shelf. Some produce may be contaminated with bacteria (from soil, water, or a picker's unwashed hands), while other produce may sport a coating of pesticides. To make sure that the fruits and vegetables that are supposed to keep your toddler healthy won't actually make him or her sick:

- Stick close to home. For one thing, locally grown produce is usually fresher than imported – which means it's likely to retain more nutrients – nutrients your toddler needs. For another, it doesn't require post-harvest

---

Chemicals Aren't Kids' Stuff

It may seem that your toddler eats next to nothing, but here's a bit of tot trivia that may surprise you: little ones eat more food – and drink more water – per pound of body weight than adults do. They also eat a lot more of certain foods, at least comparatively (like fruit), and, thanks to their picky habits, tend to eat the same foods over and over (apple slices, followed by apple purée, followed by apple juice).

What does that mean for your toddler? Potentially, more exposure to pesticides and other chemical contaminants found in the food chain and the water supply – exposure to which toddlers are especially vulnerable. Not only because toddler bodies are still developing, but because young children ingest more chemicals (in proportion to their weight) from the food they eat and the water they drink, and they absorb those chemicals more easily.

A few good reasons why it's extra-important to be extra-careful about chemicals when you're feeding your extra-special eater.

The Dirty Dozen . . . and the Clean Team

Wondering whether organic products are worth the premium price you pay for them? When it comes to your toddler, they may be, especially in some cases. Organic foods are guaranteed to be free of toxic pesticides, fertilizers, hormones, antibiotics, and genetic modifiers. While they don't promise greater freshness or improved nutritional benefits (unless they're locally grown, in which case both perks may apply), eating them will reduce your toddler's exposure to potentially harmful chemicals – definitely a big plus.

Of course, an all-organic policy comes with a big bottom line. If you have to pick and choose, here's something to consider. Certain fruits and veggies (aptly called the "dirty dozen")

have been identified as the ones *most* likely to contain pesticides if they're conventionally grown – so whenever possible, opt for organic on these: apples, bell peppers, celery, cherries, grapes, nectarines, peaches, pears, potatoes, raspberries, spinach, and strawberries. More recent studies have implicated blueberries, too, suggesting that they should be added to the list (making it a baker's dirty dozen). Blown your budget avoiding the dirty dozen? These five fruits are the *least* likely to have pesticide residues when they're conventionally grown: avocados, bananas, kiwi, mangoes, and pineapple. The vegetables *least* likely to contain pesticides: asparagus, broccoli, cabbage, sweetcorn, aubergine, onions, and peas.

---

chemical treatment to preserve it during a long cross-country or overseas journey. Try to buy fruits and vegetables in season (for the same reasons), or opt for fresh-frozen or freeze-dried.

- Go organic. Whenever it's available, affordable, and looks good, choose organic produce. It isn't less likely to harbour bacteria, but at least it won't be covered with pesticides. See the box above to find out which fruits and veggies are best bought organic.

- Switch off. Choosing a variety of fruits and vegetables guarantees not only better nutrition, but also safer eating. That's because different chemicals are used on different types of produce. Vary the produce you serve your toddler (as much as those finicky habits allow), and he or she won't ingest too much of any one chemical.

- Be as picky as your toddler. Take a good look at and a good whiff of fruits and vegetables before you serve them to your little one. Bruises are no big deal (though some toddlers turn down blemished produce), but throw away any that have traces of mould or smell funny.

- Always date your produce. Don't buy (or serve to your toddler) prepackaged produce that is close to its expiration date – or that doesn't look fresh or hasn't been well refrigerated.

- Be a clean freak. Wash the surfaces of all fruits and vegetables, organic or conventional – even those you plan to peel (otherwise the knife or peeler you're using can pick up surface germs and transmit them to the part of the produce your toddler will be eating). Don't soak produce (you'll end up throwing out many of the vitamins with the soaking water), and don't use soap. If necessary, use a small scrub brush to remove dirt or residue.

- Pick up pasteurised. Make sure you serve your toddler pasteurised juices only. Unpasteurised varieties – and that may include juice from the health food shop or market – can contain harmful bacteria, such as E. coli, that may make young children very sick.

For more information on chemical residue and pesticides on produce, contact the Food Standards Agency at www.food.gov.uk.

SAFE MEAT, POULTRY, AND FISH

Growing bodies need lots of protein, and there's no more efficient source of protein (not to mention other vital nutrients, like vitamin B_{12} and iron) than lean meat, poultry, and fish. Unfortunately, there's also no better source of bacteria (and in some cases, chemical contamination) – that is, unless you take a few protein food precautions. To make sure your toddler can cash in on the protein without tapping into the bacteria or chemicals:

- Cook it through. Raw or rare meat, poultry, or fish can harbour microorganisms (such as salmonella, E. coli, or campylobacter, all of which can cause serious illness, particularly in young children), as well as parasites. To make sure harmful bacteria don't find their way to your toddler's plate, cook meat, poultry, and fish thoroughly (see box for appropriate temperatures).

Is It Done Yet?

How do you make sure that the dinner you're serving your toddler isn't half-baked – and potentially harbouring germs that could make him or her sick? By taking your dinner's temperature (a high enough temperature means you won't be serving harmful bacteria along with that roast or that fish). The following foods can be considered safely cooked when they reach these internal temperatures:

Beef, veal, or lamb roasts, chops or steaks: medium – 160°F/71°C; well done – 170°F/77°C

Minced beef, veal, lamb: 160°F/71°C

Precooked ham: 140°F/60°C

Whole chicken or turkey: 180°F/82°C

Minced chicken or turkey: 165°F/74°C

Chicken breasts: 170°F/77°C

Stuffing: cooked in bird or alone – 165°F/74°C

Pork, fish: 145°F/63°C

Egg dishes and casseroles: 160°F/71°C

Don't have a meat thermometer handy, or you're at the mercy of a restaurant kitchen? Meat can be considered safe to eat when it's grey or brown (though if the meat was previously frozen, as in a fast-food restaurant, the colour test may not be an accurate gauge of doneness). Poultry should have no traces of pink, and juices should run clear. For fish, check to be sure that it flakes and is no longer translucent (salmon should turn opaque pink).

One Fish, Two Fish . . . No Fish?

Fishing for a healthy meal for your toddler? Fish is low in saturated fat, high in protein, and a good source of vitamin D and many of the B vitamins. What's more, fatty fish (like salmon) is full of omega-3 essential fatty acids, believed to boost brainpower.

But even with the amazing benefits of fish, it's important to choose fish wisely (so don't cast your fishing net too wide). Contaminants, like mercury and PCBs (polychlorinated biphenyls) lurk in many fish and shellfish. Some species contain very high levels, others have only trace amounts. Babies and toddlers (like pregnant women) are particularly vulnerable to the effects of these contaminants, which is why recommended restrictions on fish consumption are greater for this age group.

So what's off the fish menu completely? According to NHS Choices, you should never serve your child:

- Shark

- Swordfish

- Marlin

- Mackerel

What are some of the fish that are considered safest for young children to eat? Happily, they are ones they're most likely to enjoy:

- Pollack (the stuff of fish sticks)

- Haddock

- Hake

- Ocean perch

- Freshwater trout

- Whitefish

- Wild salmon (including tinned)

- Fish carefully. Certain fish are swimming in chemicals, such as mercury and PCBs. See the box above for more on fish safety. And skip the sashimi; no raw seafood for your little one.

- Spring for organic. If it's available in your supermarket and doesn't break your budget, opt for meat (including beef, pork, and lamb) and poultry that's labelled organic – the best way to ensure you're not serving up a side dish of chemicals with that meat stew or chicken nugget. The next best: look for meat and poultry that's raised without hormones or antibiotics (all organic meat and poultry is). Meat and poultry that's "free-range" (and organic usually is) comes with another health perk: it's likely to be leaner and higher in omega-3s than non-organic meat.

- Go lean. Not only is lean meat and poultry lower in unhealthy saturated fats, it's likely to be far lower in chemical contamination, even if it isn't organic. That's because the chemicals an animal ingests are stored in the fat (and in the skin and organs). So choose lean cuts (like extra-lean minced beef), avoid organ meats (as if your toddler would eat them anyway), and get in the habit of trimming fat and skin before cooking. Also, opt for cooking methods that allow fat to drain, and then be sure the fat doesn't end up in your little one's meal (drain fat off of sautéed minced beef or meatballs, for instance).

- Tilapia

- Flounder

- Sole

- Shrimp and scallops (though check with the GP before serving up seafood if there's a family history of allergies)

Thinking tuna mayonnaise for lunch or tuna noodle casserole for dinner? Reach for the tinned tuna, which contains considerably less mercury than albacore (white) tuna, and limit intake to no more than 25 g per 5.4 kg of your toddler's weight (so a toddler who weighs 10.8 kg should have no more than 50 g a week). Thinking of serving salmon? Keep in mind that some farm-raised salmon (the most readily available salmon in the UK) may contain high levels of PCBs. When you have a choice, choose wild salmon instead.

If your family goes fishing – or you have friends who share their catch – check with area health or fish and game departments about whether it's safe for young children to eat fish pulled from a particular fishing hole.

Once you've narrowed in on a healthy fish to serve, the way you prepare it can make it safer still. For instance, contaminants collect in the skin and fat on the fish, so if you trim away those areas before you cook, you'll lose many of the toxins. Frying seals in the toxins, so stick with grilling, baking, or poaching, which allows those chemicals to seep out and be discarded instead.

Aim to serve a variety of healthy fish two to three times a week, if you can get your toddler on board with that. And remember, toddler servings are about a quarter of a "normal" serving (read: not half a fish – about 25 g, or the size of a matchbox. And then, ahoy . . . and enjoy!

For more on meat and poultry safety, contact the Foods Standards Agency, www.food.gov.uk.

SAFE DAIRY

Most toddlers love their dairy – and that's a good thing. There's no easier way for your toddler to fill up on calcium and score some protein than by milking the dairy case. To make sure the dairy products you serve your little one – from milk to yogurt to cheese – are as safe as they are nutritious, just take these precautions:

- Pick pasteurised. Never serve raw (unpasteurised) milk, because it may contain bacteria that could make your toddler sick. This is the one time that

processed – in this case pasteurisation, the process that kills bacteria – is better.

- Be choosy with cheese. Make sure all the cheese you choose for your toddler is made from pasteurised milk, too (if a cheese isn't labelled, don't offer it). This is especially true of soft cheeses, which can be contaminated with listeria (a bacteria) if they're not pasteurised.

- Store with care. All dairy products should be stored in the refrigerator (even pasteurised products can become contaminated after pasteurisation). Don't use them after the expiration date or if they smell or look spoiled (when in doubt, throw it out).

A Mouldy Situation

Hiding in the back of your fridge – waiting to fill your hungry tot's plate with wholesome goodness – is a container of cottage cheese and a punnet of strawberries. But when you finally dig them out for a healthy toddler breakfast, a blue fuzz has started multiplying across the top of the cottage cheese, and a green one is sprouting on the strawberries. Do you scrape and serve – or throw it out? Here's what you should do when you've got a mouldy situation on your food:

- If small fruits (grapes, berries, strawberries) become mouldy, throw them out. If a few berries at the top of a box are mouldy, it's okay to eat the rest as long as you've screened and washed them carefully.

- If a hard fruit or vegetable (apple, potato, broccoli, or onion, for instance) or hard cheese has a small area of mould, it's safe to cut the mould away (plus a centimetre margin of safety) and eat the rest. Mouldy soft fruits (peaches, plums, melons, tomatoes) should be tossed.

- Dairy products (cottage cheese, yogurt, sour cream, butter) that are sprouting mould should be discarded – even if the mould is only on top. Ditto mouldy meat and leftovers.

- Mouldy bread, grains, peanut butter, nuts, sauces, and jams should be thrown away (even if the mould is only in one area).

  And always remember: when in doubt, throw it out.

- Shop organic, if you can. When it's available and affordable, consider buying organic dairy products. This is an especially good idea when it comes to whole milk – which most toddlers drink – since chemical contaminants are stored in fat and whole milk contains more fat than reduced-fat or skimmed milk. Just be sure that the organic dairy products you choose are also pasteurised.

SAFE EGGS

Scrambled or poached, fried, or boiled with toast soldiers – most toddlers enjoy eggs in one form or another. Problem is, some eggs can be contaminated with salmonella, a particularly dangerous bacteria. Happily, there are steps you can take to make sure all the eggs that end up on your tot's high-chair tray are good eggs – and safe ones:

- Buy refrigerated eggs only. Once you've brought them home, store them in the fridge; they can stay fresh for three weeks (assuming the expiration date hasn't passed – always check). And because even hard-cooked eggs can become contaminated, don't leave these out at room temperature longer than two hours.

- Check for cracks. Don't use an egg that's cracked when you buy it or that cracks on the way home – disease-causing organisms can creep in too easily.

- Cook eggs thoroughly. The whites should be set and the yolks should have begun to thicken. Runny eggs can still harbour bacteria.

- Don't serve up foods made with raw eggs. That goes for homemade hollandaise sauce or mayonnaise, mousse and cake mix – even if it's finger-licking good. Pasteurised eggs (and egg whites) can be bought for home use, and are safe to use raw in prepared foods or to serve under-cooked to your toddler (in soft scrambled form, for instance).

SAFE DRINKING WATER

Tap water. Thirsty? You're lucky to live in the UK, where tap water is considered to be among the world's best – and consistently meets the highest standards set by the EU Drinking Water Directive (98/93/C). Water quality and safety is closely monitored by independent inspectorates in England and Wales, Scotland and Northern Ireland – which means that you can most likely turn on the tap and drink with confidence. Still, there are questions you might want to consider before filling your toddler's beaker with water straight from your tap:

■ Is there leaching of lead or other metals from pipes in the water supply? This may be the case in your own home if you have old lead pipes or if lead has been used to solder the pipes. Lead exposure can lead to serious health problems for a young child, so it's essential to avoid it. If you suspect there's lead in your water, or if testing reveals high levels, changing the plumbing would be the ideal solution, but isn't always feasible. A filter is another option (though not all filters remove lead or remove it effectively – make sure you invest in one that does). A less pricey

way to reduce lead levels: use only cold water for drinking and cooking (hot water leaches more lead from the pipes), and run the tap for about five minutes in the morning (as well as any time the water has been off for six hours or more) before using cold water. You can tell that fresh lead-free water from the street pipes has reached your tap when the water has gone from cold to warmer to cold again.

Well water. If your water comes from a well, have it tested for chemicals and bacteria at least once every two years. Check with Water UK (www.water.org.uk) for information on the best way to test in your area.

Bottled water. Has your family gone bottled for convenience or for the taste? The problem is, water that comes from a bottle (or a delivered water cooler container) isn't necessarily better than water that comes from the tap (and in fact, some bottled water actually comes from a tap, too). To check the purity of a particular brand, contact NSF International, www.nsf.org, or check the label of the bottle for NSF certification.

If you do choose bottled water, you'll want to opt for one that has just the right amount of fluoride added (check with the doctor or dentist to see how much is just right to protect your toddler's teeth) – many bottled waters contain no fluoride. (Although, currently, only 10 per cent of the UK [mainly the West Midlands and North East] receives fluoridated tap water.) Always avoid distilled waters (from which beneficial minerals, such as fluorides, have been removed).

BPA in Food Containers

Bisphenol A (BPA), a chemical that may be toxic in humans and may adversely affect brain development, is found in many polycarbonate plastic products, including some baby bottles and beakers. There is some concern that BPA may have potential effects on the brain, behaviour, and prostate gland in foetuses, infants, and young children. Children, because they're more able to absorb the chemicals that end up in the various body systems, because they're still growing and developing, and because they do a lot of drinking and snacking from plastic containers, may be most vulnerable to BPA exposure. Consequently, many manufacturers are voluntarily avoiding the use of the chemical in their products and some countries are calling for an outright ban of its use. Most experts agree it's wise to avoid buying or using products with BPA until more is known. How can you tell if a bottle, beaker, or plastic container contains BPA? Simply look for a number in the triangle on the bottom. If it says #7, it likely contains BPA. Or look for the "BPA-free" label.

CHAPTER 5

Sleeping

T HERE'S NO DOUBT ABOUT IT – at the end of a long day with your toddler, you're ready for bed. Or at least, ready for a little adult-only relaxation (and a tantrum-free zone to relax in). But your toddler? Maybe not so much. Few toddlers look forward to bedtime, and most resist it pretty resolutely (like just about everything else that's good for them). How do you convince your toddler to turn in without a fight each night? And to stick with those all-important naps? All it takes is a little consistency and a lot of determination. That, and maybe, just one more story . . . and one more drink of water . . . and one more hug . . .

What You May Be Wondering About

Bedtime Rebellion

"Bedtime is a battle in our house. Our toddler doesn't want to go to bed, and once she's there, she doesn't want to stay there. It takes her forever to settle down."

I t isn't easy to go from 60 to 0, which, if you think about it, is what toddlers are asked to do every night at bedtime. From toddling around, climbing, jumping, and playing to cooped up in a cot, lying still – leaving toys, family, and daytime fun for hours of solo slumber. That's number one on your toddler's list of reasons to resist bedtime. Number two is the developmentally appropriate trouble tots have with transitions – and there are few trickier transitions in a toddler's day than the one that bridges being awake to being asleep. Add to that what may be a budding fear of the dark and of being alone, and – of course – that trademark toddler characteristic, rebelliousness (as in, "If Mummy or Daddy want me to do something, that's a good enough reason not to"), and it's far from surprising your little one, like most little ones, puts up a feisty fight when bedtime comes around.

To help your toddler brake for bedtime:

Sleepy Time

Remember when your infant slept nearly three-quarters of the day (and night) away? While you may still feel like you're in a constant state of sleep deficit, your toddler actually needs far less sleep now that babyhood's been left behind. But as the total number of hours of sleep decreases, the sleep cycles become more mature, organised into a pattern more resembling that of an adult (with a couple of naps tossed in). Still, many toddlers don't get all the sleep they need, and the proof is in the pudding . . . that was smeared all over the wall during yesterday's meltdown. Children who get too little sleep are grumpier, have more tantrums, and are less able to learn and focus – while those who get their fill of daytime and nighttime sleep tend to be better behaved, more interested in playing and exploring, and just plain happier (as are their parents). Here are some general guidelines for how much sleep the average toddler needs, keeping in mind that some little ones need more sleep and others need less:

12 to 15 months. A 1-year-old child needs about 14 hours of shut-eye each 24-hour period. Around 11 to 11½ of those hours should be concentrated during the night, with the other 3 hours split between two daytime naps.

15 to 18 months. Not much of a difference in terms of average sleep hours as your tot reaches the mid-year mark. Eleven hours of nighttime sleep and around 2 to 2½ hours of daytime sleep divided between one or two naps is the norm.

18 to 24 months. For the rest of the second year, your child should be getting about 12 to 13 hours of sleep each day. Most tots this age have given up their morning nap – especially as they approach their second birthday. Anticipate ending the year with about 11 hours of nighttime sleep and a 1½- to 2-hour nap during the day.

- Set up a regular bedtime routine and stick to it. The right evening ritual – consistently performed – will help your toddler unwind while bridging that challenging transition from awake to asleep (see box, page 134). Try not to take holidays from bedtime – instead, bring that same regular bedtime routine with you into weekends, holidays, and on trips.

- Consider an earlier bedtime – or a later one. Finding just the right time for bedtime can make all the difference. Overtired children often have trouble settling down because they're all wound up. If this might be the case with your toddler, consider starting – and finishing – the bedtime routine earlier in the evening. On the other hand, a child who isn't sleepy yet will also have a hard time settling in (can you sleep when you're not tired?). If that sounds like your toddler, putting her down a little later could help quell bedtime rebellion.

- Don't overnap – or undernap. Overnapping, or napping too late in the afternoon, could easily lead to being over-rested when it's time for bed. Undernapping may mean she's too overtired to surrender to sleepytime. Keep naptimes, like bedtimes, consistent.

- Wake up little sleepyheads. It sounds counterintuitive to ever wake up a sleeping toddler. But getting her up at the same time each morning – if you're lucky enough to have a little one who sleeps in sometimes – helps set that internal sleep clock, so she'll be more likely to be sleepy at the same time each night.

- Make comfort the object. Life's transitions are easier to make if you have someone – or something – to take along with you for the ride. Enter the transitional object, which can help your toddler transition from being awake and with you to being asleep without you (though not every child needs or wants a transitional object). That object can take many comforting forms – a stuffed animal (a large one can be used to climb on, so stick to small ones), a security blanket, even an old T-shirt of yours.

- Let her settle down solo. If your toddler cries when you leave the room, don't return immediately. She may stop crying and fall asleep on her own. If she continues to cry, treat this bedtime rebellion as you do night wakings (see next question).

- Don't lose it. No yelling, no threatening, and definitely no concessions. The more unfazed you stay in the face of a bedtime battle, the more your toddler will realise you mean business (and bedtime means bedtime).

Night Waking

"Our daughter is still waking up in the middle of the night, and we've reached the end of our tether. We need our sleep!"

She needs her sleep, too. But it's not her night waking that's keeping her from getting that sleep – and you from

---

Pillow Talk

Eager to tuck your toddler in – as in, with a pillow and blanket? Well, you can. There's no official reason to keep those comfy companions out of your little one's cot any more (they no longer pose the SIDS risk they did during the first year).

But while there's no reason to keep them out of the cot, there's also no compelling reason to put them in. Toddlers don't need a pillow for comfort (they're used to sleeping flat). They also rarely stay in one place while they sleep (you'll put your child down facing one way, and when you go in to check a few hours later, he or she is fully rotated). Which means that the pillow you've so lovingly tucked under that little head at bedtime is now acting as a foot warmer. Ditto for blankets and duvets – no amount of tucking is going to keep your toddler covered. Instead, you'll usually find a blanket or duvet crumpled up in the corner of the cot by morning.

Go for a toddler pillow and a lightweight blanket if you'd like – or if you'd rather not bother, leave it until your snoozer has transitioned to a bed. And of course, comforters are always welcome in a toddler's bed.

---

getting yours. It's that she hasn't learned how to fall back asleep on her own yet, an important life skill she's due to master – and has to master before anyone in the house can sleep through the night. After all, waking up isn't hard to do – everyone wakes up several times during the night. Nodding back off . . . now, that's the tricky part, at least for the uninitiated.

Making Bedtime Routine

Toddlers, little creatures of habit that they are, love knowing what comes next. Predictability makes them feel safe, secure, comforted, and in control (and you know how they feel about control). And that's why toddlers love bedtime routines, even if they don't love bedtime too much. The right bedtime routine helps a wound-up toddler unwind and relax, and it smooths that transition from rambunctiously awake to peacefully asleep. It can also become one of the highlights of your little one's day – and yours.

Getting the timing right (and being consistent about it every night) is essential – the trick is to begin before your tot has crossed that fine line from happy and active to overtired, grumpy, and bouncing-off-the-ceiling. Keep the routine mellow (quiet cuddling in, giggle-monster games out) and keep it just long enough (around 30 to 45 minutes). Drag it on too long and you could easily end up making a night of it. Order is important, too – being able to count on the next step (no unexpected switches, no surprises) makes it easier for a toddler to cooperate, so once you settle on a sequence that works, stick with it. Consider including all or some of the following in your tot's before-bed routine:

Brakes. Start a steady, gradual slowdown of noise and activity after dinner – not just for your toddler, but for the whole household (at least, as much as possible). Turn off the TV, dial down the stress. That way your little one won't be too tightly wound up when the unwind begins.

Bath. There's nothing like soothing, warm water to calm a little body down, making a bath the perfect beginning for the bedtime routine. (If your toddler is fearful of baths, skip this part of the ritual for now.) Using a little natural scent makes perfect sense, too (if your toddler's skin isn't too sensitive) – lavender-scented baby bath products may help enhance the relaxing properties of that warm water.

Bed clothes. Changing into pyjamas (make sure they're cosy and comfy) continues the transition from day to night. In the morning, make the change from nightwear to daywear as soon after your child gets up as possible, so that those pyjamas become a clear symbol of bedtime and sleep (lounging around in pyjamas all morning long can blur the line).

Bite to eat. It may have been a while since dinner – and it's a long way until breakfast – so give your toddler a little bite to stave off middle-of-the-night hunger pangs. Good sleepy-time snacks include a carb–protein combination: crackers and cheese, yogurt and sliced banana, a biscuit and a cup of milk. Keep it light, though (too much fuel will rev up that engine all over again), and stay away from sugary sweets (particularly those that contain caffeine, like chocolate).

Brush. Nighttime brushing is even more important than the morning cleaning – bacteria can build up at night and attack those tiny pearly whites. For tips on how to make brushing fun, see page 35.

Books. Snuggle side by side in the same special place each night and read some books together. Choose simple, quiet, soothing stories, and keep your voice more modulated than you would during a daytime reading session. The point is to lull and relax, not overexcite. If your toddler still has trouble sitting still for story time, focus on looking at the pictures instead – or skip the books and sing a few favourite lullabies while you cuddle. When your toddler begins to enjoy story time so much that there's no limit to the books he or she will sit still for, you'll have to impose a limit (and stick to it).

Bedtime. Your toddler is clean, cuddly, and hopefully even a little sleepy. You're in the homestretch of bedtime (which your little one would probably like to stretch out as long as possible – but don't forget who's the bedtime boss). To keep the bedtime mood mellow and ease that final transition from awake to asleep, add any or all of the following to the big bedtime finale:

- Use your bedtime voice. By this point in the routine, start speaking in your bedtime voice. (You didn't know you had one? Now's the time to discover it.) Reserve this voice for naptimes and bedtimes only – it should be soft, hushed, calming, no ups and downs, and definitely no fun monster imitations. Encourage your toddler, as he or she starts saying words, to use the bedtime voice, too – little ones love to imitate.

- Recap. Though your toddler's a little young to appreciate this part of the ritual now, it will become one that you'll both treasure soon – and once again, it can help bridge that gap between awake time and sleep time. So as you cuddle, spend some time talking to your toddler about the day, about what fun you had together, about how much you love him or her.

- Say good-night. To continue easing that transition, let your little one say "good-night" all around. Together,

say, "good night", to Mummy, Daddy, pets, toys, the stars and moon outside the window – even to your toddler's reflection in the mirror. Limit each encounter, though – otherwise, the Good Night Tour could go on for hours.

- Tuck in a few friends. A trusted teddy in hand and a few well-selected sentries (a row of familiar dolls and stuffed animals) standing guard over – but not in – the cot can make a toddler feel more secure about submitting to slumber. So can a picture of the family, placed where your little one will be able to see it by the glow of the nightlight.

- Hugs and kisses. Finally, leave your toddler with a big smooch and a cuddle, and say your "good night" – using a consistent phrase like "see you in the morning" (a comforting reminder that night will predictably end with the start of day). If your toddler gets upset or cries, say you'll be back in a few minutes to check in. Then keep your promise. Fingers crossed, your little one will be fast asleep when you return – if not, just try again.

- And repeat. Stick as closely as you can to the bedtime routine – doing the same things the same way, in the same order, each night. Pretty soon, your little one will know the routine and will look forward to predicting each step (even if sleep never actually becomes a favourite part of the ritual).

Is the bedtime routine so effective that it's putting your toddler to sleep before it's even over? Just move the proceedings to an earlier time slot so that your little one will be able to keep eyes open until tuck-in. Or shorten the routine.

So, time for some Sleep 101 – with classes starting as soon as possible, for everyone's sake. Getting your little one to transition from wakeful nights to restful ones won't be easy, especially now that her malleable baby ways have given way to toddler intractability, but it can be done. Here's how:

Factor day sleep into night waking. The top reason why toddlers have trouble falling and staying asleep during the night? They're sleeping too much – or not enough – during the day. Too many hours spent napping (like in that pushchair half the day), or napping too close to bedtime, can keep a toddler up at night. So can skimping on naps, since overtired kids don't sleep well, either. Keeping naptimes and bedtime consistent can help reset a toddler's internal clock and make for more restful nights.

Relax before bed. Is bedtime stresstime around your house? Even if your toddler manages to fall asleep in stress central, she may be too on-edge to sleep well during the night. Maintaining a calm atmosphere in the hour or so before your toddler beds down for the night can help her sleep better. Turn off the TV (believe it or not, she can be unsettled later by what she saw or heard earlier) and turn off the ringer on your phone, keep the lights low and your voices down (it's not the time to argue about whose turn it is to load the dishwasher), and try your best to relax – even if you just got home from work and have a thousand chores waiting. And whatever you do, hide the toy fire engine that makes that screeching sound.

Be there before bed. When you're home, make sure you spend bedtime with your toddler. Sure, you've got to go through your post, or get that load of washing in. But there's nothing like Mummy time or Daddy time – and your little one needs to store up enough of that special comfort to last the night.

Start the night right. The first goal is to get her to start the night the way you'd ideally like her to finish it: by herself, in her cot. Children who fall asleep alone (instead of with a parent keeping them company) are more likely to go back to sleep on their own when they wake at night and find themselves alone. If you've been "helping" your child fall asleep by staying with her – or if you've been letting her fall asleep in a different location (on the sofa, for instance) and then transferring her to her cot once she's out – you've also been helping to perpetuate her night-waking habit (or actually, her night-not-going-back-to-sleep habit). See the next question for better ways of getting a toddler to fall asleep.

Consider her comfort. Ever wake up in the middle of the night too hot or too cold and have trouble falling back asleep? Your toddler's sleep can be disrupted, too, by an uncomfortable room temperature, or by being over- or underdressed for bed. A room that's too bright or too dark, too noisy or too quiet, can also keep her from sleeping through the night. As needed (and the perfect recipe for a good night's sleep varies from child to child), consider adding a strategically placed nightlight, a room-darkening shade, a white noise machine or fan to generate a peaceful hum – whatever it takes to make the room just right at night for your little sleeper.

Wait out whimpering. Toddlers are noisy sleepers, and most of the sounds they make (the ones you're lying awake anticipating) don't require a response. If you rush in, you may actually fully wake your toddler (who might have only been half awake, and able to settle down again by herself).

Waking for a Reason

Waking up during the night is part of the normal sleep cycle, but sometimes it's stepped up by circumstances. Here are some of the reasons why toddlers wake at night:

Separation anxiety. Waking up alone can be tough on a toddler, especially one who's already struggling with separation anxiety (which can either reappear or appear for the first time during the second year, most often starting at around 18 months). See page 185 for ways to handle separation anxiety.

Teething pain. Those second year molars can be a real pain to cut – and that pain can wake little teethers in the middle of the night. The problem is, waking that starts with teething pain can become a habit that sticks – especially if it's met with too much midnight attention.

Illness. Toddlers are always more likely to night wake when they're under the weather – but especially if they're stuffy or in pain. Symptoms often take a turn for the worse at night, too, particularly with an earache or a cough. Unfortunately, night waking that comes on with an infection can continue long after the bug has buzzed off – that is, unless you cut off the all-night comfort supply once your little one is all better.

Stress. Any kind of stress in a toddler's life – a new child care arrangement, weaning from the breast or bottle, a parent who's away, depressed, or sick – can make a little one sleep more fitfully. Lots of attention during the day, and especially before bed, can make a stressed-out toddler feel more secure at night.

Milestones. Often, toddlers have a harder time sleeping when they're about to take a big developmental step or when they've just taken one (who wants to sleep when you've just learned to walk?).

Fears. Once a toddler's thought process becomes more sophisticated, fears can appear – especially at night. Among those that might keep a toddler from falling back to sleep are fear of the dark and fear of being alone. See page 196 for more on dealing with fears.

Nightmares. As their sleep matures, toddlers dream more – and more intensely. A scary dream can wake a toddler up, and keep him or her from settling back down without some comforting. See page 149 for more.

Offer quiet comfort. If whimpers escalate to wailing, check back in with her. Keep the reassurance low-key – the idea is to help your toddler comfort herself, not to do the job for her. Lay her back down if she's standing up (which she likely is). Without picking her up and with a few words in a hushed tone (you want to be as boring as you can), gently pat or stroke her back or chest for a moment. Set the mood with a soothing "shhhh . . ." Wait until she's calm, but not until she's asleep, and then quietly tell her that you're going back to your bed now, and leave the room.

If she begins crying again (which she probably will) or never stops crying (another likely scenario), you can try any of the sleep training approaches suggested by experts (see the next question).

Sleep Training Revisited

"We never quite got around to sleep training our son, and let's just say he hasn't trained himself – he's up three times a night. Is it too late to try now?"

While it's never too late to sleep train, you might want to consider hopping on board that train sooner rather than later. After all, the trademark stubborn streak you've probably already had a glimpse of is only going to run deeper – and those problem sleep habits you're eager to change are only going to become more entrenched as your toddler's second birthday approaches.

Need a refresher course in those sleep techniques you heard about back in the first year but never got around to implementing? Here's a quick rundown on some of the more popular getting-your-child-to-sleep tricks of the trade. Keep in mind that not every option will work for every parent or every toddler – stay flexible and move on to Plan B if the method you opt for at first doesn't work:

Reinforcing sleep rhythms. According to this technique, being overtired is the root of all sleep problems – and if you anticipate natural sleepiness (both at naptime and bedtime), you'll have a better sleeper on your hands. The theory is that the right amount of rest results in more restful sleep – that putting your sleepy head down tired (but not overtired) will allow him to drift off like a dream and sleep deeply and, more important, without interruption. If he does wake crying in the middle of the night, make a brief visit, offer a few quiet words of comfort and a quick pat, then leave the room and let your child fall back to sleep on his own. Keep in mind that this method requires a little "crying it out", but it's not as regimented as the Ferber approach (see below).

Crying it out. Also known as Ferberising (named for Dr Richard Ferber), the method works like this: at bedtime, while your child is sleepy but still awake, put him in the cot, give a gentle pat, a soft "I love you", and then leave the room. Cue the crying (you knew it was coming). And here's where the going gets tough: let your tot cry for a full five minutes (it'll seem much longer). Then go back in and repeat the original routine – a quick pat, a gentle "good night", and go. Repeat this process for as long as your little man cries, extending the time you leave him alone by about five minutes each time until he falls asleep. Stretch the times your child spends on his own by a few more minutes the second night, and again on the third. You can expect the crying jags to diminish steadily over three nights, and – drumroll, please – virtually disappear somewhere between the fourth and seventh night, replaced perhaps by

---

Active Today, Peaceful Tonight

Want your toddler to sleep better at night? Get moving during the day. A well-exercised body sleeps more soundly than a sedentary one. Adding some fresh air to the exercise equation boosts this benefit (so your mother was right!). Just remember to put the brakes on physical activity at the end of the day – too much running around (or climbing, or jumping) right before bed can keep your little one from settling down for sleep.

a bit of fussing or a short burst of tears. The next sound you're likely to hear? Nothing . . . except maybe a tiny snore.

Systematic awakening. This technique allows you to skip the potentially long bouts of crying. Keep a diary of your toddler's nighttime wakenings for a week so you will have an idea of the usual times they occur. Then, set your alarm clock for about half an hour before you expect the first howl. At the alarm, get up, wake your tot, and proceed with whatever comfort you usually offer when the waking is spontaneous. Anticipate each usual waking in the same way. Gradually expand the time between these systematic wakings and then begin to eliminate them. Within a few weeks you should – so the theory goes – be able to begin phasing them out entirely.

Breaking bad sleep habits. Have you become a human pacifier? If the answer is yes, it's time to retire and show your toddler how to pacify himself. That means no more nighttime breastfeeding, bedtime bottles, or "rock till you drop" routines. It may sound harsh, but in reality, those habits are counterproductive to your goal of getting your toddler to sleep through the night. While some children can fall asleep in your arms at bedtime and still manage to soothe themselves back to sleep without you in the middle of the night, most will demand the same parent-provided comforts, whatever the hour might be. So you'll have to revamp the bedtime routine. If your toddler's dependent on a bottle or breast to sleep, start scheduling the last feeding a good 30 minutes before his usual bedtime or nap (and consider ditching the bottle altogether; see page 97). Then, when your little one is sleepy (but not asleep) make your move to the cot. Of course, there will be fussing at first, but give it a chance.

Does a Whimper Mean Awake?

All children (and adults for that matter, too) spend their sleep in cycles. Cycles of REM (active) sleep, when dreams occur, and cycles of non-REM (quiet) sleep. Each complete cycle (active plus quiet sleep) lasts about 90 minutes (which is why a good nap should last at least an hour), and each cycle ends with a partial awakening. Just as you wake up after each sleep cycle (with a snort, an unintelligible mumble, a quick turn to the opposite side, or a fluff of your pillow), your little snoozer does, too – but his or her awakenings might be accompanied by a wail, a whimper, or even some talking. Should you rush in at that first sob? Definitely not. Just as you're able to fall back asleep between cycles (most of the time you don't even realise you've woken up), your tot can, too – or, at least, your tot can learn to.

Once your tot learns to self-soothe – perhaps by rocking back and forth, sucking his thumb, or stroking his comforter – you won't be needed at bedtime any more. And as long as your little one can drift off solo, it's fine to go in for a quick dose of comfort should he wake at night. Once the art of self comforting has been mastered, your voice and a gentle rub should be enough to get your toddler resettled into sleep.

Whichever getting-your-child-to-sleep-through-the-night-method you choose, remember that they all share two very important rules: 1, be consistent with the method, and 2, give it a chance to work. If you don't stick with it long enough to see a difference, you'll never know whether the failure lay with the method or your follow-through. Use each technique faithfully for a solid two weeks before you give up on it. Skip from method to method, or enforce the method of choice only sporadically, and your toddler's confusion will only compound his issues. For more on these sleep techniques, see *What to Expect the First Year*.

Late Bedtime

"We don't get home from work until 7 or so, and we want to play with our toddler before she goes to bed – which often isn't until 10:00. She has a hard time settling down even then. Is late bedtime the problem?"

The numbers are definitely against you. Studies show that young children who go to sleep before 9 P.M. fall asleep faster, wake up less often during the night, and get more rest overall. For 1-year-olds, the magic bedtime number is on the earlier side – most sleep best if they're tucked in by 7:30, 8:00 at the latest.

It's completely understandable that you'd want to put your toddler to bed later so you can spend more after-work hours with her – and more and more parents do the same – but it isn't in her best interest, or, ultimately, yours. Keeping your smallest family member up for that nightly reunion can take a toll all around. She won't be getting the sleep her little body needs, and you'll have a super grumpy, overtired tot on your hands – one who takes longer to fall asleep and who has a harder time sleeping through the night. Mornings are likely to be rougher, too.

A better strategy: build your schedule around hers, at least as much as you can. Try to streamline your after-work re-entry so there's a good chunk of quality together time each night. Pick a reasonable bedtime for her, say 7:30 or 8:00, and spend the hour or so you have before then easing into a relaxing bedtime routine together (which

---

Sleep by Association

We all have sleep associations (reading a few pages before bed, adjusting the pillows a certain way), but toddlers can become especially attached to them. That's why where and when your toddler falls asleep at bedtime can make all the difference in how he or she deals with waking up in the middle of the night. It's simple, really: a toddler who falls asleep on the sofa, in your arms, with the TV blaring, with the light on will expect the same conditions during a night waking – and if those conditions aren't the same (all of a sudden, your tot's in the cot, in the dark and the silence, alone), falling back to sleep will be a lot more challenging (read: crying will be involved). Which makes sense – wouldn't you have a hard time falling back to sleep if you suddenly woke up in a different place from where you went to bed? To avoid so-called sleep onset association disorder (yes, this one actually has bed cred with the sleep experts) – when a child becomes so dependent on falling asleep in a certain location (like your bed) or with a certain activity (like back rubs) that sleep will be elusive any other way – make sure you put your toddler to sleep the way you'd like him or her to stay asleep . . . start to finish.

can be one of the best bonding times of the day, anyway). Put off until after her bedtime all those other post-work essentials – like catching up on chores, returning e-mails, eating dinner, and spending time as a couple (which is also essential, after all).

Middle of the Night Feedings

"We both work all day (and need our sleep), so when our son wakes at night, we've got into the bad habit of giving him a bottle. Help!"

It's understandable that you've been choosing the path of least resistance in getting your son back to sleep. With busy schedules and a demanding toddler draining your patience and your endurance, you probably don't want to deal with any more resistance than you have to – especially during predawn hours. Bring on the easy fixes.

But you're right. Feeding your toddler in the middle of the night at this age (whether breast or bottle) isn't a good idea. And for a whole load of reasons:

- As effective as it is, feeding a toddler to coax him back to sleep keeps him from learning how to fall back to sleep on his own, a skill he'll need every night of his life.

- Nighttime feeding can lead to tooth decay if the bottle is filled with anything but water (milk and juice are full of sugar).

- Your toddler doesn't need a meal during the night any more than you do. His body is as equipped as yours to go those 10 to 12 hours of sleep in fasting mode. But just as your stomach would come to expect a midnight snack if you had one every night, his

will too – which means that he'll continue waking hungry for a meal his body doesn't need.

- Feeding your toddler when he doesn't need to be fed can lead to overweight and eating for the wrong reasons (he calls for comfort, you give him a bottle). These, in turn, can cause weight problems later on in life.

- Too much nighttime fluid results in – what else? – too much peeing, which results in uncomfortably wet nappies, and, in turn, to more waking (not to mention nappy rash).

- A bottle offered in the wee hours of the morning can easily spoil your toddler's appetite for solids at breakfast.

Clearly, you and your toddler are caught in a vicious cycle of supply and demand. You supply your toddler's tummy with a nighttime meal, and his tummy wakes him (and you) to demand a repeat each night. The only way to encourage him to sleep through the night without a feeding is to cut off the nighttime food supply and reset his internal hunger clock.

You're bound to meet up with some pretty heavy resistance (in the form of waking and crying) once you stop taking this path of least resistance. And though you'll almost certainly lose sleep in the short term, you'll eventually all sleep better for your efforts.

Exactly how do you end those night wakings and night feedings? First steel yourself – this will take commitment, not to mention at least a few sleep-deprived nights. Then try one of these two approaches:

1. Go for speed. Try the techniques for ending night wakings (suggested in the previous answer) and at the same time, stop night feedings cold turkey. If you don't cave (and that's the big "if"), you can expect at least a few nights of big-time struggle followed by acceptance of the new no-nighttime-snack policy.

2. Go slow. Get chills at the thought of going cold turkey? Gradually wean your toddler off the midnight snacks first, and then work on the night waking if it continues. With this approach, you'll substitute a bottle of water (filling it with a little less water each night) for the accustomed bottle of milk. This allows your little snacker to use the bottle as a go-back-to-sleep aid a little longer, but ends his middle-of-the-night need to feed. Eventually, the bottle of water may end your toddler's night waking, too – many toddlers (and their tummies) decide it's not worth waking up for it. But if your toddler continues to wake for the water, or if the substitution of water for his beloved milk just makes him mad, then you'll need to think about trying Option 1: cold turkey.

Early Rising

"Our daughter wakes up before the crack of dawn – usually 5:00 A.M. – every single morning. Either we go to bed super-early at night in self-defence, or we're constantly exhausted."

Does your little rooster's cock-a-doo-dle-doo come a little early for you? Pour yourself an extra-large cup of coffee and join the club. Most parents of toddlers are chronically sleep-deprived, thanks to those predawn wake-up calls. If your early bird is content to play in her cot for a few minutes while you catch a final snooze, consider yourself lucky. If she's the kind who wants out of her coop the moment her little eyes pop open, however, you'll want to find ways to encourage her to hit her own snooze button – or, at least, let you hit yours. Here's how:

Wait before you leap. Instead of rushing into her room the moment you hear an early-morning peep, wait 10 or 15 minutes. It's possible that she'll whimper, or even cry a bit, then turn over and go back to sleep – especially if you stick it out consistently for at least a few mornings in a row (think of it as early-morning sleep training).

Shut out the dawn. Some children are more sensitive to incoming light than others, so it's worth a try to darken your toddler's room in an effort to keep her eyes shut longer. Hang curtains lined with blackout fabric, or add a room-darkening blind.

Put entertainment at her fingertips. It's possible that keeping a favourite toy or two in your toddler's cot may encourage her to amuse herself when she awakes, giving you an extra few minutes of early morning peace. (Be sure she can't hurt herself on these toys or pile them up to scale the heights of the cot rail.) It's also possible that it won't work; some pint-size roosters aren't happy until they've roused some human company.

Play musical wake-up. Admittedly, it's a long shot – but it's worth a try. Set an iPod or clock radio in your toddler's room to start playing music at a decent hour (an hour when you'd feel good about starting your morning). Teach your early bird (through lots of patient, consistent repetition) to wait for the music before she begins crowing. When your toddler can recognise numbers, have her hold off on her wake-up until she sees the right number on the clock.

Push back breakfast. Feeding your toddler fluids or solids as soon as she stirs trains her tummy to wake up for that crack-of-dawn feeding. Instead, try tabling her morning meal until it's less like dawn and more like morning. Adjust breakfast by 10 minutes each

Daylight Saving Time and Bedtime

Ah, spring – when the days get longer . . . and your toddler has an even harder time than usual going to bed. After all, it isn't easy to explain daylight saving time to a 1-year-old – or to convince your little one that it's time for bed when it's still light outside. To ease the adjustment:

- Reset the clocks, then watch them. Maintain your little one's regular sleep, wake, and nap schedule, even in the face of time change (bedtime is when the reset clock says it's bedtime). Eventually, your stubborn sleepyhead will adjust.

- Stick to routines like clockwork. Don't let the time change alter your toddler's schedule. Keeping all routines at the expected times will help make the transition smoother.

- Block out the light. Use blinds or curtains to keep out at least some of the light and create a more night-like environment in your child's room.

And what about when daylight saving time ends, and the clock "falls back"? That presents another potential sleep issue: your toddler wakes up an hour earlier than usual (so much for "gaining" another hour of shut-eye, like you used to in those pre-child days). This transition is also challenging for parents of toddlers, but if you stick with the schedule, those earlier-than-usual wake-ups won't last more than a few days.

---

day, until you have breakfast time where you want it. If she's really hungry, give her a very light snack (such as a cracker or a few multigrain hoops) to hold her off until breakfast.

Change a too-early nap. If your toddler gets up at 5:00 A.M. and naps at 8:00 A.M., that early nap may be the problem. Her early-morning waking may be more like a middle-of-the-night waking, after which she completes her normal sleep span with the nap. The solution: start the nap 10 minutes later every morning until she's napping at 10:00 A.M. or 10:30. She may be grumpy until she adjusts to the new nap schedule, but once she does, she should start sleeping later in the morning.

Reconsider bedtime. Although it's counterintuitive, a toddler who's getting to sleep later than she should often ends up rising earlier than you want her to. All too often, an overtired child means

unrestful sleep – and early morning rising. So put your early riser to sleep a little earlier – it just might be the ticket to a few more minutes of extra sleep in the morning.

Sometimes a way-too-early bedtime can sabotage your chances of getting your wake-up call at a decent hour. If your toddler's currently hitting the hay at 6:00 P.M., try tucking her in about 10 minutes later each night until her bedtime is at 7:00 P.M. (and don't move it any later than 8:00). Gradually moving the afternoon nap to a slightly later time slot can help accomplish this.

Cut down on nighttime liquids. If your toddler is still taking a bottle of water to bed, a sopping nappy may be waking her up early. Stop that bottle, if possible, as well as other excess fluids before bed.

Accept what you can't change. Though your early-to-bed, early-to-rise routine may not make you feel healthier,

Keeping Track

Does your toddler's sleep pattern seem to have no pattern to it at all? Are you thinking there might be some sleep issues going on – but you're just too groggy (from lack of sleep) to remember how many times your toddler got up last night . . . or the night before? How about what time you tucked him in? Or what time she actually fell asleep?

If you're not sure about your toddler's sleep pattern, a sleep diary may be just the ticket. For the next two weeks, jot down bedtimes, actual falling asleep times, night wakings, and night feedings (if any), and keep track of how long wakings and feedings last. Also include naps: when and where they take place and how long they last. And if you have an inkling that certain high-sugar foods (especially caffeinated ones, like chocolate) or food additives might be contributing to restless sleep, consider keeping track of pre-bed consumption of those in the sleep diary, too.

Analysing the diary should give you some insight into whether your toddler has any sleep issues, and it may also provide some clues for dealing with them. If you notice that overall total hours of sleep are way under the average (see page 132), try putting your little one down to bed earlier . . . or adding that morning nap back into the mix. If your toddler is waking up three times a night, examine what, if any, enabling behaviours might be contributing to those night wakings. Are you picking up your toddler and rocking him back to sleep? Are you nursing her in the middle of the night? Putting an end to such getting-back-to-sleep crutches can help get your toddler to sleep through the night, start to finish.

Want to check in with the doctor about some sleep concerns you may have? Take the sleep diary along.

---

wealthier, or wiser – and almost certainly has you reaching for the extra-strength concealer – you may have to get used to it. Very few parents can count among their blessings a late-sleeping toddler. Most, like you, have an early bird in their nest.

Catnapping

"The only time my toddler naps is when she's in the pushchair or the car. But those naps are short, maybe 15 minutes at a time. Is that bad?"

Catnaps may be fine for felines, but they're probably not doing the trick for your little kitten. The average 1-year-old can't fill her sleep requirements at night. Most need two or more hours of daytime sleep, typically split more or less evenly between a morning nap and an afternoon nap.

There are plenty of nap equations that work (three instead of two, one longer nap and one shorter, or just one long one), but rare is the toddler who can function well on just a few snippets of daytime sleep. And if she's not having those quality naps in the cot, her exhausted little body will grab the sleep she needs when it can (like in that pushchair or car seat). Which means she catnaps, wakes up, catnaps, wakes up. Even if the total number of catnaps nets a reasonable daytime sleep total, the sum of those parts may not add up to a full-rested toddler. She may be grumpier and more prone to frustration, have less appetite and energy, and sleep less well at night. Not to mention the effect on those who care for her (no naptime for toddler means no downtime for you).

To nip a catnapper's habit and ease her into a better sleep routine:

- Start each day at the same time. Waking your toddler up at the same time each morning may prompt her to fall asleep at about the same time each afternoon. (See previous questions for suggestions on how to regulate morning waking.)

- End each day at the same time. Erratic bedtimes can lead to erratic napping patterns. Try to settle into a nightly routine that she can set her internal clock to.

- Don't make a move when she's sleepy. When you can, try to schedule trips in the pushchair or car when your catnapper is wide awake – soon after wake-up and a meal would be ideal. Keep her awake, whenever you're out, with chat or songs, or by pointing out sights.

- Beat fatigue. Instead of waiting until your toddler has crossed that line from tired to overtired (and nap amenable to nap resistant), or until a trip to the supermarket is unavoidable (and a catnap inevitable), try to head off fatigue with a real nap.

- Read those cues. Toddlers are high-energy animals (less cat, more puppy). But even the most active toddler has low-energy times of the day, usually mid-morning and mid-afternoon. When you see your little girl showing early signs of slowing down (blink and you might miss them), take advantage with a nap.

- Then, create a sleepy mood. After you've picked a sleepy time, help your toddler prep for her nap by slowing down and relaxing. Think modified bedtime routine: a snack and some milk, a cuddle and a story, peace and quiet.

- Lay her down . . . hopefully, to sleep. You can't force her to nap, of course, but you can enforce a rest period. Fingers crossed, one will lead to the other.

From Two Naps to One

"Up until last week, my 20-month-old son was a wonderful napper – he napped twice a day like clockwork. Now, all of a sudden, he refuses to go down in the morning."

It happens to even the best nappers eventually: two naps a day become one too many. You might still need his morning nap, but it seems he probably doesn't. And he's right on schedule: most toddlers midway through the second year can, and do, get by with just an afternoon snooze.

While your toddler adjusts to his new sleeping schedule, he may seem sleepier and grumpier than usual – especially around the time when he used to nap. Moving his lunch back for a little while so that he can take his afternoon nap earlier should help. You can also try establishing a "rest period" devoted to stories and quiet play during his old napping hours. That way he can recoup his energy without sleep.

Sometimes, a toddler gives up his morning nap before his body's ready – or his parents misread his signals and are too quick to put the nap to rest. If your toddler doesn't adjust quickly to his new nap schedule, consider that his body might not be on board with it. Fortunately, the switch isn't irrevocable – just add the morning nap back in for now.

A Good Night's Sleep Times Two

Just when you think you've got this whole sleeping-through-the-night thing in the bag (no easy feat with two infants), you enter the second year. And boom, boom: a whole new set of sleep issues, times two. Here's what you might be wondering about when you've got double the sleep trouble:

Different wake-up schedules. So tot A is an early riser and tot B burns the midnight oil? While the ideal would be for both your toddlers to be on the same schedule (ideal for your sleep needs, at least), the reality is that each of your children is a unique individual with unique sleep needs and sleep patterns. You can try encouraging your little rooster to sleep in (see page 142 for tips on how to do that), or at least play quietly until his or her sibling wakes up (easier said than done, but vaguely possible with a lot of reminding). If that plan doesn't pan out, and tot A still petitions for an early release from the cot each morning, think of the bright side of this predawn routine: at least you'll have some special alone time with him or her (when else do you have the chance for that?). Just make sure tot B gets some of the same later on (maybe at the end of the day, if you can get A down to bed earlier).

Different nap needs. Let's say one of your twins still needs that morning nap while the other twin is now raring to go through lunch and beyond. There goes your perfectly crafted nap schedule (the one that allowed you time off from playing twin tag team). So, now what? Again, respect each child's individual sleep patterns and reschedule accordingly. One twin goes in for a nap while the other takes quiet time. Just make sure that the twin who has abandoned the nap is definitely ready to – some toddlers just think they are. The last thing you'd want is one well-rested tot and one off-the-wall overtired tot.

Too Late Naps

"It takes me all afternoon to get my 1½-year-old to take her nap. By the time she settles down it's usually close to 4:00 P.M. When she wakes up at 6:00, she's raring to go for hours, so we can't manage a reasonable bedtime."

Late-breaking naps can definitely make a mess of your evening, but when they push bedtime to 9:00, 10:00, or even later – which they often do – they can make a mess of your toddler's sleep cycle, too. Kids who go to bed too late usually don't get the sleep they need – and they don't sleep as well.

Eating patterns may also be thrown off, which can further throw off sleep patterns (she eats dinner so late that she's fuelled up for hours to come).

The steps you'll need to take in order to adjust your toddler's schedule – so that her nap and her bedtime fall at more convenient (and age-appropriate) times – will depend on the kind of sleep pattern she's fallen into. So consider:

- Is the nap coming too late? The average toddler at 18 months needs about 1½ to 2 hours of nap a day, but timing is everything. Ideally, an afternoon nap should come earlier in the afternoon, so that it doesn't interfere with

Playing, not sleeping. Does this scenario sound familiar? You put your twins down for a nap or bedtime in the same room and instead of dozing off, they just play with each other ("partee!"). Here are some options to try (all toddlers – and all twins – being different, they may not all work):

- Let them play. Allow some back-and-forth babbling each night until they settle down – it could just be their way of unwinding. If you see playtime extending well past bedtime (or taking up all of naptime), you're probably best laying down the law – the law being: no talking to each other once you're in the cot. Like everything else you tell your toddlers, be prepared to repeat this message (calmly and firmly) over and over again until it sinks in.

- Split them up. Set up sleeping arrangements in separate rooms (if you have the space), or separate the cots with a room divider (one that muffles sound will make the back and-forth far less satisfying). Being separated for bed but together for nighttime rest. So try to bump the afternoon nap earlier by 10 or 15 minutes. Easier said than done? Maybe not if you unwind her first with a pre-nap routine (similar to a bedtime routine, but shorter). After a few days, when she seems adjusted to the earlier slot, move naptime back another 15 minutes. Continue this process until she is napping at a reasonable hour (such as from 1 P.M. to 3 P.M.).

play may help them get the sleep they need (they're already getting the play by day) – and also give them some time apart from their ever-present twin. Getting your little ones used to some separation at night can also help them handle daytime separations more easily – and minimise the separation anxiety some twins experience whenever they're split up.

- Stagger bedtimes. Try putting one twin to sleep 10 minutes before the second twin (and alternate who goes in first each night). Hopefully by the time you put your second to sleep, the first will have drifted off to dreamland. The less ideal but just-as-possible result: Twin 1 could scream bloody murder while waiting for Twin 2 to arrive in the room – so stay flexible with this plan.

Once you figure out all these sleep hurdles you're home free, right? Wrong. Stay tuned for the preschool years, when your twins graduate from cot to bed. Can you say jack-in-the-bed, times two?

- Is she napping too long? Your toddler only needs so much total sleep. A morning nap that lasts longer than an hour may keep her from napping at a sensible time in the afternoon. And an afternoon nap that lasts longer than 1½ to 2 hours can definitely cut into nighttime sleep. Waking her up from an afternoon nap that reaches 2 hours can help.

- Are two naps too many? Maybe she needs only one nap now. Try pushing her morning snooze later and later (by 15 minutes a day) until it becomes an early afternoon nap. This will probably eliminate her need for the late nap. Or, if she still seems to need two naps, move her morning one to an earlier time slot. That way, she'll be more likely to conk out earlier in the afternoon.

Weight for Sleep

Need another reason to make sure your toddler gets enough night- and daytime sleep? Researchers have found that babies and toddlers in their second year who sleep less than 12 hours a day are twice as likely to be overweight at age 3. Scientists believe the amount of sleep a toddler gets may affect levels of the appetite hormones.

■ Is she sleeping late in the morning? Late risers (and late-to-bedders are often late risers) tend to have a late napping schedule. To change this, begin waking your toddler 10 or 15 minutes earlier each morning until she's getting up at what you consider a reasonable time. As you do this, her nap (or naps) and evening bedtime should start to move towards an earlier schedule.

Too Short Naps

"My toddler takes two naps during the day but they're both only about 30 minutes long, 45 tops. How can I get her to sleep longer?"

Longer naps are definitely better for you (half an hour doesn't really buy you enough time), but they're also better for her. Since a sleep cycle is around 90 minutes, 30 minutes doesn't get the rest job done. It's better than a catnap, and definitely better than no nap at all, but still not ideal.

Can't get your wound-up child to stay snoozing long enough? Try putting her down for a nap before she starts showing the signs of tiredness (eye

rubbing, whining, grumpiness, and so on). Once your toddler is overtired, she'll have a harder time not only falling asleep, but also staying asleep. Unwind her with a pre-nap routine (it's just as hard for a toddler to go from 60 to 0 at naptime as it is at bedtime), and try to be buttoned down with your nap schedules, since erratic naptimes won't allow your toddler to set her internal clock. If she seems to need less sleep, try organising one longer nap in the early afternoon instead of two shorter ones. And don't forget to use the cot for her naps, not the pushchair or car seat (see page 144 for reasons why).

Resistance to Napping

"Our son used to take a two-hour nap every afternoon. Recently, he's refused to nap at all, no matter what I do. Is he ready to give up his nap?"

A toddler often needs his nap a lot more than he thinks he does. The problem is convincing him of that. With so much to do, and so little time in a day to do it, taking an hour or two off for sleep isn't high on his priority list. ("Are you really asking me to lie down in a dark room, when I could be climbing up the back of the sofa or splashing in the dog bowl?")

Sometimes, a toddler gives up his nap prematurely because of a one-time event that knocked his schedule out of whack – an afternoon birthday party or a trip to the museum, a weekend at Grandma's (where it's too much fun to waste time sleeping). Less often, he gives it up because he really doesn't need it. If your close-to-24-month-old child sleeps well at night, seems rested in the morning, and is happy and generally good-tempered all day, he probably can drop his nap. If, however, he seems chronically grumpy and overtired, easily frustrated and uncharacteristically clumsy at his customary naptime or in the evening, he probably doesn't know what's good for him. Ditto if he's been sleeping less well at night since calling it quits on his nap. Try some gentle persuasion to get him napping again (see page 145 for tips), giving it a week of best efforts. If your toddler resolutely resists naptime, won't even brake for some enforced quiet time (a better-than-nothing alternative), and continues to show signs of fatigue, aim for an earlier bedtime.

Snoring

"My son snores in his sleep – so loudly we can hear him down the hallway. I didn't realise small children could be such loud snorers."

It's strange but true – some of the biggest nighttime noises actually come from some of the smallest sources. Studies show that up to 12 per cent of children snore, and though snoring typically reaches its peak between ages 3 and 6, it often shows up in toddlers as well.

Snoring is the sound that is created when air can't flow freely through the nose and mouth. Often, a snoring tot's breathing is partially blocked by enlarged adenoids and/or tonsils. These bits of lymphatic tissue in the nose–throat breathing passage can swell when a child has a cold, flu, or sore throat, sometimes triggering temporary snoring. Persistent allergies and exposure to tobacco smoke may also cause tonsils and/or adenoids to become enlarged (which is why children of smoking parents are more likely to snore). Sometimes, however, the adenoids and tonsils grow excessively for no apparent reason. When this happens, snoring can occur nightly. Enlarged adenoids

may also cause mouth-breathing (both day and night), nasal speech, and noisy breathing, especially during sleep.

Snoring alone isn't cause for concern (though it may be cause for some earplugs for you). Usually, it pipes down as the tonsils and adenoids stop growing and begin their natural shrinkage (after age 7 or 8). When it's associated with obstructive sleep apnoea (a condition, rare in toddlers, in which breathing momentarily stops during snoring, sometimes triggering frequent night wakings), it requires medical attention. Mention your son's snoring to the doctor at the next checkup.

It's possible that elevating the head of your tot's cot mattress (with a pillow or some blankets under the mattress) may help him breathe more easily – and hopefully, more quietly.

Nightmares

"Last night, our almost-2-year-old woke up in the middle of the night weepy and shaken, like he'd had a nightmare. I didn't even know toddlers could dream."

Your little one can definitely dream bigger than ever – for a couple of reasons. First, his improving memory allows his brain to recall images and sounds from his busy days and recycle them realistically at night. Second, sleep cycles are longer than they were in babyhood, with more time spent in lighter "dream" sleep.

But while life can be a dream for toddlers, it can also occasionally be nightmarish. Though true nightmares are more common after the second birthday, it is possible for a younger child to have a bad dream, and to wake up from it. Chances are, however, that your son's verbal skills are no match for these late night plotlines, which means that he probably can't recount what he's

Nightmares vs. Night Terrors

Your toddler wakes up screaming in the middle of the night. Was it a bad dream or a night terror? It's easy to tell if you know the difference.

Signs. During a night terror, a child usually perspires profusely, has a very rapid heartbeat, appears frightened and confused, may call out for you, yet pushes you away. He or she may scream, cry, moan, talk, or even seem to hallucinate; sit, stand, walk, or thrash around – and though the eyes may be open, staring, even bulging, the child is still asleep. A child having a nightmare, on the other hand, may seem a little restless while dreaming, but it's not until he or she is fully awake that the panic, with plenty of crying and screaming, begins. When a parent comes to the rescue, the child is likely to cling desperately. A verbal child may try to describe a nightmare but will not recall a night terror. And there's nothing to describe with a night terror, anyway, since these episodes aren't associated with visual imagery, like dreams are.

Frequency. Bad dreams, or nightmares, typically occur more frequently than night terrors. Still, most children experience at least one episode of night terrors during the toddler or preschool years. When children have frequent night terrors, there's usually a family history at work.

Timing. Night terrors usually occur in the early hours of sleep, most often between one and four hours after a child goes to bed. Nightmares strike later, during the second half of the night's sleep, when REM (rapid eye movement, or dream) sleep is more concentrated.

Stage of sleep. Nightmares occur during REM sleep, which is the light sleep phase. Though the child sleeps through the dream, he or she awakens after it, usually terrified. Night terrors are a partial arousal from a very deep (non-REM) sleep – essentially, part of the brain is trying to wake up while the other part stays asleep. Children experiencing them usually do not awaken fully, unless they are roused (and there's no reason to rouse a child who's having a night terror).

Duration. Night terrors can last from 10 to 30 minutes, after which the child usually continues to sleep. A nightmare is usually brief, and is followed by waking. The duration of the period of panic following a nightmare varies from child to child and episode to episode.

dreamt about, even if he remembers it when he wakes up – so you may have a hard time working out if he's actually had a bad dream.

As your little one's memory and imagination grow (and as long as his imagination is unchecked by reason), those bad dreams may become more complex, and possibly more frequent (though some kids seem to have more than others). Other factors can step up bad dreams, including daytime stress (nightmares are more common when there's a parent away on business, a new child minder, or any other change in a child's life), pre-bedtime excesses (of noise, excitement, activity, or food), or an illness (certain medications or a fever can provoke a scary dream).

To help your toddler have sweeter dreams, make bedtime a tranquil time. Avoid rough play (don't pretend to be the "big bad wolf" when you put him in bed, don't play the "tickle monster" when you're tucking him in), and skip scary TV or books. Reduce the stress level around the house, as much as possible, so that your toddler doesn't take any stress to bed with him. If you sense that your little one is more stressed out than usual, step up daytime comfort, too.

When your toddler's older, he'll be able to talk about his dreams – and you'll be able to explain that they're make-believe (like in a story), not real. For now, until those kinds of abstracts make more sense, just offer quiet reassurance after he wakes up frightened – a whispered "it's okay" or a soothing back rub should help him settle back down.

Moving to a Bed

"We want to move our son to a bed. When's the right time?"

All good things must come to an end eventually, but when it comes to sleeping in a cot, this is one good thing that you shouldn't be in a rush to end so quickly. Before you decide it's out with the old (cot) and in with the new (bed), consider what most experts say: it's best to introduce a bed at about age 2½ or 3, or to switch out of the cot when a tot is taller than 89 cm. If you've got an extra-tall 1-year-old on your hands, or if your little daredevil is climbing out of his cot night after night, it might be the right time for the switch. But if all's quiet on the cot front, there's no need to rush the relocation just yet.

Got a new baby on the way? That's still not necessarily reason enough to push your tot out of his old digs. Before you do, think about what the cot means to him (it probably makes him feel secure and comfy) and how he might feel towards the new sibling who bounced him out of his accustomed accommodations (resentful, to say the least). Instead of booting your toddler out of his cot, consider borrowing a second cot for the new arrival, or keeping the new baby in a bassinet or co-sleeper next to you for the first few months (which is recommended for safer sleep, anyway).

One more thing to keep in mind if you're eager to transition from cot to bed: once you make that move, you're giving an adventure-loving tot a ticket to nighttime freedom (it's a lot easier to hop out of bed than it is to scale the cot walls) – and that opens up a whole house full of safety concerns. See the next question for ways of dealing with nighttime wandering.

Night Wandering

"We switched our very tall 23-month-old daughter into a big bed and now she wanders around the house in the middle of the night. We're worried about her safety. What should we do?"

Whether she's learned how to scale the walls of her cot or has been having an easy time escaping from the minimum security of a big bed, the toddler on the nighttime prowl is a toddler at risk. Minimise the risks by taking these precautions:

Make her room safe. Survey your toddler's room to be sure it is thoroughly child-safe – it should be anyway, even if she's not a midnight explorer. Hot radiators, electric fans that aren't child-proof, and other dangers should be covered, removed, or placed completely out of reach (remember, your toddler is a good climber). Move out of the way furniture she can bump into, rugs and toys she can trip over, cords she can stumble across (especially if they're

When a Threesome Isn't Your Speed

If you've been co-sleeping with your little one since he or she's been, well, little – and you'd like to continue the arrangement into the second year, there's no reason not to (as long as there's across-the-bed agreement – not fair leaving one parent out of the decision). Co-sleeping toddlers can be just as happy, independent, and well adjusted as those who sleep solo.

But if you've suddenly found yourself in a family bed you never intended to have (say, because your night-waking tot has worn you down, and issuing an all-access pass between your covers is the only way to get some sleep), you may want to reassess your open-bed policy. Bringing your tot into your bed may be the route of least resistance, and it may offer a short-term solution to sleep issues, but it'll set your toddler up for a long-term problem (the problem being that he or she won't know how to sleep through the night solo in his or her own bed). So instead of throwing back the covers to invite your toddler into your bed, consider putting an end to bed sharing.

Do it the cold turkey way by being firm ("Mummies and daddies sleep in their own beds and big girls and boys have their own cots") and reminding yourself that a few nights of no sleep (because your tot will resist cot-sleeping at first) is better than the unsatisfying sleep you've been getting while bed-sharing. Or, if you're not the cold turkey kind of parent, you can soften the blow by gradually withdrawing: sleeping in your child's room for a few nights (him or her in the cot, you on a mattress or in a sleeping bag on the floor), then staying in the room only for as long as it takes for your tot to fall asleep for a few more nights, then transitioning to leaving the room as soon as you've said good night and letting your child fall asleep on his or her own.

---

attached to lamps she can pull over). Make sure there are window guards on all windows, and that cords from window coverings are secured out of reach. Unless she is more likely to stay in her bed in a darkened room, add a nightlight to help your toddler see her way around in the dark and to prevent bumps-in-the-night.

Close the escape route. To keep your toddler in her room, you can either close the door or use a gate across the open doorway. The gate arrangement may be less disconcerting because it allows her to see out and doesn't cut her off completely from the rest of the family – though the odds are that a toddler who can climb out of her cot can also clamber over a gate. In that case, you can make a deal: if you stay in your bed, we will keep the door open (or the gate open). Be sure to childproof any rooms in the house she might be able to access after hours (put locks on any doors that lead to especially dangerous places, like bathrooms).

Make your return policy clear. Is her favourite midnight destination your bed? It may seem a lot easier to invite her under your covers than to take her back to her bed (especially because she'll be back before you can close your eyes). But if a family bed's not your intention, you might want to adopt a strictly enforced return policy instead. If your little one wanders out of her room and into yours at night, return her promptly, calmly, and matter-of-factly, with little comment and no wriggle room or negotiations. Sit near her bed for a bit if she seems frightened, patting her back, and reassuring her that everything's okay. But don't yell, start a conversation, turn on lights, or lie down with her. Your message: night is the time for sleeping, her bed or cot is the place for sleeping – and that is that. Repeat the firm returns to her bed as many times as you have to until that message sinks in and your toddler stays put. Consistency will pay off, eventually.

ALL ABOUT:
Establishing Good Sleep Habits

Though you may find it hard to believe after the fourth wake-up call of the night, your toddler will spend a lot of time sleeping in the years to come – about a third of his or her life, in fact. The benefits of your toddler becoming a good little sleeper now are probably pretty obvious – you might actually get to enjoy your own solid stretch of sleep – but he or she can actually reap a lifetime of significant benefits, too. Short term, getting enough sleep can boost a child's growth and development, energy, coordination, concentration, attention span, behaviour, mood, and ability to learn and solidify memories. Long term, better sleep is linked to reduced risk of obesity, diabetes, cardiovascular disease, and depression; improved immune function, longevity, cell repair, memory, and productivity; and much more. Not too shabby for an activity you can do lying down with your eyes closed.

How do you get your toddler's sleep habits where they need to be? Though sleep scenarios – and challenges – vary from child to child and home to home, there are some fundamental sleep strategies that always apply. For a better night's sleep, stick to these top 10 tips.

1. Keep routines routine. Establish or continue a soothing bedtime routine and stick to it each and every time you put your tot to sleep. On holiday? Pack up the routine and take it along. It's another special occasion? Try your best not to break from the routine (your toddler will need that unwinding more than ever after a day of festivities). Your toddler's sick or teething? The routine will be particularly comforting to an out-of-sorts sleepyhead.

2. Stay on schedule. If bedtime is 8:00 P.M. on Monday, 9:00 P.M. on Tuesday, and 7:00 P.M. on Wednesday – and naptimes are hit and miss (mostly miss) – your toddler won't be able to establish healthy sleep cycles his or her little body can rely on. And there's even more bad news about an erratic bedtime schedule: not only won't your little snoozer get enough sleep overall (hello, grumpy), he or she will also soon work out that bedtime is just a number – one that's completely negotiable. ("Last night Daddy put me to bed later because I put up a big fight. If I put up another fight tonight, he'll let me stay up later again!"). Pick consistent bedtimes and naptimes and stick to them (aim to hit the mark within 15 minutes either way every day) – you'll all be better off.

3. Wake by the clock. Erratic wake-up times are no better than erratic bedtimes, and they can also keep your toddler from developing those important healthy sleep habits. So keep wake-ups consistent, too, even if it means – yes – rousing a toddler who's taken to sleeping in, or one who's on the fourth hour of napping (or on the verge of napping through dinner).

4. Dry up the midnight milk supply. Toddlers in their second year can make it all the way from that pre-bed snack to breakfast without a refuelling. If your little one wakes up and expects food in the middle of the night, it's only because he or she has come to expect it – not because he or she needs it. Dry up the supply and you'll soon stop the demands.

5. Never underestimate the value of a nap. A tot on the run all day (and have you ever met a tot who isn't?) needs a chance to rest, regroup, and recharge. Daytime naps do just that – and more. Since toddlers typically can't get all the hours of sleep they need in one nighttime stretch, most won't fit it in unless they nap. Napping tots have an easier time settling down at bedtime, and they sleep better at night. And research shows that lots of abstract learning and memory formation takes place during daytime naps – valuable brain development that can't take place if a toddler doesn't stop during the day for a rest.

Keep naptimes as consistent as bedtimes, even if it means scheduling the whole day around them. The payoff – a more cheerful, better-functioning toddler – will be worth the postponed trip to the supermarket (plus, isn't that why they invented online grocery shopping?).

6. Beat tired to the punch. Toddlers sleep best when they're tired, but not overtired – a fine line you'll want to avoid crossing whenever possible. Make a point of starting the bedtime routine before those sleepy signs (like eye-rubbing or whining) appear, so your little snuggle bunny will be relaxed, not overwrought, by the time he or she hits the hay. Do the same at naptimes.

7. Make bedtime relaxing time. Is it getting close to bedtime? Turn down the noise, light, and activity level in your home, and relax. Slowing the pace gradually (starting after dinner) will help your toddler ease into the evening and eventually brake for bedtime.

8. Encourage self-soothing. Have you become your toddler's sleep aid? Absolutely, you might end up expediting bedtime tonight if you let your toddler fall asleep in your arms on the sofa. Or in your bed (back rub included). Or while you sing lullabies. But what about tomorrow night? And the next night? And in the middle of every night? In order to become a good sleeper, your toddler needs to be a self-sufficient sleeper – able to drift off to dreamland (and then drift off again during those normal night wakings) without any help from you. Another key factor to remember: location, location, location. If you want your toddler to sleep through the night in the cot, that's where he or she needs to nod off (not on a pillow on the floor in front of the TV).

9. Enlist a bed buddy. Yes, your toddler needs to learn how to fall asleep solo. But that doesn't mean a (small) friend can't come along for the ride. Each night and each day before naptime, ask your toddler to pick out a "bed buddy" for cot company and support. And speaking of support, don't forget to dole out plenty of hugs and kisses before bedtime – a lot of love goes a long way (into the night).

10. Be consistent. Make this your mantra when it comes to your toddler's sleep – and for that matter, when it comes to just about anything related to your toddler. From bedtimes and naptimes to wake-up times, bedtime routines to good-night rituals, sleep-training techniques to parental bed policies, staying consistent from day to day and night to night (and in the middle of the night) will help your little one develop the good sleep habits his or her little body is counting on – and you're dreaming of.

Behaviour

....

YOUR BABY – the one who went willingly into the pushchair and car seat, who cooed and squealed (but never tried to run away) during nappy changes, who hung on your every word with rapt attention, who was putty in your hands and perfectly content in your arms – is gone. In your baby's place: a toddler – one who won't take "no" for an answer (but is happy to dole it out), struggles against pushchairs, car seats, nappy changes, or anything else that confines or controls, has an uncanny ability to find trouble, uses hands more often than words, and only wants to be held when you're busy. There's no doubt about it: your toddler is an adorable little bundle of contradictions. Human Velcro, superhuman escape artist. Creature of comforting habits, habitual resister of house rules. Bear-hugger, hair-tugger. Fearless, fearful. A master of mixed feelings, predictable only in being impossible to predict. Sometimes maddening, always maddeningly cute. Yet, the more things change, the more toddlers yearn for them to stay the same. Which is why, along with the fierce independence you're glimpsing in your tot, you'll also likely see a fair amount of clinging – a sign that he or she is still pretty ambivalent about giving up those baby days (and those cuddles on your lap) completely.

What You May Be Wondering About

The Into-Everything Toddler

"Our toddler touches everything – in the house and out. Half the things he touches aren't even safe to touch. How do we get him to stop?"

He's part explorer, part scientist – and all toddler. Like a pint-size Columbus or Newton, your tot views the world around him both as his oyster and his laboratory. Everything is his for the touching, and the pulling, and the grabbing, and the mouthing – not

Behaviour at a Glance

The questions you have about your toddler's behaviour are endless. Luckily, the answers you seek are at your fingertips – right here in this not-surprisingly-large chapter. But with so many behaviours to cover, you may be wondering how to navigate through it all. Simple. Just use the index or this handy table-of-behaviour contents to pinpoint your concern and then flip to the appropriate page for the answer and coping tips. Want to plan ahead so you'll know what to do when a behaviour issue strikes? Just read through this chapter from start to finish to cover all your behaviour bases.

to mention the occasional dissecting. And even as it drives you mad, all that manipulation is how your toddler learns about his environment – one sticky fist-ful at a time.

Your toddler has probably heard the phrase "Don't touch" as much as any other – and he may even know what it means. But is he remotely capable of following those directions and hold-ing those little hands back in the face of temptation? Not until the second half of the second year at the earliest. That's because it takes impulse control, something he'll need to learn over many months.

Toddlers touch, and touch indis-criminately. Dirty? Doesn't matter. Alive? Whatever. Breakable? That's a bonus. But while a toddler's gotta do what a toddler's gotta do (touch), a parent's gotta do what a parent's gotta do (keep him from touching things he shouldn't). Here's how:

Do damage control. To protect your home from your toddler (and vice versa), make sure everything within his curious reach is safe to touch. Childproof thoroughly (see page 405) and put away breakables.

When you can, stay one step ahead of your toddler's explorations. He loves to upturn the milk cup, or toss it over the side of the table to test that theory of gravity again? Hand it to him for sips, then take it back in between. When you're shopping, keep your little man buckled in and keep his hands busy – if he has a box of cereal to hold on to, he may be distracted from trying to pull the display down. Or keep him occu-pied as your helper – have him point to the crackers you eat at home, choose between two apples and then plop the winner in a bag, and drop a loaf of bread into the trolley. And always keep an eye on those hands – that way, even if you can't stop him from picking daisies when you're at the park, you may be able to stop him from eating them.

Set limits on what's off-limits. It's not like you can put away the TV, or the cooker, or the glass bowl on a friend's table. That's why it's important to start teaching your toddler that certain things around the house (and elsewhere) are simply off-limits. It will take lots and lots of repeating that "Don't touch" refrain, and lots and lots of immediate redirection, before the lesson – and the impulse control – will sink in. When you do catch the most fleeting glimpses of impulse control (he reaches for the glass bowl but backs off when you warn "Don't touch!"), be quick to reinforce it: "Good job!"

Let him reach out and touch some things. Make an effort to provide more touchable moments for your toddler. When he reaches for something he's not allowed to touch, supply a substitute. When he goes for the freshly folded stack of washing on the bed, move it out of reach, but give him a couple of tow-els or T-shirts to drape around himself, drag behind him – or even try to fold. When he wants to program the digital box or make calls from your mobile phone, offer up a toy that has buttons to push or let him play with a remote that has no batteries or an out-of-service mobile that can't dial out (to India).

Supervise touching. He's eager to squeeze the toothpaste tube? Teach him how to squeeze it neatly and in pea-size amounts, then appoint him the offi-cial (supervised) toothpaste-squeezer for the family. He's keen on using your keyboard? Sit him on your lap in front of the computer (with your work safely saved) and let him tap away – or let him get his hands on some toddler-friendly software (see page 278). He's excited

Exploring the World . . . by Mouth

Give babies a toy, a book, a stuffed animal, even your hand, and they're sure to stuff it in their mouths – not because they're hungry, but because that's how they get to know the world around them. But a taste for mouthing doesn't end at a baby's first birthday. A young toddler, too, will often explore his or her environment by mouth. Once a toddler starts tapping into other sensory resources, that primal urge for oral gratification will diminish – usually by the age of 24 months.

Of course, while you're waiting for the oral phase to end, you'll need to be sure that whatever your toddler mouths is safe. Mouthing an object that's been lying around the house is fine (unless it's a germ-infested bathroom sponge, a mouldy piece of bread discovered under a pile of toys, or a grimy shoe that's been walking city streets). Mouthing an object that's been discovered outside isn't usually a problem, though it should definitely not be encouraged. But mouthing anything that's toxic or small enough to be swallowed or choked on (or that your toddler can bite a small piece from) is clearly dangerous – so keep such items out of reach (close the bathroom door, keep a toddler-proof lid on the bin, put shoes in the wardrobe, lock away toxic substances, and regularly sweep the house for coins and other small objects; see page 405 for more). And since no number of precautions can keep all potentially dangerous items away from your toddler, you'll also need to supervise closely. Be sure you know how to handle a choking incident (see page 469), just in case.

When you catch your child mouthing something forbidden, firmly say "No, not in your mouth. Please give it to me." If your tot doesn't pass it over, remove it from his or her hand or mouth yourself. Your toddler will soon begin to learn what's okay to mouth and what's not.

to push the lift button? Pick him up and let him push away (just make sure he pushes the right button . . . and only one button – especially if you're sharing the lift with others). He wants to pat the doggy in the park? With the owner's approval, put your hand over his and show him how to pet the dog nicely and safely. Is he fascinated by falling liquids? Give him a chance to experiment in the bath or the sink with cups of water.

Don't get touchy yourself. Of course you'll need to stop unsafe touching. But try not to make a big deal of it while you do. Instead, say "Don't touch", then quickly redirect your toddler. Major reactions – negative or positive – usually prompt encores in a toddler (which means he may reach for your mobile phone just for attention next time).

Opening and Shutting

"Our daughter's discovered how to open the fridge – and now she does it about 300 times a day."

It's an open-and-shut case: Your toddler opens it, you shut it. It may be the fridge, a kitchen cabinet, the bin – anything that has a door or a lid low enough for a toddler to reach. And it's loads of fun – for your toddler, at least. Especially when it's repeated, again and again.

Let your tot open and close to her heart's content (she'll move on to an equally annoying activity soon enough) – that is, if what's behind the door or lid is safe. When it isn't, or if she could accidentally get locked behind the door, stop her open-sesame antics by installing a childproof lock or latch. No doubt she'll find it frustrating when the fridge door suddenly won't budge (or she can't dip into the 12-pack of toilet paper you put in the bathroom cabinet), so be ready to give her another opening – like a special cabinet that's just for her, filled with plastic containers, wooden spoons, nesting metal measuring cups, and other safe treasures. Of course, if it's food or a drink she's looking for, offer a snack.

Emptying Things

"My daughter goes around the house emptying everything she sees. But I can't get her to put anything back."

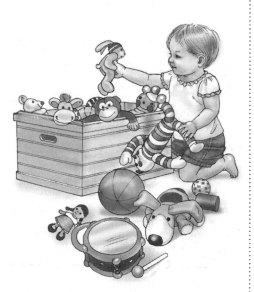

Toddlers get much more satisfaction from taking things out of where they belong than they do from putting things back in their place.

It's a developmental joke, and it's on you . . . and your floors: the ability to empty comes months before the ability to put things back. It may be something of a laughing matter, and it's definitely incredibly cute sometimes – except when you can't find the book you're looking for, or the pack of socks you just bought, or when your living room floor is littered with groceries, or your little one gets the "empties" around something nasty and potentially unsafe, like the rubbish. But believe it or not, it's hard developmental work he's up to. Your toddler is busy practising fine motor skills (developing his hand dexterity) and flexing his cognitive muscles (testing out cause and effect). To help direct her practice so it doesn't demolish your home:

Stock up on safety measures. Do a safety check and recheck around the house, and install child-resistant locks and latches as needed to make sure your toddler can't empty – or get into at all – anything that might harm her and/or be harmed by her (cleaning fluids, washing-up detergents, toxic substances, knives, matches, scissors, glass, china, and other breakables and chokeables). See page 405 for tips on childproofing your home.

Be open to emptying. Remember, your mess is her fine motor skill practice. So stay open for emptying business. Provide boxes filled with fabric scraps (no ribbons or strings, though); baskets for toys; low shelves for board books; a safe cabinet filled with plastic containers, nesting measuring cups, and spoons. At bath time and in the sand pit, bring out the plastic cups, bottles, and buckets for a little emptying fun.

Put in some put-in practice. Refilling a basket with toys is a lot tougher – and a lot less satisfying – than emptying it. But turn it into a game, and your toddler may sing a different tune (and while you're at it, come up with a "fill-up" or "tidy-up" song to entice fill-up follow-through). Keep in mind that even if your toddler does succeed at filling a container, the uncontrollable impulse will be to empty it again . . . promptly. That's okay – remember, she needs the practice. Tired of playing the pick-up part of the empty-out game? Just put the box out of your toddler's reach for a while and quickly redirect activity to avoid a fuss.

Keep in mind, too, that while most toddlers aren't big fans of putting away what they've emptied out, some quite enjoy putting away things Mummy and Daddy need – in random, hard-to-find places (like burying your wallet in the deepest recesses of the wardrobe, your keys under a pile of shoes).

Dropping Things

"Our toddler loves dropping things – from her cot, her pushchair, the supermarket trolley. And she seems to get even more of a kick from watching us pick them up."

Who knew gravity could be so entertaining? What started out as fine-motor practice for your little one is now part science experiment, part sideshow (with you as the sidekick). Her catch and release programme is fascinating, engaging stuff for her – and almost as fun as watching you stoop over to retrieve and return what she's dropped. And if what's dropped splatters or breaks on impact . . . well, that's just gravity gravy.

Clearly, dropping is tops for your toddler – whether she's rapid-firing stuffed animals over the side of her cot or lobbing a toy from her pushchair. Maybe it was cute the first hundred times she did it, maybe it's still occasionally adorable (what about your toddler isn't?). And at this age, it's always developmentally appropriate. Still, a dropping habit can wear on your nerves, not to mention your back and knees. And often, it can be more than a little inconvenient or messy. To help her drop her habit (eventually):

Let her drop in the bucket. A brick or a little beanbag into a container, a ball down a slide – there are plenty of dropping games your toddler can play that are amusing for her, but not mad-making for you. Play them often until she moves on to other activities.

Drop the reaction. Whether it's a giggle or a grumble, any rise at all from you will encourage the fall of more objects. Remember, it's not a party without you (and your reaction).

When you've had it, drop it. Not in the mood to pick up? Or she's chosen a particularly inopportune time and place to drop (you're at the park and she keeps dropping her toy into puddles)? Just say "No more dropping." Take the object she's been dropping away from her, and quickly distract her with another activity. If you're at home, place her on the floor – dropping objects from the floor isn't nearly as satisfying as dropping them from high places.

She's flinging food from her high chair? Dropping something otherwise messy? If warnings aren't stopping it, put an end to the activity.

Don't drop your guard. Those in the dropping habit shouldn't be trusted with anything breakable. So if you haven't already, do a sweep for objects that might break if they're dropped (china, glass, small electronic gadgets), and do some putting away before she can send them crashing. Be especially vigilant when breakables can't be kept out of her reach (when you're visiting a baby-free friend's house, a shop, a museum).

Hello, New Baby

Announce to your family and friends that you're expecting again, and you're bound to be greeted with enthusiastic rounds of congrats. Tell your toddler the big news, and the reaction definitely won't be such a sure thing. For starters, a young toddler likely won't have the slightest clue what you're talking about ("A baby in Mummy's tummy . . . eh?"). Even if your little one grasps the basics, the announcement could leave a lot of mixed emotions in its wake: confusion ("What does being a big sister or brother *mean*?"), excitement ("Great – a new friend!"), anger ("I have to *share* you?!"), anxiety ("Will you still love me?"), complete disinterest ("Yeah, yeah – now what about the trip to the playground?"), or all of the above. Here's how to break the news – and start getting your toddler on board with the new baby on board:

Time the announcement right. To someone who lives for the here and now, 9 months can seem like a lifetime – literally, since it's half his or her lifetime. So try not to spill the baby beans to your little one right away. Waiting until you're in the second trimester makes sense, not only because the wait for baby will be shorter for your tot, but also because your expanding belly will provide the perfect talking point – and visual aid – for this very abstract concept.

Keep it simple. Intangibles are tough for toddlers to wrap themselves around – and let's face it, there's nothing more intangible than a baby who can't be seen, heard, or touched. So keep your announcement as simple, age-appropriate, and concrete as possible: "My belly is getting big. That's because there's a new baby growing inside me. You'll be the new baby's big brother (or sister)!" Provide follow-up information only if you get follow-up questions – and don't give more info than you're asked for (your 1-year-old doesn't need to know the mechanics of reproduction). The concept of "brother" and "sister" may be tricky for a tot, too, so offer up examples: "Cousin Jake is cousin Ellie's big brother. You're going to be a big brother, too!" Since a picture is worth a thousand words to a toddler, read picture books about becoming a big sibling (such as *My New Baby What to Expect* or *When Mommy's Having a Baby*), share photos of yourself when you were pregnant with your toddler (that's *you* in there!), and show videos of him or her as a newborn.

Set a date the toddler way. Telling your toddler that the baby will be arriving in four months, six months, in May or even "soon" won't be enough. Put the due date in perspective by saying, for instance, that the baby will be born when it's warm enough to go to the beach.

Invite participation. The best way to help keep your little one from feeling left out of Project Baby is to make him or her feel included. If he's curious about what's going on in your belly, offer some basic baby facts. ("The baby is as big as this melon, but getting bigger every day. He has teeny tiny fingers that look just like yours.") If she's wondering why you're always going to the doctor or midwife, invite her along on a visit (tell her it's a "checkup" for the baby), so that she can listen to her little sibling's heartbeat and watch your belly being measured. If he's eager to practise his big-sib skills, have him sing, talk to, rub, hug, and kiss your belly (tell him that the baby can hear his voice and feel his touch – and loves both!). She has no interest in baby business? Don't push participation.

Keep it real. It's tempting to paint the rosiest picture possible of life with a new baby. And little siblings *can* be lots of fun . . . eventually. But if you talk up your newborn so much that your toddler expects the perfect playmate to pop out, he or she will be pretty disappointed when a can't-do-much lump shows up instead. Explain that newborns don't do a whole lot – that is, besides eat, sleep, pee, poo, and cry. Illustrate this, again, with film clips or photos of your toddler as a newborn. Point out how far he or she has come since those boring baby days.

Focus on what *won't* change. A new baby means a whole lot of new for the big sibling: new sights (of you breast-feeding), new sounds ("waaaaah!"), new smells (of the throwing-up variety), and new realities (you having to split your time between two little ones). In the face of all these unsettling changes, knowing that some very important things will stay the same will be very important for your toddler. So even as you're rushing around preparing for the new arrival, make time for all those special, predictable routines that make your child feel secure. That bedtime bath and story. Sunday afternoon at the playground. That morning cuddle with lots and lots of kisses and hugs.

So your tot's prepped, prepared, in-the-baby-know – at least when it comes to the baby in your belly (who's relatively undemanding). But what about when that baby comes home in your arms? And spends lots of time on your lap? Or cries at story time? Or needs to be fed at playtime? In other words, becomes competition for your attention? Real live babies can present real challenges for their older (but still very young) sibs. To make welcoming a new baby a welcome event for the new big brother or big sister in your home:

Stick to the routine. For toddlers, nothing comforts like consistency – especially in the face of big-time change. So make sure the person who's caring for your tot while you're busy giving birth – and after, when you've returned with newborn in tow – is someone who's familiar and well versed in your child's schedule and treasured rituals (crackers and milk at 10:30; story and naptime at 2:00; two rounds of "Hush, Little Baby" at bedtime). Keeping the routines routine during this time of transition will help your toddler feel secure.

Welcome your toddler first. When it's time for the big new sib meet-and-greet (whether it's in the hospital or birthing centre, or at home), let your toddler know right away that he or she is still first in your book. If you're holding your newborn, do a quick hand-off to Dad so you're completely available to greet your older child before he or she meets the new baby. Knowing you're the same old Mummy as before – full of hugs, kisses, love, and attention – will be reassuring.

Give your oldest an "I'm-a-big-sib" gift. New babies aren't the only ones who should be receiving gifts. Mark this momentous occasion with a present that makes your toddler feel included in all the excitement, yet special in his or her own right. Anything that celebrates big-sib status – an "I'm a Big Brother (or Sister)" T-shirt, sticker, or photo frame – will build your tot up.

Hope for the best, but be prepared for anything. It could be love at first sight when oldest meets little sibling. Or it could be the cold shoulder . . . or the green-eyed monster . . . or worse. No matter how your older tot responds to your newborn, be understanding, patient, empathetic, and most of all, fully accepting. Don't withhold your love or make your toddler feel badly if there's new sibling snubbing or resentment. And don't force your oldest to do anything (like hug or kiss the baby) he or she would rather not do. There's plenty of time for sib bonding in the years to come.

Play pick-up. Picking up will never be as much fun as dropping (except, of course, when she's picking up something you don't want her to touch . . . like an interesting rubbish specimen on the pavement). But make pick-up a game, and you'll make it less of a drag: "Let's see how fast we can pick up the toys!" Or play pick-up to a song.

The Little Destroyer

"Lately, every time we turn our backs, our toddler sets about destroying something. He tears up magazines, scribbles on the walls, pulls the books off the shelves. Our house is starting to look like a disaster area."

You probably expected a little mess – and even occasional property damage – from your toddler, but maybe you weren't prepared for a second-year demolition derby. Yet, what seems like destructive behaviour – believe it or not – can sometimes be pretty constructive. Those seek-and-destroy missions aren't motivated by malice, they're fuelled by curiosity, a drive to discover, a compulsion to create – and it's all part of his job description, which can be summed up as: learn as much as you can about the world, as quickly as you can. When he tears up a magazine, he's determining that paper crinkles and tears. When he upends a basket of bricks, he sees that they spill out, make a crashing sound, and scatter. When he throws the sofa cushions on the floor, he finds that they can be used as a trampoline – or a climbing structure. And there's much about the world he can only learn the hard way. For instance, with his limited comprehension about cause and effect and natural consequences, he doesn't anticipate that if he hurls a toy across the room, it might break, and that if it breaks, he can't play with it any more.

That said, taking on the world doesn't mean you have to let him take down your home in the process. In fact, one of the most important lessons he can learn – and must learn – is that destroying things isn't okay. Don't scold or punish, especially if he broke something accidentally, but let him know that you'd like him to try to be more careful next time, and why ("Coffee cups can break when you drop them" or "When you throw the remote control, it doesn't work any more"). Have your toddler help repair the damage when possible (wipe up spills, tape a page back into a torn book, scrub crayon marks off the wall).

If he destroyed due to frustration ("I can't stack these bricks, so I'm just going to throw them onto the glass table . . . oops"), give him constructive suggestions for dealing with it ("If you pile the bricks this way, they don't fall over"). If it was just the junior scientist at work again, provide plenty of opportunities for safe and acceptable experimentation and manipulation (toys to put together and take apart, for example).

Throwing

"My son has a habit of throwing everything he picks up. I'm afraid he's going to hurt somebody or break something."

The first time you saw your tot hurl a toy across the room you may have daydreamed about him being good at sport. But chances are those visions have now been replaced by nightmarish premonitions of lamps shattering and playmates' eyes being blackened. So, do you teach him, or do you punish him? A little bit of both, actually. Banning throwing will only make it more enticing (plus, it's not fair – or sensible – to keep him from doing what's developmentally appropriate). So will your throwing a fit (or stifling a giggle) when he throws. Instead, groom him for athletics without throwing safety and good sense out the (hopefully unbroken) window. Here's how:

Play ball. Given plenty of opportunities to throw or roll a ball in safe and supervised surroundings, a toddler's itch to pitch may well be satisfied – at least somewhat. Catching will still be beyond his developmental reach, since his eye–hand coordination is pretty primitive (see Milestone box, page 78, for information on when that'll likely develop). But he'll probably get a kick out of retrieving a ball that's been thrown or rolled to him.

Vary the ball. A wide range of balls are suitable for toddlers, including beach balls, tennis balls, and small, medium, and large rubber balls. Avoid hard balls, balls small enough for your toddler to put in his mouth, and balls made of spongy material that he could take a bite out of. You can also throw a beanbag or a quoit set into the mix.

Cry foul if it isn't a ball. Make it clear that some things are meant to be thrown (balls, beanbags, and so on) and others are not (toys, bricks, books, cups): "This is a ball – a ball is for throwing." "This is a book. We don't throw a book – a book is for reading." Also set appropriate limits on where he throws (outside, or only in the playroom).

One chance and he's out. The moment you see your toddler fling (or get ready to fling) an object that's off-limits for throwing, take it away from him. Explain in simple terms the potential consequences of random throwing ("If you throw a brick, it can hit someone and give them a bruise" or "If you throw the lorry, it might break"). Quickly supply your little thrower with a more appropriate object to toss; if that

doesn't satisfy, try to distract him with an entirely different activity.

Banging on Everything

"Our toddler bangs on everything in sight – the coffee table, the front door, the TV. It's so loud, and I'm scared she'll break something."

Have a mini-metalhead – who's giving you a maxi headache? Your petite percussionist is just making music the only way she knows how, and with the only instruments she has access to (unless you count the vocal cords she uses for shrieking). Banging the day away, she's experimenting with sounds and rhythm ("When I bang on a pot, it's sounds tinny – when I bang on the cot, it's more of a thud. And listen to the spoon on the cabinet . . . genius!"), cause and effect ("I bang on the coffee table, the magazines go flying. I bang on the high chair, the peas and carrots start dancing . . . and look, there goes the yogurt!"), and audience reaction ("You should have seen the look on Mum's face when I started banging in the restaurant – priceless!"). All completely normal and age-appropriate.

Still, how much jamming can you and your home handle? And what about banging that can hurt more than your head (say, that glass bowl)? Here's how to let your diminutive drummer rock on within reason:

Pull the plug on dangerous drumming. Banging on the TV, a dinner plate, or a window can lead to damage, injury, or both. Promptly end it (or, better, stop it before it starts). Stop the music, too, if banging threatens to upset a cup of hot tea or if it's being performed with a sharp implement. "No banging on the table" is a good place to begin, but remember: (A) your toddler is listening to her banging, not to you, (B) she has poor impulse control, and (C) your actions always speak louder than your words when you have a toddler, and that's especially true when your toddler's banging more loudly than you can speak. Which means it's time to end a dangerous jam session and distract your drummer with another activity.

Whatever you do, don't try to shout over the banging – that'll only make her turn up the volume. When do you use your words, keep them matter-of-fact, soft, firm. Who knows? She might even stop for a minute to hear what you're saying (though don't bank on it). Keep in mind, too, that toddlers rarely take "don't" for an answer – especially the first few dozen times. So get ready to repeat your message – and your redirection – many times to come, and for best results, without losing your cool.

Redirect the banging. Instead of banning all banging (what are the chances, anyway?) give her a chance to bang on safe surfaces. Offer her the timeless – and priceless – toddler drum set: a pot and a wooden spoon. Or a toddler workbench, with toy hammer. Or even a real toy drum. Provide other instruments that might not be music to your ears, but at least won't make them bleed – like a tiny tambourine.

Let the beat go on. Just about all toddlers love listening to music almost as much as they love making music. They relish rhythm, too. So go ahead – dance, clap to music, play foot-stomping games. Make your own family music band.

Private performances only. Of course, your toddler enjoys an audience – preferably a large one. But it's important to set some guidelines when it comes to public performances. When it's not appropriate for your toddler to bring down the house (in restaurants,

even fast-food ones; cinemas; church; museums), bring down the curtain on banging . . . ASAP. Even better, divert her before the drumming starts, with a game of peek-a-boo (use a menu or napkin), a quiet song, a picture book, or paper and crayons you've had the foresight to bring along.

Hold the applause – and the boos. When your toddler overdoes the banging at home, but there's no harm done that a paracetamol can't fix, the less attention you pay as she plays the better. Any reaction – positive or negative – reinforces most toddler behaviours.

Screeching and Screaming

"We've got constant headaches from the screeching and screaming our son does around our house."

Unfortunately, 1-year-olds don't come equipped with automatic volume controls – or, for that matter, with self-control over their volume. Your toddler has suddenly discovered his capacity for creating and broadcasting sound, and he's gleefully taking advantage of it – with ear-shattering results. Like a recording engineer with a sound control panel at his fingertips, he experiments with levels of pitch and volume. And while everyone around him is developing a headache, he's having a blast. Literally.

You could invest in earplugs while you wait for this annoying habit to run its natural course – like many toddler habits, it eventually will. Or, with the help of the following tips, you can make an effort to bring the screeching, if not to a screeching halt, at least to a decibel range that's easier on the ears.

Turn down your own volume. Keeping the general noise level in the house low (no blaring background television, loud music, or shouting matches between parents) will help – at least in the long run – to encourage your tot to turn down his volume. Shouting at him to stop shouting, on the other hand, will rev up the competition and inspire him to greater volume ("Listen, Mum . . . I can scream louder than you can!"). You'll also validate his screaming ("If Mummy and Daddy scream, screaming must be okay!"). Instead, model the voice modulation you'd like to hear him use.

Switch stations. When the screeching starts, turn on some lively music and encourage your toddler to sing instead. If you're outside the house, try engaging him in a sing-along of favourite songs or a recitation of nursery rhymes. Even if he doesn't join in, he may stop screaming, if only so that he can hear you sing. Or suggest other interesting ways your child can use his voice – mooing like a cow, meowing like a cat, barking like a dog, vrooming like a car. Making sounds with musical instruments, though not voice box generated, may also satisfy your toddler's need for noise.

Speak softly. When the screeching starts, get down to your tot's level, look him straight in the eye, and whisper to him. Seeing your lips move but not being able to hear what you're saying may make him curious enough to stop screaming and start listening. The operative word here being "may" – he might, instead, get a kick out of drowning out your whispers. Play it by ear.

Help him find his little voice. Small children have a hard time lowering their voices to a whisper (funny . . . they have an easy enough time pumping the volume up). Still, they can enjoy trying. When your toddler's vocals shoot up the decibel charts, challenge him to a

"whisper" match: whisper a word to him, then have him whisper it back. Though his will sound more like loud stage whispers for at least the next couple of years, playing the whisper game shows your toddler that there's fun not just in raising his voice but in lowering it, too.

Limit his big voice. By the time your toddler is in the second half of the second year, he will have an easier time accepting limits, including those put on screeching. At this point, he'll be able to understand (if not always put into practice) the concept of an "inside voice" and an "outside voice" – and you'll be able to enforce when and where his "big" voice can be used ("You can scream in your room, but not in the rest of the house", or "You can screech at the playground, but not in the shop"). Setting shrieking limits works better than an across-the-board ban (you know how fond toddlers are of forbidden fruit).

Hitting

"Yesterday I was mortified when my daughter swung at another child in her playgroup. She didn't hurt him, but she really could have."

When you're a year old, hitting says it all – or at least, it says a lot of the things that you can't yet say any other way. Like "Move it, mate – you're in my way!" Or "Hand over the toy, Mister!" Or simply, "I'm so frustrated right now, I need to punch someone!" At this age, hitting (and other kinds of aggressive behaviour, such as biting or shoving) can't be considered malicious or callous. Toddlers (especially young ones) aren't capable of hurting on purpose – primarily because they haven't quite worked out that other people have feelings.

Keeping Your Baby Safe from Your Toddler

Keeping a newborn safe is never easy – especially the first time around, when even holding that tiny, seemingly fragile bundle seems risky (remember how you always used two hands – just in case?). This time, you're an old pro with the safety basics (even the car seat you never thought you'd master), but there's a whole new level of baby protection you'll have to add: protecting your baby from your toddler. Handling with care – or using a gentle touch – isn't something that toddlers are known for. Toddler hands and arms aren't big enough or coordinated enough to support a newborn's heavy head and underdeveloped neck muscles. Their attention spans are fleeting, their minds prone to wandering – which means the tot who pleaded to hold his or her new sibling one moment may become bored or distracted seconds later, unceremoniously dumping the infant on the edge of the sofa to make a beeline for a pile of bricks. Then there's a toddler's

natural over-exuberance, which can turn a loving hug into a too-rough squeeze, a playful game of peek-a-boo into something dangerous. And there's potential, too, for aggression (whether it's on purpose or accidentally-on-purpose) – biting, hitting, pinching, and otherwise expressing understandably mixed feelings in unacceptable ways (trying to push the baby off Daddy's lap or hitting a colicky infant to quiet him or her down).

How do you nurture the big sib in your toddler while keeping your infant safe?

- Supervise, supervise, supervise. Stay close by whenever your toddler is within reach of his or her baby sibling – just in case hands start grabbing or fists start flying. And, of course, never leave your toddler alone with your baby, not even for a moment.

- Pass the baby. While your impulse may be to keep your toddler away

While it's too early to expect truly empathic behaviour from your toddler (she's more likely to experience cause-and-effect curiosity than empathy when her punch reduces her playmate to tears), it isn't too early to start planting the seeds. When your child takes a swing at her playmate, say firmly, "Don't hit! Hitting hurts – ouch!" When your child is the victim, comfort her and say, "Hitting hurts, that's why we don't hit." But realise that your words will almost certainly need to be backed up by actions. Supervise playdates closely and stop aggressive behaviour the moment it starts by removing the offender from

the victim and quickly distracting both with a new activity.

Whatever you do, don't respond to toddler aggression with adult aggression. Hitting a child teaches her that violence is an appropriate response under stress or in anger. So be sure to keep your temper in check when dealing with hers.

Biting

"At the playground, my son bites when someone won't share a toy with him."

The choice of weapon may be different, but the motives are usually the same for the biter as for the hitter (and

from your baby for safety's sake, preventing those sibling interactions can leave your toddler feeling left out, setting the stage for resentment – and aggression. Instead, let the bonding begin. If your toddler is interested, let him or her have plenty of closely supervised cuddles. Sit your toddler down in a comfortable armchair, then position the baby on the big sib's lap, a pillow under the arm supporting the baby's head. Stay within arm's reach, so if your toddler suddenly loses interest or the baby starts wailing or wriggling, you'll be on hand to take over. Feel your toddler needs some practice before he or she is ready for baby prime time? Show him or her how to gently hold a baby doll first.

- Pour on the toddler attention. Pent-up resentment can let loose in any number of physically aggressive ways (remember, your toddler doesn't have the vocabulary to say "I hate that Mummy-hogging baby!", so taking a swipe at the tiny competition says what words can't yet). Try to

head the aggression off by stepping up the attention your toddler craves.

- Teach the art of "making nice". Being gentle is a skill that, once cultivated, has plenty of practical applications in your toddler's life beyond keeping a baby sib safer (say, keeping dogs from nipping grabby fingers). Show your bigger little one how to stroke the baby's hand or toes (instead of pulling), how to gently rock the infant seat, how to tenderly swing the baby swing, how to cuddle, kiss, and hug without smothering. Point out how the baby likes that soft touch. Practise making nice on stuffed animals and dolls, too. Remind your toddler often, "gentle touch, please" or "make nice to baby", but don't rely on those mantras alone for impulse control (it'll take a while for them to sink in). As always, heap on the praise whenever gentle contact is made to encourage more of the same (and less aggressive behaviour). For more on squashing the hitting impulse, see page 167.

for the hair puller, and the shover). Your toddler is frustrated by his inability to manipulate his environment (for example, appropriate that bucket he's been eyeing in the sandpit) – and even more frustrated by his inability to express that frustration. Aware that his words won't have the bite he'd like them to have, he simply uses his teeth.

But toddlers sometimes bite for even more innocent reasons. For the curious toddler, biting may be just another inquisitive sensory experiment ("How will Taylor's shoulder taste? Will it taste the same as Spot's ear? Or Mummy's arm?"). For the affectionate one, biting may be his unique way of

saying "I love you". Biting may also be a case of monkey-see, monkey-do, picked up from other tots. Or a sign that boredom, fatigue, sensory overload, or hunger has set in, or that teething pain is provoking the need to nibble on something (or someone). And, as is the case with many other negative behaviours, biting can represent no more than a call for attention (which biting inevitably brings).

Probably because biting seems so primal, so animal-like, parents are often more horrified when their toddlers bite than when they hit. Yet the biter is no more vicious than the hitter. In fact, a majority of toddlers engage in some

Taming Aggression

You know why your toddler is aggressive: he or she is insatiably curious ("What will happen if I pull Grace's hair? Will she cry?"), completely self-centred ("I'll just push all those other kids out of the way so I can get to the slide first"), possessive of all possessions, even those that belong to others ("I want to play with that lorry now and I don't care that it's Noah's"), selectively empathetic ("Why not grab that toy out of Claire's hands and then bop her on the head with it?"), frequently frustrated ("I'm so angry and the only way I can let Daddy know that is if I bite him"), and unable to communicate effectively ("I can't reach my cup and I'm thirsty, so if I hit Mummy, she'll get it for me"). But knowing the reasons for this developmentally appropriate behaviour doesn't mean you have to put up with it. Problem is, your tot won't learn how to tame those primal aggressive instincts without some help from his or her civilised friends. Here's how you can help:

Pay attention to good behaviour. Hitting, biting, and other aggressive behaviours are sometimes calls for attention – and toddlers learn quickly that they're a surefire way of getting it. Paying more attention to good behaviour and as little as possible to bad (other than stopping the behaviour and disciplining appropriately) will give your toddler less incentive to act up.

Validate your child's feelings. All feelings are okay, even though some actions aren't. Acknowledge that it's okay to feel angry when you don't get your way or when a friend grabs a toy from you, but point out that it's never okay to hit.

Encourage translating feelings into words. Toddlers are capable of experiencing most feelings – from disappointment to jealousy, sadness to fear – but they're usually not capable of expressing those feelings in words yet (enter the fist or the teeth). Help your toddler find the words that will eventually take the place of aggressive action.

Banish boredom. Idle toddlers can do major mischief. Anticipate your toddler's boredom whenever possible, and respond with a challenging game or activity before all-hellish behaviour breaks loose.

Minimise frustrations. When so much is still beyond your ability and your reach, the world can be a frustrating place. Helping your toddler learn the skills needed for everyday living – social skills, dressing skills, playing skills, eating skills – may reduce not only frustration, but aggression.

Defuse with soothing activities. Take breaks each day (especially during high-stress times) for quiet cuddling, singing, reading, and other pacifying pastimes; these can help diffuse a toddler's aggression. The other plus: they're relaxing for you, too.

Provide opportunities for venting. Pent-up frustration, energy, or anger can explode in aggressive behaviour –

or it can be channelled into a variety of appropriate outlets (see box, page 80).

Change the pace. Free-play can often lead to free-flying fists. When aggressive behaviour breaks out between tots – or preferably before – restore peace by swiftly switching to an adult-supervised activity (such as painting, or a circle game) or otherwise directing the children's attention elsewhere. Ditto if the aggression is aimed at you. Simply divert your child's focus to something else ("Let's read this book together now").

Be a model of mellow. The best way to teach your toddler civilised social skills is to consistently use them yourself. So use your words (calmly, as much as you can), practise compromise over confrontation, and demonstrate empathy when your little one is watching. When you lose your temper – hey, everyone does – try to make sure your toddler sees you admit your lapse, and apologise for it.

Avoid a heavy hand. It's tempting to drag a reluctant-to-leave toddler out of the sandpit, to give a pavement dawdler a little push when you're late for an appointment, or to deliver a quick smack of retribution for kicking a playmate, but remember that aggressive parenting tactics can lead to aggressive kids. Try, instead, to handle your toddler in a firm but calm and physically gentle way, even when you're annoyed, impatient, or over-the-top stressed.

Know when to stay out of it. A few harmless rounds of shoving over a spade isn't likely to hurt anyone and doesn't require adult intervention as long as nobody's crying. Step in when you're needed, step back when you aren't. Civilised social behaviour doesn't happen overnight, but it won't happen at all without experience. It's in the trenches – and in the sandpit – that your tot will ultimately figure out how relationships work, how to make them work, and what happens when they don't work.

Know when to step in. If kids come to blows (or bites, or kicks), step in promptly to end the conflict. In a group setting, focus your immediate attention on rescuing (and if need be, comforting) the victim rather than admonishing the perp. If your child was the attacker, distract the victim with another activity, and then take your toddler aside for a little talking-to. Whether the aggression was directed at a peer or at you, calmly state that the behaviour is not acceptable, and briefly explain why ("You hurt Benjamin when you kicked him"). You can warn of consequences if the behaviour is repeated ("We'll have to go home". . . "We'll have to stop playing with this puzzle together"), but avoid threats of any kind unless you intend to follow through – or else your attempts at modifying your toddler's behaviour will be futile.

Don't be pushy – or a pushover. The most aggressive children usually have big-bully parents who discipline them harshly and physically or big-softy parents who don't discipline them at all. Middle-of-the-road discipline is the most likely to lead to well-behaved children. For practical disciplining tips, see Chapter 7.

At the End of the Day

Whoever coined the term "Happy Hour" obviously never spent 5 o'clock with a toddler. This hour – and often the hour or so preceding and the hour or so that follows – is rarely a time for relaxing and unwinding. More typically, the mood is frantic and frazzled. At the end of a long day, toddlers are often overtired, oversensitive, and overwrought, and even more prone than usual to fits of irrationality and negativity. Unfortunately, this hard-to-cope-with behaviour happens when parental patience may already be stretched to the snapping point – after a tough day at work or an average day-in-the-hectic-life-with-a-toddler. It's a time when even the coolest of heads are quick to overheat.

While nothing will guarantee peace, quiet, and intact nerves, there are ways to tame the 5 o'clock frazzles:

Unwind before you get home. It's not only little ones who tend to be high strung at 5 (or 6). With dinner to be made, a toddler-taken-apart house to put back together, and, if you've been at work all day, household chores, washing, post, and messages to get to, your stress level can also soar. Problem is, a parent's 5 o'clock frenzy tends to fuel a toddler's. So try to spend a few minutes unwinding before you pick up your toddler from nursery or walk through the front door. Get off the bus or tube a few streets from home and walk the rest of the way. Listen to soothing music in your car. Stay in the driver's seat for five minutes longer after you've pulled up to your driveway; close your eyes and take a few deep cleansing breaths. Visualise a peaceful scene (lapping waves on a beach), and imagine throwing away the day's stress (since you've got that ocean handy, you can toss the disagreement you had with your boss right into the next wave). Once you've emptied your mind, be careful not to fill it back up again with thoughts of the potential chaos that awaits you.

---

biting some time between their first and third birthdays. For most, it never becomes chronic; a few experimental chomps seem to satisfy the urge. But for some, the behaviour persists and continues to cause problems.

The following tips may help nip a nipper in the bud:

Separate the biter and the victim immediately. Offer comfort to the victim as needed (and even if it isn't needed, since this will reinforce for your toddler that biting isn't the way to get attention). Don't overreact, yell, or embark on a lengthy lecture – simply take your toddler aside and explain calmly but firmly, "Please don't bite. Biting hurts. You hurt Alysha when you bit her." When he bites out of an inability to communicate, help him find the words he needs to express his feelings: "I know you feel angry. It's okay to say 'I'm angry.' But it's not okay to hurt someone when you're angry." Not a message that will sink in or even be understood right away, but it's a good message to begin sending.

Never bite back. As with hitting back, biting back is confusing to a toddler. Your bite says that it's okay to bite someone if you're angry with him, while your words say "Don't bite". Even biting back once to show him how it feels isn't likely to help, since he probably

If you've been at home all day with your toddler, you'll probably have to do your unwinding together (see the suggestions below).

Take a time-out together. Instead of attacking your to-do list immediately, try to take a relaxing break (chances are that if you have a whining toddler tugging at your leg, nothing's going to get done anyway). Take a few deep breaths, postpone dinner preparations, put the BlackBerry aside, and settle down for a special activity with your toddler. Cuddle up together while you read some nursery rhymes or listen to some soothing children's music. Making it the same music each and every evening can provide the comfort of consistency, and may even have a Pavlovian effect – you and your toddler will come to associate the music with calming down. Or get involved in an activity that you both enjoy (resting together in a dimly lit and quiet room, taking a bath together in a tubful of warm water and bubbles, colouring in, reading a favourite book). Or, unwind with a family workout – take a walk down the street together or stretch out on the living room rug for a yoga session. If you have to get started on dinner, have your toddler "help" you in the kitchen.

Set a serene scene. Switch off the television, power off the computer and the phone, and remove any other agitating influences that might disturb the peace – it's tranquillity time. Encourage your toddler to play quietly and gently discourage high-energy activities.

Fend off hunger. You may be hungry after a long day at work – or a long day running after your little monkey – and your toddler is likely to be hungry, too. Since low blood sugar can take everyone's mood down, fight back with food. If you'll be eating later on in the evening (once your little one's asleep), sit down and have a snack with your toddler while he or she eats dinner. Or, if you'd rather dine as a family, feed your tot a healthy appetizer to hold off those hunger pangs until it's dinnertime (cooked veggies and dip are a perfect, fun-to-eat choice – and great for sharing with you).

isn't yet able to connect his own pain with the pain others feel. Being bitten may hurt or startle him, but it's unlikely to keep him from biting again.

Avoid a double standard. Some parents nibble on their child's toes or fingers playfully or allow their toddlers to take a nip of their shoulder, cheek, or arm occasionally – especially if it doesn't hurt much. Then, when their toddler bites a playmate, they scold. It's best to avoid any confusion by banning biting for everyone.

Provide a nibble to prevent biting. Once in a while a very young child bites just because he's hungry. Snack-up as needed before letting him loose in a social situation.

Take biting seriously. Can't help but laugh the first time your child takes a bite out of you? Almost nothing will encourage biting more, so repress those giggles.

Hair Pulling

"When my daughter doesn't get what she wants, she pulls hair."

For many toddlers who don't yet have a grip on vocabulary, gripping – and yanking – the closest handful of hair is a fallback form of communication. The

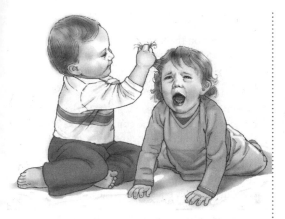

Toddlers often express their frustration, as well as demonstrate their considerable lack of social skills, with hair pulling, pinching, biting, or another form of aggressive behaviour.

reasons are the same as for those other primitive forms of expression, hitting and biting, and so are the interventions (see the previous questions).

With the toddler who pulls hair, it may also help to give her a shaggy stuffed animal to tug at to her heart's content. Try, too, to change the way she thinks about hair – from something that gets tugged to something that gets styled – by allowing her to brush your hair or giving her a long-haired doll and doll brush to play with.

Aggressiveness with Toys

"Our son seems to be very wild when he's playing. He doesn't hurt anyone, but he throws his teddy bear against the wall for fun, or pummels his sister's doll."

Ever unload tension in a vigorous game of tennis or by going a few rounds with a punching bag? Chances are, your toddler is letting off steam (and excess energy) the same way – and happily, he's not hurting anyone

in the process. Just as likely: he may just be flexing his curiosity ("I throw this teddy bear and it bounces off the wall – awesome!").

Bottom line: if there's no harm done to people or property, there's no harm to this kind of aggressive play – and making a big deal about it will just step it up. You can certainly point out to your tot that although his toys don't have real feelings, people and real animals do (though he probably won't understand that message yet). You could also encourage gentle play (make a game out of petting the stuffed animal or rocking the baby doll nicely) – not that he'll necessarily find the fun in playing along (for some toddlers, it's just not fun unless it's physical). Following the tips on fighting aggression on page 170 may help curb his wild ways. Definitely draw the line on aggressive play that damages or threatens to damage toys, furniture, or other property, or that hurts people or animals – and if he crosses that line, stop him in his tracks. Let him know such behaviour is not appropriate, ever, and immediately remove him from the object of his aggression.

Thumb Sucking

"Our daughter sucks her thumb – usually when she's tired or upset. Is this okay?"

No need to give a thumbs-down to your tot's thumb sucking. That little thumb is a big source of security for your toddler – and like all sources of comfort, her thumb comes in especially handy when she's feeling stressed, tired, or just out of sorts. Plenty of kids hang on to the thumb-sucking habit into the second year (and well beyond). And unless she's sucking her thumb every waking (and sleeping) hour, there's no reason to worry about this common comfort habit – it won't affect her teeth or her mouth development. In fact, the more you pester (or scold, or tease), the more likely she is to suck away. If she's like the majority of children, she'll give up the thumb-sucking habit by about age 3, without your intervention.

Continued Dummy Use

"Our son is so attached to his dummy, we're afraid he'll never give it up."

Have visions of your son popping the dummy from his mouth so he can answer questions in algebra class? Take heart – and a chill pill. Despite the understandable fears harboured by their parents, even persistent dummy users usually abandon the beloved plug by age 4 or 5, and most stop sucking it well before.

Still, there are some good reasons to consider pulling the plug sooner rather than later, including an increased risk of ear infections and possible slower language and social development in diehard suckers. Here are some ways to break your toddler of the dummy habit:

Establish limits. Start by limiting where the dummy can go. Begin with the house or car only; then house only; then just your child's bedroom; then only his cot. Another tactic: set time limits on dummy sessions, and gradually reduce them (from 30 minutes down to 2 or 3). Even better, require your toddler to sit or lie still when he has his dummy in his mouth. Bor-ing!

Keep his mouth busy. Ask questions, strike up conversations, and encourage your tot to recite rhymes, sing, laugh, make funny faces in the mirror, and otherwise use his mouth for non-dummy purposes. If he tries to talk with the dummy in his mouth, let him know that you can't understand him and that he has to remove it if he wants you to know what he's saying.

Don't let him go hungry – or sleepy. The child who's hungry or overtired tends to lose his ability to cope; it's then that he's likely to turn to a familiar coping mechanism, such as his dummy. To cut down on those moments, offer snacks before your little man hits a blood-sugar low and make sure he naps before he crosses the overtired line. Don't, however, get in the habit of offering him food (or a drink of juice) every time he pleads for his dummy – that will only substitute one coping mechanism for another.

Provide extra comfort. If your toddler seems dependent on the dummy for comfort, offer him other sources of solace. Heap on the love and attention, particularly when he's grumpy or upset. Before he reaches for the dummy, reach for him with a hug, or distract him with a story, or turn on some soothing music and settle down for a cuddle.

Take matters into your own hands. If you're desperate to rid your son of his dummy vice, poke tiny holes or cut some slits in the teat of the dummy – this changes the sucking sensation, making it less satisfying. You can also try "losing" the dummy – either deliberately (via the "Dummy Fairy", who comes to collect dummies from all the big boys and girls, leaving a toy in its place) or "accidentally" ("Oops, we can't find your dummy!"). Another plan: stage a "dummy-good-bye party" – pick a day to hold the festivities, inform your tot about the big bash (and remind him about it often as the special day approaches), and then, with great fanfare, help him throw out the dummy or put it in a box to send to "the babies", after which he can celebrate his new independence with a piece of cake. This plan usually works best with tots closer to age 2.

If all your efforts to limit dummy use fail, don't force the issue. While tougher tactics may be needed a year or two from now (when both peer pressure and damage to his mouth and teeth can become problems), they aren't necessary now. It may be that your toddler needs the comfort this comfort habit brings him more than ever – and that's completely age-appropriate. For further reassurance, speak to your toddler's doctor or dentist at the next visit.

A Comfort Object

"Our toddler drags a grimy old blanket around with her. When will she give it up?"

Comfort isn't just for babies. In fact, dependence on a comfort object, also called a security object or transitional object, doesn't typically peak until the second year, for a few good reasons. For one, though a toddler can't always take Mummy or Daddy along as she explores her world, she

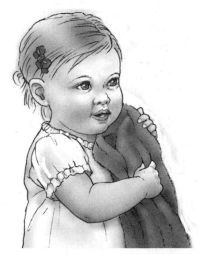

Many toddlers latch on to one comfort habit or object – and some latch on to several.

isn't quite ready to go it alone. A transitional object – whether it's a tattered blanket, a well-worn teddy bear, or a little pillow – provides a perfect, portable source of reassurance, a reliable stand-in for you. A transitional object, not surprisingly, also helps a toddler make those tricky transitions – bridging the otherwise overwhelming gap between A and B (whether A is the playground and B is home, or A is being awake and B is being asleep). That security object also offers a sense of, well, security when a toddler faces her fears. And since fears (of the dark, of strangers, of dogs, of vacuum cleaners, to name just a few) start multiplying in the second year, she begins to need that courage crutch more than ever. Toddlers are also more likely to cling to a comfort object when they're tired, grumpy, frustrated, or otherwise out of sorts (which toddlers are often known to be).

So support your toddler's right to the support of a comfort object. Let her clutch that blanket or teddy whenever she needs to – don't tease her about it or pressure her to give it up or leave it at home. But, at the same time, take these steps to keep that comforting companion from becoming her constant companion – and to make giving it up easier, when she's ready:

Try to set some limits she can live with. If your toddler isn't already in the habit of carrying her comfort object with her everywhere, try to put acceptable (to her) limits on where it can go. Suggest that it can go in the car, but not into the supermarket. Or that it can be carried around the house, but not around the playground. Offer plausible reasons for the restrictions (it might get lost at the supermarket or dirty on the swings). Volunteer to "take care" of the blanket when she climbs on the climbing frame or works on a puzzle in playgroup. With her help, find a special place where she can leave her blanket when she isn't toting it. But don't insist on limits if she's not open to negotiating any. When the timing's right for her, she'll wean herself off her beloved comforter.

Keep it clean, with regular washings. If you don't, your toddler may become as attached to the odour the blanket develops as she is to the blanket itself – and she'll protest when it comes back smelling like springtime. Since separating a child from her security object can be tough, you'll probably have to wash it while she's sleeping.

Duplicate it, if you can. Though a baby just starting out with a blanket might not notice (and probably wouldn't object) if you cut the blanket into a couple of pieces (one for you to wash, one for her to cuddle), a toddler who's clutched the same blanket for months is likely to both notice and object. Instead, try buying an identical blanket (if you can find one), washing it a few times so it won't seem too new, and either offering it to your toddler as an extra (she may or may not accept it) or putting it away for emergency use (when, for example, the original blanket is nowhere to be found at bedtime). If the comfort object is a toy or stuffed animal, purchasing a duplicate can accomplish the same objective. If your toddler is only mildly attached to her blanket, however, you might just stick with the one. Should it get lost, she can shed a few tears and then get on with her life without it.

Give her something else to do with her hands. Busy hands can't clutch a blanket or a teddy. Keep your toddler occupied with interesting toys, crayons and finger paints, puzzles, and anything else that will divert her hands, and her attention, from her comfort object – at least some of the time.

Comfort at a Cost

Not all security objects are harmless. Toddlers who get their comfort from a bottle or beaker of juice or milk can end up with tooth decay or with diarrhoea (from drinking too much juice, or from milk that's gone bad). If your little one insists on carrying a security bottle or beaker around with her, fill it with plain water. Objects that present a choking or other safety risk can also be classified unsafe and should be removed and replaced with a safe alternative.

Avoid applying pressure. Pushing your little one to do too much too soon can increase stress and her need for the support of a security object. So can overscheduling (too many playdates, too many activities). If she seems stressed-out, relax her with some cuddling, a quiet book, soft music. And don't tease or chide her for her blanket habit – that will only step up her attachment to her treasured friend.

It's likely that your toddler will be ready to leave her blanket behind – or any other comfort object she's become attached to – somewhere between ages 2 and 5, though she may continue reaching for it again during times of stress and change (plenty of kids, in fact, tote a tattered teddy to college). Until then, as long as she's happy and thriving, relax. If the comfort object becomes an obsession, however, and your child spends more time stroking and cuddling the object than interacting and socialising with others, playing with toys, looking at books, and so on, you may need to look closely for underlying causes: for instance, an unhappy

No Comfort Habit, No Problem

Just call it a case of different strokes for different little folks. Some toddlers find security in a portable, inanimate object or in a stress-releasing habit. Others find comfort is more satisfying when it takes human form (Mummy, Daddy, or another favourite person). They may enjoy playing with teddy bears and cuddling under blankets, but never develop an attachment to any particular one. That's just their style – and it's perfectly okay. There are plenty of obvious benefits to not being hooked on a comfort object or habit – no dragging around a dirty blanket, no trauma when the treasured teddy can't be located, no thumb or dummy to be weaned from. So if your tot has no comfort object or stress-releasing habit, don't object. Just consider yourself lucky.

childcare situation, too much stress or pressure at home, or an undetected medical or developmental condition. If you can't uncover and remedy the problem yourself, consult your toddler's GP.

Head Banging and Other Comfort Habits

"When we put our son to sleep he goes through this ritual where he literally bangs his head against the wall next to his cot. We also hear him doing it in the middle of the night sometimes. It seems to calm him down – but it stresses us out."

All that noggin-knocking driving you nuts? It may be hard to believe (and even harder to watch), but the very same rhythmic rituals that stress you out (head banging, rocking back and forth) are relaxing to your little rock-and-roller. These very common self-comforting activities, kinetic cousins to comfort objects, are at least three times more likely to show up in boys. They appear most often at night, when your little fireball is brimming with energy and tension that need releasing. Many tots bang only while they're falling asleep or trying to fall back to sleep, while others bang when they're bored, overstimulated, in pain (from teething, for instance, or an earache), having a tantrum, or want some attention.

Luckily, your little one's habit is unlikely to harm his head (his skull is built to take it – along with all those minor tumbles). As with most toddler behaviours, the less attention paid to it, the better – scolding and overreacting will only step up comfort habits. But you can try:

Relieving stress. The arrival of a new sibling, a change in caregivers, being weaned off the bottle, or any other adjustment can be unsettling for toddlers. While head banging does a bang-up job of destressing your toddler, so can providing plenty of hugs and kisses, some undivided attention, and relaxing activities (like a quiet story or a mellow massage).

Rocking around the clock. Satisfy your child's need to follow the rhythm action by inviting him to rock in a child-size rocker, ride one end of a seesaw, or play circle games like Ring a Ring o' Roses or Farmer in the Dell. Music can also satisfy the primal need for rhythm your tot's been filling by rocking or banging. Play lively music during the day, and encourage him to dance to it, clap to it, stomp to it, or bang on a pot to it. At bedtime, select some soothing tunes. Try rocking or swaying to the music gently as you read a bedtime story, or slow-dancing to it with your little one in your arms.

Providing release. Give your tot a big shaggy stuffed dog to wrestle with so he can release whatever he has pent up. Pounding with a toy hammer or banging on a toy drum, punching a pillow, pounding on Play-Doh, running around outdoors, and swinging on a swing can also help him get rid of excess energy. Just don't encourage these activities too close to bedtime, when you want your rocker to be relaxing, not releasing.

Making bedtime routine. Self-comforting activities generally peak in the evening because children use them to unwind after a busy day. A regular soothing and calming bedtime routine – begun well before he's bedded down for the night – may help your toddler find more tranquil routes to relaxation. Also try to keep the atmosphere around your home as serene as possible in the hour or two before bed – no blaring TV, no loud conversations, and definitely no shouting.

Setting up safe surroundings. Move the bed or cot away from the wall, try padding the cot and other bangable surfaces within reach, and if necessary, detach the wheels from the cot and place a carpet underneath so it will stay in place.

In most children, rhythmic comfort activities disappear by age 3 without parental intervention. If your toddler's head banging or body rocking is really excessive (he does it all day) and is accompanied by other developmental red flags (see box next column), mention it to the doctor, since it could be an indication of a developmental disorder, such as autism.

Rituals

"Everything's a ritual to my toddler: he always has to have his juice in the same cup, he always has to have his sandwich cut up the same way, he always has to wear the same trainers. It's driving me mad."

Everything having to be "just so" may seem just so . . . compulsive to the adults around him. But to your toddler – and to a lot of his pint-size peers – "just so" feels just right. While not every toddler craves ritual (and that's normal, too), most demand at least some predictability in their food, drink, clothing, and daily routines – and some seem to obsess about consistency. For these tots, even the slightest variation in the same-old-same-old can set off a tirade.

Like negativity and temper tantrums, clinging to rituals is a toddler's way of trying to gain some measure of control over his life, which isn't easy to do when you're less than 2 years old, less than a metre high, and hopelessly dependent on those much bigger and

Ritual Red Flags

Predictability and routines bring little kids security and comfort, but there are limits to what's normal. When ritualistic behaviour becomes so obsessive or compulsive that it interferes with daily activities (he consistently prefers to stack and unstack books instead of looking at them, for instance), or if your child has so many rituals (she must line up her dolls in a perfect line, she twirls her hair nonstop, she rubs her blanket over her arm repetitively, and so on), mention it to the GP at the next visit.

Embracing the Routines

To most grown-ups, routines are, well, routine. Predictable, boring, monotonous – same-old-same-old. Yet for most small children, routines are reassuring. Knowing what they can expect at various times during their day can make children feel more secure, in control, comfortable and comforted.

What's in a routine for you? There are actually plenty of parental perks. Routines can help toddlers handle transitions, reducing resistance as they switch gears – from story time to lunch, from playground to home, from bricks to bedtime. Knowing what to expect also helps make tots (somewhat) more compliant and cooperative, helping them anticipate and accept inevitable next steps. Plus, routines eliminate a lot of time-consuming planning (once a routine is established, you don't have to give it a second thought), cut down on last-minute panics, and generally make frenetic days run more smoothly.

Routines don't work for everyone. They can upset little ones who are by nature "irregular", and can stress out some families by cramping their spontaneous style. But most families with small children find that having some routine in their chaotic schedules – whether a single weekly routine or several daily rituals – makes sense.

Good-morning routines. Start the day off right with a morning ritual, like a cosy cuddle when your tot wakes up. Or start off with a special greeting: a kiss, a hug, and a favourite song, for example.

Off-to-work routines. When one or both parents leave in the morning, a group hug, a special parting phrase, watching and waving from the window, can all make the bye-byes easier on your little one.

Departure routines. Leaving – a friend's house, the playground, or the toy shop – is hard for many young children (as are most transitions). Establishing a regular routine for departures – singing a special good-bye song, for instance – may decrease resistance.

Welcome-home routines. No matter who is coming home – Mum or Dad from work or toddler from nursery – sticking to a predictable unwinding routine (sitting down together for a light snack, reading a book, playing a favourite game) before starting on meals, post, and other obligations can help all of you relax after a long day. Or make taking care of these obligations part of the routine – setting the table together, collecting the post together, and so on.

much more powerful than you. Being able to control some of the little things in life (which cup he drinks from, how his sandwich is sliced, which trainers he wears) means a lot to a toddler and his self-esteem. Predictability is also comforting. With a toddler's world ever expanding, it's good to know that the more things change, the more he can keep them the same.

So instead of trying to pressure your child out of the rituals he treasures, let them rule for now, at least as much as is practical. Tell anyone else who cares for him too what these rituals are and discuss how you deal with them. (Chances

Dinner routines. Knowing that if it's Monday it must be beef burgers and carrots, if it's Tuesday it must be pasta and cheese, if it's Wednesday it must be chicken stir-fry can take some of the last-minute stress out of shopping and cooking. (Of course, your toddler may have his or her own dinner routine in mind: pasta and cheese every night of the week.) If menu routine feels more like a rut to you, consider other meal-time traditions: taking turns talking about the day's activities, listening to music, saying grace.

Tidying up routines. Whether you insist on each toy being put away before the next comes out (good luck with that strategy) or call for a thorough tidy at the end of a play session or the end of the day, getting your toddler into the routine of picking up after himself or herself will pay both short- and long-term dividends.

Linking tidy-up time with a particular song ("This is the way we pick up our toys, pick up our toys, pick up our toys. This is the way we pick up our toys, so early in the evening") will help establish the routine in the first place and make it much more appealing over the long haul. So will making a predictable game of it: for example, set a timer for a beat-the-clock tidy up.

Washing routines. For the toddler who tends to resist hygiene-related activities, knowing when to expect them helps him or her accept their inevitability. So establish a predictable routine for toothbrushing, hand washing, bathing, and shampooing.

Bedtime routines. These set the tone for a happy close to a toddler's day. For tips on how to create a bedtime routine, see page 134.

Weekend routines. Since having a toddler in the house pretty much ruins any chance of lazy day spontaneity (remember breakfast and love-making in bed, followed by a film in the afternoon?), you might as well stick to weekend routines that you and your toddler can look forward to. For instance, early-morning cuddle sessions, toast soldiers for breakfast, Saturday afternoon outings with Mum, Sunday in the park with Dad.

Remember that once you establish a routine, sticking to it is important to its success and your tot's comfort level even when holidays, visitors, and other circumstances shake up the status quo. Some toddlers are easily unsettled by change, particularly the last-minute variety. So if you must break with a routine, try to prepare your toddler in advance and then muster up that extra patience to help him or her cope with the disruption.

are, he'll adapt in environments where his rituals can't be performed, like in nursery.)

Your toddler may be more open to a change if he's in control of it. So every once in a while, propose that he pick out a new cup to drink from, show him a fun way of eating a sandwich (use a biscuit cutter to cut yours into a star, an animal shape, or a heart and suggest that he do the same with his), propose shopping for sandals just like Daddy's to wear at the beach. But if he clings to the standard, don't push. With time and patience, ritual will lose its hold on your toddler.

Resistance to Change

"Any little change – a difference in the daily schedule, a new haircut on her mummy, new glasses on me – and our daughter unravels."

As far as some toddlers are concerned, there's no such thing as a change for the better.

Like so many toddler trademarks, rigidity has its roots in the toddler's compulsion to try to control her environment as much as a tiny person can. She feels comforted by predictability and sameness, unnerved by newness (unless it's her idea – like a new toy she picked out).

While not all toddlers unravel in the face of change, most resist it at least some of the time. Understanding that inflexibility is normal and age-appropriate for a toddler (and that flexibility may be at least a year away) should make this phase easier to survive. For now, try to go with the flow – or rather, the lack of flow. Keep the status quo as is – at least, as much as is practical, at least as it relates to your toddler. If a change is coming, whether she'll like it or not – you need new glasses or want a new haircut – help your intractable tot adjust with lots of reassurance ("I'm still Daddy. I just have a new pair of glasses"). When a truly major change that can't wait is on the horizon – a new child care situation suddenly becomes necessary, for instance – take extra pains to prepare her for the change and to help her get acclimated. Anticipate that she will be feeling unsettled while she adapts to her new environment or schedule, and that she'll need extra support and understanding from her stabilising source (you), but that pretty soon different will be the new same – and all will be right again in her world.

Clinging

"My toddler seems so dependent on me. Every time I leave his side or start paying attention to anything else, he starts to cry or pull on my leg."

It's flattering to know that even as your little man's universe expands, you're still the centre of it. But it can also be something of a drag. Literally. Like when you're trying to get dinner ready with a 11-kg weight on your leg, or listen to voicemail over howls of "Muummmmy!"

While your toddler's in this tricky trademark transitional phase – giddy at the prospect of facing the world on two feet, conflicted about leaving the cosy confines of your arms ... excited about his newfound independence, but ambivalent about giving up the trappings of babyhood – you'll have to walk a fine line (not easy, with your toddler still clinging to your leg) between providing too much comfort and providing

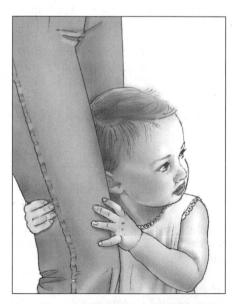

Torn between a hunger for independence and a craving for security, many toddlers still feel the need to cling.

too little, between supporting and stifling, protecting and overprotecting. With just the right balance of reassurance and encouragement, your tentative tot will gain the confidence he needs to let go of you . . . and your leg. In the meantime:

Play peek-a-boo. Really. Your toddler – and others his age – most likely understands the concept of object permanence (if something isn't visible, it still exists). In theory. But he still likes to be reassured that his favourite object – you – is permanently by his side (fast-forward 15 years, not a chance). The peek-a-boo you've played with him since his baby days can still help reinforce your permanence. But try taking the game up a notch, to help him learn that when you leave, you come back. Hide behind a door or the sofa and say, "Where's Mummy?" Then poke your smiling face out and say, "Here I am!" Gradually extend the hiding time from a few moments to a minute, as long as he doesn't seem to get worried. If he doesn't handle the game well at first, go back to hiding your face only – or hiding a teddy bear instead of you. Once he's enjoying your disappearing act, encourage him to try his own (in the house, that is – be clear that these games are not to be played outside). Then move on to hide-and-seek.

Make time for togetherness. Have you been busy, busy, busy? That might be one reason he's clingy, clingy, clingy. Try to sit down more often for one-on-one time (not fair counting one-on-one plus the TV, or one-on-one plus your phone), even if it's just 15 minutes of stories or car races. When you're on the run, swoop down for frequent hugs and kisses. Of course, the idea is to get him to loosen his hold on you . . . eventually. But a little extra togetherness may help him feel more secure on his own.

No Clinging Here

Not all toddlers are clingy. Some seem to make the leap from dependence to independence without a second thought – and they never look back. These independent types don't cling, aren't needy, show no separation anxiety, and love doing things on their own. And that's just as normal.

Make time for independence. If you're a hovering heliparent, you may be unintentionally sending a mixed signal: "Play on your own. . . . no, wait, playing on your own isn't a good idea!" Keep a close eye on your little one for safety's sake, but also encourage him to go it alone with his bricks or shape sorter. Taking a step away from your toddler once in a while may help him feel more secure in taking baby steps to independence.

Set him up. Before you walk away from your toddler – even if you're just walking to the other side of the same room – give yourself a head start by getting him busy with an activity. Set him up on the kitchen floor with a doll and an empty bottle and let him feed his baby while you get lunch ready for your big boy. Underfoot is better than stuck to your leg, isn't it?

Keep in touch. Chat with him occasionally while you work. Reach over and pat his head, or help him fit a challenging shape into the sorter if he's having a tough time.

Underreact. Does this scenario sound familiar? Your toddler starts to unravel the moment you get up to check office e-mail. You react with exasperation: "Can't you be alone for two seconds?" Or with pity: "Oh, you poor baby – Mummy's right here!" He's emotional,

Cutting Those Strings Safely

Whether your toddler's the clingy type or independence-plus, there will be times when you'll both want your space. Just remember, as you provide it, that no tyke is ready to go it completely alone. Never leave even the most self-reliant toddler alone in a room where you can't keep a close eye – unless the room is 100 per cent childproofed and you're within ear-shot (and checking in visually every minute or two), or if your little one is asleep in the cot. Make sure your little one can't leave that safe room and wander down the hall, either. If you want your toddler to get used to staying in a room without you for longer periods of time, attempt basic training only when another adult or responsible child over the age of 8 is present.

you're emotional – and you both wear it on your sleeve, and not well. You end up giving up on the e-mail and leaving it unchecked until he's napping or in bed. And of course, the scenario keeps playing out like it's on a loop – day in, day out.

Instead, try this script. He starts to cry. You nonchalantly say "It's okay, I'll be right back." Or just as matter-of-factly say "Here, you can sit on the floor with this lorry. Mummy's busy now." He keeps crying (of course), you keep checking your e-mail. Calmly, coolly. Finish up, then re-enter your toddler's world – just as calmly, just as coolly. With a smile, say "Here I am. Mummy's back! Did you have fun while I was working?" Of course, you know the answer is "no" – at least right now. But that's not the point. With practice, he'll get the hang

of keeping it together when you leave his side – and your comings and goings will become a nonevent.

Let him follow you. If your toddler insists on following you around the house, even into the bathroom, it's fine to let him. He has a whole bunch of temporarily conflicted feelings (Do I want to be independent? Dependent?) – but, for now, no need to add rejection to the mix. If he insists on grabbing your leg, try to make light of the load you're dragging around: "Is there a monkey on my leg? Where did that monkey come from? I better get a banana for the monkey!" But also know when to draw the line. If he's keeping you from getting important stuff done, calmly explain why that's not an option: "If I don't get the chicken cooked, we can't eat dinner." Then get back to business.

Leave the leaving to him. Separation is probably only traumatic for your toddler when it's your idea – not when it's his. If the two of you have been playing together at home and he wanders off to do his own thing, let him (as long as you can see he's safe). He needs to know it's okay to leave your side (at home).

Make sure you're not the dependent one. Everyone likes to be needed, right? But sometimes, parents like to be needed by their kids just a tad too much. They'll hover over a puzzle that's getting done slowly, barge in on a stuffed-animal birthday party uninvited, anticipate clinginess before it happens ("Don't cry – I'm just going to wash the dishes"). Stuck in a cycle of neediness? Make an effort to break out, and be codependent no more.

Hang in there. You've heard this before – and you'll hear it again (and again and again over the next 20 years or so): your child's going through a phase. Clinging comes and it goes (and sometimes it comes back – like when preschool starts . . . or college). Some kids cling more, some less. As long as you know your toddler is otherwise happy and getting enough love and the right amount of attention, you're not doing anything wrong, and neither is he. So hang in there as he hangs on.

Separation Anxiety

"Our daughter cries when we leave her at nursery. Shouldn't she be over this separation anxiety already?"

Growing up is hard to do. From the moment the cord is cut, life is full of separations – including plenty that you probably can't imagine yet (first day of preschool . . . first sleepover at a friend's). And all of them will be challenging, potentially for both of you (let's be honest: how well do you really think you're going to handle driving away from summer camp without her?)

Here's that phrase again: it's only a phase. Separation anxiety comes and goes many times as a child walks (and yikes! . . . later drives) that long road to adulthood. You may have glimpsed this anxiety for the first time when your little one was about 9 months old, or sooner, or later. Some toddlers aren't good at separations (as you may have noticed at nursery drop-off, when your toddler's tiny hands adhered to your neck with the tenacity of a pro wrestler). Others, often to their parents' secret chagrin, hardly ever look back. Some little ones initially have an easier time, then get unexpectedly clingy later on (sometimes not until age 2 or 3 – and sometimes not until 5 or 6). Others have a tougher time at first, then gain the confidence they need to sprint away from their parents' side. There are children who separate more easily from Dad, others who cling less to Mum. Sometimes a stress

in a child's life, like a new child minder, Mum going back to work, teething, even an oncoming cold, steps up clinginess.

There's no predicting when Operation Nursery Drop-off (and other separations) will start running more smoothly. Until it does, keep these tips in mind:

■ Let your toddler lap it up. Attention is like a chocolate bar – when you know you can have one any time you want, you're not as likely to crave twelve at a time. If your toddler knows that your love and attention are always there for the taking (at home and away), she won't be as needy for it – and in time, she'll feel more comfortable venturing away from it at separation times. She'll just want more and more of it if you give that attention only grudgingly – admittedly not hard to do when you're late for work already, and you're desperate to pry her fingers off so you can get out the door.

■ Don't give her any ideas. Even if you're dreading the worst while you're on the way to nursery, pretend you expect smooth sailing. Don't mention the separation – instead, talk about the fun things she'll be doing in nursery or when you'll pick her up ("after nap time" or "before dinner"). Or talk about the leaves flying around, the little dog passing by, or the big green lorry stopped at the traffic light.

■ Play it cool, but not too cool. Your toddler is screaming bloody murder. Your watch is ticking (late again!). Your nerves are shot, and speaking of shots, you haven't had your coffee yet. The impulse is to lose it – to do a little screaming yourself, be over-the-top exasperated. Or to be so stressed out that you resort to putting your toddler's feelings down ("You're acting so silly!"), or even catering your

The Long Good-bye

Parting's all sorrow (and not the sweet kind) at your house? The following tips can help you get out the door . . . without the drama:

- Don't be a sneak. Tempted to slip out when your toddler's not looking or is fast asleep? A sneaky retreat from your home or the nursery may avoid a scene short-term, but it'll also put your toddler on high front-door alert in the future – not to mention introduce all kinds of trust issues. Knowing you could leave at any time will just step up anxiety (and round-the-clock clinging), adding to those good-bye melodramas. If your toddler and child minder leave for the playground or a play-date or errand before you head out, let your toddler know that you'll be gone when they return.

- For a shorter good-bye, slow it down. Last-minute rushes are stressful for you and your toddler. When you can (and you won't always be able to), slow down the pace before you make your exit. Plan to arrive at nursery a little early, so you'll have time for a quick story. Devote the last 15 minutes before the child minder arrives to building a brick castle (instead of frantically trying to locate your left shoe). Even a few moments of uninterrupted togetherness can help your toddler transition to apart time.

- Get your toddler busy. Here are the rules of engagement: before you pick up your work briefcase or your handbag, engage your toddler in an absorbing activity. Being busy won't necessarily keep your little one from making a big scene when you do leave, but it'll give him or her something to go back to once you're gone, a win-win scenario.

- Leave a Mummy or Daddy memento. Whether it's a T-shirt of yours to clutch, a photo of you in a mini soft frame to keep in a pocket, a lipstick-print kiss, or a dab of aftershave or perfume, having a little piece of you to carry around can help your toddler bridge the parent gap while you're gone.

- Ditch the drama. Stop the long, dramatic good-byes, and aim to be a no-drama Mama or Dada. Rewrite the script (the one where your tragic hero or heroine is anchored to your foot, wailing as you struggle to walk out the door), and direct it with a light, upbeat touch (even a little humour – but no laughing at your little one's tears). Keep to the four Cs: casual, cool, calm, collected. Choose a parting phrase that reinforces going and coming back, and use it whenever you leave your toddler. Like "See you later, alligator. In a while, crocodile." Or even a simple "Later, 'gator." Pretty soon, your toddler will be able to join cheerfully in the refrain. A wave or two is fine, but try not to go overboard. This isn't the send-off of the *Titanic* – you're just going out for the day or evening.

toddler's pity party ("Awww, my little baby wants her mummy!"). Instead (and this is another recurring theme), make "matter-of-fact" your mantra. Act like the crying doesn't stress you out in the least (as if). Be upbeat, confident, all smiles, annoyingly cheerful, if you have to. Kids tend to take their emotional cues from their parents, so the calmer you are about the separation, the calmer she'll become – in time.

- Leave quickly. You don't want to convey to your toddler the message that "the longer you cry, the longer I stay". So once you've made a speedy handover to the child minder or nursery, plaster that teeth whitening advertisement smile on your face, say your bye-bye, and hightail it out the door. Whatever you do, don't look back.

- Hold the guilt. Learning to separate is hard for some little ones, but it's an important life lesson. You're actually doing your toddler a favour by helping her learn it. If she's in good hands, feel good about stepping away from your toddler.

- Take a good look in the mirror. Yes, to make sure you don't have blueberry yogurt on your suit. But also to see (be honest now) whether your own separation anxiety is rubbing off on your toddler. Maybe it's that pesky guilt again, maybe it's ambivalence about working or child care, maybe it's just pre-drop-off stress (you anticipate a scene, you get one). Children have a sixth sense when it comes to reading their parents, so be careful what your little one sees in your face. Check that mirror of self-reflection – and then check those anxieties at the nursery door (or before you leave your toddler with a child minder or otherwise face a separation).

- Take a good look around you. Chances are you're only noticing the kids without separation anxiety at nursery: the ones who toddle or run off to start playing as soon as they're unbuckled from the pushchair or the car seat. Well, look again – you'll see there are lots of other little ones with big separation issues. That's because . . . it's normal.

A Preference for One Parent

"Our toddler won't let anybody else do anything for her when I'm around, not even her father. It's tying up all my time, and it's making him feel like he's not needed."

As far as most toddlers are concerned, nobody does it better than Mummy (though for some children it's Daddy who's up there on the parent pedestal). Nobody pours a drink, makes toast, puts on shoes, changes nappies, or pushes the pushchair in just the same way as Mummy does, and as long as Mummy's around, nobody had better try – that is, unless they're fans of rejection.

It's understandable that Mummy, being all the wonderful things Mummy is, tops many toddler A-lists – especially if Mummy's been the primary need-filler (and food-fixer) from early on. Still, if you're your tot's one-and-only, it's sometimes hard to feel all that flattered about this attention – and easy for you to feel a little put upon (or a lot, especially after a hard day). As for Daddy, it's tough to compete with Mummy worship (or vice versa, in homes where favouritism is flipped) – and sometimes it may not even seem worth the trouble.

A little perseverance will help, along with a lot of perspective. Playing favourites is just a toddler's way of demonstrating her right to choose – just as she does when she clamours for a certain cup at snack time or a certain book at story time. It's also her way of maintaining the sameness that brings so much comfort (Daddy may get an "A" for effort with the toast, but maybe he forgot to trim the crust like Mummy always does – or to add the jam smile). It's not a sign that one of you is a better parent or the parent who's better

TWINS

When Twins Turn Green with Envy

Have your twins' baby blues (or browns, or hazels) been taking on a decidedly green hue these days? Some jealousy's bound to happen – and happen often (make that daily) when you're parenting twin toddlers. After all, there's one of you – but two of them, each competing for your full and undivided attention and affection. And compete they will. You're giving twin A a cuddle on the sofa, and twin B clamours for a spot on your lap – even if it means he has to shove his sib unceremoniously off that coveted perch. You hand out the first cracker to twin B, and twin A stomps her little feet in fury. You help twin A negotiate the successful upending of a bucket of sand, and twin B retaliates by throwing her bucket at her brother. You pick up twin B for a hug, and twin A tries to pull her right out of your arms.

But jealousy between toddlers isn't just about a competition for you, your lap, and your love. It's also about a toddler's normal, developmentally appropriate out-size sense of self, which demands centre-of-the-universe status, at least in his or her little world. While a singleton tot doesn't have to vie for that pre-eminent position, a twin toddler does. It's tough to share when you're a toddler, but twin toddlers have to share just about everything (and everyone). It's hard to wait your turn when you're a toddler, but twin toddlers have to wait their turn all the time. Sometimes, it's enough to make a child mad – and jealous.

So now you know why sweet little twins can turn into green-eyed monsters (albeit very cute ones). But what can you do to keep the competition from getting ugly? Try these strategies:

Divide and conquer. You'll never be able to devote as much one-on-one time to your twins as a parent of a single tot can. And that's nothing to stress about (after all, the two of them get plenty of stimulation, not just from you but from each other). But it is important to try to carve out some alone time with each of your little ones, as challenging as that goal will sometimes be. Since cloning yourself is out

loved. What's more, it's bound to end sooner or later. Many children switch from being mummy's girls (or boys) to daddy's once they hit the preschool years – leaving Mum on the outside looking in.

In the meantime, with some effort on the part of both parents, some of this single-minded mummymania can be minimised. Here's how:

- Don't ask for it. If you've got a "she likes it better when I do it" mind-set, you could be inadvertently feeding the favouritism – not to mention dumping all the childcare on yourself.

- Let Dad do his thing. His way may be different, but your tot will get used to the variety in sandwich-making techniques and story-reading style.

- Share the good jobs. Sharing the responsibilities of parenting fairly means sharing both the tedious and the fun. If you dole out to Dad only those jobs that you don't feel like doing (or that your toddler hates – like getting her shoes on her), and

of the question (how many times in a day do you wish you could?), try the divide and conquer approach: Mum takes twin A, Dad takes twin B (then reverse). Occasionally enlist help, too, if you can (from a child minder or a family member), so while you're spending solo time with one twin, the other one is getting attention from another adult. Just make sure you switch off – especially important if they share a parent preference right now (it's all Mummy – or all Daddy – all the time).

Distract and occupy. Before you single out one of your tots to spend some alone time with, set up the other twin with crayons and a big sheet of paper, a pile of Play-Doh, or a favourite toy. You may be able to sneak in a few minutes of one-on-one before it becomes two-on-one again. Or try a game of one-on-one. Use a timer to set aside five minutes per twin – and alternate who gets first dibs on you each time.

Separate but equal. Daddy and Mummy are in the house at the same time? Well, then the math is definitely a lot easier – one parent takes one tot, one takes the other. But that alone time will be even more special to your toddlers if you take them on separate, but hopefully somewhat equal, excursions: Mum takes one to the playground, Dad takes the other to playgroup. At this stage, neither will know what the other one is up to, so there won't be anything to be jealous about (even if Dad's excursion turns out to be the supermarket and the dry cleaner). They'll just enjoy getting some of that undivided attention they're always hankering for.

Respect and validate. All siblings have their green moments, and twins – because they're the same age, the same size, and at the same stage of development – can have more. Sometimes it helps just to validate those feelings of jealousy: "I know you're mad that I'm spending time with Sophie, but when I'm done reading to her, you'll get a special turn with me." As your little ones improve their verbal skills, encourage them to use words to express what they're feeling.

If your twins are pretty much always happy as a package deal – and even protest when they're separated from their sib – there's no need to push the alone-time agenda. Just take your cues from your twin team.

hog the ones that are fun, he's going to have a hard time competing.

- Step to the sidelines. Given a choice, your tot will opt for Team Mummy, true. But step off the field altogether on a regular basis (go for a walk, take care of some business, soak in the bath, run to the shops), and she'll have the chance to discover Dad's winning ways. Leave without second thoughts about her – or a million last-minute reminders for him – and whatever you do, don't call in every five minutes to check on how they're doing without you. They'll not only survive without you, but they'll bond on a whole new level (and she may even discover that Dad's shampoo sculptures beat the suds out of yours). What starts out as Daddy-by-default time may become Daddy-by-choice time.

  Make an effort to step back when the three of you are together, too. Say: "I'm busy now, but Daddy will pour your milk (or put Paddington's boots on, or help you with the puzzle, or read you a story)."

When Baby Makes . . .
One Too Many for Your Toddler

Little kids *really* love their mummy and daddy and they're usually not too hot on sharing them – especially with a red-faced, bald-headed, lap-stealing home wrecker. Sure, the actual homecoming may be exciting for a day or two ("Your new brother is here!"), but once your toddler realises that this baby thing is for keeps – and that he or she will no longer be the centre of your universe – the novelty (and good will) may well wear off. There'll be jealousy for sure, and maybe even some emotional manipulation – especially if your tot is close to the second birthday. Your toddler may revert to baby behaviour (the "regression" you've heard so much about) to try to recapture the attention that's suddenly being showered on the baby of the house ("hey, if it works for him . . ."). Clinging may climb off the charts. Acting up or acting out may heat up. Or your tyke may decide to dote adorably on that little sib – that is, until treasured trips to the playground become scheduled around baby naps, Mummy's lap is monopolised by baby feedings, and early-evening routines are disrupted by baby colic.

Concerned about the road ahead? Use these tips to help you navigate the bumps – and potholes – of two under 2, so they won't trip you and your toddler up:

Put yourself in your toddler's shoes. A little perspective goes a long way in helping you understand your older baby's new baby ambivalence. Imagine, for a moment, how you would feel if your husband walked in the front door with another woman, and cheerfully announced (fully expecting you to be happy about it): "Look, darling – this is our new wife! We're all going to live together, and be happy together . . . and by the way, isn't she gorgeous?" Well, it's the same thing for your toddler when you step in the door with a new baby. A little suspicion about this new situation – and some resentment – is perfectly normal. Something else to keep in mind: your tot may be older, but he or she is still very, very young. Despite his or her new designation as big sib, your toddler can – and should – be expected to act that very young age.

Enlist a helper. To make the new and needy competition less threatening, appoint your toddler Big Helper – a full-fledged member of Team Baby. Show your tot how to kiss without smothering, hug without squeezing, hold (carefully seated and supervised) while supporting the baby's floppy head. If your toddler wants to play with the baby, have him or her hold out a clean finger for the baby to clutch, or shake a rattle softly while the baby watches (be nearby to make sure the shaking doesn't turn into baby-rattling). Encourage your toddler to entertain the baby with songs, dances, and funny faces. If your toddler is clamouring to take on baby-care duties he or she isn't quite ready for – like burping, bathing, and nappy changing – hand over a baby doll to practise on (and fully control) instead. Meanwhile, look for age-appropriate tasks that'll make your little big sib feel competent and proud – even a 1-year-old can become an expert fetcher of nappies, dummies, flannels, and rattles.

Make three company. Those endless feeding sessions will be easier for your older little one to cope with if he or she isn't on the outside looking in. So invite your toddler to cuddle up beside you for a story or a quiet game while baby feeds.

Let your toddler be a baby. Let's face it – babies have the life. No responsibilities or expectations (beyond eating, sleeping, and nappy-filling), needs met instantly (no questions asked or strings attached), Mummy and Daddy on call 24/7 – it's pretty cushy. So don't be surprised if your toddler decides to act like a baby, hoping to cash in on the same cushy (and seemingly preferential) treatment. Taking a few baby steps backwards (a.k.a. regression) is nothing to worry about, and definitely nothing to show disapproval over. It's just a natural response to the new competition (as in "I'll have what she's having"). Instead of chiding "That's just for babies!" when your toddler tries to commandeer your newborn's dummy, offer a drink from a big-kid cup and a special snuggle close to you. Instead of teasing "Only babies cry" when your tot fake cries for your attention, offer the hug he or she is craving more than ever. Reassuring your tot that he or she is still your baby, too – with all those extra cuddles and all that extra lap time – may actually help the baby act run its course faster.

Play the big kid card. Even as you let your toddler know that it's okay to be a baby (especially given his or her tender age), take the opportunity – often – to point out "I love my big girl (or big boy)!" Reinforce big kid behaviours whenever you glimpse them – piling on the praise when your toddler shows patience (waiting without wailing while you change baby's nappy), cooperativeness (handing you that nappy instead of flinging it at the wall), or empathy (letting you know the baby's hungry). And play up the perks, every chance you get, of being the big kid in town – point out all the cool things he or she gets to do that the baby can't (like walk and climb, swing and go down the slide, paint and Play-Doh, eat real food).

Build in one-on-one time. Newborns need a lot of care, true – but they're generally not too picky about who provides that care. Your older one, on the other hand, is picky and – no surprise – picks you. Making sure you build some just-us time into every day will reassure your toddler that you love him or her just as much as you always did, and just as much as the new baby. Make a collage together, bake biscuits (which the baby can't eat – another bonus), or read stories while the baby naps.

Don't push the sibling bond. One minute your oldest will be in love with the baby – the next, he or she will want nothing to do with the tiny lap invader. That's partly due to his or her understandably mixed feelings, partly due to a toddler's fleeting attention span, partly because a newborn's not a whole lot of fun to play with yet, and partly because, unlike you, your toddler isn't programmed to adore the baby – especially not unconditionally or around the clock. The sibling relationship evolves over years, not days, so if your tot turns down your invitation to a group cuddle session or could care less about your newborn's newest trick, don't push it. Give your toddler time to grow into the big sib role.

"My toddler won't let me do anything for him. He only wants Daddy, Daddy, Daddy – and frankly, I'm insulted."

In many toddler homes, Mummy can do no wrong . . . and Daddy can do nothing at all. In other homes, like yours, Daddy rules. As with mum favouritism, dad bias is sometimes a product of circumstance (Dad's around more), sometimes one of personality (they're just made for each other). Either way, try not to take it personally – it's not a reflection on your mummy stuff. Instead, use these tips to help you get through the snubbing phase:

- Be patient. "It's just a phase" is something you'll be saying a lot throughout the second year (and the third, and the fourth, and the fourteenth . . .), and it holds especially true in this situation. Before you know it, it'll be your turn to shine.

- Be cool. If you're not the chosen one (this time around), don't make a big deal out of it. Show that your toddler's preference bothers you, and he's sure to stick even closer to Dad (remember, full-on empathy's not a 1-year-old's thing).

- Be positive. Try to warm your toddler up if he's been giving you the cold shoulder. Play his favourite game with him, or read his favourite book, or fix his favourite lunch. You'll be more likely to score points with your tot when the two of you are alone, but don't let that stop you from trying when you're all together, too.

- Be different. Carve out some activities that only you and your child do together – and that the preferred parent isn't already known for: cake baking, Sunday morning brunch, a stroll through the park to see the ducks, making Play-Doh.

"Our son seems jealous. Every time my husband tries to hug me, he pushes us apart and complains. At first we thought it was cute, but it's getting annoying."

Your toddler's not the only little Oedipus on the street. Many tots have a fierce, possessive love for the woman in their lives. And these feelings are both normal and normally transient – by the time they reach age 3 or 4, many boys start keeping Mum at arm's length, rejecting the hugs and kisses they used to clamour for.

While you're waiting for this jealous phase to pass, try not to react with annoyance (spurning your toddler for Daddy will only fuel jealousy and confirm his fear that Daddy poses a threat) or too sympathetically (spurning Daddy for him will only confuse his notion of family dynamics). Instead, try some good humour (but no laughter – he won't appreciate your making fun of his feelings). Include him in your hugs when he seeks to pry you apart, so that he won't feel left out, and remind him "I love you and I love Daddy. We all love each other. Group hug!"

Stranger Suspicion

"Every time someone outside the immediate family approaches my toddler, she hides behind me. Isn't this fear of strangers a little extreme?"

Extremely age-appropriate is more like it. So-called stranger suspicion is very common during the second year – and it's actually a much more mature and rational fear (rational to your tot, at least) than the "stranger anxiety" that many babies experience in the first year. Think of it as a thinking child's paranoia. Because your toddler is capable of more complex thoughts than she used to be, she's also capable of more complex fears. During this often intensely apprehensive time, every grown-up who isn't Mummy or Daddy may be viewed with suspicion: a neighbour, a babysitter, a friend; even a once-well-accepted grandparent or other relative may receive the distrustful treatment. While this fearful reaction may sometimes embarrass you and upset others (especially Grandma), it's actually not an altogether bad trait. In fact, if you think about it, knowing that your toddler isn't likely to walk off with the first stranger who offers her a sweetie should be somewhat comforting.

But fear probably isn't the only reason that your toddler stays hidden behind your legs in the face of strangers – there may be an element of annoyance, too. Consider how you might react towards a stranger, or someone you barely knew or recognised, who came right up to you and helped themselves to a hug, a tummy tickle, a pinch of your cheek, a pat of your head – who tried to pick you up or barrage you with silly questions you didn't even understand. It's likely that even you, a grown-up, might have a tough time minding your manners. For a toddler, who hasn't been around the social block, whose grasp of manners is shaky at best – well, it's no wonder she rebuffs the advance and dives behind your legs for protection.

Stranger suspicion, like most phases of toddlerhood, will inevitably come to an end – sooner in some children, later in others. While you're waiting for wariness to run its developmental course, there are ways you can help her (and yourself) cope more effectively with it:

Cut strangers off at the hug. Try intervening before a stranger makes a move towards your toddler. As with a suspicious animal, a suspicious child will be less fearful if the newcomer approaches her gradually. Without labelling your child as "shy" or "scared" (kids tend to live up to their labels), explain to the wannabe hugger that slow's the way to go.

Support her all the way. If your toddler wants to be held while in the company of strangers, hold her – for as long as she needs and wants to be held. If she wants to hide behind you, let her. When and if she's ready to go it alone, she'll let you know. In the meantime, offer your reassuring support and understanding unconditionally, and without demeaning comments ("You're acting like such a baby") or teasing ("You silly girl").

Try more exposure. Your toddler will thaw faster if she's exposed to a wide variety of familiar and unfamiliar people on a regular basis. So take her to the supermarket, shopping centre, museum, zoo, playground, and social gatherings. Travel on buses and the underground, go for walks down crowded streets. But be careful not to push your child to interact with the people she'll meet during these outings – always let her take the lead. Just being around strangers is achievement enough for now.

Don't push it. Often parents worry more about the rejected stranger's feelings than those of their child, especially if the "stranger" is a friend or relative they don't want to see rebuffed. So they may push a reluctant tot towards an exuberant stranger, with toddler tears the invariable result (and how's that going to go down with Grandma?). The strange truth about stranger suspicion is that the more you respect it, the faster it will fade. Push those interactions and you'll push your toddler farther behind your legs. Worried about the stranger's feelings (especially if he or she is no stranger)? Simply explain that the reaction shouldn't be taken personally – your tot's just at an age when only Mummy or Daddy will do.

No Fear of Strangers

"Our toddler is very outgoing and he'll go up to any stranger indiscriminately. That makes us a little nervous."

Some toddlers are fearless in the face of strangers – possibly, a little too fearless. Maybe it's because they're extra-extroverted by nature, maybe it's because they've had extra exposure to different people in different settings, maybe it's a combination of both. Because your toddler's judgement is no match for his outgoing nature yet, your vigilance in public will be his protection. Never let him out of your sight, even for a moment, when you're out and about. If he tends to wander, see the the next question for tips on keeping him close at hand.

Though it's too soon to expect your people-loving tot to be a good judge of strangers – or a good exerciser of impulse control – it isn't too soon to start building those skills, which will keep him safe in the future. When your toddler heads for a smiling stranger without your go-ahead, say: "If you want to say 'hello' to someone, you have to tell Mummy or Daddy." If he takes something from a stranger (like that sales assistant who hands him a piece of chocolate), remind him to check with you before accepting. The concept probably won't sink in yet, but repeated often, it will eventually. Meanwhile, you – and other caregivers – will be there to protect him from his own outgoing personality.

A word of caution about these precautions: as you gradually educate your toddler about stranger safety, be careful not to send the signal that strangers are universally menacing – most strangers are well-meaning, after all – or to stress him out about being sociable. Keep your stranger rules simple, and avoid incorporating scare tactics (don't warn that "strangers might be mean" or that "strangers might steal you"). The ultimate goal is to make your child appropriately cautious, not unreasonably fearful.

Wandering Off

"Whenever we go out with our 1½-year-old, she wanders off to look at this or that or runs ahead of us towards the street. We're constantly chasing after her."

Your toddler goes left when you want to go right. She turns right when you're facing left. She plows full speed straight ahead if there's a busy intersection on the horizon. She takes off the minute you put her down. And she puts you on notice the minute you step outdoors: the chase is on, Mum and Dad.

There's definitely a bit of catch-me-if-you-can sport in her wandering ways (and it's always entertaining for her when you run after her, waving your arms wildly and screeching for her to stop), but believe it or not, she's not just trying to annoy you or exhaust you. She's also trying to discover as much as she can every time she's out. Safety? Proper outdoor behaviour? Not on her list of priorities.

Balancing her outing agenda with yours isn't easy, but it can be done. To encourage your toddler's explorations while keeping her safe, teaching her some basic street sense, and even occasionally running an errand or two yourself, you'll need to begin thinking in terms of two kinds of outings:

- Parent-in-charge outings. Some places can be dangerous to explore: a crowded pavement, the middle of the street, a busy shop. When safety is at stake or when you've got a lot to do in a little time, your toddler's curiosity

Teaching Street Sense

Toddlers are brimming with energy, burning with curiosity, driven to discover. And they're also completely lacking in judgement, impulse control, and the ability to keep themselves safe. Having no danger radar of their own, they count on an adult's to keep them safe at all times. But while there's no substitute for constant vigilance, teaching your toddler some basic rules of the road (and the pavement) can be a great way to supplement your supervision – and groom him or her for a safe and responsible pedestrian future. There's lots to learn: never run out into the street. Always hold Mum or Dad's hand in a crowd. Stop, look, and listen at every corner. Stay in one place when a parent says so.

Of course, the only way for your toddler to learn this essential street sense is for you to give him or her the occasional, well-supervised opportunity to pound the pavement – those lessons can't be learned from a pushchair or your arms. So let your toddler loose (loosely speaking) sometimes.

Another lesson your toddler needs to learn: walking is a privilege that comes with strings attached – and most of the time, your hand. One chance (he tries to bolt into a crowd, she insists on running off when you've mandated her staying at your side), and it's back into the pushchair, your arms, or a firm handhold. Calmly explain that "there's no walking on your own if you break the rules", and then be consistent about enforcing those rules. Teaching a toddler to be reasonably street-smart takes a lot of patience, and resolutely repeating the same rules, outing after outing, but it's well worth the effort.

has to take a backseat (or a seat in the pushchair). Make it clear in such situations that she can't run ahead or lag behind, that she must hold your hand or ride in her pushchair. She may be more willing to agree to these road rules if you keep her occupied with questions, challenges, or observations about what you see around you, or with a round of silly songs or nursery rhymes.

- Toddler-in-charge outings. When time permits and the route you're taking is reasonably safe, let your toddler guide the expedition (always well within your sight, of course), dawdling to kick a mountain of leaves or rushing ahead to see a squirrel scamper up a tree. Just lace up your running shoes and be ready to take off when she does. She will get infinitely more satisfaction (and gain more knowledge) out of her explorations if you play co-explorer with her – pointing out that the acorn she found came from that oak tree, or that the dandelion she's smelling is yellow, or that the rock she's proudly displaying in her palm has some shiny spots in it that are called mica. Don't, however, monopolise her investigations or overdo the commentary (especially if she's tuning you out). Remember, she's leading the excursion.

And, of course, provide constant supervision – it takes only a second with your head turned away for a toddler to run off into a crowd at the shopping centre or dart into the street.

Fears and Phobias

"Every time I turn on the vacuum around my toddler, she starts screaming in fear. What can I do about it?"

Things that go bump in the night. Things that go woof. Things that get plugged in, make loud noises, suck up everything in sight, or loudly flush down the drain. To an adult, they're just a part of everyday life. To a toddler, they can be downright terrifying.

Topping the fright-worthy list in the second year are sudden, loud noises (like the vacuum), animals, and doctors. At age 2, fear typically comes in the form of the toilet (usually coinciding with potty training), the dark, and people in masks and costumes (such as clowns at the circus and Father Christmas at the shopping centre). But, as always, your one-of-a-kind toddler is likely to have her own one-of-a-kind set of fears.

What brings on those fears? Growing up, actually. Your toddler knows more and thinks more than she did as a baby, giving her more mature mind material for countless frightening scenarios. She's able to grasp cause and effect, but without the experience to sort out the reasonable from the un-, she thinks up consequences that might seem absurd to an adult. If a vacuum cleaner sucks up dust and dirt, could it also suck up me? If the dog on TV snapped, won't all dogs bite? If water goes down the bath drain, isn't it possible that a person – especially a small one like me – could, too?

Also contributing to fears are a growing imagination, a realisation that she's smaller (and thus more vulnerable) than those around her, an expanding memory ("I remember going too high on that swing and I didn't like it"), increased mobility (which allows her to toddle into fear-provoking encounters – with a meandering dog, a dangling spider, a lawn mower at work), and suggestibility (if a playmate or a sibling displays a fear of escalators, she may become afraid, too).

To help your toddler deal with fears:

- Realise the fears are real. They may seem irrational to you, but they are real to your toddler. Though ignoring many other kinds of behaviours may discourage them (think tantrums, whining), ignoring fear doesn't usually make it go away. In fact, not validating a fear can magnify it and/or make it the foundation of a lot of other fears (a fear of birds may grow into a fear of all animals; a fear of spiders may lead to a fear of all insects). Laughing it off can backfire, too. While a little playful teasing may work wonders on a toddler who's stubbornly refusing to get dressed for nursery, teasing a toddler who's terrified of dogs by getting on all fours and barking like a terrier may only feed the fear.

- Don't make your toddler face fears. Forcing a toddler who's afraid of dogs to pet the neighbour's collie, dunking a toddler afraid of water in the swimming pool, or insisting that a toddler afraid of the vacuum stand close to it when it's on could turn a fear into a long-term phobia. Admonishing "Be brave" or "Don't act like a baby" is also bad medicine. Instead, follow a fear-reduction programme that combines sensitive support and understanding with gradual exposure (see box, facing page).

- Keep your fears in check. If your toddler sees you take charge of your fears calmly, she may eventually learn to do likewise, based on your model. If, on the other hand, you jump high in the air every time you spy a spider, you'll be showing your toddler how to let fear take control.

- Let your toddler lean on you. Fearful toddlers need a strong, supportive hand to hold. Approach potentially challenging situations confidently and calmly, reassuring your toddler that you won't let anything hurt her. Try not to go overboard with coddling, though, or you may reinforce your toddler's fears ("If Mummy's giving me a whole lot of comfort, that dog must be a monster!")

- Steer clear of scares when you can. You can't avoid every dog, but it makes sense to cross the street so you won't walk close to the snarling dog's house. You can't avoid all loud noises, but it's a sure bet you should stay out of situations where thunderous applause or fireworks can be expected. If you and your tot come across an unexpected scare, offer reassurance, then distract your toddler right away – don't dwell on the fear.

- Try not to anticipate fears. Or to create them where they hadn't existed. Warning "Don't be scared" when a cat approaches you may introduce a fear of felines. Better to say "See the pretty kitty. She wants to say hello to us."

- Be a booster. Self-confidence can go a long way in overcoming fear. So praise every bit of progress your toddler makes over her fear (no matter how small) and avoid criticising steps taken backwards (no matter how big).

Fear of Dogs

"Whenever my toddler sees a dog, even if it's far away, he clings to me in terror. It's getting so bad we can't even take a walk any more."

Being a little cautious around dogs isn't such a bad thing, if you think about it. When toddlers are totally fearless, the consequences can be serious for little fingers and faces, as well as for fluffy tails and floppy ears. But while a little fear can go a long way in protecting your little one from the neighbourhood canines (and vice versa), it can definitely keep you both from exploring the neighbourhood – or any place where dogs roam. Not to mention, deprive him of the many benefits of having four-footed friends.

Facing Fears

Fearful that your little one's fears will last a lifetime? Fear not. As toddlers mature into more confident, rational, and worldly preschoolers, most fears fade (though others do persist throughout early childhood – and let's face it, sometimes through adulthood). In the meantime, you can try helping your little one face those big fears with a gentle, reassuring desensitisation process. Holding a toddler who's afraid of the vacuum cleaner at the other end of the living room while Daddy vacuums or standing with a drain-fearing toddler at the doorway of the bathroom while the bath empties may help him or her face the threat at a safe distance. Similarly, it may help to let a dog-fearful toddler watch a playmate frolic with a neighbour's dog, near enough to hear the giggles and see the glee, but far enough so that there's no perceived threat. Experimenting with turning a vacuum cleaner on and off may also ease a child's fears by allowing him or her to see that the control lies in the human hand, not the demon dust-sucker. Riding on the vacuum when it's unplugged may be reassuring, too. Your toddler doesn't handle desensitisation well? Don't push the programme. Just continue giving your little one the support he or she needs, and wait out the fear.

Is It Time for a Pet?

Like toddlers, pets are cuddly walking photo ops. But also like toddlers, pets are a major responsibility – particularly if they're (like toddlers) young and untrained. So you'd be smart to consider the responsibility pet ownership entails before you succumb to the irresistible selection at the local pet shop or shelter. Whether this is the right time to expand your family by one furry member will depend on several factors:

- Is your toddler comfortable with animals? Some toddlers are afraid or tentative around dogs and cats. If this is the case with your child, wait until he or she becomes more relaxed around animals before bringing a four-legged friend home.

- Is there enough room in your home for pet and toddler? Pets, especially puppies, need space to play in (just as toddlers do) – and feed in (you definitely don't want your toddler tucking into the kibble). Consider whether there's enough space in your home for child and pet to run around in without having a run-in.

- Is there enough time in your day (and night) for both a pet and a toddler? As you know if you've owned one before, pets need care, attention, and guidance – just like toddlers do. And unless you acquire a pet that's already obedience-trained, both have a whole lot to learn. Think about whether you have the time to feed, groom, entertain, clean up after, and teach them both. An even more critical consideration: will you be able to provide constant supervision for safety's sake? Since toddlers are much more likely than an older child to unknowingly provoke a pet, they are much more likely to become the victim of an animal attack. In other words, if you get a pet – especially one that has free run of the house – you'll have to watch your toddler even more carefully than you otherwise would.

Next, you'll need to decide what type of pet to get. Dog or cat – or bunny? Great Dane or mini schnauzer? Purebred or from the pound? Male or female? Frisky newborn or settled senior? Choosing the right pet isn't just about choosing the cutest one. You'll also need to consider the following before proceeding:

Species. Whether you've always been a cat lover, a dog lover, or a bird lover, your perspective may have to change to accommodate your toddler's needs. Here are some good choices for tots:

- Dogs. A dog can be not only a toddler's best friend, but also a good teacher. With the right dog, a young child can learn about animals and nature, about responsibility, about empathy, caring, and sharing, about getting along with others, about unconditional love and loyalty. And since dogs, especially young ones, like to run, jump, frisk, and frolic just as toddlers do, they can join in the toddler games long after parents have run out of energy or enthusiasm. Unlike parents, they're rarely too busy for a romp or a cuddle. Of course, not every dog lives up to this companionable description, so choose wisely (see the next page). Another less obvious bonus with getting a dog: researchers say that children who grow up around two or more dogs (or cats) may have a reduced risk of developing common allergies. While it's not known for sure why a houseful of flying fur seems to prevent allergies in children, scientists believe that early exposure to antigens carried by dogs and cats stimulates a protective response in the body's immune system, making it better able to resist allergies later. Of course, filling the house with furry friends solely to prevent allergies you're not sure your child will develop doesn't make sense.

- Cats. In general, cats may not be as naturally compatible companions for toddlers as dogs are. Though some cats (particularly those raised in a family with children) are very affectionate and fairly patient with toddlers, many felines prefer the more sedate company of adults. They may be less likely to run around with a toddler than to run away from one. They may also be less tolerant of a toddler's rough play, and that can prove frustrating – and possibly dangerous – to the toddler. (Keep in mind that some dogs, especially small or high-strung ones, may be just as impatient and just as potentially dangerous.) If you choose a cat as a pet, screen candidates carefully with your toddler in tow.

- Birds. Most birds, ensconced in childproofed cages, can be an interesting-to-watch (if not safe-to-play-with) pet choice for a toddler. The bird will also be safe from the rough and tumble toddler who won't be able to ruffle its feathers (literally). Potential perk: if the bird talks, your tot may pick up some words. A potential pitfall: many birds bite.

- Fish. Young children love watching fish swim around a tank, and it's actually a great way for a wound-up toddler to unwind. Just be sure your little one knows that fish are for watching, not petting or touching – and no hands in the water.

- Hamsters and guinea pigs. Both are low-maintenance pets that will delight your toddler (especially if you outfit the cage with an exercise wheel), but remember that most hamsters and gerbils are nocturnal animals (something you're hoping your human little one won't be any more). Guinea pigs, who play by day and sleep by night may be the better bet. No matter what rodent you choose, make sure the cage is high enough that your toddler can't unlatch it on his or her own, or make the latch toddlerproof. And remember that these balls of fur can bite – especially when they're poked or prodded.

You're best off not bringing members of the reptile family into your home when you've got a toddler, since they can carry disease. Rabbits, while temptingly cuddly and cute, should probably be left in the pet shop for now, too. They tend to be biters.

Breed. Not all dog breeds are equally patient and playful with children, so do your homework before you start your search. Often, mixed breeds are less high-strung, more easygoing, and easier to train than purebreds. But more important than breed is the personality of the individual animal, so spend some time getting to know a prospective pet with your toddler before you seal the deal. The right pet will be friendly and affectionate, won't shy away from young children, and will not snap or scratch if an ear is poked or a tail pulled.

Gender. In general, female dogs are gentler than males, while male cats are often more people-loving and affectionate than females. Neutering tends to make both dogs and cats less aggressive, more gentle, and easier to handle. But, again, individual temperament should be the overriding consideration.

(continued on next page)

(continued from previous page)

Age. The advantage of buying a puppy or kitten is that it can grow up with your toddler. The disadvantage, of course, is that you'll have two babies in the house, both of whom require a lot of attention and training. A mature animal will usually be housebroken or litter-trained, a definite plus. But it will also be set in its ways and may have a difficult time making friends with your toddler (unless it was raised in a family with small children) – and it may lack the energy it'll need to keep up with your two-legged tyke. Consider, too, that a pet on the brink of old age may require more time-consuming care than you can give.

If you do decide to go ahead with your plans for a pet (or you already have a pet and need to step up safety now that your toddler is mobile), consider the steps you'll need to take to get your pet toddler-ready (and your toddler pet-ready):

- Pets need to be toddler-trained. A toddler's high-energy style can take getting used to, especially if your new pet isn't used to young children. Even if your new pet lived with children previously, have it spend time with your toddler at first only under close supervision. Keep these getting-to-know-each-other sessions brief at first so that neither the animal nor your toddler will be overwhelmed. Closely monitor the pet's reaction to your toddler's actions and antics.

- Toddlers need to be pet-trained. Often overly exuberant toddlers can hurt or alarm a pet when they actually mean to show affection or get a good game going. See the box on page 202 for tips on training your toddler in pet sensitivity and safety.

Pets and toddlers may need to be protected from each other, at least at first. Since both can be unpredictable – and both, frankly, can act like animals – the potential for harm, intentional or not, is there on both sides. Always supervise your toddler while they're together and provide a separate safe play space for each (seal off areas with a closed door or a gate – if neither can scale it – so neither can get access to the other's space). A large crate might be a good refuge for a dog that's tired of toddler antics.

- Pet bowls and toddlers don't mix. Feed your pet when your little one is sleeping, busy in another room, or not at home. Pick up the pet bowl after each meal, unless it's in a space that's inaccessible to your toddler. These steps will not only keep your toddler from nibbling on the kibble but also keep your pet from nibbling on your toddler when it catches his or her fingers in the chow. Even friendly animals tend to turn hostile when their food or water is threatened. Another reason to keep your toddler away from the pet food bowl: pet food (and the bowl it's been in) can harbour salmonella.

- It may also make sense to keep your pet out of the room when your toddler is eating – especially if more food tends to end up in (and on) your pet than in your toddler.

- Keep your pet healthy. From vaccinations to flea, tick, and worm prevention, be sure your pet is up-to-date with immunisations and other preventive care. Some pet health problems can spread to humans, especially little ones.

No need to aim to eliminate your toddler's fear entirely. Just modify it, so that he can approach dogs with sensible caution, not senseless panic. Here's how:

- Make nice to make-believe dogs. Spend some time acclimating your tot to furry friends who can't jump, lick, or bite: cuddly toy dogs he can pet, hug, and control; battery-operated dogs that bark and romp; picture-book dogs of all sizes and breeds. Read stories that centre on friendships between children and dogs and that depict dogs as playmates, as helpers, as heroes.

- Demystify dogs. Explain that barking and tail-wagging are a dog's way of talking, and that dogs sometimes jump on or bump into people to say hello. Also show – on a stuffed pet – the proper petting protocol (see box, next page).

- Seek out mellow mutts. Check with friends, neighbours, and relatives to locate a real live dog who's good tempered (older dogs and dogs who have been spayed or fixed are usually more placid than puppies, but temperament can also vary with breed and within breed), friendly (but not over-the-top friendly, since jumping and slobbering can frighten a toddler as much as barking and biting), and accustomed to children (some dogs are as wary of young children as young children are of them). Then you can do some doggy desensitisation.

- Start with a snapshot. Before the face-to-snout introduction takes place, show a picture of the dream dog to your toddler, and give a little back story ("The dog's name is Ralph – isn't he cute?").

- Arrange the meet and (hopefully) greet. Do the introductions from a distance at first – your toddler in your arms, the dog held securely by its master. Wave to the dog, talk to it and about it by name, and encourage your child to do the same. If he seems nervous, try to reassure him. Make a point of asking the owner for permission before moving forward, even if you know you have it.

- Give him space and time. If he doesn't seem ready to make contact during the first visit, schedule these not-too-close encounters until he warms up. As his comfort level increases, decrease the distance between him and the dog until he's finally near enough to touch it (but keep him in your arms at first to give him a sense of security and a height advantage). Don't force him, or even urge him, to pet the dog at this point. Instead, pet the dog yourself. Say "See, I'm petting the nice doggy. He's so soft. Do you want to pet the doggy, too?" If he shows interest, have him pet the dog as you hold his hand and show him how to stroke fur gently. If he refuses, let him know "That's okay. Maybe next time you'll pet the doggy." Give him an opportunity to change his mind each time you visit with the dog – and keep up the visits until he finally summons the courage to reach out and pet his new pal.

With lots of patience, no pushing, and a desensitisation process where he sets the pace, your toddler should be able to overcome his fear of dogs eventually – maybe he'll even become a dog lover.

Since little children can pick up stress signals from their parents like a white sofa picks up dog hair, he won't buy your "There's nothing to be afraid of" line if you've got some dog fears of your own. You'll have to overcome yours before you can help your tot conquer his.

Pet Prescriptions

Whether or not they have four-footed siblings at home, toddlers should be petproofed as early on as possible. Teach your toddler the following pet etiquette:

■ Let sleeping (and eating) dogs (and cats) lie. Don't touch or go near pets when they're napping or eating. And never touch their food. Curious fingers can easily be perceived as a threat – even a mellow animal may retaliate.

■ Never poke an animal's eyes, pull its tail, or tug on its ears. Always pet with palms down and fingers curled inward. (Show your toddler how to do this.) Avoid holding its paws and don't pat a dog on the head – it implies domination. Instead, pet gently under the chin.

■ Always ask the owner before you pet or touch any animal.

■ Never go near any pet you don't know, especially one that's not on a lead, unless there's a grown-up with you. Same goes for members of the wild animal kingdom, such as squirrels and birds.

■ Stay away from dogs or cats when they're fighting.

■ Stay away from a mummy dog or cat who is with her babies. She'll fight to protect her offspring.

■ Always move slowly when you approach an animal. Don't run towards an animal or ride a riding toy up to an animal. It can get scared by sudden movements, including jumping.

■ Never put your face near a dog's face. (Because toddlers are small, they are most likely to be bitten in danger areas – face, head, and neck.) The same goes for cats (since a feline's teeth and claws can do a lot of harm to tender young skin, too).

No Fear of Dogs

"Not only isn't my toddler afraid of dogs, she's completely fearless, even with animals she's never met. And that worries me."

Dogs and toddlers have a lot in common – they're frisky, exuberant, volatile, impulsive, unpredictable, cute, and often hard to control. Put them together and you've got the stuff that Hallmark moments are made of – or a disaster waiting to happen.

To keep her dog-loving ways safe ones, start instilling a little caution now. Whenever she runs up to a strange dog or one you know well enough not to trust, stop her before she gets too close. Without scaring her (you don't want to turn her from fearless to fearful), calmly explain, "You can pet a dog only if Mummy or Daddy is with you and says it's okay – and the dog's owner says it's okay, too." Repeat the message every time she encounters a dog. Also begin making your toddler familiar with the pet prescriptions in the box above.

Negativity

"No matter what we tell him or ask him, our toddler has the same answer: 'No!' Sometimes it's cute . . . but most of the time it's frustrating."

It isn't always a toddler's first word, but "no" quickly becomes a favourite word – the one-size-fits-all response to just about everything you've got to say. Even when you've just said something you're sure he agrees with, or offered something you're sure he wants, he'll respond with a resounding "No!"

Some of this negativity has to do with physiology, especially early on ("no" is less challenging to say than "yes," shaking that little head side-to-side takes less coordination than shaking it up and down). A lot more of it has to do with psychology. More specifically: mum and dad psychology.

And it's pretty easy to analyse. "No" is, simply put, one syllable that speaks volumes about your toddler's emerging identity, his struggle for autonomy. It's his declaration of independence, primarily from you, his parents, and it states: "I am my own little person. I may only be a metre tall, but I'm the boss of me, and whenever possible, the boss of you, too. I'm nobody's baby (unless, of course, I need a cuddle . . . or a drink of milk . . . or a toy from a shelf I can't reach)."

Maybe your toddler's negativity will be halfhearted and short-lived . . . but more likely, not. For most 1- to 2-year olds, negativity is just getting rolling. As he picks up negative steam – and sharpens that trademark toddler stubborn streak – you can probably expect your little naysayer to say "no" more often and mean it more consistently (though he may continue to say "no" when he means "yes," just for negative effect). He'll say "no" to your limits, "no" to your requests, "no" to your offers, and of course, "no" to your questions. You can expect him to put up more of a fight, too, in that toddler-typical war of the wills (and will nots). Sometimes it'll be cute, sometimes it'll be exasperating, but it'll always be age-appropriate.

Though such negativity is just your toddler being a toddler, you'll still need to know how to deal with it:

Limit your "nos". Is your toddler learning "no" from the best – you? Understandably, it's a word little ones tend to hear a lot – especially before impulse control kicks in, and particularly from their parents. Of course there are times – plenty of them – when you'll find that no other word but "no" will do: "No hitting," "No emptying out your juice," "No throwing sand," "No walking outside unless you hold my hand." But too many "nos" may

Hug It Away

Have you hugged your toddler today? Daily hug therapy – squeezing as many squeezes, and cuddles, and snuggles, and nuzzles, and back rubs into your toddler's day as possible – is really one of the best strategies for managing those typically negative tot behaviours. Hug when the impulse strikes, but also when it doesn't (like when your tot's lost it in aisle 6, and you're about to lose it, too).

A rub on the neck, a stroke on the cheek, a sudden and unexpected embrace can often miraculously dissipate anger and bad feelings, heading off a tantrum or turning an afternoon gone awry onto a happier new course, and magically improving both your moods. It may not always work, but it's always worth a try.

Of course, since some children don't like to be held as much as others, tailor your touch therapy to your child. If he or she squirms out of your hugs, maybe a high five or some verbal "stroking" would be more appealing.

When to Say "Yes" to a "No"

Should you ever give in to your toddler's "no"? Actually, yes. It's simply a case of learning how to choose your battles.

Here's how it works. When "no" means "no" – not "maybe", and definitely not "yes" – your rules rule. So, for instance, there's no negotiation, no wriggle room, no exceptions to your rules when car seats must be buckled, medicine has to be taken, or walking-outside protocol must be followed (no walking unless an adult hand or the pushchair is held onto at all times). Not to say that your toddler will always give up without a struggle when you enforce certain rules – just to say that you won't back down on them, ever, no matter what.

But what about when a war of wills isn't worth fighting? When there's no real downside, and potentially an upside (a happier toddler, a less stressed you) to bending or breaking a rule – to letting a toddler "no" turn into a "yes" from you? That's when giving in can be a win–win. Let's say you and your toddler have run three errands already, and someone (besides you) is hungry and grumpy and has had enough. You arrive at the dry cleaners, and that someone shrieks, "No! Home!" (or maybe just "No!") If the dry cleaning can wait for another day, now would be an excellent time to give in and let your toddler win. Your toddler calms down, the shrieking that threatened to explode into wailing stops, and the rest of your afternoon could actually be more pleasant than it would have been. Most important, you'll have sent an important message: sometimes you'll win, sometimes you'll lose – and for now, I'll decide which is which. Just remember to choose your battles with care. If not picking up the dry cleaning means you'll have no clean clothes for work tomorrow, your toddler will have to deal with no deal.

---

dilute their effectiveness, as well as your authority – even egging your toddler on, when what you're really trying to do is head him off at the pass (to the remote control . . . to the dishwasher . . . to the stagnant pool of park water). What's more, it can threaten his brand new sense of self and step up negativity (which means the more times your toddler hears "no", the more you may hear it). So say "no" when you need to, by all means, but try to avoid playing it on a loop.

Be careful what you ask for. When you'd rather not take "no" for an answer, be crafty with your questions. Instead of asking "Do you want to put your jumper on?" or even saying "Let's put your jumper on", offer up a choice: "Do you want to wear the jumper with the bear on it or the jumper with the stripes?" Hold them up, and your toddler may actually point to his sweater of choice. Instead of "It's time to wash hands for dinner", try "Where do you want to wash your hands, in the kitchen or the bathroom?" Realistically, your toddler may sometimes answer even multiple-choice questions with "no" – or with a stubborn shake of his head. But it may also surprise you, now and again, how a little power in your toddler's hands can take some of the power struggle off yours. Just make sure you offer that power only when it's appropriate – and that choice only when it's available. When there is no choice, don't offer one. Asking "Do you want to go home now or go down the slide again?" when going home is the only option is asking for trouble (and a "No!"). A better exit strategy: "It's time to go home now. When we get home, should we draw a picture or play with your cars?" Stay away from other hot-button questions that have non-negotiable answers, too, like "Do you want to get ready for bed?"

No giggling. Of course, a sense of humour can help keep you sane on those days when your toddler's testing your limits – and trying your patience. Plus, keeping a straight face in the face of toddler cuteness is never easy, so an occasional giggle is understandable. But always cracking up at your toddler's negative antics can backfire: first, by annoying him (nobody likes being laughed at when they're trying to make a serious point); second, by reinforcing the negativity ("Mum and Dad giggle when I say 'no'. This behaviour's a keeper!").

Be the boss, but don't be bossy. You're the parent; you're the boss. And now that this important point is cleared up, here's the "but": but, good bosses try not to be bossy. In charge, for sure, in control, without a doubt – but not bossy. As you go about parenting your toddler, the good-boss model (hopefully you've had one or two along the way) is the one you should try to emulate when you can. You may elicit less negativity if you engage your toddler in cooperating, instead of commanding cooperation. So instead of "It's time for bed. No more playing", try "Let's get ready for bed. Can you help me find the bedtime book?"

Keep your cool. Another trait that good bosses have in common: the ability to stay calm, even when things take a turn for the tense – which, in turn,

keeps everyone else in the workplace from losing it. The toddler application: your toddler's negative, you're calm, your toddler eventually calms down, too, and everyone's happier sooner. Obviously, toddlers being toddlers, a calm approach won't always turn a negative into a positive – but it'll definitely have a better chance of working than the bad-boss model (boss loses it, whole team loses it, nothing gets done, everyone's mad).

Stay positive. Negativity won't last forever, no matter what. And all other things being equal (some toddlers – like some adults – are just more naturally negative, or more naturally high strung, or more naturally stubborn), the worst of it will pass more quickly if you stay positive. Reinforce your toddler's cooperative behaviour instead of highlighting the not-so-cooperative and you'll gradually see more of the former and less of the latter.

Not Listening to Your "No"

"My toddler loves to say the word 'no', just not to comply with it when I say it. What should I do?"

You probably like to get your way – everybody does. But by this point in your life, you've also come to terms with the fact that you won't always get your way. That you'll win some, you'll lose some.

It almost goes without saying that this particular realisation hasn't checked in with your toddler yet. To your little one – with her very small perspective but her very oversize ego – her way is still the only way. At least, the only way that matters. Which is why saying "no" isn't a problem for her, but accepting "no" is.

Testing authority is part of gaining autonomy, which is to say it's part of growing up. It's normal and age-appropriate. And for you, the parent (and to a lesser extent, other authority figures in your toddler's life), it's frequently frustrating.

To help your toddler learn (eventually) to take "no" as well as she dishes it out:

Avoid "no" overload. Too many nos can easily lead to toddler tune-out. So try to find a happy balance, saving "no" for when you mean it, saying "yes" when there's no compelling reason not to. You can avoid some nos with thorough childproofing – put a lock on the bin, say, and you won't always be warning her to stay out of it.

Expect the best. Anticipate a misdeed and that's what you're guaranteed to get. Even if your toddler is clearly making a beeline for your laptop, wait until those chubby little fingers have made contact with the forbidden buttons before you say "No touching the computer". Who knows – maybe she'll get distracted by a dropped toy and never wind up touching the computer at all . . . which means you'll save yourself (and your little one) an unnecessary "no". Or she'll end up touching it, and you'll end up saying "no" – but not before the misdeed has actually been done (for your toddler to become trustworthy one day, she'll have to know she's worthy of trust). Maybe she'll try to touch the buttons again and again, but she'll be less likely to push them just to push your buttons. Of course, if she's on her way to something dangerous, redirecting her up front isn't only a good idea, it's the best idea.

Make a switch. Turn lose–lose situations into win–wins by following up a necessary "no" with a satisfying "yes".

She goes for your book, so you say "No, you can't play with Mummy's book. But, yes, you can look at yours." Quickly put away your book, substitute hers, and everybody's a winner.

Be a spin doctor. The prescription for getting a more cooperative toddler? A more positive parent. "Please stay on the pavement" is somewhat more likely to cash in on compliance than "No walking in the mud!" Spin it positively with a little distraction, and the odds of her tuning in and cooperating increase exponentially: "Let's stay together on the pavement. We can look for birds. There's a bird!" Asking for help invites compliance, too. So next time she throws your papers on the floor, try "Mummy's papers need to stay on Mummy's desk. Please help Mummy pick them up and put them back."

Mean it when you say it. If "no" is ever going to mean something to your toddler, she has to know it means something to you. When you see her dipping into the dog bowl, "No eating Darwin's food, please" is a good place to start. But you're not finished without a thorough follow-through. If you turn right back to stirring the pasta sauce, she's more likely to tune you out – not only this time, but next time. Instead, put down what you're doing, remove the dog bowl along with another "No eating Darwin's food" to reinforce your point, then distract your toddler promptly. Do it calmly, matter-of-factly, without anger, pleading, or giggling, and your "no" – and your authority – automatically have more credibility, and possibly better results.

Keep it short. Sometimes, children don't listen to their parents in self-defence. If you have a tendency to drone on and on, that's just another excuse for your toddler to tune out your directives.

So offer an explanation but keep it short and sweet. Knowing that there's a reason for rules makes rules easier to follow, eventually, but remember that easy does it. "If you wash your hands, you won't get dirt on your cheese stick" is easier to swallow than "No hand washing, no cheese stick!" But you'll lose your toddler with a 10-minute explanation about germs, dirt, a cheese stick that tastes bad, dirt that gets in your teeth . . . and so on . . . and so on. When there's no time for an explanation, or you're just not in the mood, or you're pretty sure your toddler won't understand anyway, it's fine to pull out the timeless "those are the rules", "because I said so", or "no means no."

Commend compliance. Your toddler backed away from the hot cooker top without a second – or third – "no"? Time to bring out the positive reinforcements: "Good job!"

Whining

"My son's constant whining is driving me nuts. I usually end up giving in to everything he whines for just so he'll stop."

Forget a dripping tap, fingernails on a blackboard, or squeaky brakes. A young child's whining (which is really a kind of low-grade crying) tops the list of irritating sounds – and whining can get under a parent's skin faster and more effectively than any other behaviour. A tantrum? At least that erupts and subsides. Whining is steady, unrelenting, nerve grating, maddening.

What brings on the whine? Tiredness, hunger, boredom, overstimulation, frustration, lack of attention – to name a few triggers. There's no sure cure for whining, but it's sometimes possible to prevent an attack or to deal with it more effectively when all

fails and whining begins (it's bound to happen):

Pay attention. Toddlers often whine after they've tried and failed at other ways of attracting attention. So no matter how busy you are, or how many tasks you're juggling, listen when your toddler talks to you and try not to take too long to respond when he asks for your help (you're good at multitasking . . . right?). If possible, take a few moments to read a story, do a puzzle together, or just sit quietly and cuddle.

Eliminate triggers. He's hungry? Feed him. He's got a pooey nappy? Change him. Tired? Nap him. Bored? Involve him in an activity before the whining begins. If he seems generally out of sorts, consider that he may be coming down with something or might simply need some extra attention or comfort, so bring it on. Sometimes all it'll take is a quick cuddle or a back rub to relax your toddler out of a whiny mood (and as a bonus, it may make you feel better, too).

Fend off frustrations. Some frustration is a necessary part of learning new skills (and for that matter, of life). But too much frustration can bring on the whine. Make sure you aren't pushing your toddler to perform beyond his skill set or giving him toys that are not age-appropriate. When you see your toddler becoming overly frustrated, offer a helping hand.

Distract. Distraction – that all-purpose parental ploy – can allow a toddler to stop whining without losing face. He's whining for a toy you've passed by at the shops? Overlook the request and say "Let's get home fast so we can make a picture for Grandma!" Hopefully, the diversion you create will take your toddler's mind off the toy and switch off his whining.

Feeling Down

Having one of those down days – and worried about your true blue colours bleeding through while you're with your toddler? Don't be. Among the many important life lessons that your toddler needs to learn is that everyone feels down sometimes, even parents – and that it's okay to show you're blue, too. Always keeping your sad feelings under wraps can give your child unrealistic emotional expectations – after all, no one can be happy all the time. It can also lead your little one to believe that repression is the better part of valour (which it definitely isn't). Healthier by far is to grow up knowing that sad feelings are valid and that sharing them (or even asking for help in dealing with them) is one of the best ways to turn a frown upside down ("I bet a hug would make me feel lots better"). Which means that along with teaching emotional coping skills, you'll also be encouraging the development of your little one's empathy.

That said, your mood matters to your toddler. If you've been feeling down a lot, it's time to take some positive steps to lift your mood:

Figure out why you're blue. Try to get to the bottom of what's getting you down. Maybe it's not having enough time to yourself or with your spouse. Maybe it's the stress of work, or stress over not working (What if your career falls behind? What if you can't pay the bills? And what if you're finding yourself bored?). Maybe it's from feeling overwhelmed and under-helped. Once you've identified the source, try to do something about it (consider getting a part-time job, ask for more help around the house, plan a date night, schedule in some "me time").

Take care of yourself. Is taking good care of your toddler keeping you from taking good care of yourself? That's understandable (you're a parent, after all), but in the long run, not a smart strategy. Good health habits don't only do your body good, they benefit your mind, too. So make sure you're getting a reasonable amount of sleep, eating regularly and well (blood sugar crashes take your mood down, too), and getting plenty of exercise (the endorphins released during a workout actually do generate an exercise-induced high). You may also get a lift from mood-boosting omega-3s (take a supplement or make sure your diet gives you a healthy dose; see page 92), or from time spent outside, especially when it's sunny (even five minutes of outdoor exercise can fade the blues). And, yes, from a little chocolate, preferably dark.

Have a good cry. Feel like crying? Go ahead, and make your day. Believe it or not, some research has shown that crying helps improve mood by ridding the body of depression-triggering chemicals, which exit with the tears. So let them flow. When possible, do your crying away from your toddler, but don't worry if he or she happens to catch you mid-cry. Just dry your tears, segue into a hug, and quickly move on to a fun activity to distract you both. You can also say "I was sad, now I feel happy."

Get silly. Injecting a little silliness can sometimes switch off the whining. You could pretend, for instance, not to know where the whining is coming from ("Do you hear that squeaky sound? Where do you think it's coming from?"). Proceed to check under the sofa, behind the television, and in the closet

Have a good laugh. Laughter's the best mood medicine – and it's easier than you'd think to administer. Researchers have found that smiling and laughing, even if it's completely forced at first (as in, the last thing you feel like doing right now) can literally turn a bad mood good. In other words, plastering on a happy face can literally make you feel genuinely happy. Can't think of anything to smile about? Close your eyes for a moment and recall the cutest thing your toddler did this week.

Cheer up with your toddler. Even a toddler whose food fights and tantrums have gotten the best of you lately can become part of the solution. Go somewhere fun with your toddler – the zoo, the children's museum, the playground. Ideally, go with another parent–child duo so you will have some adult companionship, too.

Cheer up without your toddler. Whatever it is that gives you a lift, indulge yourself – do it, enjoy it, and don't feel guilty about it. Get a babysitter (or exchange-sit with another parent) and head for the gym, a dance class, some retail therapy, the cinema, the nail salon, lunch with a pal, a date night.

Unwind with your toddler. Try sharing some quiet time – relaxing on the front lawn and watching the clouds pass or the stars twinkle in the sky, cuddling on your bed and listening to soothing music. And don't forget the best therapy of all: a hug from your love bug.

Unwind without your toddler. Does time never seem to be on your side? Stop the clock once in a while – or at least, slow down the pace – and steal that just-for-you time. Let that pile of washing wait (where's it going, anyway?), and use your toddler's afternoon naptime to soak in a bubble bath, do a little yoga, read a book (one with more than four words on a page for a change) . . . or all of the above.

Talk it out. Share what you're feeling with anyone who will listen – your spouse, a pal, your Facebook friends. Often, just unbottling what's bogging you down can help you rise above it. If you don't have some communication time built into your day, add it now – everybody needs to have an adult conversation every now and then.

Get help if you need it. An occasional down day, or even a few down days in a row, is normal, especially during times of high stress. But slumps that come often – and that you can't easily bounce back from – can start to take an emotional and physical toll on you and your little one (children of depressed parents are often depressed themselves). If feelings of sadness interfere with your functioning or your relationships (including your relationship with your toddler), and/or if your depression is accompanied by sleeplessness, lack of appetite, loss of interest in yourself and your family, feelings of hopelessness or helplessness, thoughts of hurting yourself or another, and/or lack of control, don't wait for it to pass. Get the professional help you need – and that can help – right away. Need help finding it? Speak to your doctor or visit www.nhs.uk.

before stumbling upon the source of the squeak (your toddler's mouth, of course). If that hasn't stopped the whining and started the giggling, offer to "fix that squeak" (blowing raspberries on the belly usually does the trick). For older toddlers and preschoolers, a dose of good-natured reverse psychology may also reverse the whining process ("I don't think you're whining enough. I think you'd better whine more"). If your tyke becomes more upset at the slightest hint of teasing, though, skip this one and try another tactic.

Don't give in. When your toddler starts to whine, matter-of-factly make it clear that it won't get him anywhere – you'll listen only if he uses his "normal" voice. Then avoid eye contact and don't respond to the whines (stay firm, Mum and Dad). If your tot changes to his normal voice, try to satisfy his request or offer options: "I can't give you a biscuit now, but you can have a banana or some grapes." If the whining continues (and even if it threatens your sanity), don't buckle. Giving in after 20 minutes of incessant whining teaches your toddler that persistence is the key to successful whining – that if he simply whines long enough, he'll always get what he wants.

Get him talking. If your tot is verbal enough, encourage words instead of whining: "I know you're upset about something. Let's see if I can help you say what it is."

Provide voice lessons. Children often don't realise the negative effect of whining on other people until they hear it for themselves. Point out when another child is whining – your toddler may agree that the noise is hard to take. Reinforce by explaining, "Whining hurts my ears – ouch!" With that realisation fresh in his mind, make a game out of practising your normal voices together – and then don't forget to reinforce how much better a normal voice sounds: "I like when you talk in your normal voice. It makes my ears happy!"

Avoid labels. Don't label your child a "whiner" – children are notorious for living up to parental expectations.

Unreasonableness

"I know that my daughter is too young to reason with, but her unreasonableness makes it really hard to get her to cooperate."

It's definitely hard to see it from your rational adult perspective, but your toddler actually has good reasons for being unreasonable. The most obvious reason, of course, is that she's a typical toddler, struggling for independence. She wants to make her own decisions, even if they're clearly (to you and the rest of the reasonable world) wrong. Why doesn't she know they're wrong? Because she hasn't yet acquired reasoning skills – and that's reason number two. No coat on a cold day? She's not yet able to anticipate consequences ("If I don't wear a coat, I'll be cold") and weigh them against her whims. Need more reasons? Being hungry, tired, frustrated, overstimulated, or feeling out of sorts can all trigger or step up unreasonableness. (Think about it: you're not at your most rational, either, when your blood sugar's plummeting or you're running on too little sleep.)

Reasoning with your unreasonable toddler is not realistic. Neither is arguing your point (arguing with a toddler will get you nowhere, even when she's at her most rational) or opening the floor up to debate (ditto). Instead, try these techniques:

Let cause have its effect. The best way to learn consequences is to experience them firsthand. It's called learning from mistakes – and it's particularly valuable when you've got so much to learn. So when the consequence of an unreasonable choice won't do anyone (or anything) any harm, let her live with it and maybe even learn from it: when she doesn't put her boots on, she can't play in the mud; when she throws her biscuit in the dirt, she can't eat it. It'll take plenty of trial and error (and tears) on her part, but eventually she'll begin to realise that parents sometimes have a point – and there's a reason for reason.

Hold the "I told you so"s. It may be tempting, after your toddler has disobeyed the injunction not to step in puddles, to rub her nose in her wet trainers – figuratively, at least. Resist that temptation. The consequence – cold, wet feet – is punishment enough for her faulty judgement, and she doesn't need your insults added to her injury. Instead, underline the lesson matter-of-factly: "Oops, wet feet. That's why we don't step in puddles without boots on."

Don't let irrationality rule when it comes to rules. If your toddler refuses to get into the car seat, and your efforts to cajole, distract, or humour haven't helped, you'll have to strap her in kicking and screaming. Likewise, if she tries to unshelve all the books at the library, her whim will need shelving.

Try a little Mum or Dad magic. You probably already have a stash of distraction tricks up your parental sleeve – pull some out and see if you can work some magic. Try a change of activity, a silly incongruity (the old boots-on-the-hands routine), reverse psychology, an ad-lib song, or a little fast-talking ("Do you know what we're doing after lunch today?").

Treat with food or rest. If it's been a while since her last meal or snack – or since her last nap – it could be hunger or tiredness inciting her irrational behaviour. So give her a snack if she's hungry, or pack her in for a nap if she's sleepy. And while you're at it, make sure that you've had something to eat recently, too – unreasonable toddlers are less exasperating to deal with when you're not grumpy with hunger yourself.

Laugh it off inside. Instead of letting your toddler's irrational behaviour drive you up a wall, look for the humour (and the cuteness) in it. Remember, she's just acting her age. Of course, keep your smiles under cover – even a tiny tot knows when she's not being taken seriously.

Impatience (Now!)

"No matter what it is, my toddler has to have it 'now'! I'm losing my patience with his impatience."

With no understanding of how time passes, no concept of past or future, your toddler lives for the moment – in other words, for "now". "Now" is when he wants a snack or a drink, when he wants a story read, when he wants to go on the swings (even though they're all occupied). He hasn't yet learned that good things come to those who wait. To him, good things come to those who demand immediate delivery.

It isn't until around the second birthday that the typical toddler begins to realise that there are times besides the present – and at that point, he'll be able (if not always willing) to comply when asked to "wait a minute". For now, you'll be hearing a lot of "now".

Be patient while you wait for your toddler to develop patience. To make that wait easier on you, you can try the following:

Make sure it's worth making him wait. Of course, on principle you'd like your toddler to wait for something he's asked for ("he's got to learn to be patient"), but it's not always fair or reasonable. Hunger and thirst, for example, are very pressing problems to him that need immediate resolution. If it's a half hour until dinner and he's hungry right now, offer a light, nutritious snack that will take the edge off his appetite without zapping it entirely.

Create a diversion. If the wait is legitimate and necessary, try to make the time pass more quickly with entertainment. Say you're in the car en route home and he wants his lunch "now!" A song, some favourite nursery rhymes, or an impromptu game – like "What does the cow say?" or "Can you see a doggy out the window?" – may buy just enough time to get you home.

Set a timer. If you need five more minutes on the computer before you can take your toddler to the park, set a timer and let him watch it until it dings. Or turn over a sand-filled egg timer and let him watch the sand sift through. This will give him some sense of control over you and over time, while making a very abstract concept a little more concrete. Just make sure that when the timer goes off or the sand's all sifted through, you'll be ready to keep your part of the bargain. Otherwise, he won't trust your deals in the future.

Move it. If you can't get it out of mind, get it out of sight. If your toddler wants something he can't or shouldn't have now (the riding toy on which he wants to scoot across your just-mopped, still-wet kitchen floor), physically separate him from it and stow it some place where he can't see it (like in the garage or spare bedroom).

Be willing to wait yourself. If you think about it, your toddler probably spends a lot of time being rushed ("Hurry up – we're late!"). Be a little more patient with him when you can (give him two more minutes to finish his project in the sandpit, an extra five minutes to dawdle on the pavement before rushing him along), and who knows? Maybe your patience will rub off on him . . . in time.

Demanding Attention

"Every time the phone rings or the doorbell rings, it's like a signal for my son to start whining for attention."

Toddlers, you might have noticed, don't like to share. And that doesn't just go for toys – it goes for attention, too, particularly yours. Anything or anyone that competes for your attention, from the phone conversation you're trying to have to the work you're trying to do, is not okay in his book (and speaking of books, Dad, don't even think about picking up that one unless you plan on reading it to me!). He'll fight for your attention with everything he's got, and as you've seen, he's got quite an effective arsenal (whining, carrying on, clinging to your leg like a baby chimp).

In your toddler's magical world, Mummy and Daddy would never be otherwise occupied. In the real world, there will be times when your attention can't be on-demand. To keep those worlds from colliding:

Don't give him any ideas. Anticipate a cry for attention before he's issued one, and you're sure to get it, in spades. Skip the warnings ("Now, don't cry while I'm on the phone!"), and instead just calmly go about your business. It's possible he won't even notice you've answered the phone.

Don't blow a fuse. Understand (and try to remember during times of stress) that your toddler's need for attention is age-appropriate, and that he'll respond better to empathy than to anger. As always, keeping your cool will help your toddler keep his.

Multitask. Staying in touch with your toddler as you chat on the phone or answer e-mails will help him feel less cut off, and may also take some of the edge off his phone or computer envy.

Let him know you're still there for him, even though you're busy with something else. Rub his arm or shoulder, cuddle him, bounce him on your lap, hold his hand, or get down on the floor and stack bricks with him. Granted, it's hard to concentrate on a conversation when you're being whisked from the bricks to the lorries, but that's better than no conversation at all.

Put him on the line. If you're on the phone with a friend or family member, invite your toddler to join in the conversation, either by handing him the phone or putting him on speaker. Granted, he'll have no idea where the disembodied voice is coming from (that's not Aunt Olivia!), and he probably won't know how to respond, but at least you'll have somewhat demystified the competition. If he pushes the phone away, don't press him. You can also allow him to "type" a few of his own e-mails if it's your screen time he's not happy about (obviously, make sure he's not online, or he may send who-knows-what to who-knows-who).

Add another line. Having his own play phone or computer may make your toddler feel less threatened by yours – plus it'll capitalise on his budding love of imitation. When you have to use your phone or computer, hand him his and suggest he call or send a message to someone special – Grandpa, his cousin, someone in his playgroup, a favourite storybook character. It doesn't matter if he doesn't speak many words yet – carrying on a one-sided babble or typing a pretend message may keep him happily occupied, at least for a few minutes.

Call in the positive reinforcements. Ultimately, of course, your goal is to get your toddler to recognise that you have rights, too – among them, the right to talk on the phone or pay bills or answer texts, if only for brief sessions at a time. The best way to work towards that goal is to share your appreciation when he shares your attention. Add a bonus, too: "Thank you for letting me talk on the phone. Now we can do something special together."

"Whenever I'm trying to talk to someone, whether it's a friend I've run into or a repairman at the house, my daughter starts screaming for attention."

Most toddlers not only demand centre stage, they also prefer that the rest of the stage be empty. When you focus on someone besides your little one – whether it's a friend or relative you'd like to chat with or a plumber you need to show the leaky sink to – she'll do everything in her power to regain the spotlight of your attention. Among the many tricks in her repertoire, she may glue herself to your leg and turn on the whine, crawl all over your lap and pull your hair, screech and scream, or even clamp her hand over your mouth to keep you from speaking to someone else.

At this age, when a toddler's own wants and needs are the only wants and needs that matter to her, it's particularly difficult to teach her to respect the wants and needs of others. But while respect is a lesson that may take years to learn, there's no time like the present to start teaching it. With a lot of patience, understanding, careful choreography – and the following tips – your toddler and your visitors may come to share the stage successfully, at least sometimes:

Try not to interrupt her. You can't focus on your toddler all the time, and it's important for your sanity and her development that you not try to. But for her to learn how to respect your time with others, she'll need to see that you respect her time with you. So try (whenever possible, and obviously it won't always be) not to interrupt playtime with her to take care of something you can just as easily put off until she's independently occupied or asleep. Instead of popping up every 30 seconds to check the washing or update your Facebook status, try to provide your undivided attention. When a chore can't be put off, try involving your toddler, too (let her stack tins on the kitchen floor while you start dinner, have her doodle in her notebook while you return a text). If someone drops by while you and your child are at play, invite your guest to join the fun for a minute or two before you switch focus.

Time the entrance. If you can, try to schedule visitors to arrive during your toddler's usual naptime. If you can't, at least aim for a time of day when she's generally most cheerful.

Bring her on stage. If she's comfortable being sociable (don't push her if she's not), getting her involved may help her feel less left out. Ask her to show her favourite book or doll to your friend. Take her along to "help" show the plumber the leaky tap and let her watch the plumber open the pipes under the sink. If you're expecting a special visitor, your tot can help prepare. Clean up the living room together, bake or shop for biscuits, and decorate with pictures in honour of the visit (her ego will get a boost when her artwork is admired).

Provide special props. If you're having company, set up a special play area so she can be entertained while you're entertaining. Pile up some picture books and bricks, tape a piece of paper to the coffee table so she can scribble with crayons or pencils. If she likes pretend play, make arrangements for her own tea party so she's more likely

to keep out of yours. Or appoint her "cleaner-upper" and equip her with a feather duster and a play broom while you chat. Just be prepared to stop every now and then to encourage her on her brick tower, compliment her on her doodle, have a "sip" of her tea, or admire her dusting job.

Break for intermissions. There's only so long you can realistically expect your toddler to stay independently busy (and happy). Once it's clear she's about to reach her limit, excuse yourself from your company and take a toddler break. Make it clear what the limits of the intermission are before you begin ("Now I'm going to take a break and read you one book. When I'm done, I'll go back to my friend and you can do a puzzle"). When the break's over, set your toddler up with that puzzle or another activity before returning to your guest. Make time for physical contact, too. If she's playing at your feet, lean over frequently to squeeze her shoulder, rub her back, or pat her head.

Remember who's running the show. That would be you. Problem is, that's not how your toddler sees it from where she's sitting (and tugging on your leg). Help her see the light. Be understanding, be empathetic, be friendly, be calm, but be firm. Distract her, involve her, hold her, cuddle her, matter-of-factly remove her hands from your mouth as many times as you have to – but don't let her think that making a scene steals the show.

Applaud cooperation. Even if your toddler was only marginally cooperative while company called or you chatted with that friend (she whined just 75 per cent of the time), reinforce that little bit of positive behaviour instead of calling attention to that whole lot of negative behaviour ("I like the way you played nicely when I was talking to Jessica. Now you and I are going to do something special together!"). A trip to the park, an uninterrupted period of play with you, a collaborative art activity are all good ways of letting your toddler know how much you appreciated her patience, and how much patience can pay off. Of course, if she did whine 100 per cent of the time, hold your applause – but skip the commentary. Just reinforce the behaviour you'd like to see in the future ("Next time I talk to my friend, you'll play nicely").

Car Seat Conflict

"Our toddler hates riding in the car seat. Whenever we put him in it, he arches his back so that it's almost impossible to strap him in."

When you're born to be wild (and isn't every toddler?), being strapped into a car seat can really cramp your style – not to mention your sense of adventure. That's why most toddlers aren't easy riders. Still, whether you and your toddler are heading out on the motorway or driving around the corner, strapping in is a must. Not only is the car seat required by law in the UK, it can also make the difference between life and death in even a minor crash (see page 432 for more on car seat safety).

Clearly, in the battle of the buckle, you must come out the winner – no ifs, ands, buts, or negotiations possible. The following strategies should make winning that battle easier on you both:

Do a comfort check. If the car seat straps are too tight, the plastic is sticky, the padding is inadequate, or the seat is cramped, your tot may be protesting because he's uncomfortable. Correcting these problems may help change his tune.

Divert and conquer. Instead of starting out with "Now we have to strap you into your car seat", words that will quickly incite a struggle, distract your toddler with casual chatter ("Look at the sky – see how pretty it is", "Let's go to Meghan's house this afternoon", "We're going to have such a yummy lunch when we get home"). Or challenge him with questions ("What does the doggy say?", "Where's your nose?") as you quickly carry out the dastardly deed. Try a silly made-up song or rhyme that your toddler can begin to associate with being strapped in: "Let's strap in our belly and eat all our jelly!" Whether these ploys actually make him forget what's happening or simply allow him a graceful way out of having to make a fuss doesn't matter as long as they work. And they may, at least some of the time.

Add some music, maestro. Always have a supply of engaging children's tunes ready to soothe your toddler once he's been strapped in.

Strap in some entertainment. Diversion doesn't always work, but it's always worth a try. Have a few favourite toys at the ready to distract your child and occupy both his mind and his hands. Keep a rotating selection of toys that can be snapped, Velcroed, or tied (with plastic rings or a ribbon or cord no longer than 15 cm) to his car seat.

Let him strap in his "baby". If there are enough seat belts to go around, let your toddler help strap in a teddy bear, a doll, or a favourite toy before he gets into his car seat. Or, use a makeshift belt to tie the doll to your toddler's seat. Explain that safety belts are meant to keep his toys from falling out or getting hurt – and that's why people need to buckle up, too.

Buckle up together. The buckle-up rule should apply to everyone in your car, including the driver – in the interest not only of following the law and setting the right example, but also of safety.

Know how to fold him. A rigid, arching back can definitely stand in the way of getting him seated. To loosen him up so you can settle him in, tickle his belly, blow a raspberry on it, or be a kissing monster attacking his midsection – he won't be able to help folding.

Allow no exceptions. Even one "Okay, no car seat just for today" could be a tragic mistake. And surrendering once could undermine your authority on the issue, raising the hope in your child's mind that you can be persuaded to surrender again . . . and again. As every experienced parent knows, this is a tactical error.

Pushchair Problems

"I can't get my daughter into the push-chair without a fuss, and since I live in a city, that's the only way we get around."

Put yourself in your toddler's trainers, and you'll see why she fights being put in the pushchair. For someone who's just discovered the joys of life on two feet, having to sit it out is, after all, one of life's biggest bummers. Especially when everybody else on the pavement is walking.

Of course, understanding your toddler's perspective on the pushchair won't get the grocery shopping done. Or the dry cleaning dropped off. For that, you'll need your toddler in the pushchair – at least part of the time. To increase cooperation, it's worth trying the following tips. But ultimately, it's also worth accepting one of the realities of life with a toddler: getting there is rarely twice the fun, but it generally does take twice the time.

Arch Enemy

Back archers, whether they're in the form of pushchair strugglers or car seat mutineers, don't stand a chance against the old belly-button push trick. As you put your toddler in the seat, playfully push or tickle his or her belly. He or she will reflexively retract that arched back and lean forward, allowing you to strap him or her in. Presto . . . the deed is done. Score one for Team Parent!

Make sure the pushchair's fully packed. Bring along and attach to the pushchair a rotating supply of playthings designed specifically for the pushchair (if you use a ribbon or cord, make sure it's no more than 15 cm long; better still, use plastic links).

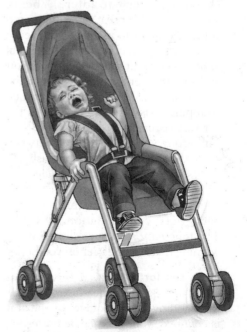

Many toddlers resist being cooped up in a pushchair – that is, unless Mum or Dad has asked them to walk instead.

Be distracting. From the moment you approach the pushchair, engage your toddler in a song, a conversation, or with a toy – she may be strapped in before she knows it. Strolling along, point out dogs, pretty flowers, displays in shop windows, cement mixers, and lorries. Chat about where you're going and what you're going to be doing. Break into a rousing chorus of "The wheels on the pushchair go round and round". Keep the distractions coming, and you may (at least sometimes) keep your toddler from complaining.

Empathise. When your toddler starts grumbling "No pushchair!" or, once in, yells "Get out!" be understanding. Respond with "I know you don't want to ride in the pushchair, but we don't have time for you to walk right now." Then dangle a carrot to (hopefully) keep her satisfied: "You can walk when we get near the house (or the shop, or the playground)."

Try a raspberry. Is she stiffening up on you when you try to sit her down in the pushchair? Arching her back? Try blowing a big raspberry on her belly – it'll reflexively collapse her rigid stance so you can ease her into the seat. Hopefully it'll put a smile on her face, too.

Be calm. It's a law of toddler nature: the more it seems to mean to you, the more your child will fight you on it. So try to come across unruffled by your toddler's pushchair struggles.

Let her walk. When it comes to car seats, there's no negotiating – not strapping in is not an option. But when it comes to pushchairs, there's usually more wriggle room. If it's feasible and practical (even if it means leaving a little earlier or arriving a little later), let your toddler walk. Having her "help" you push the pushchair (assuming she'll let

---

A Ride to Obesity?

Can't imagine life without a pushchair? Maybe you should, some of the time. As indispensable as they are for toddler-toting parents on the run, pushchairs may, according to some experts, be contributing to a less active lifestyle for young children – and, consequently, to increased rates of childhood obesity.

Does that mean you'll have to hide your pushchair? Not at all. Even experts who point out the pushchair's pitfalls can't argue with its compelling convenience, especially when you've got exactly 10 minutes to get in and out of a crowded shopping centre. But they do recommend that toddlers spend more time walking and less time riding – and that pushchair use be reserved for times when safety's an issue or time's really tight.

Now all you'll have to do is leave two hours early for that appointment two streets away.

---

you share the job) can keep her in step with you, as will holding hands. Let her walk as long as her little legs hold out; if she gets tired enough, she may even ask longingly for that pushchair.

"My son doesn't want to ride in the pushchair any more – he only wants to push it. This wouldn't be so bad, except that he pushes it into everyone and everything. When I try to take it away from him, he has a screaming fit. What can I do?"

The drive to gain control propels a toddler – whether it's control over what's served for breakfast, over when he goes to bed, or over who gets to steer his pushchair. In the latter case, this

Shopping with Toddlers: Mission Impossible?

Remember when running to the supermarket actually meant sprinting in and then out with what you needed in 10 minutes or less? When the greatest challenge posed by a shopping excursion was finding a dressing room that wasn't occupied (and a pair of jeans that actually fit)? Well, having a toddler certainly signals the end of shopping as you knew it. If a toddler isn't disappearing down the frozen-food aisle, he's trying to knock over a carefully stacked display of cereal boxes. If she isn't vanishing behind a sale rail, she's trying to go up the down escalator. If he isn't loudly demanding that you buy a treat or toy he's just spied on the shelf, he's throwing a full-blown tantrum in front of a sea of strangers. If she isn't hungry ("right now!"), she's thirsty ("right now!"), and if she isn't either, she's pooed in her nappy (and you forgot to bring a spare).

Yet shop you must. Following these tips won't make the process entirely painless, stress free, or a logistical piece of cake, but they may help you get the job done:

- Shop solo. Unless a fitting is necessary (as it is with shoes), even shopping for toddler clothing is better accomplished without the toddler.

Seize the opportunity to shop whenever there's someone else around to stay with your little one. Or organise a babysitting/shopping co-op with a friend who has a toddler, so you can take turns getting shopping done. Or alternate shopping duty with your spouse – one of you stays home with your toddler, and the other goes off to the shops. Or, don't leave home at all: do all your shopping (from groceries to clothes to nappies) online.

- Put timing on your side. There's no predicting toddler behaviour, but there's no point in writing a script for disaster (suggested title: "Mayhem at the Market") by taking your little one to the shop hungry, due for a nap, or overstimulated. Time your shopping trips accordingly.

- Don't go it alone. Even a tween who isn't old enough to babysit alone can do a good job of looking after and entertaining your toddler while you shop.

- Put it on paper. Before leaving home, make a detailed shopping list. Not only can this dramatically cut down on your actual shopping time, but it can eliminate the last-minute dash during checkout for the carton

drive can propel him (and the pushchair) into the heels of a pedestrian, the trunk of a tree, the dairy shelf at the supermarket, the flower bed in the park – annoying, destroying, and potentially putting himself at risk.

Although in some areas where toddlers crave control, it's possible to hand it over, it clearly isn't appropriate in the case of the runaway pushchair. Instead:

Leave home without it. Getting around without a pushchair may not be easy, but it may be easier than trying to get around with a toddler pushing his own pushchair. If necessary, put off walking trips that can't be accomplished without a pushchair, or make these trips using a car or public transportation.

Help him sit it out. If you make riding in the pushchair diverting enough (see

of eggs you forgot – as well as an extra trip to the supermarket when you forgot the eggs entirely. Plus, it can help you say "no" to toddler-generated impulse buys ("I'm sorry, but those crisps are not on my list").

- Spin it. Use a positive approach when telling your toddler about the behaviour you expect. For example, before going through the automatic doors at the supermarket, say "You're going to ride in the shopping trolley. You can help me find the foods on our list and put them in the trolley," not "You can't walk around inside, and no touching anything!" And don't forget to give positive reinforcement when your shopping companion has exercised even a modicum of cooperation.

- Provide transportation. You may be able to cut your shopping time if you can persuade your toddler to ride in the shopping trolley (strapped in for safety) at the supermarket rather than toddle down the aisles. Some supermarkets and shops have specially designed trolleys with cars or firetrucks for tots to sit in, which may help entice your toddler to climb in for the ride. Others have pint-size shopping trolleys for tots to fill and push.

- Make a run for it. Focus on getting everything you need in as short a time as possible. Leave label reading, comparison shopping, and careful scrutiny of produce for solo trips to the supermarket. Take the time to analyse a unit price, and your toddler could be two aisles away.

- Steer clear of trouble. If you know your regular shopping destinations well, it should be fairly easy to circumvent or at least speed by potential hot spots (such as the toy department, the fine china and crystal section, or the biscuit aisle). Some supermarkets have a sweet-free checkout counter to eliminate (at least in theory) the threat of toddler tantrums.

- Put your toddler to work. Idle hands are bound to reach out to pull breakable jars off the shelf, idle heads will think up ways to empty the contents of your purse while you're distracted. So keep your toddler busy "helping" – carrying a box of favourite crackers, loading (unbreakable) items into the trolley, pushing his or her own mini shopping trolley, counting out three containers of yogurt, spotting circles, or picking out apples. Though shopping will probably take a little longer with this kind of help, at least you'll have a chance at getting it done. Plus, your little one will likely love being a "big helper".

the previous answer for tips), he may not press so hard to push it.

Push together. If he won't take "sit" for an answer, offer a compromise alternative: you push the pushchair together. Instead of saying "I have to push because you're not big enough," emphasise teamwork – he's helping you and you're helping him. If he protests (and he probably will), explain matter-of-factly but firmly: "We can push the pushchair together, or you can ride in the pushchair."

Let him push something his own size. A child-size pushchair or shopping trolley is much easier for a toddler to keep on course than a full-size one (and both are wonderful for imaginative play at home, too). And since toy pushchairs and trolleys are lighter, they're less likely to inflict damage when pushed across someone's toes or into a shop display. (Remember that he'll still need a hand pushing it across the street, for safety's sake.)

Dressing Dilemmas

"We have a very active, always busy toddler, and getting him dressed in the morning is like running a marathon. I chase him from room to room trying to get his clothes on him."

On the plus side, your little one's helping you get your daily workout (who needs a step class?). On the minus side, too much running around and you'll be running late by the time both his legs are in his trousers.

Running from the hand that dresses him may be your toddler's way of getting attention when everyone is busy (and maybe stressed-out) preparing for the day. If you think that might be the case, try to work a little "quality time" into the morning schedule – read a story, play a quick game, have breakfast together. Or use one of these special activities as a carrot: "If you hurry up and get dressed, we'll have time to read your favourite book before we have to leave."

Is it over-the-top toddler energy that has him on the morning marathon circuit? Try dressing him as soon as he gets out of bed, before he has a chance to kick himself into high gear. Or, if time and patience allow, you could go along with this daily dressing marathon for a while and make a game of it: "Okay, we'll get your first sock on in the bedroom. . . . now where do we go to put the other one on?" Your willing participation may take some of the fun out of the chase for your toddler and might even lead him to abandon it. If all else fails, and time is of the essence on busy mornings, simply hold your child down gently but firmly and calmly dress him.

"Our toddler struggles with us every morning when we try to get her dressed. It's such an ordeal that we'd leave her in pyjamas all day if we didn't have to get her to nursery."

By now, you may have noticed a recurring theme in typical toddler behaviour: you (the parent) want her to submit, she (the toddler) wants to resist. Getting dressed is a common source of conflict – after all, it requires a whole lot of submission – and since it has to be repeated daily, it can be especially challenging. But since clothing's not optional (at nursery or anywhere else outside the home), it's got to get done. One reality: you've got to get to work (or to an appointment, or to the shops). Another reality: your toddler is kicking and screaming naked at your feet, rejecting your pleas for cooperation, dodging your every dressing manoeuvre. What to do? Try these tips on for size:

Start while she's sleepy. Try to get her dressed as soon as she's up, before she's even rubbed her sleepy eyes – definitely before she starts running around (moving target and all), and absolutely before she eats breakfast (the less energy she has to fight you off, the better).

Begin with a cuddle. A hug before the dressing process can mellow both your moods. If your toddler becomes really overwrought during dressing, have another cuddle to help her calm down.

Tame with a game. To reduce resistance, try making a game out of dressing. "Where are you? I can't find you!" can often turn a potentially upsetting shirt-over-the-head moment into a gleeful round of peek-a-boo. Likewise, a "What happened to your foot?" or "I can't find your fingers. Where could they be?" is likely to produce squeals and cooperation rather than tears and opposition.

Try a little humour. Pretend to put her shirt over your head or her shoes on your feet, on her teddy bear, on her ears, or on her hands, then let her correct you – her giggles may get the better of her grumpiness.

Try a little reason. Point out to your toddler that everyone wears clothes and shoes – the teachers at nursery, her friends at playgroup, Grandma and Grandpa, cousin Sam, Aunt Jodi, and of course you. Explain, "Without clothes, we could get cold. Without shoes, we could get sore bits on our feet when we're outside." Your reasoning may sail right over her head at first (besides, toddlers aren't exactly known for their reasoning skills). But, in time, your point will be taken, and even accepted.

Change the subject. Instead of focusing on the dreaded dressing, distract her with conversation about what she will be doing in nursery or her playdate in the afternoon, or about the rain outside the window. Or keep her busy with a special dressing song or a small toy. Keep in mind that distraction probably won't work if her tantrum's already in full swing, so start distracting before you start dressing.

Let her dress herself. As with everything else, your toddler may be much more amenable to dressing if she can do some of it herself. So do everything you can to make dressing a cinch (it'll make it easier on you, too). Choose easy-on trousers with an elastic waist, help her to step into them, get them pulled up halfway, and then challenge her to pull them up the rest of the way. Shirts will be tricky at this stage of development, but she can probably yank a jumper down once you've navigated it over her head. Avoid clothes with a lot of buttons or poppers she can't manage (do you

really want to be messing with those while she's struggling to get away, anyway?). Provide shoes that are easy-on – she won't be able to get them on herself, most likely, but she may enjoy sticking the Velcro in place.

Let her dress someone, too. Your toddler may feel less persecuted by the process if she's allowed to inflict it on someone else. So make the dressing-of-the-doll or teddy bear part of the morning ritual. Chances are she'll have considerable trouble getting the clothes on the doll herself, but she can get the project started, and you can finish it up (after you've dressed her).

Be sensitive to touch-sensitivity. Toddlers can't usually express discomfort in words, or even work out what's making them uncomfortable, so they simply struggle and cry when a scratchy jumper, a stiff pair of jeans, or a too-tight shoe is bothering them. Some toddlers are more touch-sensitive than others, and some are super touch-sensitive. If that seems to describe your toddler, opt for soft, comfortable, loose-fitting clothing. Avoid polonecks, scratchy wool, stiff synthetics, and starched cotton, and buttons, poppers, seams, or tags that can rub against bare skin. Select soft blends or prewashed cottons (and always wash the clothes a few times before your toddler wears them, to soften them up some more).

Try a lot of patience. Of course you're stressed and pressed for time. Just try not to let it show. Nothing fuels a toddler tirade like a confrontation with an exasperated parent. Instead, plaster that carefree smile on your face and keep your voice cheerful (yes, even above the screeching). And so that you don't run out of time or patience (or both), try to get an earlier start tomorrow.

"My daughter never wants to wear what I've picked out for her – I seriously didn't think I'd have to deal with this until she was a teenager."

Are the wardrobe wars wearing you down . . . already? Though some little ones choose other battles (and some make everything a battle), there are many who make their stand in the wardrobe. Problem is, you needed her to get dressed (five minutes ago) and she's lying prone on the floor, shrieking because you selected the pink jumper (how could you?) and she wanted to wear something else (you're not exactly sure what – but she's gesturing wildly at it). So how do you deal with a dressing diva?

Let her choose. While giving your daughter complete control over her daily outfit isn't practical or sensible (she's liable to select a swimming costume and a pair of sandals on a freezing winter day or a snowsuit and mittens in July), even a little sway can go a long way in preventing dressing disputes. So offer your toddler a chance to choose between two or three outfits (no more, or she'll be overwhelmed). If she comes up with a wild idea of her own (that swimming costume, in January), come up with a compromise when possible (she can wear it under her tracksuit). To reduce the chances of wrong-for-the-weather choices, pack away out-of-season clothes.

Compliment her choices. Praise your toddler's selections when they make the suitability cut (she actually opted for a jumper on a blustery day). But avoid critiques of her style sense (or glaring lack of), and don't worry if her socks and trousers clash. She has plenty of time to learn good taste – and let's face it, your personal style and hers may never match (and neither may her socks and trousers). But, don't worry: the fashion police don't ticket toddlers.

Take the long view. Look at it this way: you can have clash of the outfits (pink flowered shirt, red striped dungrees), or clash with the toddler (complete with tantrum). In that context, is forcing your fashion statement really worth the struggle? Think big picture and you'll realise that her fashion faux pas are no reflection on her (or on you) – and that her pint-size peers won't be judging her on these outfits for years to come. As long as her selections are safe (no sandals in the rain) and borderline appropriate (no pyjamas to church), let it go – and let her exercise her freedom of clothes choice. Keep your sense of humour, too – now and later. Though the wardrobe wars tend to wane as the preschool years approach, they tend to return – with a vengeance – during adolescence. Remember, this is only a glimpse into the wardrobe of your daughter's future ("You're going out like *that*???").

"My toddler wants to wear the same pair of dungarees and T-shirt every single day. Not only is washing them a problem, but they're getting really tatty and we're getting really sick of seeing them."

The same-old-same-old outfit may be boring (and a tad gross) to you – but it's comforting to your toddler. He likes to know that no matter where his day takes him, his familiar dungarees and T-shirt will be along for the ride, representing the security of sameness. The simplest way to deal with a case of clothes monotony: accept it. Buy duplicates of your toddler's faves (if you can), wash them a few times so they won't be noticeably new, and try substituting them for his usual on alternate days. Continue to offer your toddler a different option alongside his old standby, but don't be surprised if he stands firm with the familiar.

A Toddler in the Buff

Is your toddler's favourite outfit his or her birthday suit? Many toddlers are happy to bare it all – no matter where they are or who they're with. What makes letting it all hang out so appealing to little ones? For starters, being naked just plain feels good – allowing the ultimate in freedom of movement. And then there's the fun in showing off a newly acquired skill – undressing. Shedding their clothes is also a way of asserting control and testing boundaries (a common theme in the second year). By taking off the outfit (or part of the outfit) you painstakingly put on, your little streaker is sending the message: "You might be able to dress me, but you can't keep me that way!" Finally, toddlers have no inhibitions and no concept of modesty or appropriateness (or what's public vs. what's private). Taking off clothes at bath time, or taking off clothes at a playdate – it's all the same to a toddler.

The more fuss you make about your toddler's clothing-optional lifestyle, the more appealing it will be. So keep your cool, stifle the giggles, and try these tips instead:

- Say yes sometimes. When temperatures and circumstances allow, let your child go bare (but with nappy). When clothes must go on (and stay on), try dressing your tot in togs that are a challenge to take off – shirts with small buttons, dungarees, trousers with a belt.

- Tell it like it is. Explain: "You won't be able to go to the playground if you don't have clothes on" or "No clothes, no playdate." Point out that Mummy and Daddy wear clothes, friends wear clothes, people outside wear clothes, people who come to your home wear clothes.

- Provide other undressing opportunities. Give your toddler a doll or stuffed animal with easy-off clothes to strip to his or her heart's content. And of course, when it's time to get undressed for the bath, let your toddler go to town.

Is it the nappy that keeps getting yanked off? Since toddler minus nappy can equal pee or poo on the living room rug, you'll have to step up the steps. Try putting the nappy on backwards so your little stripper can't peel open the tabs. If you're really desperate, use packing tape or duct tape to secure the nappy.

"Every time we try to get shoes on our son, he has a tantrum – he kicks and struggles so that we have to practically pin him down to get them on him."

Well, of course he does. Having his shoes put on represents just about everything a toddler resents and resists: being confined, being controlled, having done for him what he'd rather do himself, and if he's touch-sensitive, submitting to restrictive clothing. Add a dose of normal toddler negativity and it's not surprising that your toddler bucks like a bronco every time you approach him with a pair of shoes. To break out of this daily rodeo routine, try the tips on page 220 and:

- Stay away from laces. And buckles. And any shoe that's tricky to put on. Opt instead for slip-ons, Velcro closures, and other easy-on styles. The exception to this rule: if you have a toddler who likes to take his shoes off anywhere and everywhere, stay away from easy-on styles – they're also easy-off.

■ Let him find out the hard way. If your toddler absolutely refuses to wear his shoes, let him venture out in the push-chair or car seat in socks – but take his shoes along. When his feet get cold, or he wants to get out and walk, pro-duce the shoes – and matter-of-factly say "Oops, you forgot your shoes! Let's put them on fast so you can get out and play." Don't try this tactic on a bitterly cold day, though.

■ No shoes needed? No reason to force them on your shoe-averse tot. Though it may not be practical (or safe) to go barefoot in the park, let your toddler go shoeless at home and anywhere else it's possible. Not only because sparing the shoes spares the conflict, but because feet develop best when they're bare.

"My toddler seems to have a problem with socks – she complains as soon as I put them on her, and I can't figure out why."

Like the heroine of "The Princess and the Pea" (remember, she couldn't sleep with even the tiniest pea under her stack of mattresses), your toddler is probably touch-sensitive. Anything next to the skin that is not extremely soft and smooth can feel uncomfort-able to a touch-sensitive child – whether it's a pair of hugging arms or a pair of wrinkled socks. Realising that this sen-sitivity is something that a toddler can't control is the first step in helping her cope with it. The second is anticipating and minimising those articles of cloth-ing that might bother her. Avoid bulky socks that can bunch up inside shoes and socks with thick, rough seams or seams that run across the top of the

toes (look for seams that run across the base of the toes instead). Choose soft socks that are smooth-fitting, but aren't too large (extending beyond the tips of your toddler's toes) or too snug (leaving red marks or lines on her feet). Be sure to pull up your toddler's socks so they are completely smooth before putting her shoes on. Choosing socks with fun designs and appliqués may also help (as long as the designs won't rub her sensitive skin the wrong way).

As soon as your toddler is able to put on her own socks (it'll be a while), she'll be able to get them to feel "just right" more easily than you can – plus, by then touch sensitivity will prob-ably ease up. In the meantime, practise patience – and let her go without socks at home (bare is best, anyway).

"I can't get my daughter into her snowsuit without a struggle, no matter how cold it is."

When you've just started getting the hang of moving around freely, free-dom of movement isn't easy to give up – but that's what happens to your toddler every time you dress her in a snowsuit or coat. Bundled up in inflexible winter wear that keeps her arms and her legs stiff, your little one becomes madden-ingly immobilised – sort of like a turtle on its back. No wonder she struggles.

The problem is, when a snowsuit or coat is necessary, it's necessary. So how can you get your toddler dressed for winter weather with less of a struggle?

With the right stuff (and stuffing). Some snowsuits make it almost impossi-ble for walkers to make their moves. So next time you buy a cold-weather coat look for one that's not too bulky, too itchy, too heavy, too tight, or otherwise too restrictive. Choose lighter-weight insulating materials over heavy pad-ding. And when snow wear is absolutely necessary, opt for a two-piece if possible – it'll give her a tad more flexibility.

With a choice. No, she can't have a wardrobe full of coats to choose from. But next coat around, look for one that's reversible. That way, she'll be able to choose which side she wants to show off on a particular day. And when the weather is mild enough, give your toddler the option of wearing an extra layer over a heavy jumper instead of the coat.

With a challenge. Sometimes, if you're very lucky, a challenge can make toddler dressing less challenging. Try "Let's see how fast we can get our coats on!" or kneel down so she can "help" you put on your own coat (after which, you'll "help" her put on hers).

With distraction. Talking fast (and working even faster), distract your toddler with conversation and/or a few props (a toy, your keys) before approaching with the coat.

With the unexpected. Do something silly with your toddler's coat before attempting to put it on her. Put it on yourself (which should look silly enough) and announce "Okay, I'm ready to go out." Or drape the coat over her toy dinosaur or the lamp. With any luck, your toddler will find you so amusing that she'll forget to protest when you help her into the coat. She may even become so possessive of the coat that she'll insist you put it on her.

With a little logic. Before your toddler reaches the point of tantrum, try a little reason. If you have a window that offers a view of pedestrians, put your toddler in front of it and point out people passing by: "See how cold it is outside. Look at all the people wearing coats. Brrr. Let's get our coats so we can go outside!"

When no number of playful ploys convinces your child to put on her coat willingly, you'll have no choice but to put it on her anyway. Be firm, but understanding ("I know you don't like to wear a coat, but when it's cold out, you have to") and try to stay as cool as the weather you're about to step out into – if you get angry, she'll get angry. Once the deed is done, quickly distract her ("Let's hurry outside and find out if we can see our breath today").

"No sooner do I put a hat and mittens on my son than he yanks them off. This goes on for streets, and he always ends up the winner."

Almost every toddler has an on-again-off-again relationship with hats and mittens. Fortunately, though bare fingers and a bare head may make a child feel colder (particularly the bare head, since most body heat escapes via the head), they won't make him catch a cold – only a virus can do that. And on most days, there's no need to worry when the hat and mittens come off.

On very cold days, however, when the windchill factor is below 32°F/0°C, frostbite is a distinct possibility – which means your little kitten will have to don those mittens (and a hat), and you'll have to keep replacing them when they come off. You may also want to consider:

- Comfort. A hat made of a soft synthetic (such as fleece) instead of something scratchy (such as wool) may be more appealing, as might a roomy hood (it won't be as confining as a tight knit hat). A hood-type hat that slips over the head, covers the neck and chin, doesn't need tying, and eliminates the need for a scarf can also be a winner. Knit gloves, because they're less bulky and allow more hand movement, may be more acceptable to your toddler than bulky mittens – plus, a little tougher to yank off. The downside: they're not as warm.

- Fun. Try a hat with a fun shape (with puppy ears, for instance). Likewise, mittens shaped like animal puppets (show your child how his hands can chat and play with each other) or adorned with sparkly stars, favourite characters, or emblems may do the trick.

- Perseverance and patience. If it's not too cold, don't push the hat and mittens. If it is, let your toddler know that they have to be worn – even if you have to replace them every time he pulls them off. Avoid making it a game or a source of attention (you know how toddlers love those) by doing your replacing matter-of-factly and without exasperation or giggles (just a business-like "It's cold and you have to wear your hat and mittens"). Then try distracting your toddler with a song or by pointing out a squirrel scampering by. Or, if your outing is optional, opt to end it: "No hat, no playground."

Self-Dressing Frustrations

"My daughter wants to dress herself, without my help – but she gets so frustrated that she ends up having a meltdown instead."

Life for toddlers is a series of challenges – most of which they're eager to take on, but some of which they're just not completely able to handle, as hard as they try. Among the most challenging of those challenges: self-dressing. With chubby little fingers, fine motor skills that still need fine-tuning, and a shaky sense of balance, getting those clothes on solo is an uphill battle

for a 1-year-old. In fact, most tots can't master self-dressing until closer to their third birthday.

The result in the meantime: frustration, and lots of it. It isn't possible to protect your toddler from all of life's frustrations – and it's not a good idea, either, since a certain amount of frustration motivates little ones to achieve and develop. But it is possible to set your toddler up for dressing success while limiting her frustration, with these steps:

Make it easy. When you're buying clothes or making selections from her wardrobe, look for easy-to-pull-on trousers, shorts, and skirts with elastic waistbands, roomy-necked jumpers and sweatshirts, and dresses that won't get stuck halfway down (or up), and clothing without zips, buttons, buckles, and poppers.

Emphasise teamwork. She needs the practice and the self-satisfaction that comes with doing it herself . . . while you need to get her dressed and out the door, pronto. Instead of taking over the job entirely, let her know that getting dressed is a team effort: "Let's get you dressed together!"

Let her finish what you start. If getting the clothes into position is too tricky for her (she always gets both legs into the same trouser leg, for instance, or puts her dresses on backward), set her up then let her finish. Get the sweatshirt over her head and let her pull it down. Get the trousers halfway up and let her pull them the rest of the way. This can be particularly satisfying for her if you pretend that you need her help ("I can't get these trousers up. Can you do it for me?").

Blame the clothes, not her. When she runs into dressing trouble, criticise the

Having Fun Getting the Job Done

Does your little one put up a big fight when it's time to have a shampoo . . . get dressed . . . put away toys . . . wash up . . . buckle up . . . and more? Of course – after all, it's in a toddler's job description to struggle against you and the things you want to get done. In your job description? Being clever enough to get the job done by making it fun. Here are some winning ways to give your toddler's resistance a rest:

Laughable lyrics. You don't have to be a pop star to entertain a toddler with a song. An impromptu chorus of "I'm going to wash those elephants right out of your hair" or "This is the way we dress our feet" or a parody of your own making is a great opening act. The more silly the lyrics, the more likely your toddler will be distracted by them. For best results, sing the same song each time you perform an unpopular task.

Mistake making. As someone small who's always being told what to do and how to do it, nothing's more fun for your toddler than showing you up. The object of this game is to give your child that pleasure while giving you the pleasure of his or her compliance. When you want a cup of milk downed, for instance, you might say "Yum, yum, *my* milk. I think I'm going to drink it." After you've run the bath and your toddler is about to draw a battle line, announce "I'm all ready for my bath," and proceed to take off your socks and pretend to get into the bath. Your toddler will get a kick not only out of correcting you with "My milk!" or "My bath!" but out of the silliness of the situation. And you'll get a kick of your own when your child (you hope) takes the cup and drinks the milk or scrambles into the bath before you do.

Situation-saving sillies. In this ploy, you get silly (rather than angry) when trouble is about to erupt. You pretend, say, to put the boots on the doll when your toddler refuses to don them, or to struggle into your toddler's coat when he or she is resisting getting dressed to go outdoors. With any luck, the game will yield not only giggles, but results, too: "No, my boots! My coat!"

Silly voices. High, low, squeaky, creaky, mouse-like – the sound of a silly voice can often distract a toddler. If you're one of those talented parents who can produce realistic sound effects (a buzzer, horn, siren, animal imitations), use them to catch a resisting toddler off guard.

Funny faces. Again, it doesn't take much to amuse a toddler. Puffed-out cheeks, a scrunched-up mouth, a stuck-out tongue – improvise until you tickle that funny bone.

An imaginary setting. An older toddler who's resisting a pair of shoes may relent if you play shoe shop. Line up a few pairs that are obviously not toddler-size and suggest "Let's try these on." After giggling his or her way through a couple of wacky misfits, your toddler may relish trying on a pair that's "just right". Likewise, play beauty salon at bath time, clothing shop at dressing time, restaurant at mealtime.

Giggly games. Hold a hand-washing contest (who can soap up faster?); a mitten-donning race (who can get their mittens on first?); a pick-up party (who can put away more toys?).

Reverse psychology. Turning the tables sometimes turns the tide: "Whatever you do, don't smile . . . no, don't – oh, oh – I think I see a smile!"

clothes instead of her efforts: "This jumper is being so silly today. Let's see if we can get this silly jumper on you together."

Challenging Toddler

"It was hard enough having a 'challenging' baby – I'm sure he holds the world's record for colic and crying. But now that he's a toddler, he's not just challenging, he's impossible."

Sometimes, it's not easy to tell a normally challenging toddler from an especially challenging one. After all, many parents of toddlers would describe their tantrum-throwing, negative, rebellious, change-resistant offspring as "challenging" at times. But some toddlers take their behaviour beyond what's normally challenging. They're even more prone to tantrums and to more negative, more rebellious, more ritualistic behaviour. Often, these extra-challenging toddlers were, like yours, challenging babies who cried and fussed a lot more than other babies did (though far from every colicky baby ends up a challenging toddler). Many were tough to handle as infants, and they're even tougher to handle as toddlers.

Knowing you're not alone – that some 25 per cent of parents of toddlers are in the same rocky boat – may not help a whole lot, but commiserating with these parents, swapping stories, and exchanging tips may. (Look for parents who can relate on the message boards at WhatToExpect.com.) Learning what makes your child so challenging and what you can do about it is also helpful. The box starting on the next page describes different types of challenging temperaments, as well as some techniques for coping with them.

Even more helpful will be a little perspective. Keeping these points in mind will help you deal with – and look past – the challenging behaviour:

- Inborn temperament is inborn. When he behaves true to his personality, he's not being "bad" – he's just being himself. That doesn't mean his behaviour can't be modified, channelled, or even changed – just that it's not anyone's fault.

- Personality extremes can pay off (eventually). The very qualities in a toddler that drive his parents to distraction at age 2 (perfectionism that just won't stop, for instance) may make them exceptionally proud of him at 22. Extremely challenging children, with the right support and encouragement, often end up becoming extremely motivated, hardworking, successful adults.

- The right nurture can enhance nature. Accepting and appreciating a child for who he is, instead of trying to change him into someone you'd like him to be, can help shape a potential liability into an asset. It will also help boost his self-esteem (it feels good to know you're loved just the way you are) – and make home life happier for everyone.

- It may be just a phase. Sometimes challenging behaviour is less a matter of temperament than development – which means your toddler may grow out of it completely. Other times, it's a combination of temperament and development – which means that your little one may become gradually less challenging in the years to come (you may still glimpse the behaviours, but less often and in a less intense form). Remind yourself that this, too, may pass – or at least become a lot easier to deal with.

Living with a Challenging Temperament

Life with even the easiest toddler presents some daily challenges, but life with a challenging toddler presents a (sometimes) seemingly endless series of them. The stress of coping with a child who won't sit still, who loses it completely when faced with the tiniest of changes, who's hypersensitive to sound or touch, or who can't be quiet, ever, can be daunting and draining for parents. Struggling to find ways to help their toddlers and themselves, even with the best of intentions, it's hard not to feel frustrated, at least once in a while.

Determining which children are unusually challenging and which are age-appropriately challenging is probably subjective. Behaviour that may seem typical and manageable to some parents may seem unusually challenging to others (especially if they've parented an easier child in the past). Sometimes, the challenging behaviour is due to an inborn temperament – which means parents are in it, to some extent, for the long haul. Other times, it's just due to development – some children become temporarily challenging as they pass through transitional stages of childhood, or as a result of illness or stress. Either way, there are steps you can take to help you meet the challenges of your challenging toddler.

Whether your challenging toddler fits neatly into one of the following categories or exhibits behaviours from two or more, these tips can help:

The super-high-activity toddler. These children make the average active toddler seem to be operating in slow motion. They won't sit still, resolutely resist confinement (in a car seat, a high chair, even a cot), and tend to behave "wildly" and to lose control easily.

Best techniques for managing:

- Allow plenty of opportunity for outdoor play and for burning off energy, but insist on and enforce specific limits for safety's sake and for your own sanity (no jumping on beds, climbing on sofas, running down a busy street, and so on).

- Try to stop high-energy behaviour from escalating into out-of-control behaviour. If your toddler seems to be working up to a feverish frenzy, take him or her aside and quietly explain: "You're getting too wild. If you don't calm down, you will have to get off the slide." If the frenzy continues to build, follow through with your warning and insist on a "cool-down" period, trying one or more of the techniques for handling very active children on page 77. Or, substitute an acceptable excess energy outlet for the unacceptable one (see page 80).

- Respect your child's inability to sit still, and try to avoid situations that require church-mouse decorum.

- Ask the doctor about the latest research linking overactivity in children to diet, food additives (especially artificial colours), and sugar excesses. Try keeping a food diary to see if you can find a link between diet and behaviour in your toddler: did switching to naturally coloured ice lollies or weaning from neon-coloured cereal to multigrain hoops seem to slow your tot down? Did those three post-Halloween days of wanton chocolate-gobbling turn your active toddler into a wild child? Adjust accordingly.

(continued on next page)

(continued from previous page)

The distractible toddler. Toddlers typically have fleetingly short attention spans, but the distractible toddler seems to have none at all – flitting from activity to activity, distracted by a different pursuit before engaging in the first. The distractible toddler seems unable to listen or pay attention to parents or caregivers – especially when he or she isn't that interested in what's being said or done.

Since most toddlers are pretty distractible, the highly distractible toddler may not need much in the way of special attention at this age. You may, however, be able to gradually extend your child's ability.

Best techniques for managing:

- Avoid forcing your distractible toddler to stay focused longer than he or she is able to (story time may be over in a flash, and that's okay).

- Engage your toddler in fun activities you can do together, like finger painting or Play-Doh. It's easier to stay focused when you have focused company.

- Keep the house quiet and calm to help your child be able to pay attention longer. Minimising clutter may also help your toddler concentrate, since fewer distractions from other toys may help him or her focus on one at a time.

- Eliminate or limit TV watching, which can make all kids more distractible. Don't use the TV as background noise.

- Make eye contact when you speak to your toddler to help him or her shut out the distractions long enough to listen. Say, "Please come here and sit down with me. I want to talk to you." Then, with your toddler next to you or on your lap, assume a face-to-face position, and say "Look at me and listen to what I'm going to say." Or, get down on your toddler's level to make that attention connection.

The slow-to-adapt (or slow-to-warm-up) toddler. Even more than the typical toddler, this child craves routine, ritual, and the status quo, plays favourites with clothes, foods, and toys, and finds everyday transitions and even minor change seriously unsettling and disturbing. When faced with new people, places, situations, food, or clothes, this child withdraws, cries, becomes clingy, and if pushed, may have a tantrum. He or she can also be stubborn and persistent, prone to prolonged tantrums, and whine incessantly. Once adjusted to a change, however, these children tend to cling to the new situation fiercely (there's a meltdown when it's time to go to nursery, then another one when it's time to leave nursery).

Best techniques for managing:

- Try not to spring surprises. When it's possible, prepare your toddler for transitions by giving some notice: "After lunch, we're going to Angie's house to play." Then, when it's close to the time you'll be leaving the playdate: "You can throw the ball one more time and then we'll go home." Give your tentative tot plenty of time to acclimate to a new situation or an unavoidable change of plans – and while you're waiting for acceptance, be as supportive, patient, and understanding as possible. If your toddler is extra clingy in new situations, gently encourage him or her to loosen up that grip on your neck or leg, but don't push it.

- Use a timer to give your slow-to-adapt child a chance to adjust to a change ("When the timer rings, it's time to take a bath").

- Try to stick with old favourites when you can (visit the familiar playground instead of the new one across town, dish out the same cereal instead of a brand-new one).

- Ease a transition by choosing the most opportune moment to make it (wait until your toddler has tired of playing with the shape sorter before moving on to dinner, for instance).

- Instead of buying all new colours and styles of clothing when your little one moves up to the next size, select those that are as similar to the old familiars as possible. Let your toddler wear the same outfit over and over if that brings comfort – even if it means buying a duplicate (one to wash, one to wear).

- Serve up the same foods every day, if that seems to provide your toddler with much-needed security.

- Offer new options – a bite of the stew you're having for dinner alongside that must-have pasta, or a different jumper to wear over the same old shirt – but don't push a change agenda.

- Avoid major changes that can wait. Thinking about replacing the family room sofa, the kitchen tile, the bathroom carpet? If you can, consider waiting until your toddler grows more open to change. If you can't, try not to bring on more than one change at a time.

- When changes must be made – say, that beloved pair of trainers must be replaced by a new pair in a different style – try to give your slow-to-adjust

toddler time to adapt. Talk about the new trainers for a few days before shopping for them. Allow some time for getting to know the trainers (looking at them, handling them, carrying them around), instead of insisting they be put on fresh out of the box.

The high-volume toddler. This child is always heard. When a high-volume child is happy, miserable, angry, frustrated, or tired, everybody knows it.

Best techniques for managing:

- Teach your child to have a relatively quiet "indoor" voice and a less restrained "outdoor" voice. Challenge him or her to whisper games.

- Provide your toddler with plenty of opportunities for exercising his or her vocal cords in a socially acceptable way – singing along with music, making animal noises, reciting nursery rhymes.

- If your toddler can't seem to modulate volume at all, try some soundproofing strategies at home.

The unscheduled toddler. As infants, these children never settled into a regular feeding or sleeping routine. It was always anybody's guess when they would wake up, go to sleep, nap, or be hungry, grumpy, or cheerful. When they become toddlers, the guessing game continues. These children, not surprisingly, often have trouble settling into schedules, such as bedtimes.

Best techniques for managing:

- Don't count on getting the unscheduled child into a completely predictable schedule. Keep routines where you can, especially if schedules are important to you, but bend them

(continued on next page)

(continued from previous page)

as necessary. For instance, if your toddler isn't hungry at dinnertime, invite him or her to join you for a snack, but don't force the issue of a main meal. Offer the meal later, when your toddler is finally hungry. If your toddler won't nap at the same time each day, don't push him or her to sleep at prescribed hours (but do make sure he or she is getting the right amount of sleep overall). Instead of insisting on a bath each evening right after dinner, keep the timing fluid – one day the bath is before bed, the next day it's right after playground time, another day the bath comes after breakfast.

- At night, maintain a bedtime routine, but when you tuck your child in, don't insist on sleep – just tell your toddler he or she needs to lie quietly. Provide a few books, toys, or a playlist of lullabies to enjoy until sleep comes.

The low-sensory-threshold, highly sensitive child. The socks are bunched up, the jumper itches, the collar is too tight, the coat is too warm, the clock ticks too loudly, the lamp is too bright, the dog is too smelly, the apple purée is too "bumpy", the broccoli is too bitter, the ice cream is too soft. While most toddlers are finicky about some things, low-sensory-threshold children (and children with sensory processing disorder or sensory integration dysfunction; see page 478) are finicky about almost everything. These children may be supersensitive to light, sound, colour, texture, temperature, pain, taste, and/

or smell. They're disquieted by things that other people may not even notice.

Best handling techniques:

- Understand, accept, and validate. To your toddler, the bunched-up socks truly are uncomfortable, the jumper really is itchy, the broccoli is intensely bitter. Acknowledge this in what you say to your child: "I know you don't like it when the street noises are so loud" or "I know that rubbish smells really bad to you."

- Acknowledge this high sensitivity in what you do, too. Buy stretch socks that fit well but not too tightly and that have no bulky seams at the toe; choose soft cotton clothes that are less likely to itch and wash them several times before the first wearing to soften them up even more; avoid clothes that have scratchy inner seams, rough linings, and high or binding necklines, and remove all labels that might rub against your toddler's supersensitive skin. If tying and retying shoelaces to get them "just right" takes too long in the morning, opt for Velcro closings on the next pair.

- Be respectful of your child's tender taste buds: don't push the broccoli, serve smooth apple purée instead of chunky.

- If your child always complains when it's time to put on outerwear, try to use layers that are less confining and coats that are easier to move in. If certain colours make your toddler see red, avoid those colours when shopping for clothes or when decorating.

- If smells are a problem for your toddler, opt for unscented products (from shampoo to bathroom tissue to laundry detergent), and skip your perfume or aftershave.

- Try, if possible, to adjust the levels of light and sound in your home to your sensitive toddler's comfort. For example, substitute a digital clock for one that ticks, put a dimmer on the living room lamp, keep the volume low on the TV, and consider using soundproofing techniques, wherever practical.

The serious toddler. As infants, these children didn't smile as much. As toddlers, they may whine and complain more than others, and they may seem much more serious, sometimes to the point of glum.

Best techniques for managing:

- Deal with other temperament issues your toddler may have at the same time (such as poor adaptability), which may be contributing to the apparent unhappiness.

- Smile a lot, inject humour into everyday situations, use laughter to lighten up (but never laugh at your toddler's seriousness). Maybe you can rub the edges off your child's negative moods.

- Try to determine if there are any extra stresses in your toddler's life that may be upsetting him or her (including stress you're experiencing, since little ones can be very quick to pick up a parent's mood). Do what you can to reduce or eliminate these stresses.

- Check with the doctor if your toddler seems very sad. While a "serious" nature can be due to temperament, being extremely unhappy isn't normal – especially if a once happy child has turned consistently unhappy. Though it's uncommon, clinical depression can occur in toddlers, too. Besides being chronically sad, a depressed toddler may be withdrawn, irritable, lethargic, and show little interest in activities. If you think your little one might be depressed, getting the right diagnosis is essential, so ask for an evaluation by a qualified mental-health care provider who specialises in the treatment of young children. Age-appropriate therapy can make an enormous difference.

No matter the temperament of your challenging toddler, there is a light at the end of the tunnel. Though your challenging toddler may well turn into a challenging preschooler and a challenging teenager (though aren't all teens challenging?), you'll probably be facing the worst of it in these next couple of years. Modify what you can, lovingly accept what you can't, and most of all, hang in there. You'll probably be able to ease up on these management strategies as your child matures.

ALL ABOUT:
Taming Tantrums

Look up the word "tantrum" in the dictionary and you'll see it defined simply as "a fit of bad temper". But to parents standing by as their cheerful toddler, one moment all sweetness and smiles, suddenly transforms into a writhing, flailing mound of unrestrained rage, tantrums defy such simple definitions. Just what turns little cherubs into mini-monsters?

Normal toddler behaviour, that's what. Tantrums are a fact of toddler life, a behaviour that's virtually universal among members of the sandpit set – beginning for some tots as early as the end of the first year, peaking for most some time in the second year, and continuing in many children beyond age 4. Toddlers aren't "bad" when they're having tantrums – they're just acting their age.

WHAT'S BEHIND YOUR TODDLER'S TANTRUMS?

There are a number of reasons why tantrums are developmentally appropriate for toddlers and are a normal part of growing up:

- The need to release frustration. It isn't easy being a toddler. A little one's attempts to achieve (and achieve independently) are always being blocked, either by the adults around them or by their own limitations. Being unable to finesse a puzzle piece, button a shirt, ride an older sibling's bike, say what they mean – that's frustrating stuff.

- The need to communicate. Most toddlers don't yet have the language skills to do this effectively. For them, a tantrum speaks louder than words.

- The need to assert themselves and establish their autonomy. "I am my own person, on my own two feet. I am important. What I want matters. I am toddler, hear me roar!"

- Lack of control over their lives. With adults always telling them what to do and what not to do, a tantrum is often the only way toddlers can say "Enough! This is my life – I'm the boss of me!"

- Lack of control over their emotions. Toddlers are inexperienced at checking their emotions. When emotions get out of control, so do toddlers.

The "Terrible Twos" Start Now

Thought you had another peaceful year before the so-called terrible twos struck? Probably not. This normal (and arguably unfairly named) phase of development is more likely to begin when your tot is still 1 and usually continues until age 3 or 4. Understanding why your angel's actions aren't always angelic (it's about independence and control – or lack of it) can help you get through this sometimes trying time. It can also help you thoroughly enjoy the sometimes frustrating – but let's face it, always more terrific than terrible – little person your toddler is. The tips on these pages and in Chapter 7 will help, too.

- Hunger, exhaustion, overstimulation, boredom.

- Too many choices, too few limits – or vice versa.

Though just about every toddler has a tantrum now and then, some children are especially tantrum prone. About 14 per cent of 1-year-olds and 20 per cent of 2- and 3-year-olds have what are considered "frequent" tantrums (that is, two or more a day). These children are also more likely than other children to continue having tantrums well into the preschool and early school years.

HEADING OFF TANTRUMS

Unfortunately, there's no way to prevent all tantrums (if you've got a toddler, you've got tantrums). But it is possible to head off some tantrums before they come to a head. Start your prevention programme by keeping track of your toddler's tantrums for a week or two, noting when they occur (time of day, before or after naps or meals, following a particular event) and why, if the cause is apparent (hunger, fatigue, restrictions, frustration). After a time, you'll be able to uncover your toddler's most common tantrum triggers. Then set out to modify or eliminate them, using the following principles:

- Keep a regular schedule. For most toddlers, regular meals, regular naps, and regular bedtime routines will reduce the risk of tantrums. For those irregular tots who seem to be stressed by schedules, however, watching the clock less may help more.

- Don't let your toddler get overtired. Toddlers who don't get the naps they need or enough hours of sleep at night are much more disposed to meltdowns.

FOR PARENTS

Don't Be a Cave-Mum

You don't always have to say "no" to your toddler. But sometimes you'll need to – and when you do, it's best to stick with it . . . even once the kicking and screaming have commenced. Give in to a tantrum – you buy the toy because you can't handle the disapproving stares at the checkout queue – and the message to your toddler is clear: throw a fit and you'll get your way every time. If you're going to change a "no" to a "yes", make sure you do it before the tantrum's under way.

- Don't let your toddler run on empty. Offer nutritious snacks as needed to head off hunger-fuelled outbursts.

- Say "no" only when you have to. A parent's negativity is often the trigger for a child's tantrums. Reduce your need to say "no" by childproofing your home and setting clear and consistent limits.

- When possible, say "yes". Are you on "no" autopilot? Sometimes, saying "yes" – or offering an acceptable alternative ("You can't have ice cream, but you can have some yogurt") – can spare you both a tantrum. Don't change a "no" into a "yes" once a tantrum's begun, though, or you'll be reinforcing the wrong message: you can get anything you want if you just scream long and loud enough.

- Don't overcontrol (or undercontrol). Heavy-handed parenting (controlling everything a child eats, wears, does) can lead to rebellion. On the other

Being Held Hostage by Breath Holding?

It starts as a regular tantrum. Whining. Then crying. Then more crying – and screaming. Soon, your toddler's turning red in the face with fury. Then, suddenly, the screaming stops – not because the tantrum's over, but because your toddler has started holding his or her breath. Lips begin turning blue from lack of oxygen. If the breath is held long enough, the skin turns blue or pale and your toddler might even pass out. Terrifying for you, but believe it or not, it's not so dangerous for your child. This loss of consciousness is actually the body's protective response, allowing normal breathing to resume. No harm done.

The only potential downside to breath holding (besides the wear and tear on your nerves): it's such a scary behaviour that you're more likely to give in to your toddler just to avoid the confrontations that might lead to it. It won't be long before your tantruming tot has that "aha" moment: "Holding my breath gets me my way!" So treat breath holding as you would any regular tantrum. If your toddler passes out, offer a hug when he or she comes to – but don't offer that treat he or she was howling for in the first place.

If breath holding that results in blueness or a loss of consciousness is frequent, check with the GP. Sometimes, it's a sign of an iron deficiency, which means that an iron supplement can help put a stop to those scary sessions. Also check with the doctor if breath holding isn't triggered by a tantrum or other fit of frustration or temper.

---

hand, too many choices, too much freedom, too few limits, or limits that aren't consistently enforced can also step up tantrums. Try to strike a happy medium.

- Provide choice. Having opportunities to make some decisions ("Do you want me to read this book or that one?" "Do you want to wear your jeans or your dungarees?") helps a child feel more in control – and that can reduce the need to rise up angry. But avoid offering open-ended choices ("Which shirt do you want to wear?") because your toddler is sure to either pick an entirely inappropriate one (a tank top in January) or to be overwhelmed by the options. Also remember to make it clear when there is no choice (being strapped in, holding hands on busy streets).

- Fight frustration. Listen to your toddler and try your best to understand those attempts at communication. Step in when one of life's little challenges is turning into a major frustration for your toddler – but instead of taking over completely, help only as much as is needed (turning the triangle ever-so-slightly so your toddler can fit it into the shape sorter). Keep your expectations and standards age-appropriately realistic – not so high that your toddler is frustrated in an effort to achieve what he or she can't.

- Teach the fine art of venting. Before that little pot of simmering emotion boils over, encourage your tot to let off steam in other ways. Provide words to express and work out frustration and anger ("I see that puzzle is making you angry – silly puzzle! Let's try again later"). Show how to vent those angry feelings in more acceptable ways: punching a pillow, jumping up and down, hammering on a workbench, pounding on Play-Doh.

- Keep your toddler from going over the edge. When you see your child tottering on the brink of frustration, exhaustion, overstimulation, boredom, or anything else that might fuel a fit, divert attention towards something calming, soothing, or particularly interesting: a hug on your lap, a special song, a special place in the house, a special toy, a special book, a special activity.

- Notice and note good behaviour, and even behaviour that's neutral. Your toddler's been out for an hour of errands without a tantrum? Let him or her know you appreciate the cooperation.

- Try to be a model of calm. It's hard not to lose it when your toddler's throwing a tantrum – especially in public. But being the calm centre in your toddler's storm can help the storm pass faster and less intensely.

TANTRUM DOS AND DON'TS

There is no miracle elixir you can give your toddler (or take yourself), no patented parenting technique that magically makes tantrums disappear. Like most of the more trying behaviours of childhood, tantrums pass when they're outgrown, and usually not before.

But while it isn't possible to eliminate tantrums altogether, it is often possible to moderate or minimise them. The following suggestions for handling tantrums are just that – suggestions. You're likely to find that some

will work better than others, and some won't work at all. Once you've discovered which ones are most effective, pull them out whenever your toddler begins to unravel.

DO:

- Do stay calm. Nothing fuels a toddler's fire like a fired-up parent – seeing you lose your cool will only make it harder for your child to regain his or hers. A parental fit can also terrify a toddler. Already off-balance and out of control, a mid-tantrum toddler needs your calming influence and the reassurance of your unconditional love. And though the even-tempered approach may not be immediately rewarding and certainly won't be easy to pull off (the temptation to throw your own tantrum in the face of your toddler's will always be there), you may eventually see your efforts mirrored in your child's increasing self-control. If, during a particularly bad tantrum or on a particularly bad day, you find yourself unable to maintain your composure when the screaming starts, don't feel guilty – like all

---

Time-Outs for Tantrums?

Think it's time for a time-out (especially after the third tantrum in two days)? It isn't. Time-outs are best reserved for pre-schoolers and older children, who can understand why time-outs are being used and what they're supposed to accomplish. For more on discipline techniques appropriate for toddlers in their second year, see Chapter 7.

Keeping Your Cool

Nobody can stay calm, cool, and collected all the time – especially not when there's a toddler in the house. But since your toddler looks to you as that model of mellow, that anchor of stability during stormy times, your blowups can be unsettling, especially if they're frequent. To help you keep your cool:

Don't tempt temper. Blowups are much more likely when you've got problems at work or have had a fight with your spouse, mother, or best friend; when you're PMS-ing or you're sick; when the washing machine's given out in the middle of a load and the repair person can't make it until next week. When it's "one of those days", try to avoid activities that are likely to add to the stress quotient (a trip to the shoe shop comes to mind). Instead, take time for an activity or outing that promises to be relaxing for both you and your little one (a trip to the park or reading a story with your feet up).

Choose your issues carefully. Instead of squaring off with your toddler on everything, save the showdowns for the stuff that matters. Having fewer battles with your toddler will save your emotional strength for when you need it most.

Take a time-out. When you feel you're about to boil over, step away from the situation before you do (keeping your toddler in sight while you regain your composure). Count to 10 (or 100, if you need to), take a couple of deep, relaxing breaths, think about something pleasant or look at a picture of your toddler at a cheerful moment, and repeat over and over to yourself a phrase you find comforting (such as "I am calm and serene") – until you've stopped simmering.

Mind your words. There's nothing wrong with getting angry once in a while – it's an emotion that comes naturally to humans. But knowing how to express anger without inflicting physical or emotional pain doesn't always come naturally, especially on "one of those days". So try to put into practice what you're always preaching to your toddler: use your words, and use them with care. Express your feelings, when you can, calmly and rationally, without using hurtful words or threats. Instead of saying "You're such a bad girl – you never listen to me!" say, "When you don't listen to me, I get angry" (and take a break first if you need to). Too late – the wrong words have already left your mouth? That's okay – just apologise and move on.

parents, you're only human. Take a quick time-out yourself (with your toddler safely in view) and find ways to cool down (see box, above).

- Do speak softly. Trying to scream over all that screaming will only up the screaming ante for your toddler, as he or she vies for centre stage (and an award for Loudest Vocals). A quiet, gentle tone of voice, on the other hand, says you're in control, which should help your toddler regain composure . . . eventually.

- Do protect your toddler (and others). The toddler who does a lot of kicking and thrashing during a tantrum could get hurt (on a sharp corner, a hard floor, or an overturned chair), hurt

Let it out. If you're so angry you want to hit someone or something, move away from your child immediately and find a less vulnerable target for your aggressive feelings – mangle a stress ball, jog in place, do a set of star jumps, take a few power laps around the room. Explain to your toddler: "I'm really angry now. I think I'll walk around the living room two times so I won't be so angry." Remember to model only the behaviour you'd want your toddler to imitate during an angry outburst – don't slam doors, punch walls, or throw dishes. And don't leave your toddler alone.

Settle it with music. Music can be therapeutic, soothing the beast in both of you. Ditto for fresh air.

Embrace. Not the moment, but your toddler. Hug therapy can magically melt away feelings of anger and help you both regain control of your emotions. For best results, hug tightly, enveloping your toddler in your arms. But don't try hug therapy on a toddler who doesn't like to be held – that won't make anyone feel better.

Remember the good times. When you lose your temper, try not to lose your perspective along with it. Keep handy a photo of your toddler at his or her most endearing – and reach for it to remind you of the good times during the not-so-good moments. When a tantrum is in progress, or whining has reached an ear-piercing pitch, close your eyes for a few seconds and summon up a favourite memory of your toddler – offering you a lick of ice cream, splashing gleefully in the play pool, smiling ear-to-ear from the top of the slide, or angelically sleeping.

Vent as needed. Need to let those angry feelings out to someone who understands them? Once your toddler is down for a nap or is asleep for the night, look for empathy on online message boards, or call a friend or relative who's a good listener. Sometimes just venting those angry feelings can make them disappear. If you're so angry with your toddler that you're afraid you might lose control, pick up the phone immediately and contact your most available support person – whether that's your spouse, your mother, your sister, or your best friend.

Don't be a mummy or daddy martyr. Always taking care of your toddler, but never yourself? It's hard not to get a little resentful. But resentment can escalate into hostility, which means you won't be doing either one of you a favour by ignoring your own needs. Take time for you and you'll find time with your toddler is more pleasant.

someone else (a younger sibling or a playmate nearby), or do damage to property (by throwing a plate, kicking a door, tearing a book, pulling down a display in the supermarket). So move the child who is physically out of control to a setting that's safer for everyone and everything. If you're at home, the middle of your bed is a good location. If you're out, try moving back to the car or the pushchair (and strap your toddler in), step outside of the shop, or bench your toddler at the playground. If that's not possible, you may simply have to hold your toddler snugly to prevent injury to self, to others, or to property.

- Do try holding your toddler. Being held tightly during a tantrum helps

Public Tantrums

It doesn't take too long for most toddlers to figure out that tantrums are particularly effective when they're thrown in the most inconvenient and inappropriate locales (the shops, the supermarket, the middle of a crowded pavement).

What's a parent to do? Pretending you don't know the child who's sitting in your shopping trolley, wailing for the giant "Happy 50th Birthday" balloon that's hovering over the checkout stand, is always a tempting option, but who would you be fooling? Letting your tot cry it out – a reasonable plan of action at home – becomes impractical with dozens of spectators staring (and, in your mind, judging).

Is the only alternative to giving in to the demands of public tantrums never going out in public with your toddler? Not at all. Here are some ways you can prevent or minimise public tantrums:

Take preventive measures. See page 235 for ways to head off a tantrum before it starts.

Reinforce good behaviour. At the end of a successful outing (even marginally successful), thank your toddler for being well behaved, and tell him or her how much fun you had together. Don't, however, use bribes or material rewards to exact good behaviour, or your toddler may begin expecting a treat every time he or she behaves well in a public place.

Attempt distraction. If, in spite of your preventive efforts, your toddler starts to melt down when you're out, try a quick change of subject ("Let's go see if we can pick out a box of your favourite cereal right now!"). Or implement an out-of-sight, out-of-mind manoeuvre by removing your tot from the trigger, whether it's a bag of crisps he's campaigning for or the tins of tuna she's trying to rearrange, and diverting to another activity. Distraction may allow your toddler to exit gracefully from the tantrum – saving face for him or her and saving you from a scene.

some toddlers "keep it together" when they're falling apart, and can also help dissolve anger (in both the toddler and the parent), with the hold often turning into a hug as control and composure are regained. Other toddlers, however, will only flail more furiously when an adult tries to restrain them during a tantrum. If your child resists being held, don't force it.

- Do express empathy. When your toddler is carrying on about something he or she can't have, say "I know it's hard when you don't get what you want."

- Do try distraction. Many young toddlers can be cajoled out of a tantrum – some easily, some not so easily. Others only get angrier if an adult tries to divert them. If yours is receptive to distraction (and it always works best before a tantrum has picked up serious steam), get out a favourite book or a toy your tot hasn't seen in a long time. Suggest a fun activity. Turn on a favourite song and start dancing or singing. If your toddler doesn't seem offended by your responding to an oh-so-serious tantrum with humour, you might want to try a little silliness (stand on your head, put your shoes on your hands, make funny faces). Or, perform a song and

Resort to isolation. If distraction doesn't work, try to get your toddler to a relatively private place as soon as possible. Firmly, but calmly, pick your toddler up and carry him or her out (never yank or drag by arms or hands). Speak to your child softly as you leave, which will give you the appearance of being in control – something that's good for both your child and your pride. Move to your car, a toilet, a dressing room, or your home if it's nearby. (If you're out with others, it may be more productive for a well-liked friend or relative to be the one to take your child out for a break – this strategy can distract your toddler from the parent–child tug of war.) Wait until your tot is completely calm before attempting to continue your outing. If calm clearly isn't in the cards, consider ending the excursion and trying again later or another day. But don't regularly cancel errands or outings your child doesn't like or mission tantrum will be accomplished – and repeated.

Tune out the audience. Your toddler's tantrum is between the two of you – even if it's taking place in the middle of a packed department store. Concentrate on the task at hand – calmly and firmly manoeuvring your toddler out of the tantrum – and mentally block out those around you. Try to take your toddler's public displays of temper in stride (or at least pretend to) – after all, tantrums are a normal, predictable part of early childhood, and anyone who's ever cared for a toddler knows that. If you can't help being embarrassed, at least don't let on – your child might take advantage of this weakness (guess who can embarrass you even more in a flash?). And don't bother with the "you're embarrassing yourself" line parents turn to so often – at this stage in life, your tot couldn't care less about appearances (otherwise, he or she wouldn't be having a public tantrum in the first place). This exercise will take practice – but then again, you're bound to have plenty of practice over the next year or two.

Don't give in. Always a tactical error, it's an especially big mistake in public. Give into a tantrum and you'll just be asking for another one next time.

dance (with original lyrics) based on the situation ("Twinkle, twinkle little Zoe, this for sure you know-y know-y. You can't play with playground rocks, if you do not wear your socks"). It's clear that comedy just steps up the drama with your toddler? Forget it.

- Do ignore the tantrum. Often the best course of action is no action at all – a toddler who is ignored during a tantrum may get it out of his or her system faster. With your toddler safe and in sight, continue to go about your business. Make it clear you're not paying attention to the tantrum (you can sing to yourself, hum loudly – but keep moving, since you'll be a less easy target for your tot's thrashing if you're not a sitting duck). When you begin to systematically ignore your child's tantrums, they may intensify for a while. Eventually, however, as your toddler discovers that it's just not worth getting all worked up when there's no audience, tantrums will likely become less frequent.

Don't use the no-attention approach, however, on a child who's particularly sensitive, is going through a difficult time, is under some special stress, or seems to get very upset by being ignored (or if it bothers you too much).

If you can't ignore the tantrum because you're in the middle of a shop or somewhere else in public, see the box on page 240.

DON'T:

- Don't have a tantrum of your own. Your toddler needs you in complete control.

- Don't punish. A tantrum is beyond your little one's control – and isn't his or her fault – so there's no point in punishment, during or after. Physical punishment – hitting, slapping, shaking, or otherwise hurting a child – is never a good idea, but it's an especially bad way to deal with a tantrum. It's just too easy for a parent to lose control when faced with an out-of-control child, and when force is involved, even unintended, consequences could be dangerous.

- Don't try to reason or argue with your toddler during a tantrum. Out-of-control toddlers are simply beyond reason. Logic ("You don't need that doll – you have one just like it at home") is lost on them. Save the rational explanations for more rational moments.

- Don't stress. If you're unable to stop a tantrum in its tracks, don't worry – it probably just needs to run its course. When your toddler has released the pent-up tensions, the tantrum will taper off and end.

- Don't rehash. Once a tantrum's over, let it be over. Offer a hug so your toddler knows your love's as strong as ever, then divert him or her into a fun activity.

AFTER THE STORM

When the tantrum's over, let it go. If your child manages to end a tantrum quickly, offer praise: "You did a good job of calming down." But don't rehash the episode or lecture your child about it, or insist on an apology or admission of guilt. And don't administer punishment of any kind (such as taking away a toy or cancelling a trip to the park). Your toddler's been through enough, and besides, he or she didn't do anything wrong – just something that was developmentally appropriate.

For-Parents-Only Tantrums

Wondering why your toddler behaves like a perfect angel with the child minder or the nursery staff, but as soon as you're back on duty, the tantrums start? It's a simple case of love (for you) and security (for your toddler, in your presence). That you're the target of these outbursts suggests that your toddler feels secure enough with you to lose control without worrying that you'll walk out. And after a full day of behaving for someone who clearly doesn't love your toddler as unconditionally, a fit or two of temper is letting off steam that's been held in for hours: you love me, I feel safe with you . . . now I'm going to scream for a while.

Remember, too, that meltdowns of all varieties are more common at stressful times of the day (and is there really a more stressful time of day at your home than after work?). For tips on minimising those after-work frazzles, see page 172.

Join the Club

You've got to be the only parent who ever had a toddler collapse, kicking and screaming, in the middle of a busy pavement. You're definitely the only parent whose toddler ever refused to wear shoes or a coat on a winter day. You certainly must be the only parent whose toddler yanked down an entire tray of apples at the supermarket.

Or, at least, that's the way it feels sometimes. But the truth is, toddlers can be a handful and a half. They may be personality-plus – and they're definitely cuter-than-cute – but most 1-year-olds test parental patience on a daily, if not hourly, basis. Look beyond your own always terrific but sometimes terribly behaved tot, and you'll realise you're not alone in your toddler trials and tribulations. In other words, join the club.

Recognising that you're not alone won't stop those middle-of-the-street or checkout tantrums – but it may give you the perspective you need to keep your cool in the face of them (and in the face of all those head-shaking onlookers). Knowing that your toddler's behaviour is normal and age-appropriate won't make that behaviour go away – but it can help you cope with it more effectively. Remembering that every phase of childhood is fleeting may help you ride out the stormy moments and savour the magical ones.

If it was hunger, fatigue, or frustration that triggered the tantrum, deal with the cause (with a snack, a nap, or help). If a request from you sparked the tantrum (you asked your child to put away the bricks), you might suggest that the two of you take care of the task together (and try to have fun with it). If it was your refusal to cave to a demand that sparked the fire, don't give in now that the flames have died down. You don't want to give your toddler the impression that tantrums work.

Move swiftly to a diverting and enjoyable activity – preferably, one that won't be frustrating (you don't want to risk another tantrum). Find something to reinforce in your toddler's behaviour as soon as you can – that fledgling ego is likely to have been shaken by the recent power struggle and needs your vote of support. Many toddlers appreciate being held after a tantrum, as reassurance of their parents' continuing – and unconditional – love.

Keep in mind that there are tantrums . . . and then there are tantrums. If your child's temper tantrums occur very frequently (two or more times a day), seem to be accompanied by feelings of intense anger, sadness, helplessness, aggressive or violent behaviour, or other behaviour problems (sleep disorders, food refusal, extreme difficulty with separation), or if you are having trouble handling the outbursts (especially if you are responding in a way that's physically or emotionally violent), talk to the doctor. You may need some extra support, reassurance, and advice yourself (which GPs are used to offering to beleaguered parents).

Disciplining Your Toddler

....

SOMETIMES IT WILL BE CUTE (your tot unravels a roll of paper towel around herself, toga-style – or applies your lipstick . . . on her tummy). Sometimes, maybe not so cute (he dunks your purse in the cat's water bowl, or whacks a playmate with a spade). Sometimes it'll be minor (a washable marker leaves its mark on the coffee table), sometimes it'll be major (it's the permanent marker this time . . . on the freshly installed living room carpet). But if there's one thing you can count on when it comes to your toddler's behaviour, it's this – it won't always be perfect. Rules will be broken (along with your glasses), boundaries will be tested, buttons will be pushed (yours, plus the ones that were recording your favourite show), and mischief will be made (often where you didn't think it could be – toddlers are nothing if not resourceful).

Misbehaving, whether it's intentional, accidental, or accidentally-on-purpose, is something your toddler will do a lot – in fact, it's a toddler's job to do it (a job most toddlers do very well). Your job? Setting and enforcing limits, teaching right from wrong, helping your little one learn and practise self-control. In a word, disciplining. While it's way too early to expect your toddler to play completely by the rules, or even to remember what those rules are (especially when impulse strikes), it's not too early to start laying a foundation for a future of good behaviour. It'll take time, it'll take patience, and it'll take flexibility (not all discipline techniques work effectively for all children, and not all are effective at every age). Most of all, it'll take lots of the one ingredient that every effective discipline technique is dished out with: love.

What Discipline Is . . . and Isn't

Discipline – it definitely isn't the best part of the parenting gig (that would be being on the receiving end of those yummy hugs), or the one you look forward to most (does anyone really daydream about setting limits?). It may be a word with less-than-happy connotations from your own childhood (who has fond memories of losing privileges, being screamed at, or maybe even being smacked?), and it may already be filling the softie in you with dread (how can you take away a toy when your little cutie's pouting in that adorable way that makes you melt?).

Well, it's time to take another look at discipline – and to start thinking of it in a whole different way . . . beginning with what the word really means. Though it's often associated with punishment, the word "discipline" gets its roots from the Latin "to teach". And that's what good discipline is ultimately all about: teaching your child – who, as you might have noticed, has a lot to learn. Teaching all about right from wrong (it's hard to see the error of your ways when you have no idea you did something wrong in the first place). About self-control (it'll be a while before your toddler can slam on those impulse brakes and start thinking before acting). About the rights and feelings of others (that they exist, and how to respect them). About rules and why they need to be followed (essential preparation for life in the real world, where rules rule).

Many of these lessons can be considered long-term, of course. But just as your toddler can be considered a long-term work-in-progress, there's a significant short-term perk in teaching them, too: good discipline will protect your toddler, those around your toddler, your home, and your sanity – now and in the mischief-making years that lie ahead.

DISCIPLINE BASICS

There's more than one way to discipline effectively, even when it comes to toddlers – but all good discipline techniques and strategies share some basic principles. To best guide your little one from behaviour anarchist to stand-up (most of the time) citizen:

Do it with love. Of course you love your child unconditionally, but it's admittedly easier to show the love when your little one is behaving well than not-so-well. Still, "I love you always – even when you throw a massive fit at the supermarket" is the underlying message of all good discipline. It's that love that gives your toddler the rock-solid foundation on which to build good behaviour. On the other hand, withholding affection as retribution for a misdeed ("You drew on the wall, so I'm not going to play with you") or criticising your child instead of your child's actions ("You're bad" instead of "Hitting is bad") can eventually shake that foundation. For best results, dole out discipline with as much love as you do cuddles at bedtime.

Stick to the middle ground. The most effective discipline isn't strict or lax – it strikes a happy medium. Harsh discipline that relies on parental policing rather than on encouraging the development of self-control usually turns out children who are obedient around their parents, but out of control once

Staying on the Same Page

Maybe your toddler isn't playing the "But Mummy said . . ." card just yet. But there are bound to be differences in Mummy and Daddy's discipline style – and your little one is bound to be noticing them already. Some minor parenting policy differences are inevitable, and easily handled by even very young children (Mummy's a little more uptight when it comes to toy throwing, Daddy's a little more sensitive about screeching). Parental temperaments vary, too (all parents, like all children, are different – and that goes, also, for parents in the same family). Which means that Daddy may be a yeller, while Mummy's more mellow, or the other way around.

That said, it'll pay compliance dividends if you present a united parenting front, and if you stay on the same page as much as possible when it comes to discipline. It also prevents the pitting of one parent against the other (which can get ugly – and which makes it much easier for your child to manipulate the system). So, try for consistency in your household. If you disagree over discipline – like any other aspect of parenting – talk it out, but not in front of your toddler.

they're out from under the heavy hand of authority. Clueless about right and wrong, they behave only to avoid punishment. Overly permissive, indulgent parenting isn't likely to turn out well-behaved children, either. With no rules to fence them in, no moral compass to guide them, the free-ranging offspring of laissez-faire parents tend to be rude, selfish, quick to argue, slow to comply. For a better behavioural bottom line, aim for balance. Be the boss, but not the dictator. Maintain control, but don't be controlling. Stand firm on rules, limits, and the values that you value – but don't run a police state. When it comes to discipline, try to be a mum or dad in the middle.

Remember the individual. Every child is different, every family is different, every circumstance is different. Although there are universal rules of behaviour that apply to everyone, every time (after all, you don't get to ignore stop signs because you're in a hurry, or pay your bills late because you're a procrastinator by nature – that is, without

consequences), there's no one-size-fits-all discipline approach. In figuring out what discipline works for your little one, you'll have to factor in temperament (yours and your child's), circumstances (discipline in the supermarket may be different from discipline at home, discipline when your tot's down with a cold may be different from when he or she is feeling frisky), and what feels right for your family (just as rules will vary from home to home, how those rules will be enforced will vary, too).

Have more than one child? Then you have probably already noticed differences in their personalities – differences that were likely apparent from birth. You may have even noticed how those differences have influenced the way you discipline each child or which kind of discipline works best for each (one needs a gentler approach, the other a firmer one; one listens the first time around, the other benefits from reminders). And that's how it's supposed to be.

But even the same child may respond differently to the same discipline approach on different days – which means you'll have to tailor your discipline style to the situation, too. Is your toddler unusually stressed? Under the weather? In the middle of mastering a challenging skill and feeling particularly frustrated? You may need to take a more tender tact than usual when it comes to discipline.

And then there's you and your family. Discipline that works well for one family won't necessarily work for the family next door. Some parents – and households – are more laid-back, some strive to run a tighter ship. As long as the approach you take in your home is appropriate and predictable (see below), those variations are fine.

Be consistently consistent. Though they fight them every chance they get, limits are comforting for children. Knowing what to expect and what's expected of them makes little ones feel grounded, secure, and loved. But just as important as setting those limits is consistently enforcing them. If there were no shoes allowed on the sofa yesterday, but Mum's looking the other way today, or if hand washing was a predinner must-do last week, but this week it's being mostly skipped, the only lesson your child will learn is that the world is confusing and rules are meaningless (so what's the point of trying to follow them?). There goes your discipline credibility, there goes your parental authority, there goes your toddler's compliance. Jumping on the bed is a no-no on Monday? Then it has to be a no-no on Tuesday, and Wednesday, and Thursday – and it has to be a no-no whether Mum's in charge, Dad's in charge, or the child minder's in charge. If your rules are all over the place, behaviour's bound to be, too. It doesn't mean you can't sometimes bend nonessential rules or even break them once in

a while, it just means that a consistently inconsistent approach to discipline can be predicted to fail.

Keep age in mind. The same standards of behaviour don't apply to a 5-year-old (who's developmentally capable of impulse control and reason) and a 1-year-old (who clearly isn't), and neither should the same disciplinary approach. Time-outs, for instance, aren't effective for young toddlers – they don't yet have the attention span, memory, or cognitive ability to "sit there", never mind "sit there and think about what you've done". Rules should factor in the limitations of age, too. You can expect a 5-year-old not to interrupt you when you're on the phone (at least most of the time) or to put away toys before bed (most likely with a reminder), but expecting either of a 1-year-old (or even a 2-year-old) isn't realistic. Set limits that are age-appropriate and you're more likely to get the compliance you're looking for.

Be persistent and patient – it'll pay off. Young toddlers have limited memories, minimal attention spans, nominal impulse control. You can't expect your 1-year-old to learn a lesson the first time it's taught, or to practise the kind of self-discipline that prevents an older child from doing something he or she has been told not to do. Be patient, and be prepared to repeat the same messages – "Don't touch the TV" or "Don't throw your food" – every day for weeks, or even months, before they finally sink in. Even once they do, that itchy trigger finger may not be able to exercise restraint when your toddler is faced with temptation (the remote's right there on the coffee table, practically begging to be pushed). Don't give up, don't give in – but do give it time.

Tone it down. It's tempting to raise your voice to your toddler, if only to be heard over the din of screeching and screaming. But paradoxically, your toddler is more likely to pay attention to a firm yet more modulated tone. Besides, too much yelling loses its effectiveness – and when it's angry yelling, it can be scary and hurtful.

Be the calm in the storm. So here's why you lose your temper: you're only human, and you're the parent of a toddler who's only human. Here's why you should try not to lose your temper: anger doesn't work. When you're over-the-top angry, you lose patience and perspective, two qualities you need lots of when you're disciplining a toddler. You model a behaviour you're always trying to curb in your toddler (loss of control), instead of one you're always trying to encourage (practising self-discipline). You may even frighten or humiliate your child and, if you're angry a lot, bruise that just-emerging sense of self.

And here's another important reason why uncontrolled anger is ineffective: it teaches nothing about good behaviour versus bad behaviour. Screaming or hitting in the heat of the moment may give you a quick release – and may even temporarily stun your little one into submission – but it doesn't further your long-term goal of promoting good behaviour. In fact, it promotes just the opposite (screamers

and hitters tend to raise screamers and hitters – check out any playground and you'll see).

So be the calm in the storm, as much as you can. When your toddler has done something that makes you angry, take a few moments to cool down before you attempt a disciplinary action. Then, respond. Calmly explain the error of your toddler's ways and what you plan to do about it ("You threw the lorry. Lorries are not for throwing. I am taking the lorry away"). A good example modelled, a teaching moment seized, an action connected with a consequence – and, best of all, effective discipline issued. Plus, you behaved like an adult.

A little too late for that – you already lost your cool? Don't worry if you can't always slam on the temper brakes. Again, you're only human, which is actually important for your only-human child to know. As long as the tirades are relatively few, far between, short-lived, and aimed at your child's behaviour, not your child, they won't interfere with effective parenting, or even with your overall discipline strategy. When you do lose it, however, be sure to apologise for it: "I'm sorry I yelled at you, but I was very angry." Adding "I love you" will let your toddler know that sometimes we get angry at people we love and that's okay.

Discipline Strategies That Work

While there's no one right way to discipline a toddler, there are several ways that work well. Which techniques you choose, and when you choose them, will depend on your toddler's personality, your personality, and the specific set of circumstances.

DISCIPLINE METHODS

Here are some discipline methods you can try during this sometimes trying second year:

Win-Win Solutions

The best solutions to disputes allow everyone to emerge a winner – and that's especially true with toddler–parent disputes. For example, if your mischievous tot tests you by first touching the flower arrangement on the table, then giving you a challenging glance and backing off, enough said. Your little one got to touch something off-limits (which is what he or she wanted), but didn't go any further or do any damage (which is what you want). You both end up winners.

You can create win–win situations by using distraction (he or she goes for your Kindle, you go for the crayons and paper), humour, reverse psychology, and other creative approaches (such as setting a timer that will ring when the five minutes to dinnertime are up, signalling that it's time to put down the bricks and come to the table). Everybody can end up a winner, too, when you do a little negotiating: "Take your bath right now, and then we'll read your favourite book." Just don't let negotiations cross the line to bribes or threats. If your toddler is steadfastly refusing to get into the bath, don't promise reading in return for cooperation or, conversely, threaten to revoke reading. When your child's old enough to understand, you can explain that actions have consequences: "If you waste a lot of time now and take your bath late, there won't be any time to read a story."

Catch your child being good. Most children learn early on that behaving well usually earns them far less attention than behaving naughtily. Mummy's not looked up from the bank statement she's been trying to make sense of for 15 minutes? It's time to start decorating the wall with felt tips. Daddy's had his nose in his BlackBerry since the moment he walked in the door? He'll notice me if I bang on the glass table . . . with his keys. Your toddler's thought process may not be as clear as all that – but his or her actions definitely are.

So the next time your toddler acts up, avoid overreacting (a strong reaction, even a negative one, is just what your toddler is vying for). But when your child turns the pages of your book carefully, or plays quietly with a puzzle while you wash the dishes, or picks up a scrap of paper from the floor and hands it to you, make a point of paying attention – and offering praise.

By recognising good behaviour, you'll be encouraging more. Just remember to keep raising the standards of good behaviour as your toddler's capacity for it grows – too much positive reinforcement for too little effort loses its effectiveness, plus it doesn't give your toddler any incentive to try harder. Also keep in mind that positive reinforcement on its own may encourage good behaviour, but it won't guarantee it. You'll have to include in your discipline a mix of techniques that address bad behaviour, too.

Make the discipline fit the crime. It's virtually impossible for a young toddler to understand that playground privileges are being revoked because of a crayon masterpiece drawn on the living-room wall. Your child is much more likely to get the point if you take the crayons away immediately and don't return them until after lunch (and with

FOR PARENTS

Take a Time-In

Does your toddler's behaviour typically take a turn for the worse when you're really busy? That's his or her way of calling for the attention that's been in short supply. Pre-empt some of that behaviour by periodically taking a moment – in the midst of whatever you're busy doing – to reach over for a hug, commend the progress of a brick project, or even look at a book together. Your little one will feel less compelled to propel that book through the air to get your attention.

a piece of paper, to reinforce proper use of them). That's making the discipline (or consequences) fit the misbehaviour – and that teaches right (drawing on paper) from wrong (drawing on walls).

There is almost always a way to fit the discipline to the crime. If a cup of orange juice is turned over intentionally, your toddler can participate in the clear up (and forgo a free refill). If bricks are thrown around, they can be confiscated for the rest of the day. If a swipe is taken at another child in the playground, the swiper can sit out the next 5 minutes.

Let natural consequences do the teaching. One of the more important lessons of life is that all actions have consequences. Feed your biscuit to the dog and you have no more biscuit. Tear pages out of a favourite storybook and Daddy can't read that book to you any more. Drop your teddy in a mud puddle in the playground and you can't play with it until it goes in the wash. Let your toddler learn from natural consequences instead of trying to protect him

or her from them (supplying a new biscuit to replace the dog-devoured one, for instance). Reinforce the teachable moment by explaining what just happened: "You gave your biscuit to Molly, and now you have no biscuit." The long-term effect (lesson learned, eventually) will far outweigh the short-term effect (a probably brief meltdown). The exception: if the action was unintentional (Molly the dog grabbed the biscuit right out of those chubby little fingers), it's fine to intercede (in this case, with a new biscuit).

Divert attention. For most toddlers, especially young ones, what's out of sight is quickly out of mind – making distraction an especially sensible discipline strategy now. She's getting her kicks out of pulling blossoms off a bush? Divert her (fortunately limited) attention to two squirrels playing on a tree. He's decided it's really fun to fish around in your bag? Close your bag, but open a box of toys he hasn't seen in a while. A playdate pushing match has broken out over a coveted doll? Pull out an activity that doesn't require as much sharing, like crayons and a giant sheet of paper. With distraction, everyone wins (just say "no" and you're only asking for a challenge). Your toddler keeps returning to the scene of a crime? Divert as often as you need to, or, if possible, make the source of conflict inaccessible.

Time-outs. Is it time for a time-out for your toddler? Probably not. Time-outs aren't really about discipline, since they don't teach anything. They're about giving a child the chance to cool off and regain control (something that toddlers, admittedly, need to do on a regular basis). In a true time-out, the child is removed from the scene of a crime-in-progress, placed out of the action, and told to sit still in a prescribed spot for a prescribed amount of time without

Smacking: Don't Do It

Nothing brings out the child in a parent like a toddler – especially when that toddler is misbehaving. Even for the ordinarily cool and collected, the impulse to lash out physically can be strong, sometimes overwhelming.

There's nothing wrong with feeling this impulse – most parents experience it at least occasionally. But there can be problems with acting on the impulse. Of course, smacking as a means of discipline has been passed down from generation to generation in many families, but nearly all experts agree that it's not an effective disciplinary tool, for a number of reasons. For one thing, it sets an example you don't want your child to follow (numerous studies show that children who are smacked are more likely to use physical force against peers, and later against their own children). For another, it represents the abuse of power by a very large, strong person (in a sense, a bully) against a very small, comparatively weak one – definitely behaviour you don't want modelled in the playground, ever. Smacking can be humiliating and demeaning to a child, often chipping away at self-esteem and morale. It can even, in the heat of a moment, escalate into more serious child abuse. Keep in mind, too, that children who are smacked may refrain from repeating a misdemeanour rather than risk a repeat smacking, but they obey only out of fear – not because they've developed self-control. Instead of learning to differentiate between right and wrong, they only learn to differentiate between what they get smacked for and don't get smacked for.

And the same goes, even more emphatically, for shaking a toddler. Many parents who would never consider hitting feel that shaking is an effective and safe alternative. But shaking a toddler is extremely dangerous. Although a toddler's neck muscles are stronger than an infant's, shaking can still cause serious injury to eyes and/or brain during the second and third years of life.

If once in a while your resolve not to hit dissolves in a moment of stress (say your toddler rips up your £10 note) or fear (he or she dashes into the street) and you lash out with a slap on the bottom or hand, don't feel guilty – that was your human side showing. But do apologise right away ("I'm sorry I hit you. That was wrong") and then give your toddler a reassuring hug. If the smacking was out of concern for your little one's safety, you can offer an explanation along with the apology: "I'm sorry I hit you. You scared Mummy when you ran into the street. Remember: no running into the street."

If, however, one slap leads to another; if the slap is hard enough to leave a mark on your child or is aimed at the face, ears, or head; if you use a strap, ruler, or other object; or if you strike out under the influence of alcohol or drugs, you should talk about your feelings and actions with your child's doctor, a family therapist, or another helpful professional. Or talk to someone at the NSPCC (0808 800 5000) as soon as possible. Lashing out physically at a child in anger is a danger sign. Though you may not have seriously hurt your child yet, the potential for physical or emotional damage is there. Now, before angry outbursts lead to something more serious, is the time to get some professional help.

If your spouse shows violent tendencies, he or she also needs help from a professional. So call now for that help – *before* these tendencies get out of hand.

any attention (negative or positive), entertainment (no toys or books), or company (not even a teddy pal). The problem is, 1- to 2-year-olds have a hard time sitting still (especially when they're riled up), a hard time staying in one place, and a hard time being isolated. What's more, they may not have the slightest understanding of why they're being isolated (it's not like they can reflect on their misbehaviour at this age). For those and other reasons, time-outs are best reserved for children over the age of 2 (and time-outs involving a set amount of time – a concept that's beyond comprehension for the very young – shouldn't be used until a child is at least 3). When your little one has lost control, take a time-out together (break for a hug or another soothing activity) so he or she has a chance to settle down again.

MAKING DISCIPLINE EFFECTIVE

Once you've chosen a method (or a few methods) of discipline that fits your family, your next challenge is making sure that you implement it as effectively as possible. These tips can help:

Make sure the rules are clear. Toddlers are novices at following rules. What's more, still-limited comprehension skills sometimes make it hard for them to understand the rules. You know what you mean when you tell your toddler that hitting isn't acceptable, but you can't assume that your toddler knows what you mean. So spell it out using simple, straightforward words. Explain: "No hitting. Hitting hurts."

Try a little prevention. If you think about it, there's no better form of discipline than prevention. But preventing misbehaviour doesn't mean anticipating

it (warning your toddler "No hitting Jacob today" before a single fist has started flying). It means equipping your little one with the skills he or she needs to behave well. Start by showing your toddler how to touch someone gently, then offer positive reinforcement ("You're playing so nicely with Sean!"), and finally, issue reminders as needed (when a smack seems imminent).

Go face-to-face. Especially for little ones with little attention spans and limited ability to focus, correction becomes far more effective when it takes place face-to-face. So rather than call from the other side of the room "Please stop that banging" (for your toddler, you're just background noise), walk up to your toddler and get down to his or her level. Looking your little banger squarely in the eye, tell him or her to stop. Let your body language, tone of voice, and expression make it clear that you mean business.

Give fair warning. When you catch your toddler in a mischievous act, it's legitimate to warn, "If you don't stop by the time I count to 3, I will . . ." Then, of course, you must keep your word – or your warning won't mean a thing. In situations that involve dangerous consequences – such as hitting, approaching a roaring fire in the fireplace, or banging on the window – forgo the warning and intervene immediately.

Explain the sentence. Even a young toddler can understand, albeit vaguely, that you're confiscating the toy because he threw it at his sister, or that she's being taken out of the playground because she angrily pushed the swing right at a playmate. But a simple explanation can reinforce your message as well as the discipline's effectiveness. "Simple" being the operative word: drone on and on and you'll be tuned out.

Life with Limits

Don't look now, but your toddler craves limits.

That's right, your toddler – the same little rebel who seems to live just to resist your rules, actually loves to live by them.

The reality is that living with the right kind and number of limits – balanced by the right kind and amount of freedom – is comforting for children, especially young children. Toddlers have (you might have noticed) precious little control over their impulses, which, left unchecked, can drive them to do some pretty uncivil and dangerous things. Those just-right limits certainly keep toddlers safer (shoes protect little feet from cuts, holding hands on the pavement prevents curious tots from wandering into trouble), and those around them safer, too (say, "No hitting"). But here's a perk of those parameters that's a little less obvious: limits also offer little ones a soothing sense of security during a sometimes unsettling period of development. In the face of so much that's new and different, challenging and exciting, limits are a constant comfort, helping toddlers know what to expect – and what's expected of them. And what's good for your toddler is also good for you, since a healthy serving of limits cuts down on negativity and tantrums.

So bring on those limits your toddler subconsciously craves – but struggles against with every fibre of that sweet, stubborn little being. But as you do, try to keep your limits:

Age-appropriate and fair. Rules aren't always fair, but they're easier to comply with when they are – especially for someone just learning about limits. So aim for fairness and, most important, for age-appropriateness. Expect what your little one can deliver, and

remember that at this point, it won't be a whole lot. Expecting a 1-year-old to put toys away unasked and unhelped, for instance, is futile – it isn't going to happen. Expecting that same little one to join in as a member of a toy-pick-up team (particularly if that team has a fun-to-sing theme song) may happen.

Consistent. Rules change every day? Guess who won't be able to keep up with them, never mind follow them.

Good fit for your family. Few limits are one-size-fits-every-family. Beyond the across-the-board basics (safety and health first; being respectful to others; no hitting, name-calling, or other physically or emotionally hurtful behaviour), there's a wide range of what may feel right – or wrong – when it comes to family rules. Maybe in your home, no shoes on the sofa and bedtime by the clock will be ironclad. Or maybe those won't matter at all, but no touching Mummy's desk or Daddy's mobile phone are sticking points. Pick the limits that work for you, your toddler, and your home.

Limited, but not too limited. Set too many rules, or rules that are too strict, and your toddler may not even bother trying to follow them (because expectations are always out of reach), or may tune them out altogether. A life with too many limitations can also be frustrating for a toddler who's trying to explore and discover (like toddlers are supposed to do). On the other hand, setting too few rules, or rules that are too lax, means your expectations may always be too low – another setup for "why bother trying", not to mention a recipe for chaos. Either scenario comes with the potential for even more rebellion, and who needs that?

Don't delay. Often, by the time you've finished a tirade or taken away a privilege, your in-the-moment toddler has forgotten what sparked the fuss in the first place. So be sure to react quickly to a misbehaviour. Eliminating story time before bed because of an infraction that occurred before dinner pretty much assures that there will be no link whatsoever in your toddler's mind between the misdeed and its consequences. The result: discipline loses its effectiveness.

Follow through. If your threats are empty, or your follow-through is weak, your tot will soon figure out how to work the system. Does your toddler throw a tantrum when you try to discipline? Proceed as planned anyway.

Give in and you give the impression that discipline is negotiable. For more on coping with tantrums, see page 234.

Forgive and forget. Once the discipline has been issued, it's time to move on. Completely on. No grudges, no lingering resentment, no lectures. And, just as important, no special perks intended to make amends for the discipline doled out – you don't want to send the message that disciplining your toddler was a mistake (after all, you were just doing your job as a parent). If you lost your temper, apologise as needed, but don't plead dramatically for forgiveness – that will only be unsettling to your toddler. Instead, give your little one a hug and transition promptly to an activity that's fun for you both.

ALL ABOUT:

Right and Wrong

Toddlers are the new kids in town – inexperienced in the ways of the world, yet eager to take it on. With so much they don't know – but are itching to discover – they're curious, fun loving, impulsive, and sometimes painfully naive. They're lacking that mature moral compass of right and wrong we adults call a conscience. And that's where you come in – to show your young toddler the way.

It's you who'll tell him that slugging a playmate over a toy is wrong, and that waiting his turn when three other children are lined up at the slide is hard but right. You're the one who'll prod him to thank Uncle Elliot for the gift he brought, and you're the one who'll take away her bowl when she starts flinging

Weetabix. And until your child develops a fully functioning conscience of his or her own (and some impulse control to back it up), you'll need to be your toddler's moral GPS.

But guidance alone isn't enough (when you get hooked on GPS, do you ever really learn the way?). Your toddler isn't ready to navigate the world without your input about ethics, but he or she is ready to learn some of the basic principles of being principled.

Here's how to teach right from wrong:

Explain that actions have consequences. While it's important to tell your toddler that it's wrong to throw sand, it's also important to add a simple explanation why it's wrong ("When you throw sand, it can get into someone's eye, and hurt them"). And while it's important to tell your toddler that it's right to wait your turn instead of pushing your way to the front of the queue at the slide, it's also important to add why it's right ("When you wait your turn, all the children get to go on the slide, and everybody has fun"). You'll be helping your toddler make sense of the rules, and also nurturing empathy – key to developing a conscience.

Start a dialogue. Get your toddler thinking about behaviour – both good and bad. After your child shoves a playmate, ask "How do you think Abigail felt when you pushed her?" When a character in a book has done something obviously right or wrong, comment "That boy made his friend happy when he gave her a hug" or "The girl made her friend cry when she grabbed the toy. That's why it's nice to share." It's not time yet for a deep, philosophical conversation about morality, but it is time to get the dialogue started (even if it's just one-sided for now).

Fault behaviour, not people. Try to criticise your toddler's behaviour (which can be changed), not your toddler: "Throwing that brick was bad," not "You are a bad boy." Avoid passing judgement on others, too, when evaluating their behaviour, and encourage your toddler to do the same. Instead of "The girl in the story is bad because she didn't share her sweets", try "Not sharing isn't nice. The girl should share her sweets." Will you always remember to critique this way? Definitely not – especially when you've encountered something that really strains your patience (a cupful of blackcurrant juice on your beige sofa, perhaps?). No problem – just try not to make a habit of making sweeping

(and hurtful) statements about your toddler's character.

Don't take sides. Some parents tend to side with their offspring in battles with other children, others side with the playmate, and still others try to figure out who threw the first punch before they assign blame. All well-intended approaches – the problem is, none of them really works that well. Always picking one side over the other is inherently unfair (and fairness is an important part of the right-and-wrong equation). Assigning blame when toddlers fight is tricky, too, since (A) you're unlikely to get a confession, and (B) the first punch you saw may not have been the first one thrown. So even when intervention is called for, try to play mediator rather than defender or judge and jury. It doesn't matter who started the fray, it's up to you to see that it comes to an end – civilly. Moral lesson: physical fighting is wrong, no matter who started it.

Skip the lecture. Teaching takes some explanation. But keep it short and simple. Droning on after a playdate ("You didn't play nicely at all . . . You were so mean to your friend . . . Your friends won't like you any more if you're so mean") or issuing long-winded warnings before you even get there ("Now, don't forget, no pushing. Make sure you share. No hitting or biting") – will only teach your toddler that when you start talking, it's time to stop listening. Turn on lecture mode, and there goes your lesson.

Be a moral model. As always, an ounce of example outweighs a pound of instruction. Let your conscience be your guide – and, for the time being, your toddler's – and eventually your child will develop a conscience of his or her very own.

CHAPTER 8

Talking

....

S O, MAYBE YOUR TODDLER CAN WALK THE WALK (or is well on the way to those momentous first steps). But when will he or she start talking the talk? When will that frustrating communication gap – the one that stands between you, your toddler, and the unknown toy he or she has been pointing at insistently but futilely for the last five minutes – finally close up? Listen carefully, and you might be surprised to hear who's talking. Whether your tot is already stringing words into phrases (or even basic sentences), or still hasn't uttered word one (at least as far as you can tell), there's one thing for sure: language development is in full swing.

What You May Be Wondering About

Not Talking Yet

"My son babbles a lot – so why doesn't he say anything anyone can understand?"

J ust because you can't understand a word your toddler is saying doesn't mean he isn't saying a word. Your beginner-talker's language may sound like gibberish to you, but if you listen carefully, you may notice that it actually has rhythmic patterns and inflections similar to that of your speech (they don't call it the "mother tongue" for nothing). This practice language – known as "jargon" – may mean nothing to you, yet it speaks volumes to him, enabling him to start filling the language gap (letting him chat to himself, to you) even before he can say real word one.

Is your tot babbling more than just jargon? Maybe he's moved up one step on the language ladder from jargon to single- or double-syllable sounds that mimic real words (though they'll probably still be hard to decipher). "Ba" may mean bottle, "uh" up, "da" that. Until you've broken the code (and you will), you may feel like you're in a round-the-clock game of charades ("sounds like . . ."), especially if your toddler combines those sounds with gestures, which he likely does. But at least it's a start.

Making it even more difficult to interpret these early "words": single syllables may also stand for complete, if primitive, sentences. "Ga" could mean "Give me that" or "What is that?"

Confused yet? But wait, there's more: those first words may also be multipurpose. "Da-da" may mean Daddy, but it might also be used to call Mummy, the child minder, even the dog – or a random man on the street. "Ma-ma" could, at different times, mean "I want Mama", "That is Mama", "Feed me, Mama", or "Pick me up, Mama." Or it could refer to Daddy or anyone else in a little one's life. Or a one-size-fits-all label for any woman, any time.

It takes years of practice to perfect speech, but it won't be long before the communication gap between you and your toddler starts to narrow. He'll get better at speaking, you'll get better at understanding. Sometimes it'll seem like the verbal floodgates are opening, sometimes those language skills will seem to lag – especially when a busy toddler is busier than usual building on physical skills, or when he's sick or out of sorts (aren't there times when you don't feel like talking, either?).

"I've heard other 1-year-olds talking, but my daughter doesn't seem ready yet. What's going on?"

The average child says her first word some time between 10 and 14 months – and whether her parents understand it or not, that word counts. But once in a while, a little one will start speaking up when she's younger (as early as 8 months) or older (as late as 18 months). Exactly when your toddler first opens up to say "Ah" (as in apple), or "Mmmm" (as in Mummy), or something equally cute, if incomprehensible, depends on:

Heredity. Were either you or your spouse an early verbal bloomer, or a late one? Or did both of you get an "A" – for average speech development? Obviously, you won't remember when you first started talking, but your parents might. Kids may follow in their mum and dad's verbal footsteps – thanks not only to inherited natural acumen (or lack of it) . . . but to inherited mouth and tongue muscles (believe it or not).

Birth order. A first child often speaks early because she has no siblings (yet) competing for Mum and Dad's attention and verbal encouragement – or for airtime. The more sibs a tot has, the less opportunity she may have to get a word in edgewise. Plus, she may not be in as much of a hurry to speak, since her needs may be filled quickly by a household that's now more accomplished at picking up on nonverbal cues. Of course, this pattern doesn't hold up in every home. Sometimes words are contagious – which means a subsequent child may catch the talking bug faster (much as they catch the colds older siblings bring home from school or playdates). Or she may speak up sooner, just to get heard.

Gender. On average, girls say their first word sooner. Chromosomes may contribute to this verbal edge, but environment almost certainly does, too (parents tend to chat to their female offspring more, right from the start). Of course, averages are just that – an average. Some girls are slower talkers, and some boys are the first in their playgroup to string together sentences.

The language background. Whether she ends up speaking on the early side or the later, a child will speak sooner if she's spoken to – so speak up. If there's more than one language spoken at

Talking

Your toddler is an individual when it comes to everything – including language development. So try not to compare number of words (or number of words in a phrase, or number of phrases in a sentence) against other children your little one's age. As long as your toddler is plugging away at verbal skills, and making steady (not necessarily speedy) progress, all is going according to plan – your toddler's genetic plan, that is. As always, if you have any concerns – or just that gut feeling that something's not quite on target – check in with the doctor. Most likely you'll get reassurance, but if a little something else is needed, it's always best to get that early on.

12 to 15 months. It's pretty remarkable how much a 12-month-old can get across without speaking a single recognisable word. Like a resourceful little caveman (or cavewoman), your young toddler hauls you by the jeans into the kitchen, pushes your legs in the direction of the back door, grunts or nods in response to questions, points to the cup he or she wants. And as long as your tot's actively trying to communicate, you can be impressed by that communication ingenuity. By the first birthday, most toddlers will be able to use one to five words meaningfully. By 15 months, that number could jump up to 5 to 10 real words for some.

15 to 18 months. Most toddlers age 15 to 18 months old can say 10-plus words – usually "Mama", "Dada", and other nouns (like "ball", "cup", "baby") – as well as some action words ("up", "down", "eat"). Some gifted gabbers may be able to use 20 to 30 words by this point. There may be other sounds (or "words") your little one makes – and makes meaningfully (at least to him or her), but at this stage, it's likely only you (and others close to your toddler) will be able to recognise their meaning.

18 to 24 months. Get ready . . . get set . . . go. The second half of the

home, your child may learn to speak each one more slowly than if only one language is spoken, but if there is a lag it'll be temporary. And you can't beat the ultimate pluses of a strong bilingual background.

Child care. Children who are talked to early and often speak sooner than they would without a language-rich environment, that's a given. But other factors come into play – including where a toddler plays. A child in nursery may learn to speak up sooner just to get her needs met, or may shut down when she isn't listened to. Little ones who do a lot of socialising with other children – especially older and more verbal ones – may pick up language skills earlier. What's clear is that regularly receiving verbal reinforcement – whether it comes from parents, childcare providers, babysitters, grandma, other children, or a combination – is what matters most in a child's speaking future.

The schedule. Her schedule, that is. You already know this, but it's worth repeating: your toddler is one-of-a-kind. Incomparable to every other child in every way – including in the language department. Without a doubt, every word that's said to her can nudge her

second year is when a toddler's language engine really gets revved up. Vocabulary will likely increase by leaps and bounds now – and you may find your little one using anywhere from 50 to 200 words by the time he or she reaches 24 months. Even more exciting (for both of you) is your toddler's use of primitive two- or sometimes three-word sentences: "No milk", "Aiden up", "Mama kiss".

Be on the lookout: If your 1-year-old doesn't gesture or point to things he or she wants, or try to communicate with you using nonverbal language, mention it to the GP. The same goes if by 16 months you still haven't heard your toddler's first word. Some later talkers just take their sweet time to speak, but the doctor might recommend a hearing test to see if a problem as simple – and as simple to clear up – as residual middle ear fluid that lingered after a cold or ear infection or an excessive buildup of earwax is limiting clear hearing and thus clear speech. Ask the doctor, too, if a formal assessment of language skills by a certified speech

and language pathologist is a good idea if your toddler:

- Isn't using more than one or two words by the 18-month mark.

- Seems to have poor receptive language (he or she should understand simple questions, be able to follow simple requests, and respond to simple statements).

- Is unable to communicate nonverbally (by pointing at a toy that's out of reach, for instance).

- Doesn't mimic simple words and sounds (if you "moo", your toddler should be able to "moo" back, for example).

- Has underdeveloped mouth muscles (a more-than-typical amount of food drops out of his or her mouth when eating, he or she regularly rejects food that requires chewing, or there's excessive drooling).

If a problem is found to account for your child's slower verbal skills, therapy can make a tremendous difference and help him or her catch up and even zoom ahead.

---

towards speedier speaking, but try to remember this isn't a race. Perfectly normal toddlers speak their first word before they can walk, others do it the other way around. Today's late talkers can become tomorrow's chatterboxes. Your toddler's timetable, like your toddler, is unique.

Also remember that before a toddler can say a word, she needs to understand many words. Call it by its official term (receptive language) or just call it comprehension (that's all it really is) – it's the first step in learning to speak, and a step that your toddler is probably taking without you even noticing it.

When she points to the cereal after you ask what she'd like for breakfast, when her whole body shakes with excitement after you announce a trip to the swings, or when she grabs her favourite book when you suggest storytime, your busy preverbal bee is telling you that she's in the language loop. What's more, she's building vital verbal skills she'll tap into big-time once she takes the next step: speaking (or, as it's officially called, expressive language).

If your child doesn't attempt to vocalise at all, and especially if she doesn't seem to understand or hear what you're saying, bring your concerns to her doctor.

The General Idea

Wonder why your brand-new talker just pointed to the man behind you in the supermarket queue and called him "da-da" – and expected you to be proud, not mortified? It's because young toddlers tend to lack the experience they need to be specific in their word choices. So they overgeneralise (in expert-speak: "overextend"). If the grey-haired lady in a toddler's life is "ga-ma" ("grandma"), then all grey-haired ladies, wherever they're encountered, are "ga-ma". If one animal with four legs and a tail is "dah" (or "dog"), then that holds for cats, too. And the man in the supermarket queue? Your toddler wasn't talking paternity, and wasn't confusing Daddy with random men, either. With only a few words to work with, your resourceful little one is using da-da to identify a whole category (people of Dad-like appearance).

What should you do when your toddler gets the general idea – choosing a word that's close, but not quite on the money? Praise the effort and move on? Make a correction? Try a little bit of both: "That's a man.

Daddy's a man, too. This is a different man. Look, there is another man. And another man." Or, "That's right. It has four legs and a tail, like a dog, but this animal is called a cat. Cats say meow." Gradually, your toddler will start to pick up more words, along with the ability to be more specific with labels (skills that will come with their own set of potentially cringe-worthy public moments, like "Why does that man have such a big belly?" or "Why does that girl have so many bumps on her skin?").

Some tots reverse overextension, in what's called "overrestriction". Instead of being general about specifics, these beginning speakers are specific about generals. So, all books will be labelled "G-nite Moo" (*Goodnight Moon*), the favourite bedtime book. All dogs are called "Sam", like your dog. Just like overextending, overrestricting is normal and disappears as a child builds verbal skills. In the meantime, you can help demystify the general idea for your toddler: "Yes, that's a dog, just like Sam is a dog."

Conversation Frustration

"We know she's trying to talk to us, but we don't have the slightest idea what our toddler's trying to say. We're frustrated – and she's frustrated, too."

If only toddlers came with subtitles. Or translation software on their hard drive. Or even a phrase book.

Of course, they don't. Instead, they come with primitive verbal skills that evolve at an impressive rate – but never

quickly enough to satisfy a toddler in a hurry to be understood, and parents in a hurry to understand her.

That challenging transition period between happy babbling and successful communication is frustrating on both sides of the conversation, yet it's completely normal. As her age-appropriate jargon progresses to syllables that sound more like words, single words, clumps of words, and finally, sentences, she'll start speaking your language and you'll start understanding hers. She may have a meltdown when you won't stop for ice cream, but not because you can't figure out that she's asking for ice cream.

While you're waiting to close (or at least narrow) that communication gap, try to keep in mind that she just wants to be understood. Also be sure to:

- Listen carefully. Sometimes there's a consonant clue in there, sometimes it's a vowel, sometimes a combination. "Eh" might be egg. "Ohg" might mean yogurt. She may not use labels consistently (cheese might be "eeeezzz", but it may also be "eee", which to further confuse things may also be a pet name for a blanket), but attention to those patterns may at least help you narrow down the field.

- Look while you listen. Don't understand your toddler's verbal language yet? Her body language can speak volumes. Look for hints in those adorable smiles, pouts, raised eyebrows, drooping shoulders, stomping feet, folded or outstretched arms. Obviously, pointing fingers are going to be your best go-to clue.

- Make talking interactive. She needs all the help she can get, so offer up tools. Invite her to "Show me what you want. Point to it with your finger" or to "Take me where you want to go", and encourage her to take your hand and direct you.

- Let her take her time. Yes, your watch may be ticking, reminding you that you both should have been in the car

---

Signing In

For the not yet-verbal, a finger is worth a thousand words. Toddlers will do just about anything to narrow the verbal divide (grunt, stomp, throw themselves on a display of stuffed animals). But resourceful ones – and is there really another kind of toddler? – usually realise pretty quickly that the most effective forms of preverbal communication are in their own hands . . . and in those chubby little fingers. A toddler who can't say "I want a cereal bar" may lead you by the hand to the cupboard where the stash is kept. One who's thinking "sandpit" may point to the bucket and spade at the door. But some toddlers – and the parents who try hard to understand them – get even more creative with their hands-on communication by "signing".

Certain signs are universal and timeless (you probably used a few of them yourself in your own preverbal days): waving to signify "I want to get out of here", cupping a hand to the mouth to say "I want a drink", rubbing a round belly to announce "I'm hungry". Other signs are less intuitive, but are easily taught (a hand tilted under the head for "sleepy", a finger touched to the nose for "smell"). Whether you sign your little one up for a formal baby sign language system or just develop a handful of your own homegrown signs, research shows that you won't be slowing down your toddler's speech development when you sign. In fact, by easing frustration and boosting communication confidence, you may be stepping up those early verbal efforts. Just make sure that you supplement signs with words (it's fine to sign "sleepy", but also say "You're sleepy. It's time for a nap.") For more on baby signs and how to use them, see *What to Expect the First Year.*

TWINS
Double Talk

Can't wait for your tots to start talking in tandem, but wondering if you'll have to wait longer than a parent of one? Twins (and other multiples) are often on a different – and usually somewhat slower – talking track than singletons. Here's why:

Slower speech development. Research shows that twins exhibit speech delays more often than singletons do – especially twin boys, who can lag behind in the language department by months. Sometimes those delays are due to prematurity, low birthweight, or birth complications (all of which are more common in multiple births) or gender (even singleton boys develop speech at a slower rate, on average, than singleton girls). But, more often, there's a surprisingly simple explanation for speech delays in twins: they're spoken to less frequently. Studies show that parents of twins talk directly to each twin less than they would to a single child – and for an obvious reason: they'd have to talk twice as much (and there just aren't enough hours in the day to do that). The result of being exposed to less targeted language than a singleton toddler is? Somewhat slower language development.

Fewer words. Research also shows that even when twins do start talking, they tend to speak up less – with fewer words and, later, shorter sentences. That probably has something to do with the fact that twins don't need as many words to communicate with each other – since one's needs and wants are often so similar to the other's, they can rely on intuition, hand gestures, eye contact, and so on. Consequently, they're often toddlers of few words, at least in the early language-development stage.

Secret language. Do your tots have "twinese" on their tongues – a seemingly secret language all their own, unintelligible to outsiders listening in? There's actually a medical term (or two) for this extremely common twin phenomenon: cryptophasia or idioglossia. Are your twins using their secret language to plot late-night escapes from the cot, a car seat rebellion, or a breakfast-time biscuit coup? Probably not. Experts believe that twin talk is less about keeping their communication private and more about their mimicking each other's rudimentary (and often incorrect) attempts at language. While the language models for a singleton are usually those who speak the language well (parents, older siblings, care providers), twins often model their emerging speech after each other's emerging speech – complete with word-mangling mispronunciations and butchered grammar. One twin hears the other say "ooh-ide" for "good-bye", so he or

20 minutes ago. But try to take a few minutes to calmly figure out what she's trying to ask for. The calmer you stay, the less frustrated she'll be. Plus, you'll be giving her the ultimate positive verbal reinforcement: "When I talk, they listen."

Loss of Vocabulary

"For a while, our son was using a wide variety of words, but in the last week or so, he seems to be using fewer. Shouldn't he be adding to his vocabulary instead of losing from it?"

she copies it. Pretty soon, both twins are waving "ooh-ide" when someone leaves. Can't crack the code? Not to worry – twin talk is both normal and temporary. By the time your twins reach age 5 or 6, their "secret language" will all but disappear.

Designated speaking. When you're a twin, someone's always got your back. And that's a good thing – except if that someone is always doing the talking for you. In some cases, one twin may take the verbal responsibility for the other (asking for the milk they both want), leaving the other twin speechless (and possibly, slower in speech development).

To encourage language development in your twins, check out all the tips in this chapter, but also:

- Talk it up with each twin. Though you can't reasonably expect yourself to double talk (talking twice as much, so each twin gets a targeted earful), try to spend time every day talking to each of your toddlers individually. Some one-on-one interaction and communication – combined with the usual team talk, which also counts – can help each twin beef up his or her language development.

- Encourage each child to speak up. Is one of your twins a spokes-tot for the other one? It's bound to happen to some extent; even identical twins have different personalities, so one's likely to be more outspoken than the other. But if you notice that one twin is always taking the communication lead for the other (and never letting the other one get a word in edgewise), try to break up the talking monopoly: "Aisha, Nahla told me you want something. Can you please tell me what you want?" Be sure, too, to give each twin ample airtime – even if one is easier to understand or more verbally advanced than the other.

- Branch out. Provide your little ones with opportunities to interact with other children, not just with each other. Joining a playgroup or visiting other tot hangouts, like the sandpit, will give your twins a chance to mimic – and learn from – other language models.

- Don't talk their talk. Even if you're able to decipher your twins' secret language, don't adopt it as your own (as cute as it might be). Follow up their twin-speak with your adult-speak so they'll learn the real words.

- Give it time. Most twins catch up on their communication skills by the time the preschool years roll around. But if your twins aren't combining two simple words by age 2, or if they have a vocabulary of fewer than 10 to 20 words by the time they hit their second birthday, mention it to the GP and consider getting a speech evaluation. Ditto if by age 2 your twins aren't able to be understood at least 25 per cent of the time by someone who's not a family member.

Before you assume your son is losing his vocabulary (he's most likely not), take a step back to look at the whole developmental picture. Ask yourself: what skills has he gained in the last week or so? Has he learned how to kick a ball? Paint with a paintbrush? Climb up stairs? Has he mastered using a fork? Is he trying to figure out how his new lorry works? Or how to fit the puzzle pieces together? The truth is, he's probably so focused on polishing a new skill-of-the-week ("Watch me kick that ball!" "Look . . . I can stick this fork right into

The Gift of Gab

Is your not-yet-2-year-old yapping up a storm? Can he speak in four- or five-word sentences? Has her vocabulary passed the 400-word mark – or does she have so many words that you've lost count? If so, your child may be what experts call a "precocious talker".

While precocious talkers can talk with the best of them, it's important to keep in mind that there's probably a large gap between what your child can say and what he or she means or understands. In other words, just because your toddler is able to say "I won't spill the juice" when wielding that orange juice container doesn't mean he or she is truly developmentally ready to pour it spill-free. Also remember that being able to suck up words with the power that would do a Hoover proud means that your toddler may hear and repeat words and phrases that you might prefer he or she didn't – at least not in public. So watch what you say, too.

my pasta!") that he's neglected to practise the others (including adding more words to his growing vocabulary). And that's typical of toddlers – one week they concentrate on verbal skills, the next week physical skills, the following week social skills, the week after that verbal skills again, switching back and forth in an attempt to master as many different skills as possible.

It's also possible that your tiny talker is taking the same hiatus from speaking that many young toddlers take after they've mastered their first few words. The break allows beginning speakers the time they need to consolidate their gains and strengthen their receptive vocabularies (words they understand), so that they can prepare to start learning a whole new list of words.

It could be, too, that he's been feeling a little too much pressure to perform his newly acquired verbal tricks, or to add to them. If your cheering has crossed that very fine line into pushing (however well-intentioned), try easing up a bit. Encourage – but try to avoid the kind of verbal hard sell that could lead him to clam up.

A cold virus that's just started to take hold can also temporarily slow speech (talking can seem too much like hard work). So can a change or disruption in your toddler's routine or his life. If so, bring on the hugs, extra cuddles, and reassurance – all of which will help get him talking again.

If your toddler's loss of language skills seems to be more than just temporary, mention your concern to the GP at the next visit.

Unclear Speech

"Our toddler has been talking up a storm lately. But I don't think there's a single word she pronounces even close to correctly. Is that normal?"

Imperfect (yet always achingly adorable) pronunciation is standard during the second year – even for a serious toddler motormouth. Often, only Mum, Dad, and maybe another regular caregiver will be able to translate that totspeak (and not always with 100 per cent accuracy, either). In fact, it's usually not until closer to age 3 that most little ones stop mangling language and start mastering proper pronunciation – and even then it'll still be far from perfect.

And it's easy to understand why your little one is still so hard to understand, particularly given the age-appropriate limitations of her mouth.

The manipulation of tongue and lips necessary to produce most consonant sounds – a skill you probably aren't even aware of having – is a manoeuvre she can't yet manage (try reading this paragraph out loud without using either your tongue or lips and you'll see what your toddler is up against). When she can't produce a particular sound, she resourcefully replaces it with one she can handle. So a child who gets tripped up on "d" but has no difficulty with "g" may call her father "gaga". Another may say "dute" for "cute", "ditty" for "pretty", "hewwo" for "hello", and "mappy" for "nappy." Consonant blends spell trouble, too, so "flower" may become "fower"; "tree", "tee"; "shoe", "soo".

Clarity isn't the name of the game now for your little garbled gabber. Learning how to express herself is. Eventually, clear speech will take the place of those precious mispronunciations (though you'll probably never forget the cutest of them – and you'll almost certainly share a few with your daughter's future boyfriends, much to her teenage horror). In the meantime, don't drive her crazy with corrections – there's plenty of time for English lessons later. And besides, are you really in a hurry to stop hearing "I wuv you"?

Only One Word at a Time

"My son has a pretty big vocabulary – maybe 100 words – but he mostly uses just one word at a time, maybe throwing in an occasional two-word phrase. When will he start using sentences?"

Imagine if you moved to a foreign country where you didn't speak the language . . . at all. First, you'd communicate with the native speakers using gestures, smiles, pointing, an awkwardly pronounced word or two tossed in here and there. As your vocabulary picked up, you'd start stringing two, maybe three words together – phrases without much in the way of structure. But full, spot-on sentences? Since grammar's always tougher to conquer, that would take far longer. It's the same for your novice English-speaker. He may be accumulating words at an impressive clip, he may have mastered a few two-word combinations (such as "go out" or "more milk") – and if he's truly precocious, he may even be closing in on three-word phrases that combine nouns with a verb ("Daddy read book"). But constructing even the most basic sentence isn't likely to happen until he's closer to 2, and if you're waiting to start hearing complete (if not consistently grammatical) sentences, think third birthday, or thereabouts.

Of course, the more sentences your little talker hears, the faster he'll start speaking them. So talk him up in full – though simple – sentences, and avoid baby phrasing (say "We're going to leave now" instead of "Justin go bye-bye"). Add on to his one- or two-word comments. When he says "car", respond: "Do you want your car? Here is your car." When he exclaims "Swing up!" help him expand on the thought: "It's fun to go on the swings. Do you want me to push you high up?" Read simple rhyming books to him, and once he's heard one several times, let him finish the final rhyming word on each page. Then move on to letting him fill in the last two or three words of each rhyme, then finally let him say the whole last line.

As always, however, don't let encouragement slip into pushing. Keep up your side of the conversation – and before you know it, your toddler will start to make sense out of sentences . . . and you'll never hear the end of them.

ALL ABOUT:
Getting Your Toddler Talking

Babies are born communicators – and, at first, crying says it all: "Feed me!" "Clean nappy over here!" "Cuddles, now!" But as the urge to connect with others – especially significant others, like mummies and daddies – gets stronger, babies add smiling to their communication tools. Then cooing. Pouting. Breathy sounds. Vowel sounds. Vowel sounds combined with consonant sounds. Sounds strung together. Word-like jargon, followed by real words, groups of real words, and, finally, grammatically complete sentences. In the space of about two years, a crying infant goes from 0 to 250 words – fully half the 500 used in a typical adult conversation. Fast-forward a year, and a 3-year-old's vocabulary is closing in on 1,000 words, a number that's likely to double again within a few years.

Some tots are fast talkers, while others take their talking time. But no matter what verbal timetable your toddler's running on, you can help him or her reach destination communication if you:

Expand the world. It may be a small world after all, but for your little one it's getting bigger by the day. Expand your toddler's environment and experiences and your toddler's vocabulary of words expands, too.

Take a trip to the zoo, then reinforce the concepts learned there by reading a book about the zoo ("Remember the monkey we saw at the zoo? The monkey was swinging on the tree!", "That's a giraffe. We saw the giraffe at the zoo – remember its long neck?"). Take a trip to the park, and point out the flowers growing (have your toddler take a sniff, too), the birds singing, the children playing. Even that dreaded trip to the supermarket can provide more than milk and bread – it can offer up aisles of vocabulary and concept building. The ice cream is "frozen", the fresh brownies in the bakery "smell sweet", you have to be "careful" with the carton of eggs so the eggs "don't break", that box of cereal is "big" and that one is "little". Turn your toddler into a mini-meteorologist ("It's hot today.", "Look at the rain!"), scientist ("If we put that ice cube in hot water, it melts!"), architect/contractor ("When you mix sand with water, you can build a sand castle."), and mood reader ("That little girl looks happy.", "That man is sad.").

Talk the talk. There's no overstating the importance of the obvious: the more you speak to children, the faster they'll speak back. So keep talking. Even the mundane is compelling to your toddler when it comes from your mouth: "We're going to have carrots for dinner. Carrots are yummy!" Showing while you tell will help increase comprehension: "Look, carrots! First I peel the carrots. Then I chop the carrots. Now I'm cooking the carrots. Mmmmmm, carrots!"

Repeat, repeat, repeat. Don't forget the oldest trick in the language teacher's book: repetition. Hearing a word or a phrase once doesn't work. For language to start making sense, your toddler has to hear the same words and phrases over and over.

Sound like a grown-up. Out of the mouths of toddlers come the cutest mispronunciations (if you haven't heard them yet, you will – and they're worth the wait). It's tempting to mimic those endlessly endearing attempts at words, but your little language learner's better off hearing the word the way it's supposed to sound. So when your toddler says "baba" for banana, reinforce the effort while making the proper pronunciation clear: "That's right, banana." Adding a "y" to certain words ("kitty", "doggy") to make them more toddler-friendly won't confuse – and let's face it, diminutives and little ones are a natural combination – but use grown-up words most of the time.

Be animated. You may have sworn you'd never talk to your child with that over-animated tone of voice parents naturally seem to adapt as their own. But (A) you know you want to and (B) that up-and-down inflection makes it easier for your toddler to pick out words as familiar. Plus, it gets and holds your little one's interest longer than a monotone does.

Label if you're able. Identify everything in your toddler's environment, so your little sponge can absorb new words. Point to and label what (and who) you see on the street (lorry, girl, bicycle, traffic light, dog, pushchair, tree), at home (table, spoon, cup, sofa, lamp, pot), in the queue at the supermarket (a man, a woman, a baby with a balloon). Labelling what you see in books also gives you a chance to identify things your toddler might not otherwise encounter on a daily basis (elephant, boat, forest, caterpillar, aeroplane).

Book it. Story time is everybody's favourite time, but it's so much more than just one-on-one fun. Of course, picture books are full of pictures, but they're also full of words. And even if your toddler doesn't know all of those words yet, pointing to the pictures as you say the words can help make that comprehension connection. See page 271 for more on reading to your toddler.

Sing a song. There's a reason why certain songs stay child crowd pleasers for generations: they're musically catchy, verbally simple, and use repetition – over and over again. So sing those children's favourites, and learn some more, too. Sing along to a CD or an iPod, or just sing without musical backup (your voice is always music to your toddler's ears, even if to others . . . not really). Topping the charts for young listeners: songs that involve hand clapping or finger play or other interaction (including those golden oldies, like "Wheels on the Bus", "Ring a Ring o' Roses", "Incy Wincy Spider").

Tune in. You appreciate being listened to, right? So try to be all ears when your toddler's babbling your way – and all eyes, too, since eye contact is a vital part of satisfying communication. On the phone? In the middle of something important? No need to drop everything. But next chance you get, try to give your toddler's efforts at conversation the attention they deserve. Keep in mind, though, that toddlers also like to talk to themselves, to toys, and to pets. Unless you're the object of your little one's babble, there's no need to barge in.

RSVP. It's French for "respond, please", and it's a good toddler mantra to live by. Try to speak when you're spoken to by your little one – even if you haven't made out a single word. Think about it this way: if someone who didn't speak English came up to you and tried to speak, you'd try to understand – and you'd make an effort to respond, too (with the old smile-and-nod, at the very least). Well, your little one's new to English, too, and definitely far from fluent. Understand what you can, piece together what you can't (read that body language, invite your toddler to "show me what you want"), but even if you end up drawing a blank, RSVP anyway – with that warm smile and a convincing "Hmmmm, that's interesting. Tell me more", if nothing else. Any positive feedback is positive reinforcement for your toddler's verbal efforts.

Hand over the mike. Sometimes, especially in busy homes with other children hogging the stage, toddlers hardly ever get the chance to flex their communication muscles. So be careful to leave some airtime for your littlest speaker. Eventually, it'll get filled with words of his or her own.

Don't make it too easy. Good communication is hard work. If you anticipate your toddler's every need, there won't be as much incentive to work those verbal skills. The results aren't so much what matters, but you do want your little one to strive for an "A" for effort.

Ask away. Your toddler may still be short on answers (that you can understand), but asking questions is one of the best ways to get little ones talking. So ask away: "Do you want a snack?", "Which book do you want to read?" Answers can come in all forms at this age – in a shaking head (though if your toddler hasn't worked out the nodding kinks yet, "no" can still mean "yes"), a grunt, a point, and more gestures and noises. All of them count – and any response lets you know your toddler is listening, understanding, and trying to communicate. After your little one has answered in his or her way, follow up with the words: "Oh, you want the book with the bunny in it!"

Get your words' worth. Clear and concise (and animated) is the best way to speak to your toddler. But once comprehension is starting to add up, you can try working a word into a couple of different contexts: "See the bicycle? The boy is riding the bicycle" or "Yes, that's a flower. The flower smells good." Once this word use sinks in, try using the word in a sentence, injecting an adjective: "Let's smell the pretty flowers.", "Daddy is singing a funny song." You can also add an adverb once a verb is conquered: "We are walking fast.", "That man is talking loudly." But try not to overload your toddler conversations. The idea is to keep it simple and layer it on gradually. And speaking of adverbs (like "slowly" or "quickly" or "gladly"), it's fine to use them, but remember they're a pretty nuanced part of sentence structure. You'll want to work up to pronouns, too ("me", "we", "I") – using them in tandem with proper nouns when possible: "Daddy is hungry. I am hungry." Or "Isabella is in the bath. You are in the bath."

Be a translator. No UN experience necessary – just the willingness to serve as translation go-between for your toddler and others. Maybe the woman at the checkout says, "I have some balloons for nice little boys. Would you like one?" Give your toddler a moment to respond, and if he's drawing a blank, or is mumbling something that someone who doesn't speak his language would never understand, step in and translate. You: "Would you like a balloon?" Your toddler: gives an excited yelp, jumps up and down, and reaches for the balloon. You: "Say thank you for my balloon." Toddler, possibly: "Ta." You: "He says thank you." Communication established – the checkout lady's happy, your toddler's happy, you're happy.

Remember those earmuffs. Since toddlers are sponges for language, they pick up just about anything they hear. Including words you might not want your toddler to hear – or repeat at family gatherings.

Don't believe every word. Another warning: toddlers don't necessarily mean what they say, any more than they say what they mean. Not just when it comes to . . . ahem . . . inappropriate words, but also when it comes to words that are conceptually way over that little head. So when your toddler says: "po-mis" (promise), well – let's just say a promise probably won't be a promise.

Support free speech. Your job is to encourage talking, not to push it. So nurture verbal development, but also let nature (and that timetable of your toddler's) take its course. Cheer, challenge, but don't turn life into an endless English lesson (boorrring!). Or a praise-fest, either. Conversation is also its own reward, so hang on to your toddler's every word – or attempt at a word – but no need to give every syllable a standing ovation.

Know when to push "pause". Getting that glazed-over look from your little listener? Your toddler may have reached conversation saturation. Or may just want some quiet time to think or babble to himself or herself. Give it a rest for a little while, then start up again later.

CHAPTER 9

Learning

....

I T MAY GO WITHOUT SAYING, but toddlers have a lot to learn. Fortunately, your little one is not only up to the job, but at this particularly impression-able age is uniquely qualified for it. Skip ahead a dozen years or so, and you may have to nag, badger, and harass in order to get algebra homework finished and essays written (or started . . . at least before Sunday night) – but for now, that naturally insatiable curiosity and dogged determination to discover drive your toddler's yearning for learning. In this second year, learn-ing of all kinds is taking place at a mind-boggling pace – and yet, if you're like most parents, you probably can't help but wonder if it's happening fast enough (or as fast as it seems to be happening for the rest of the playgroup . . . and wait, was that child a month younger than yours really just reciting the alphabet?). Is there more you should do, teach, schedule? And what about TV, computers, and classes – do they have a place on your little learner's educational agenda? Forget the three Rs – there's only one R you need to keep in mind: relax. School time is scheduled for when your busy, inquisitive toddler is awake.

What You May Be Wondering About

ABCs and 1-2-3s

"A few of the kids my daughter plays with can recite some of the alphabet and count up to five. My daughter is almost 2 and doesn't seem interested in learning any of this. Is she going to be behind when she starts preschool?"

No need to pull out the flash cards. Or sing the alphabet song until you're "B" – for "blue in the face". Or count until you're both crazy. Though there's probably nothing wrong with a toddler having an academic head start (unless, of course, the toddler is pushed into that head start), there's absolutely nothing necessary about it, either. While children who've had some pre-preschool letter and number prep may enjoy a temporary edge, studies show they don't necessarily stay at the head of the class. What's more, even those who start out somewhat behind the pack usually catch up.

So, no need to start worrying about the reports yet. Just because your toddler doesn't have much interest in an academic agenda at this very tender age doesn't mean she's not scholastically inclined. It means that she's busy building other skills that are more important (and interesting, and fun) to her at the moment. Let her – there's plenty of time for academics (and besides, are you really in a hurry for homework?). In the meantime, instead of pushing the ABCs and 1-2-3s (she's bound to tune out if you do), just incorporate them into life's everyday experiences. Talk to her. Read to her. Share some brightly coloured, simple ABC books together. Write her name in clear block letters on her crayon scribbles before you put them up on the fridge, and point out "A is for Akira, and it's also for apple."

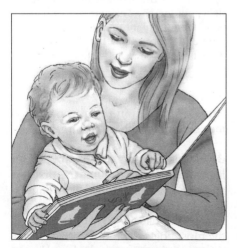

Reading books with your toddler will help to foster a love of reading.

Count out stairs that you're climbing or crackers you're doling out. Show her "this is more cereal" and "this is less cereal". Cut sandwiches into triangles, squares, rectangles, and circles, and tell her the names of the shapes. Most of all, instead of comparing your little one with the apparent overachievers in her group (who may be overachieving because their parents are overinstructing), appreciate her just the way she is. Nurture your toddler's natural love of learning – no matter what form it takes right now.

Raising a Reader

"I try to read books to my toddler as often as I can, but he doesn't really pay attention. How can I get him to be a book lover?"

Is your toddler more wriggly worm than bookworm? Few 1-year-olds have the attention span to sit out an extended story time, and many can't make it through page two of book one before distraction sets in and the squirming starts. That's more an indication of your tot's age than of his future as a reader. Still, it's possible to nurture a love for reading well before he knows an "A" from a "Z" – and yes, even with his concentration limitations. Here's how:

Be selective. Choose books with large, clear, bright, and cheerful illustrations (stay away from abstract images for now – it's harder to engage a toddler if he can't identify the pictures) and short, simple text that includes familiar words. Though most toddlers prefer rhyming books (even if the words don't mean much, the rhythm is appealing), now is a good time to begin introducing some very simple stories in prose – no more than one or two short sentences on a page to start. Heavy board books are

The ABCs of Ps and Qs

They grab and push and barge into the queue. They eat with their fingers and chew with their mouths wide open. They never say "thank you" without prompting, or "please" without prodding (and even then, it's dicey). They kick and scream to get what they want and kick and scream when they don't get what they want.

In short, toddlers break every rule of social etiquette ever written and just about every code of conduct as we know it. Yet, believe it or not (and you may find this particularly difficult to believe as you watch your toddler snatch a playmate's spade or use clean trousers as a napkin or bang on the refrigerator to obtain a drink), inside every pint-size barbarian is a mini Mr or Ms Manners, just waiting to be groomed for life in the civilized world.

So let the grooming begin. Yes, it'll be months before the pushing and shoving subside, years before you'll be able to count on an automatic "please" or "thank you" or on dinner table habits that don't turn your stomach. But toddlers who get a head start learning the ABCs of etiquette do have an excellent chance of growing up well mannered. To start your toddler on the road to civility now:

Lay the right foundation. Good manners aren't just a matter of being versed in your pleases and thank-yous, knowing when to sit and when to stand, and locating the correct utensil to use with each course. The underlying principle of good manners is consideration for others. In other words, saying "please" and "thank you" should mean that you care, not just that you're well bred. So to raise an authentically well-mannered child, teach the why of etiquette along with the how. The objective: to foster manners that come intuitively from the heart, instead of by the book (you offer your guest the plate of biscuits first, or help an elderly woman by picking up the coins she dropped not just because it's considered the polite thing to do, but because it's the kind thing to do). The fact is that a child who's raised to be considerate can't help but grow up to be courteous.

Set an exemplary example. The best way to teach manners to your toddler, of course, is to use them yourself. So say "thank you" to the bus driver, say "please" to the woman behind the deli counter, say "excuse me" when you bump into another shopper in a crowded shop; eat with a napkin on your lap and chew with your mouth

ideal for your toddler to "read" alone; keep the more delicate paper books (especially those with pop-up features) for supervised reading sessions. Vinyl books are fine for the bath (bath time is often a good time to get a little reading in), but be sure to dry them thoroughly after each dunking to prevent mildew from taking hold. And your toddler will definitely get a lot of mileage out of books that have squeakers or sound

chips embedded in them (though you may get a headache in the bargain).

Be persistent (but not pushy). Your little one loses focus after the first few pages? Release him from the reading session, but don't give up on the next one. Persistence usually pays off, even with the most fidgety of toddlers. Establish a daily story time (after the bath and before bed is ideal, since he's likely not to be

closed, and ask that the pepper be passed to you rather than reaching across someone's plate for it. But probably most important of all, remember to mind your Ps and Qs when dealing with your toddler. Say "please" when you've asked your toddler to come to the table, say "thank you" when your toddler picks up a book as asked, and say "I'm sorry" when you've accidentally knocked over a brick project. To teach respect and consideration, try to respect and consider your toddler's feelings at all times.

Set the table. Really. A toddler can't possibly learn how to use a napkin if one never finds its way in front of his or her booster chair at mealtime, or a fork if you never provide one. Taking the time to set the table neatly with the proper utensils and napkins says a mouthful to your toddler about mealtime decorum. Even if your toddler eats like a savage now, consistent exposure to civilised eating conditions will eventually instil an appreciation for them.

Speak for your toddler. Toddlers don't know enough to say "good-bye" to Grandpa or "thanks for coming" to a visitor or "thanks for having me" to the host of a playgroup. So it's up to parents to say it for them until they can say it themselves. Hearing you use the "magic words" over and over in social situations at home and away from home will teach your toddler much more about common courtesy than any amount of nagging. Gentle reminders will encourage your little one to speak for him- or herself once the words come more easily.

Keep the campaign on. Pressure isn't appropriate, but reminders are. When you're alone and your toddler forgets to say "please", ask "What's the magic word?" When he or she omits a "thank you", try "What do you say?" If you get the appropriate response, fine. If not, fill in the blank for your child. You've at least made clear you think politeness is a priority. Again, wage your campaign with a light touch: "What's this? What do we do with a spoon? Wave it in the air? Wear it as a hat?"

Have age-appropriate expectations. Most toddlers can't keep their elbows off the table. Or keep their fingers out of the mashed potatoes, their hands out of their cereal, their napkins on their laps, or their juice in their cups. Getting into food (literally) is part of the fun of eating for toddlers, plus it's really developmentally difficult for them to avoid. From remembering to say "thank you" to being willing to share, it will take many years of etiquette exposure (and as many years of reminders) before your child matures into polite company.

quite as wriggly then). If you have time in the morning – before his motor is fully revved up – a cuddly reading session in a comfy chair or in your bed can be nice, too. Even if it doesn't last long, and even if your toddler's more interested in petting the cat or climbing on and off the chair, story time will ultimately become a cherished ritual – one that you'll both continue to treasure long after your child becomes capable of reading to himself.

That is, if you're not too pushy. Holding your toddler hostage on your lap until a book's finished, long after listening has become too much like hard work, can create a reading rebel.

Be creative. You know what interests your toddler better than any author does. So if your child seems confused or frustrated by the language, don't feel obliged to read the words as written.

Doing a little creative editing can greatly enhance your toddler's comprehension and interest level (and you won't be breaking any copyright laws). Cut a paragraph down to one sentence, swap simpler words for those your toddler doesn't understand, drop in commentary and explanations as needed. If the text of a story seems to be leaving your toddler in the dark, focus on the illustrations ("Look at that big dog and that little dog" or "I wonder what's in the little girl's basket").

Be interactive. Long before your child can read, he can participate in the reading process. First by pointing to characters you've asked him to find ("Where's the kitty cat?") and objects in the illustrations ("Where's the cat's hat?"), later by filling in the blanks in sentences or rhymes in books you've read over and over. When you read a story for the first time, look for characters, objects, colours, and ideas your toddler isn't familiar with, and take the opportunity to introduce them – pretty soon he'll be able to identify those, too. Ask questions, and supply answers if your toddler isn't equipped or inclined to answer them this time (or even next time): "What does the cow say?" "Where are the doggy's ears?" "What is the boy eating?" Prompt participation, too, by reading books that are interactive: touch-and-feel books, books with surprises hiding under little flaps, books that have dials to turn, and so on.

Be expressive. Nobody likes listening to a reading robot (except maybe another robot), so if you're prone to a monotone, it's time for a makeover. To a toddler who's just picking up the nuances of language, an expressive reading style makes listening not only more enjoyable, but also more understandable. So ham it up.

Be repetitious. Toddlers love to hear the same story over and over and over again. And though the repetition may drive you to distraction (see the next question), it's incredibly satisfying to young ears. After a while, you may even be surprised to find that your toddler has memorised some of the text (especially if it's in rhyme – always verbal music to little ears).

Be brief. Short books and short reading sessions sit best with a toddler who can't sit still. Go from page to page and idea to idea quickly – to keep restlessness from setting in, and your audience from wandering off. And be ready to end story time after just a few minutes, if need be.

Be cuddly. Even tots who aren't too excited about story time will most likely love – and look forward to – the cosy comfort of being curled up on Mummy or Daddy's lap. That feel-good association will continue feeling good long after your little one has outgrown your lap. That said, if your toddler's a fidget who regularly resists confining spaces (even cuddly ones), let him sit – or not sit – however he'd like. Freedom of movement may increase listening time.

Be a reading role model. Children of readers are much more likely to end up readers themselves. Try to set time aside each day for your own story time (yes, it's okay to read something other than a four-word-a-page picture book once in a while) – even if you manage just a page or two per sitting. If you can't fit this into your schedule, or if reading's not your thing, make sure your toddler catches you reading at least occasionally. And minimise the amount of television time that's clocked in by your toddler and by you. Experts agree (though it doesn't really take an expert to do the maths on this one): families that watch less, read more.

A Taste (Literally) for Literature

Nobody devours literature or tears through a pile of books or magazines like a toddler. Turning the pages and looking at the pictures is diverting, yes, but maybe not quite as tasty as nibbling, or as fascinating as shredding and ripping. To nurture a love of reading while protecting the reading material in your home:

Invest in the indestructible. Sturdy board books can withstand almost any assault by teeth, gums, saliva, and rip-happy hands, plus they're easy for little fingers to flip through (and at this age, turning the pages is at least half the fun). Keeping a large selection of colourful, age-appropriate board books within easy reach will invite your toddler to pick up and peruse them frequently – and may somewhat discourage a search-and-destroy mission of your bookshelf or magazine rack.

Shelve the destructible. Put books and magazines you'd like to preserve intact on a high shelf, or wedge them so tightly into bookshelves that your toddler can't pry them loose. But don't make any reading material (with the exception of the very valuable) completely off-limits. An open book policy encourages the opening – and eventually the reading – of books. So let your toddler examine and touch your books under close supervision.

Stop destruction entirely. Allowing your toddler to shred some magazines (for instance, those you've read) but not others sends a confusing message. Since a child this young can't possibly distinguish between reading matter that's ready for recycling and reading material that's hot off the presses, stop the ripping or chewing of either.

Redirect interest. You don't want to give your toddler the impression that reading material is a "no-no", just that tearing and eating it is. When you catch him or her in an act of destruction, don't scold your tot. Instead, just say "Please don't hurt the book. Books are for reading and looking at." Then say "Let's look at it together." Sit down and read the book with your little one. If the text is way over his or her head, simplify the words as you read or take the opportunity to bring out a book that's more age appropriate.

Redirect the impulse. If your toddler's interest in the books he or she is manhandling is definitely not literary, try moving on to an activity that might approximate the satisfaction he or she gets from ripping (tearing lettuce up for tonight's salad, sliding a zip up and down, or opening and closing a Velcro closure on a doll's shoe).

Reading Repetition

"My daughter wants to hear the same book every single night. Not just once, but two or three times. I'm so bored reading it."

Many toddlers just can't get enough of a good thing – whether it's a favourite food, a favourite blanket, or a favourite book. What seems monotonous to adults is the height of toddler happiness, for several reasons:

- Same is safe. This may seem like a recurring theme, but that's because it's endlessly true. Little ones feel more comfortable, secure, and in control with the familiar and the predictable – the book read over and over again becomes a trusted friend, just as that teddy bear becomes a constant companion.

- **Repetition builds comprehension.** The first time you read a book to your toddler, she may not understand every word. With each subsequent reading, she'll pick up more and more words – especially if your explanations have helped her crack the code. By the time you've had it well past your ears with that book, she's likely mastered every word. For someone who's learning the language, that's productive *and* satisfying.

- **Familiar is fun – and fulfilling.** For you, reading the same story (or watching the same rerun) over and over is boring. For your toddler, it's exciting. Knowing a book well – even by heart – allows your little one to play an active role in story time, anticipating what comes next, filling in words here and there, pointing out what's familiar in pictures.

In other words, the familiarity that breeds boredom in you breeds contentment and spurs learning in your toddler. To keep her content – and learning – you'll have to resign yourself to the repetition. While she'll eventually tire of her current favourite story (and likely adopt another immediately), let it be her idea to end the repetitive reads.

In the meantime, try to make the rereading even more fun for her (and less mind-numbing for you) by channelling your inner storyteller. Though it's tempting to switch onto auto-pilot, you'll both enjoy the story more if you read with animation, experimenting with voices and style, injecting dramatic flourishes or over-the-top silliness. Share the job of story reader with her, too – letting her fill in as many blanks as she'd like (at the end of a line, at the end

of a page, and so on). Ask her to predict the plot ("Who goes into the barn next? That's right, it's the cow!"). Even though you both know it cover to cover, she'll get quite a thrill out of being so clever. Challenge her to identify characters or objects, and try to point out something as yet unnoticed (the red collar on the puppy, for instance, or the squirrel hidden in the tree), then ask her to find it the next time.

Indulge your daughter's reading rut, by all means, but also help her think outside the book box. Each night, suggest (but never insist on) an alternative storybook. Even if she's not willing to give up her usual, she may be open to hearing a new one, too. Try a new book that's a sequel to her favourite, or has the same characters, the same author, or the same illustrator. Help broaden her literary horizons, also, by taking her to the library or attending story hour at a bookshop.

Your toddler just won't turn the page on her favourite book? Let her stick with her favourite for now. Her commitment to consistency – in everything from books to blankets to breakfast foods – won't last forever.

What's This? What's That?

"About 300 times a day, my toddler asks 'Wha dis?' She'll ask even when she knows the answer!"

Sounds like your daughter has caught what's-this-itis – a condition that's pretty much universal among toddlers in the second year, for a few reasons. First, and most obvious: because toddlers are curious. Propelled by a need to know – about everything and anything in their ever-expanding world – tots are driven to discover. Asking you "What's this?"

is an easy way for your little one to make some of those discoveries (at this point, your toddler still thinks you know it all). Second, because they're eager to practise their language skills. To your brand-new talker, using a phrase such as "What's this?" or "What's that?" is more satisfying than using single words – and using the phrase over and over is satisfaction-plus (even if she knows the answer to her question).

There's also another reason why toddlers persist in asking "What's this?" – it's sure to get a response. While she might not get more than a distracted nod when she calls out "Doggy!" you're bound to offer her a full-fledged answer to a question. Result? She's successfully started a conversation – and that's satisfaction-plus-plus.

Eventually, your toddler will tire of playing the what's-this-what's-that game and move on to a more challenging question: "Why?" (so you might want to start Googling why the sky is blue). In the meantime, do your best to patiently play along. Supply her with the answers to her endless string of questions (which will encourage her to keep asking them as she grows) – even when you start feeling like a human search engine. Pretty sure she already knows the answer to the question (it's a bird, and it was a bird the last 30 times she asked)? Try turning the tables with "What do you think it is?" This may spare you some tedious repetition, while challenging your toddler to work things out for herself (plus, she still gets the satisfaction of getting the conversation started).

Toddler Classes

"There are loads of classes for toddlers offered in my neighbourhood. Should I sign my son up for some of them?"

From music and art lessons to gymnastics and mummy-and-me classes – there's certainly no shortage of programmes aimed at the pre-preschool set. While enrolling your toddler definitely isn't a must-do (skipping classes now definitely won't keep your little one from moving to the head of the class – or the top of the lineup – later on), it can come with its perks. These organised activities allow your toddler to socialise and try out games, toys, materials, and equipment he doesn't have access to at home (or that you'd rather not try at home – like certain art projects). And there's even something in it for you, if you're the one attending class with your toddler: getting to spend some adult time with other parents.

How can you choose the best programme for your toddler? Keep these tips in mind:

- Ask around. You're sure to have friends-with-toddlers who have been-there, done-that when it comes to toddler classes, and if you don't, you can check out local reviews online. So poll before you enrol – ask other parents which classes are winners and which ones you're better off avoiding.

- Try one out. Many programmes will allow parents and tots to try out a class once for free to determine if the fit is right. If not, ask to observe a class – you'll be able to get a sense of whether your toddler will enjoy it or not.

- Make fun your first objective. You want an age-appropriate, lighthearted, and unstructured introduction to a subject, not the first step to a master's degree. An art teacher, for example, should embrace messy creativity, not try to teach brushstrokes. The music instructor should encourage all sorts of ways to make melodies and rhythms, rather than instructing in notes or scales. Classes shouldn't stress a certain skill set, because this can stress a toddler out. Instead, they should take a whole-toddler (and a whole-lot-of-fun) approach, one that encourages overall physical, cognitive, and social development . . . and a good time.

- Keep it short and sweet. A toddler's attention span isn't very long, so look for classes that are no longer than 45 minutes each and that never restrict movement or demand quiet (though a programme that incorporates snack time, circle time, free play, and different activities can be a little longer).

- Keep it small. Put 25 toddlers in one room and you've got a large-scale meltdown waiting to happen. Look for classes that are limited to 12 pint-size pupils. On the flip side, a too-small class might lack energy.

- Keep it age-appropriate. Make sure the class is geared to your child's age. Make sure, too, that the equipment, supplies, and instruction are all scaled to your child's developmental level. For instance, structured football (and other sports) classes, while offered for the under-2 set, often put too many physical demands on still-developing joints – potentially setting up a toddler not only for athletic burnout, but also for early overuse injuries. Such classes are fun for some tots, too much pressure for others – but either way, a risky proposition.

- Keep it in perspective. Classes can be an entertaining break for both of you, especially if the dog days of summer or the frigid days of winter have you running a cabin fever. They can even teach your child some new skills. But if you enrol your toddler in classes, do it for the fun and the diversion – not to put him on an academic, athletic, or artistic fast track.

Computers

"Is it too early to introduce the computer to our toddler? I keep seeing programs and games designed for her age."

Wonder whether you should try turning your 1-year-old into a technotot? While there's no doubt that there's technology in your child's future, it's less certain that it should play a significant role in her life right now. In fact, most experts advise that children under age 3 are better off left unplugged and unwired – hooked up with other humans (especially you) instead of anything electronic. It's through that direct human interaction that toddlers learn best about everything from language skills to social skills. Even bricks, dolls, lorries, and other tangible toys can teach your little one more than any screen can – and that goes for those computer and online games marketed specifically to the tiny tots, too. And not only does a toddler have less to gain by spending lots of time in front of a computer, she may have a lot to lose. There are plenty of documented drawbacks to computer overuse for the 2-and-under set (as there are from excessive TV watching; see page 281), including stifled creativity, hampered social skills, lagging language skills, eyestrain, limited physical activity, and overweight, to name a few.

If you do decide to let your toddler go digital:

- Limit the time. For a toddler this young, 5 to 10 minutes in front of the screen is more than enough – she'll likely lose interest quickly anyway (and if she seems endlessly entertained by the games, you should still power off after 10 minutes – she has better, more active, and more creative things to do). If your little one doesn't seem interested in it at all, there is no reason to push it.

Teaching Time

To toddlers, there's no time like the present. In fact, there's no time but the present. The past and the future are still far too abstract to wrap their little minds around – instead, they're age-appropriately focused on "now". "Now" is when they want lunch, want Mummy to come home, want to go out, want to get to the playground. But as the second birthday approaches, there's a big jump in time savvy, and toddlers begin to understand what you mean when you say "soon" or "later". As your toddler turns into a preschooler, there's further progress, as such concepts as "today", "yesterday", and "tomorrow" become separate (though fuzzy) entities, but a complete comprehension of time doesn't usually become clear until about age 6. In the meantime, you can help this learning process with these timely tips:

Give time a context. When talking time with your toddler, use more than one way to describe the same time whenever possible: "We'll go to the playground in the afternoon, right after your nap." Or "Dahlia is coming over to play this morning, after breakfast."

Work on order. Present your toddler with your planned schedule of activities in order: "First, we'll go to the shops, then we'll go to the library, and then we will have lunch." Or, "First, we'll have a bath, second, we'll have some crackers and milk, third, we'll have a story, and last, you'll go to bed." You can also begin introducing the concepts of "before" and "after" ("We'll have a snack before we go to the park", "Henry and his mummy will come over after breakfast") and "soon" and "later" ("Soon, it will be time to clean up the bricks in your room"

or "Later, we'll go outside and play catch"). But don't expect your toddler to comprehend the nuances of these timely words just yet.

Use visual aids. Concrete examples will help put the passing of time in perspective for your toddler. Show your toddler pictures of him- or herself as an infant ("Before, you were this little") and now ("Now, you're this big"). When you've read a story, go back and outline it in chronological order ("First, the little boy went swimming. Then, he played at the park. Later, he went home and ate ice cream"). When your toddler is going to have to wait for something, try setting a timer to illustrate the passing of time ("I'm going to set the timer for five minutes. When the timer rings, I'll be ready to paint with you").

Take the daze out of days. The days of the week will be less of a blur to your toddler if he or she associates each with a particular activity: "On Monday, we have playgroup. On Tuesday, we go to the library. On Sunday, we go to Grandma and Grandpa's." A large weekly calendar with pasted-on pictures or other visual reminders of regular activities may also help get the idea across. Make a point of discussing the tangible events of yesterday ("Yesterday, we had lunch in a restaurant. Remember, we had yummy pasta!"), today ("Today, we had fun at the museum."), and tomorrow ("Tomorrow, we'll go over to Zachary's house."). If your toddler is anxiously awaiting Daddy's return from a business trip, try to make that abstract arrival day a tad more tangible: "Daddy will come home after two bedtimes."

- Share the time. As tempting as it may be, using the computer as a babysitter isn't a great idea. Instead, plonk yourself down beside your toddler and share the screen time, interacting with her just as you do when you're reading her a book. Ask questions about screen images and words ("Where's the sun?"), add insights ("The sun is yellow. The sun is a circle"), and later, connect the computer images with her real world ("Look at that ball on the floor. It's a yellow circle. Just like the sun!").

- Choose the right games. Look for games with simple pictures (forget those that barrage your toddler with fast-moving graphics) and simple songs. Sample a program at a friend's house, read reviews of software online, or visit websites that rate software. The same goes for online games. Check them out yourself to see if they're appropriate before letting your tot log on.

- Treat it like a toy. Though software companies definitely market computer games as learning devices, being a tech-savvy tot won't make your little one smarter or more academically successful. Yes, software and online games can introduce your child to numbers, letters, opposites, colours, and shapes, but so can puzzles, shape sorters, books, and a whole lot more interactive activities, from painting to visiting a museum to taking a nature walk with you. So use it for fun, once in a while, not because you're hoping to give your toddler an academic advantage.

- Don't force it. Just because your neighbour's tot has been a techie since infancy doesn't mean yours will be, too – or should be. Keep your toddler unplugged until she shows some interest (Does she pound on the keyboard or move the mouse all over the desk? Does she perk up when you turn on the screen?). Remember, there's no rush to introduce her.

Educational DVDs

"The mums on my message board all seem to swear by those baby-brain-boosting videos. Should I have my son watch them, too?"

Even though there's an entire school of DVD products marketed to stimulate babies' and toddlers' learning, the science behind those educational claims isn't very solid. In fact, studies show that these products may do more harm than good by actually delaying language development instead of beefing up brainpower. Researchers believe that the screen time tots spend on Baby Einstein, Brainy Baby, and other "educational" DVDs preempts valuable one-on-one time with Mum and Dad, which is when babies and toddlers learn language best. Bottom line: reading books together, singing songs, or channelling your inner child by improvising silly dances or getting on your hands and knees to play a game of "Name This Animal Sound" are all better ways to boost brainpower and language skills. More effort for you, but far more rewarding for your little learner.

If you do decide to turn to these baby and toddler videos every now and then, there's no harm done – as long as the viewing comes in small, infrequent doses. Remember: when it comes to DVDs or educational TV for your toddler, less is more. And when it comes to helping your child's brain grow, nobody does it better than you do.

TV Watching

"I know all the reasons why I shouldn't let my toddler watch TV, but realistically, sometimes I just need a break. Is it really so bad to turn on the TV for her once in a while?"

You've heard all the negatives of plonking your toddler in front of a TV, as backed up by the experts and the research (see box, page 282). But you've also, not surprisingly, encountered the positives – at least the ones a little toddler TV time offers you. And so have most other parents of toddlers. Despite the studies that suggest they shouldn't, the reality is that over 70 per cent of children under the age of 2 watch some television – and it's the rare parent who doesn't turn to *Waybuloo* or *In the Night Garden* for an occasional sanity-saving break. Like when you need a breather from bricks. A few peaceful moments to pick up the mess, pay some bills, or catch up on work. Or just . . . because.

Another reality here. A little carefully selected TV in the context of an otherwise busy, active, and stimulating day (the day you probably provide every day without even trying) definitely will not devastate her development, not by a long way.

Can't get on board with banning TV, but can't help feeling guilty when you switch it on? Forget the guilt (if you're going to take a TV break from your toddler anyway, you might as well enjoy it). Instead, follow these basic tenets of toddler TV watching to give your little one the most benefits with the least downside:

- Time it. Does your TV have a way of staying on once it's on? With the availability of round-the-clock children's programming, it's easy for TV to become a fixture of your toddler's day. Before it does, start setting serious limits. For children under 2, 10 to 15 minutes per day is plenty. If you find 15 minutes turns into 30, set a timer so you'll know when to turn off the TV. Even 30 minutes of TV a day is just too much for a young toddler (and more than that is exponentially worse). Stand firm on the limits you set. If your tot is clamouring for more TV time, divert attention to another activity, now.

- Time it right, too. TV time should not coincide with mealtime, which should be reserved for eating and talking. Keep the TV off during playdates, as well, when children should be practising social skills. And avoid making TV part of the bedtime routine – all those flashing images and all that noise can keep your little one from settling down for the night, even if she's not actively watching.

- Watch together. When you do turn on the set, try to make it a do-together activity instead of a babysitting session. Talk about what you see ("That doggy looks just like Aunt Kaylee's dog!") and explain what's happening ("The boy is painting a picture – that is a pretty blue colour") to prevent your child from slipping into a TV trance. Keep in mind that TV togetherness doesn't have to keep you side by side on the sofa – and you don't have to keep your eyes glued to the screen (you can pipe in just periodically and actually get something else done at the same time). Of course, there will be times when you'll need (or want) to use those 15 minutes to accomplish something that needs your full attention – enter the electronic babysitter. Just don't make solitary watching a habit for your tot.

The Trouble with TV

Must-see TV? Maybe more like a must-not when you're talking about toddlers. Though there's definitely no shortage of television programming aimed at young toddlers (and even babies), most experts recommend that the under-2 set tune out entirely. Research shows that little ones get little out of TV watching, even programming marketed as educational. In fact, they're more likely to lose out on the kinds of stimulation their growing brains need most. As mesmerised as young viewers might be by the bright, flashing images and captivating sounds, toddlers are not processing what they see and hear the way they're supposed to. Television overloads their senses, but doesn't motivate learning, achievement, creativity, imagination, or social development the way real-world interactions with parents, other adults, playmates, and toys do.

Clearly, TV has an impact on a young child – and much of that impact isn't positive. Here's a rundown on the downside of toddler TV watching:

Less physical, intellectual, and social activity. Too much time spent in front of a TV is too little time spent running around, interacting with adults and other children, looking at books or listening to stories, drawing or playing, or exercising the body or mind in productive ways.

Less (and less effective) exposure to language. Every hour a child is exposed to the television translates to 770 fewer words heard spoken to them by an adult, say researchers. At a time when language development should be fast-tracked, every word matters. Missing out on thousands of verbal interactions a day can lead to a delay in language development. And if you're wondering whether all those words spoken on TV can stand in for your words, they can't. Studies show that words heard from a television do not increase a toddler's vocabulary or help promote language skills.

Future obesity. Too much TV watching, studies show, is one reason why obesity among children is becoming an epidemic (over 1 in 10 UK children over the age of 2 are obese). The explanation is simple: TV watchers of all ages consume more calories (they tend to snack while viewing) and burn fewer calories (obviously fewer than when they're running around, but also fewer than when they're sitting down doing absolutely nothing).

- Encourage audience participation. Keep your little tater tot from becoming a passive couch potato by making TV watching an active and interactive experience. Draw characters she saw on the screen, talk and get your toddler talking about action and story lines, try activities you've just seen on a favourite programme. Motivate your toddler to sing or dance and do projects along with TV characters.

- Don't switch on the TV to switch off your child's mood. As tempting as it might be to turn to TV when your toddler's out of sorts, grumpy, wound up, or just driving you to distraction, there are much better ways to calm, soothe, or cheer up your little one. Instead of using TV as a quick fix for regulating feelings, opt for higher-effort but lower-tech solutions to life's ups and downs: a quiet story to calm

What's more, TV adverts tend to promote processed foods (have you ever seen an advert for bananas?), another known contributor to obesity. Little ones see (and are enticed by) these foods on TV, then clamour for them at the shop and too often end up convincing Mum or Dad to bring them home – a cycle that makes it even more difficult to raise healthy, lean kids.

An increase in aggressive behaviour. Mounting evidence supports what many parents have long suspected: watching TV (and even indirect viewing in the home) may foster aggressive, uncooperative behaviour in some children – even very young children. And the longer little ones sit glued to the TV, the worse behaviour can become.

An increase in attention problems. Researchers have found that every hour per day of TV watching a toddler does boosts his or her chances of developing attention problems later in life by about 10 per cent (in other words, a 2-hour-per-day TV habit translates to a 20 per cent greater risk of an attention disorder). After all, it's hard to sit still for a book or a class when you're used to the much faster pace of TV.

More fears. Very young children find it impossible to differentiate between what's real and what's not. For them, what they see on TV is as real as everything else that happens in their living room – and that can be unsettling. Your toddler may not seem stressed out while watching a show about a scary giant, but anxiety can creep up later, prompting bedtime fears and nightmares.

Less room for creativity. TV paints the whole picture for a toddler – which leaves less to imagine, to envision, and to create. While interactive shows – which encourage child participation – may be somewhat more engaging, far better are activities that let your toddler's mind fill in most of the canvas (playing with a doll, dressing up, constructing a brick building, working out how to piece together a puzzle, racing a car, scribbling with chalk).

Less play. When stimulating entertainment is always just a remote control (or a mouse click) away, play may seem a whole lot like hard work. What's the motivation to make your own amusement when it's being made for you? TV can make little bodies and minds sluggish and less resourceful. Presented with free time and free reign over a room full of toys, a TV-dependent toddler may draw a blank.

a wound-up tot, a hug and song to soothe a sad one, a little problem solving to get a frustrated one back on task.

- Don't offer TV as a bribe or a reward. If you make TV watching a perk, associating it with good behaviour ("You shared your bricks today, so you can watch CBeebies") or dangling it as a carrot for cooperation ("If you stop crying now, you can watch *Bob the*

Builder"), you're sure to make it that much more tantalising. Instead, try incentivising with an activity that's good for your toddler, like story time or a run around the playground.

- Be selective. The quality of what your toddler watches is just as important as quantity. So be a picky TV critic. Preview programming, screening for age-appropriateness (you can check out TV ratings and reviews on commonsensemedia.org), and remember to choose programming designed for young children, with simple language and short segments. Anything your little one watches should also be slow moving, encourage interaction, have music and singing to keep a toddler engaged, and have some level of educational value.

- Skip the adverts. You'd be surprised how early children can fall for a sales pitch – and how good little ones can be at spotting at the shops less-than-wholesome products they've seen on TV (and eventually, demanding them). So stick to advert-free programming.

- Set TV viewing limits for yourself. As always, children are much more likely to do as you do than as you say. Keeping the TV on for your own around-the-clock viewing sets a double standard your child is eventually likely to challenge. Plus, it'll result in your toddler logging in way too much TV time and (unless you're always tuned in to a preschooler channel) being exposed to inappropriate images and language. So try to save the bulk of your TV viewing for after tuck-in hours. If you typically keep the TV on for background noise, try playing background music instead.

ALL ABOUT:
Cultivating Curiosity

What happens if I turn my cup of juice over? Where's that line of ants headed? What's under that rock? Why does wet sand stick to my fingers, but dry sand doesn't? A toddler's inquiring mind wants to know – and itches to find out. And this naturally burning curiosity does more than lead toddlers into mischief. It propels them to learn.

To cultivate your toddler's curiosity so it can blossom into a lifelong love of learning:

- Be the Answer Parent. With so much to learn, it's not surprising that young children ask so many questions – starting with the all-purpose toddler favourite, "Wha dat?" – or just "Wha?" or just "Dat?" And though it may be tempting to ignore the fiftieth "Wha dat?" after a long day of being

grilled, try to resist. All of a young child's questions deserve answers, and it's the answers that keep the questions coming (and how do you know, unless you ask?). A toddler who doesn't receive answers to his or her questions, or receives unsatisfying ones (such as "Uh-huh" or "You don't need to know that"), may be discouraged from asking them. Of course, your answers should be tailored to your toddler's tender age and limited comprehension: keep them short and simple.

- Encourage exploration. A toddler's explorations may turn into a parent's mess to clean up, true. But it's through those explorations that toddlers make their discoveries – the world is full of fascinating things that your tot has to experience firsthand in order to understand. Try to restrain your little one's explorations mainly when safety's at stake, not in the name of cleanliness or tidiness. And when you're out with your toddler, try to build in time for exploration. If you're always in a rush, he or she won't have the chance to follow that trail of ants or find out what's under that rock.

■ Encourage experimentation. The average toddler conducts more experiments in a morning than most labs do. What happens when I pour water over the side of the bath? When I squish a banana chunk or submerge cereal with a spoon? When I poke my finger into the bubble Daddy just blew? When I fling this toy against the wall? The idea is to support the experimental impulse without allowing your budding scientist to destroy your home while he or she is making discoveries. When experiments take a turn for the destructive or the dangerous, stop them, but make it clear that you object to the result of the experiment, not the process: "I know that you wanted to see what would happen if you poured water over the side of the bath, but the water has to stay in the bath." Then redirect that inquiring mind: "Let's see what happens when you pour water into this boat." Devise experiments that can be conducted under controlled conditions: blow the fuzz off a dandelion, pour sand through a strainer, mix food colouring with sudsy water in the kitchen sink.

■ Go out and about. Let your little one experience a variety of environments, up close and personal. Museums, playgrounds, parks, zoos, a busy city pavement – there's something new to discover, explore, and learn in even the most everyday locales (yes, even the supermarket). Most toddlers pick up plenty through their keen powers of observation (and endless pointing and choruses of "Wha dat?"), but your tiny sponge will soak up even more information if you add some questions, answers, and observations of your own.

■ Mix it up. Every day is an opportunity for new experiences. Swinging on a swing, sliding down a slide, splashing in a wading pool, planting flowers or pulling weeds, playing ball, stirring flour into cake batter, scribbling with a crayon, ringing the doorbell, pushing the lift button, stacking tins in the cupboard, lining up shoes in the wardrobe. The possibilities are endless and everywhere. The experience alone is valuable, but your commentary ("See, the harder you push the swing, the higher up it goes" or "Watch when you push the button – the light goes on") adds even more.

■ Have fun with fantasy. For a toddler, there's as much to be learned from fantasy – in books and make-believe play – as there is from real life. In the world of imagination, your child can be a grown-up at a tea party, a frog in the rain forest, a doctor in a hospital full of sick teddies, the Cat in the Hat or Bob the Builder – just about anyone or anything he or she would like to be.

■ Set a curious example. Show your toddler that you're never too old to explore and discover – it'll be easy to do if you start to see the world through those curious little eyes (you've probably walked down your street a thousand times – but did you ever notice that birdhouse, those blue flowers, the little garden ornament hidden in your neighbour's bushes until your tot pointed them out?). Try to learn something new every day, and share your excitement when you do – curiosity is contagious.

Playing and Making Friends

W HETHER IT'S A PUPPY CHASING ITS TAIL, a froglet leaping onto a lily pad, or a toddler hosting a teddy bear picnic in the middle of the living room, the name of the game is play – and it's a universal part of growing up. Not to mention, the best part of growing up. Though your toddler has certainly come a long way since those days of swatting at mobiles and shaking rattles, there's still plenty to sort out play-wise. Like how to play alone for more than two minutes at a time – and how to play with others for more than two minutes at a time (without grabbing a toy or bopping a pal on the head with a book). How to get the paper to cooperate with the crayon, instead of sliding all over the table. How to turn that bucket of sand into a castle (like the big kid at the other end of the sandpit just did), and how to keep that brick tower from tumbling over before it's finished. Play, like everything a toddler does, is full of exciting discoveries, frustrating challenges, satisfying accomplishments, and lots and lots of important life lessons. That's why playtime is never a waste of your toddler's time.

What You May Be Wondering About

The Power of Play

"I know play's supposed to be important for little kids. But I always have the nagging feeling that I should be doing something more constructive with my daughter."

D oesn't matter what, or how, or with what, or with whom – there's no better use of your little one's time than playing. Child's play is fun, for sure, but it's also your toddler's work – work that's never done (which is why play is a full-time job). In other words, it's the most constructive thing she can do, and the most constructive thing you can do with her. Play helps your toddler:

Discover the world. Play is your toddler's search (and find) engine. As small as a little one's world seems from the outside looking in, it's actually huge – filled with challenges that need to be tackled and discoveries that need to be made. Through play, your toddler can discover that world: sort out shapes and sizes (and figure out how they fit into spaces); explore cause and effect; make inferences and test theories; imagine, dream, and scheme ("Look out world, here I come!"). How else could a zoo end up in your living room? A construction site in the sandpit? A king (with a bubble beard) in the bathtub? A bowl of magical soup on the coffee table? In a word: play.

Self-discover. At play, your toddler learns about the special little person she is – and can become. With endless opportunities to try new things (and try them again, even when they don't work out the first time), play is an ideal testing ground for your toddler's emerging identity ("Who am I? What do I like to do? Who would I like to be?"). A perfect – and perfectly safe – petri dish for that developing sense of self.

Become a social animal. See your toddler in the corner over there, babbling away to a stuffed elephant who's helping her out with a puzzle project? That's social interaction – the kind your little one gets every day through play, even when there aren't any playdates on the schedule. Play – whether it's with a human playmate or a stuffed playmate – helps your toddler work out how relationships work (and don't work), how feelings (and eventually empathy) factor in, how friendships are formed (and maintained). Your toddler's first

and still favourite playmate, the most influential model for all things social, the very safest person in your little one's world to have those early social experiments with? You, of course.

Feel safe about feelings. Every feeling on your toddler's emotional grid (and 1-year-olds are a lot more emotionally complex than they're usually given credit for) can be expressed and, as needed, worked out through play. Is your toddler stressed about those doctor's visits? A chance to diagnose an ailing doll with a toy stethoscope or patch up a teddy bear cut with a plaster might be just the prescription. Has a business trip you've taken recently left your toddler feeling a little ungrounded? Don't be surprised to see your little one taking an imaginary trip (complete with a packed-up shopping bag suitcase). This kind of play is one very healthy way a toddler learns to deal with life's ups and downs.

Explore new roles. In a world widened by play, your little one can grow larger than life, taking on roles otherwise reserved for the grown-up crowd: from fireman to doctor, lorry driver to dancer, farmer (or farm animal) to zoo keeper (or zoo animal), reader of books, builder of buildings, designer of roads, maker of music, racer of cars, painter of artwork, flyer of airplanes . . . and, because there's no role model like you – and no bigger or better shoes your toddler can try to fill than yours – a parent.

Go from puppy to top dog. It isn't easy always living by someone else's rules, inevitable and necessary as that is when you're just a year old. For your toddler, play is a safe way to try running the show, making the choices, even setting the rules. A big-time self-esteem booster, absolutely, but also a welcome

Fine Motor Skills

Playing doesn't only stimulate the mind and imagination – it also helps toddlers finesse their fine motor skills (activities and skills that are accomplished using small muscles – for instance, those in the fingers). Brick building, shape sorting, tea pouring, doll dressing, car racing, crayon colouring, Play-Doh squeezing, water pouring, and almost any kind of hand-manipulative playing activity will strengthen those fine motor skills and encourage the development of eye–hand coordination. Here's a look at when you might see some fine motor skills making their appearance.

12 to 15 months. Your toddler is likely a pro at banging objects together and probably has begun to perfect the pincer grasp (grabbing small objects between the thumb and index finger) – a skill learned back in the first year. During the early months of the second year, your little one will learn to use a crayon to scribble, put objects (like bricks) into a container, and turn the pages of a book. Head outdoors to blow some bubbles and watch as your tot claps his or her hands together to "catch" them. Or introduce pavement chalk and let your pint-size Picasso create a masterpiece (see page 299 for art milestones).

15 to 18 months. As the middle of the second year approaches, building with bricks may become your tot's favourite

pastime. First your toddler will master the art of stacking one brick on top of another, then he or she will try using three bricks to make an even taller tower (watch out – knocking down that tower will be as much fun for your little construction worker as building it!). Finger play is great for both fine motor and language skills, and your toddler will delight in rounds of "Incy Wincy Spider", "Five Little Monkeys", and "Wind the Bobbin Up" now that he or she can play along.

18 to 24 months. During the second half of the second year, physical coordination will improve, allowing your maturing tyke to try out impressive new finger feats: puzzles, stacking five to six bricks, shaping clay, scribbling and painting, taking toys apart and putting them back together. Watch how your toddler plays with musical instruments – all that shaking, banging, and pressing will reward those fine motor movements with a cacophony of sounds (and music to his or her ears).

Be on the lookout: If your child isn't able to deliberately release an object he or she is holding by 12 months, if he or she still uses a fisted grasp to hold a crayon at 18 months, if your 18-month-old doesn't use a pincer grasp, or if your 24-month-old can't imitate a drawing of a vertical line, mention it to the GP.

chance to wield some of the power and control your toddler craves, while easing some of the frustration that comes from being a guppy in a pond of big fish.

Learn the language. There's a word for everything in the world of play, and your little player will learn loads

of new ones: lorry, doll, car, bricks, jump, swing, slide, climb, draw, dance, down, up, under, on, go, stop, stay. And who doesn't like to have fun while they learn?

Motor up. Of course, your toddler's motor's always running – and active play is a great way to burn up some of that endless fuel. But that running, jumping, dancing, climbing, skipping, riding, swinging, pushing, pulling, rolling, throwing, and catching also develop those large motor skills, building coordination along with strong muscles and bones, and — because the best time to nip a future couch potato is while she's still just a spudlet – laying the foundation for an active future.

Fine-tune. Play develops those all-important fine motor skills – the same skills those tiny fingers and hands (which may now seem all thumbs) will one day use to write, draw, doodle, paint, sculpt – and, of course, make just about every high-tech move (from computer use to texting, gaming, and beyond). It also hones eye–hand coordination, which your little one will need for all of the above and more (catching a ball, swinging a bat, cooking a meal, putting together a puzzle).

So play away!

Toys for Toddlers

"What toys should my 1-year-old son be playing with?"

Fun's number 1 when it comes to toys, of course. But the right kinds of toys do so much more than offer your toddler a few minutes of entertainment. Some will help him flex his brainpower, others will flex his muscles. Some will help him practise motor skills, others will help him hone his social skills. Most toys have something to teach your toddler, from cause and effect to hand–eye coordination, from taking turns to recognising patterns. And just about all good toys will spark curiosity, discovery, and imagination. Whether you're buying, borrowing, or passing down, keep these toy-selecting guidelines in mind:

Play it safe. Of course, you're in a hurry to race Hot Wheels with your toddler, or to open the doors to Barbie's Dream House. But toys designed for older children are difficult for still-clunky hands to negotiate and play with without breaking (Barbie is likely to be headless before you can say Ken), and they also may not pass the safety test. Choosing age-appropriate toys (check the packaging for age labels) will help prevent potential safety pitfalls – such as toys with small pieces your toddler could choke on or toys that can cause injury. You'll probably also have to set aside your own nostalgia when it comes to vintage toys, antique toys, or toys you're itching to unpack from your own childhood. Ditto for toys from countries where safety isn't well monitored. See page 421 for more on safety.

Get personal. Some toddlers love to role-play the day away, others prefer to roll a ball or scoot on a riding toy. Some like to get crafty with crayons, paper,

Presenting Fewer Presents

Do you – or a certain overindulgent relative (Grandma, you know who are are) – tend to overdo the gifts to your toddler? Not only is that a pricey present precedent to set (the toys are only going to get more expensive as the years pass – and sooner rather than later, too many gifts may spoil the child *and* break the bank), but more than one present presented at a time can be overwhelming to a 1-year-old. If there's more than one gift – Grandma filled an extra suitcase, for instance – consider staggering them to avoid overload (and underappreciation).

Clutter Control

You're pretty sure your floors are still there somewhere, but maybe it's been a while since you've seen them under the carpet of bricks, dolls, puzzle pieces, stacking rings. If there's a downside to toddler play, you've just stumbled upon it (or tripped over it . . . or picked it up for the sixth time in two hours): toys, toys everywhere.

A neater day will dawn, when your toddler will be able (if not always willing) to pick up after play. In the meantime, you can help contain the clutter with:

A play space. Realistically, any place your toddler spends time is a play space. But, ideally, there should be a play headquarters – a central area where your family hangs out together a lot, and where your toddler can play safely and supervised. Clearly, there will be multiple satellite locations for toys (from the back garden to the car to your bedroom), but if you can, it's good to try to define the spaces where toys are encouraged and where they're not, where they're stored, played with, taken from, and returned to. Maybe you're lucky enough to have a separate playroom or family room, or maybe size or layout dictates that your entire home is your toddler's play castle. Either way, setting some early play boundaries can help keep clutter from fully invading (though it won't prevent toys being dragged from room to room and activity to activity).

Anxious to carve out some space for a play mission control (or mission-try-to-control)? If you can, include a comfy place for cuddling up at story time (an armchair or easy-to-negotiate sofa); toddler-size chairs and a small table for puzzles, art projects, and stuffed animal tea parties (a coffee table can stand in); and an efficient, safe, easy-to-reach storage system. The area should be thoroughly childproofed, even if you're always supervising, and

---

and paste, others prefer music, still others busy themselves with building projects – and some are jacks of all toys. So as you fill the toy box, try to remember who's the boss of the play workplace . . . your toddler. Keeping your tot's play preferences in mind when shopping for toys will help narrow down those sometimes overwhelming toy shop options.

Look at what develops. Having fun is the top play priority for your little tyke, but he will get the most developmental value for toy money if you also look for toys that:

- Build large motor skills. Pretty much any toy that's active flexes those large motor skills: balls of all sizes; pull toys; push toys; age-appropriate riding toys; climbing equipment, slides, swings.

- Build fine motor skills. Choose some toys that challenge those little fingers and hands: nesting and stacking toys; simple wooden puzzles (particularly those with knobs for easier put-in and take-out); shape sorters; building bricks and systems (pieces should be large enough so your toddler can handle them easily and won't choke on them if mouthed); boxes and containers for filling and emptying; activity boards and pop-up toys with dials, knobs, and buttons to manipulate

designed to withstand the abuse it'll get from your little one. For flooring (toddlers are fondly referred to as rug rats for a reason; they spend much of their time on the floor), think durable, cleanable, and not slippery.

A place for everything. Of course, everything won't be in its place often, but it's good to know it can be, sometimes. A clever storage system for toys should be designed with your player (and playmates) in mind. Think function over form (though child appealing is a plus): easy out, easy back in. Baskets stored on low, deep shelves are best. They should be large (but not so large that you and your toddler lose track of what's in them), with each assigned a category of content. You can organise by colour (your toddler won't recognise colours yet, but most likely will by age 3), or with pictures or stickers that let both of you know what's inside.

A clear-up routine. Seems like the definition of pointless, but a clear-up routine at the end of the day (or the end of a play session, if it's been an especially messy one) can keep clutter from completely controlling your home. It can also make playtime more fun, since you and your toddler will have a better chance of locating toys and books you're looking for. And, in time, it can even get your child in the clearing-up habit, not to mention teach him or her responsibility (as in: I take care of my stuff). Like all things, your little one will learn best about clearing up by doing. At first you'll be picking up most of it after your tot, but inviting involvement now can pay cooperation dividends later. Challenge your toddler, focusing on one toy type at a time to prevent overload: "Let's see if we can pick up all the bricks and put them in this green basket." Singing a special tune can make the clear-up time feel like it's part of the playtime. Pretty soon, you'll be able to add game-show elements: "See if you can pick up the doll dishes before I count to 10" (be sure to count slowly enough) or "by the time the buzzer rings" or "by the time the music stops". Or "Who can pick up the toys faster?"

(a buzz, a ringing bell, or an animal sound are all bonuses, since toddlers are result-oriented). Just about all creative and imaginative play (from scribbling to pretend cooking) fine-tunes fine motor skills, too.

- Inspire imagination. This is the stuff that early childhood dreams are made of: stuffed and plastic animals; dolls and size-appropriate play people (while dolls that can be bathed, fed, put nappies on are always a favourite, avoid dolls that have extensive wardrobes, since 1- to 2-year-olds can't yet manage to dress a doll, and make sure shoes and other accessories don't pose a choking risk); cars, lorries, and aeroplanes; simple dollhouses and car garages; basic building systems; play dishes and pots (or real ones that are safe for pretend cooking); a play telephone, shopping trolley, broom, baby pushchair; play doctor's kit, workbench, or tool belt; dressing-up clothes and role-playing accessories (bags, hats, a briefcase – plus costumes and pseudo-professional gear such as a firefighter's hat, police officer's hat, sailor's hat, dancer's tutu).

- Create. For that art start (and a fine-motor bonus): chunky washable crayons and felt tips, and paper; Play-Doh; collage-making materials; finger paints, bath paints, and poster paints,

Righty or Lefty?

Watch your toddler reach for his or her favourite toy. Does she grab it with her left hand? Does he manipulate it with his right hand? Or does your little player use both hands interchangeably? The truth is, the majority of toddlers don't start playing hand favourites until about 18 months at the earliest (it's common for young children to appear ambidextrous, freely alternating between hands until they decide which is more ... handy), and most don't settle on a preference until at least the second birthday – though some children keep their parents guessing for several years beyond that.

Statistically speaking, your toddler (and 90 per cent of his or her toddler counterparts) will probably end up preferring the right hand – only around 5 to 10 per cent of people are lefties. A lot of it has to do with genetics – when both parents are lefties, there's more than a 50 per cent chance their children will also be left-handed; when just one parent is left-handed, the chance of a left-handed child drops to about 17 per cent; and when neither parent is left-handed, it's down to 2 per cent. In a set of mirror-image twins, one will be naturally left-handed and one will be a born righty – no matter what Mum and Dad's genes hand them.

Wondering if you should try to encourage your little one to use one hand over the other? Hands off. Since it's nature, not nurture, at work here, that strategy won't work. Research suggests that pushing a child to use the hand he or she isn't genetically programmed to use can lead to problems later with hand–eye coordination and dexterity. (Have you ever tried to write with the "wrong" hand? Imagine how tough it would be if you had to use that hand consistently). Time will tell whether you've got yourself a righty or a lefty – all you need to do is sit back and watch nature take its course.

If your toddler strongly favours one hand before he or she turns 18 months old, let the doctor know. In rare cases, such an early and consistent preference can signal a neurological problem.

---

along with easy-to-use brushes and large sponges; thick chalk and chalkboards (for more on art, see page 298).

- Make music. Every toddler has an inner musician, dancer, and marcher just itching to get out. So bring on the drums; tambourines; maracas; horns and other wind instruments; xylophones; simple keyboards; toddler CD players and sing-along songs. Favour instruments over music boxes and musical toys that require only the push of a button and offer no real musical challenge (for more on music making, see page 300).

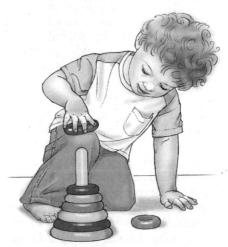

It looks like it's fun – and it is. But for a toddler, play is also work.

- Teach. Just about all toys teach something, but certain ones have an educational edge (and deserve a gold star for not getting pushy). Best are those that tap into your toddler's love of learning, with books topping the list. Thinking computer games? Simple, colourful software that encourages learning (of shapes, colours, patterns, numbers) but not a specific learning agenda (reading, maths) can also teach the right stuff – as long as it's used the right way (see page 278 for more on toddler software).

- Drive discovery. Your toddler's inquiring mind wants to know about cause and effect, shapes and sizes, filling and emptying, and more. Look to shape sorters; pegboards, with pegs of varying shapes and sizes; unbreakable mirrors; water toys (floaters, squirters, fillers and emptiers); sand toys; toys that help toddlers learn relative size (stacking and nesting toys do that).

Value versatility. Gimmicks and gadgets make a splash in the toy shop – and they'll certainly get your attention, and your toddler's – but interest in them often fizzles out quickly. Instead of fancy features, look for toys with numerous play possibilities – even as your little one grows. Simple does it for your young toddler – that budding imagination will (and should) do the rest.

Rotate your selection. Some toys are keepers from day one. Others have a limited shelf life when it comes to your toddler's limited attention span. Still others will fall in and out of favour. A great way to have more toys for your little one's playing pleasure and a rotating selection that keeps interest up, without breaking the budget or overindulging: share and share alike. Try borrowing and lending toys, or consider a toy co-op (this is especially useful for those big-cost items, or toys that are outgrown before they're worn-out). Does your toddler have a staggering selection of toys? Consider stashing some, then pulling toys out in rotation – not only so your little one isn't overwhelmed by the choices, but so there's always something "new" to play with.

Have a free-for-all. Don't forget that some of the best toys in life are free: plastic containers, cups, measuring spoons, pots and pans; a sheet thrown over two chairs to create a tent; handmade paper-bag puppets; and of course, the box that pricey toy came in (it can become a playhouse, a dollhouse, a garage, a table for tea parties, and more).

Toy Safety and Older Sibs

"Our older son, who's 5, has loads of toys with small parts, and we can't exactly ban him from playing with them. So how do we keep his little brother safe?"

When your toddler is your only (or your oldest) child, keeping him away from toys (at home, at least) that are potentially unsafe is as simple as not bringing them into your home. But when your toddler is a younger sibling, childproofing the toy box is a little more challenging. After all, you can't exactly demand that your older child give up toys that he enjoys just because they're not appropriate for your tot – at least not if you want to avoid having an uprising in the playroom. But you can try to safeguard your toddler by taking the following steps:

Enlist your older child's help. Explain to your older child the dangers that "big-kid toys" pose to toddlers. Show him what's small enough to pose a

Playing

Remember when playtime for your little one meant watching the pattern the sun made on the wall? Or giggling while you played "stinky feet"? Or cooing at a stuffed elephant? Well, that was baby stuff. Your toddler's play skills have grown – and will continue growing – along with your toddler, keeping pace with all sides of his or her development. After all, only a walker (or near walker) can play with a push toy. Only a tot old enough to recognise that his or her pretend pot is just like Mummy's real pot can role-play as a chef. And only a child who's worked out that other little people have feelings can really start to get the hang of playing as part of a team. Here's what you can expect during the second year when it comes to play:

12 to 15 months. Toys with bright reds, blues, greens, yellows (any bright colour for that matter) and toys with lots of patterns will be especially appealing to toddlers this age. With an improved grasp and more finely tuned fine motor skills, your little one will also enjoy manipulating toys that twist, spin, turn, crank, dump, and fill, and toys that can be banged, clanged, pushed, and pulled. It's a sure thing, too, that your young toddler will gravitate towards toys that have blinking lights, spinning wheels, and engaging sounds. Push toys – which offer balance to new walkers – are a favourite diversion (baby pushchairs and shopping trolleys that can be loaded up with toys and other belongings score extra points with pint-size pack rats). And though your 12- to 15-month-old definitely hasn't mastered true social play with children his or her own size (sharing a toy with a pal, for instance), he or she will delight in social games played with you, like peek-a-boo, patty-cake, and escape-from-the-tickle-monster.

15 to 18 months. Put tots this age in a room together, throw in some toys, and watch how they immediately start to play – though not necessarily with each other. Parallel play is still the name of the game these days: toddlers will sit side by side but play mainly on their

choking threat (you can even teach your child how to do a choke-tube test; see page 422), what might be broken off of a big toy and swallowed, what toys might pinch his sibling's curious little fingers. Then make your older child a member of the "small parts patrol", a helper in scouting for unsafe toy parts and keeping them safely packed away (you can provide him with a toilet paper cardboard roll of his own to test toy sizes). Also start teaching your big kid to completely close toy boxes and cupboards after taking toys out or putting them in. Just remember, as you implement this safety campaign, that a 5-year-old isn't capable of being reliably responsible and can't be counted on yet to carry out his part of the campaign consistently. Remind, but don't scold, when he forgets to put away an unsafe toy or misjudges a toy's safety.

Store unsafe toys out of your toddler's reach. If your toddler can go anywhere your older child can, store potentially dangerous toys where only you can reach them, and have your older child ask when he wants to use them. You can also store some of these toys

own (though they will often glance at each other to see how the other half plays – and of course, grab a peer's toy when it catches their eye). And now that your little one has a better handle on long-term memory and is flexing those budding verbal muscles, you may start to see the beginnings of make-believe or pretend play (real pretend play won't start in earnest until 18 months or so). You'll get a kick out of watching your little monkey ape what you do (though remember that it'll take on a rudimentary form) – talk on the phone, eat pretend food, push a doll in a pushchair. Providing simple toys that encourage pretend play (dressing-up materials, dolls, cars and lorries, a play kitchen, and so on) will open up a world of imagination for your mini make-believer.

18 to 24 months. Toddlers in the second half of their second year are starting to give other kids their size a second look, but they're still pretty primitive in the social department – which means you'll still see plenty of survival-of-the-grabbiest behaviour at playgroup. Socially evolving, your tot will need plenty of time and playdate

practice before he or she can exhibit – never mind perfect – such developmentally challenging skills as sharing and taking turns. In fact, parallel play still trumps cooperative play for 1½- to 2-year-olds. Pretend play will become more sophisticated, and may become your toddler's favourite activity: she'll drive her car, go shopping with her kid-size shopping trolley, put her teddy to bed. Role-playing is also beginning to emerge: your tot might make his stuffed animals or dolls assume roles, expecting them to eat pretend food or sing along or get examined by a "doctor" (this allows toddlers to run their own shows – something they always love to do). Improving large motor skills and the physical confidence that comes with that will lead to more active play: jumping, running, kicking, climbing, and throwing a ball (see Milestone boxes, pages 69 and 78). Riding toys are sure to be a favourite, too. More developed fine motor skills (see Milestone box, page 288) will help your tot manipulate smaller toys with finer details: puzzles, sorting games, and fitting together simple objects (like putting a square peg in a square hole).

in containers that are difficult for your toddler to open (your older child can always ask you for help, if necessary). If toys are stored in low cabinets, use child-safe cabinet latches (the kind usually used in kitchens) and show your older child how to open and close them (assuming he can be trusted with the contents of similarly latched kitchen cabinets). A hook-and-eye installed out of your toddler's reach may slow down access to toys stashed in a cupboard, but once your toddler has figured out how to drag a chair or box over to climb on, it's no longer effective. A safety gate to

block access to your older child's room (if he doesn't share with his little sib) may be helpful – but, again, only until your little one learns how to scale it.

Keep unsafe toys out of sight. Toys stored on high shelves that are visible to your toddler may tempt him to try scaling those shelves – which can itself be dangerous. Keeping the toys behind closed cupboard doors or in opaque bins may help discourage interest.

When your older child plays with unsafe toys in the same room your toddler is in, try to get your littlest one

Toddler Game Tedium

Bored silly playing silly toddler games? Dreading another round of Ring a Ring o' Roses? Terrified of another tea party? No more patience for pretend restaurant? And feeling guilty about it to boot? No guilt necessary. Many adults find toddler play a tad tedious – and that's not surprising. After all, you're not a toddler any more.

But laying off the guilt doesn't mean you can let yourself off the hook – at least not entirely. Sharing in your child's play lets your tot know that you value and enjoy his or her company – a very important esteem- and confidence-building message. Here are a few tips to help make toddler playtime more fun for you, too:

- Give child's play a chance. When it's been decades since you've been a toddler, it's tough to play like one. Tough, but not impossible – if you plop down on the floor with the right attitude. So instead of joining in convinced that you'll be bored, try shaking your staid adult ways. Allow yourself to wander into the world of childhood innocence and imagination, and you may actually find yourself enjoying those toddler games. Of course, it'll be hard to get lost in playtime if you've got one eye on the open magazine that's lying on the coffee table and the other eye on Twitter. So when you do play with your toddler, try to devote your complete attention to it.

- Learn how to play your toddler's way. Just because you've been invited to join the game doesn't mean you get to make up the rules. Toddlers and small children have very definite ideas about how they'd like their play to progress (or not

involved in an engrossing activity. If your older child prefers to play in his room (again, if he has his own room), that's fine, too. If your firstborn is old enough not to need supervision, he can close the door. If not, putting up a gate can let you keep an eye on what your older child is doing while keeping your toddler out.

Be vigilant. No matter how careful everyone in the family is about keeping potentially dangerous toys from your toddler, bite-size game-playing pieces are sure to be left under the sofa and tiny building-set pieces are certain to be forgotten behind the bed. So always keep a close eye out for any hand-to-mouth actions on the part of your toddler, or for chewing motions when he hasn't been eating – especially when your older child is playing with tiny toys. And make sure you're familiar with the emergency treatment of choking incidents (see page 469) – just in case.

A Short Attention Span

"One minute our toddler's playing with bricks, the next minute he's moved on to a stuffed animal, then 10 seconds later, he's pulling cushions down from the sofa. Attention span? What attention span?"

Your toddler may seem like he's living life in fast-forward, but in fact, time moves a lot more slowly on his watch. For a 1-year-old, a second can feel like a minute, a minute like an hour, an hour – well, that's not even on his timetable.

progress), so it's important to participate without interfering. If play gets unbearably boring, casually suggest a new game plan – but if your toddler resists your suggestions, don't push your agenda. In the world of play, toddlers rule.

- Know your limits, and let your tot know them, too. Short periods of your whole-hearted participation are more rewarding to your toddler than longer periods of grudging attention. If you start fidgeting and yawning after 15 minutes of "mummy cat–baby cat," stop it before it shows. But give your toddler a warning first. Say "The mommy cat and the baby cat can have just one more snuggle, and then the mummy cat will have to start dinner."

- Pick and choose, when you can. Some parents don't enjoy playing make-believe, but savour science experiments. Some relish reading,

but have little patience for racing cars. Some appreciate a good drawing session but are bored to tears by brick building. When your toddler wants to play but hasn't got a game in mind, suggest the kinds of things you enjoy doing. Your toddler will probably be happy to go along most of the time.

- Turn the tables. Once in a while, invite your toddler to play with you. Give him or her a pair of work gloves, a plastic trowel, and a pile of dirt to weed and cultivate while you do some serious gardening alongside (just watch carefully so weeds and dirt don't end up as a snack); provide a stack of old magazines to flip through while you read a new one; teach an exercise routine to do while you do yours. Your toddler may be delighted to participate in your games of choice – or bored. But that's okay. After all, those tea parties aren't always your cup of tea, either.

Spending more than a few minutes on any activity – except maybe sleep – is way too challenging for a young, easily distracted toddler, his age-appropriate fleeting attention span, and his normally restless nature. So he flits from one pursuit to another, one toy to the next, taking life one moment at a time. To the adult observer, this pattern of play may seem unfocused, even unproductive, but to a toddler it's just right for him and his development.

As your toddler matures, so will his attention span (though it may seem to grow at a snail's pace – and he won't really have much stick-to-itiveness until he's 5 or 6). For now, try not to expect much when it comes to focused play. He's learning no matter what he's doing or how long he's spending doing it. His

powers of concentration may occasionally surprise you (often when he's concentrating on some activity that's not house-approved, like pushing buttons on your smart phone), but for now, most play activities will hold his attention for only a few minutes, or until he's distracted by something else.

Independent Play

"My toddler always wants me to play with her. How can I get her to start playing by herself once in a while?"

Feeling just a little too . . . in demand? Parents are definitely popular – and typically preferred – playmates for young toddlers. And if you think about it, there are good reasons why. After all, what playmate her own size would have your patience? Your ability to share without grabbing her stuff? Your skill sets (handy when she wants a doll's outfit changed, a toy on a shelf reached, a book read, or a castle built)?

Of course, while playing with your toddler is one of the best ways of boosting her social development (it's through you that she'll pick up give-and-take, empathy, cooperation, and more), being her round-the-clock playmate keeps her from learning how to enjoy playing independently (and you from getting anything else done). Not to mention, it's actually good for her to know that you sometimes have something to do besides tend to sickly teddy bears. Here's how to help her transition to more "me" time:

Teach her a thing or two. Children are born to play, but they aren't born knowing how to play. They often need help working out how to use a particular toy or play a game – whether it's advice on how to stack those bricks so they won't tumble, how to turn that triangle so it will fit into the shape sorter, or how to get started on that puzzle. The more time you spend orienting your toddler to the joys of her own toys, the sooner she will be able to enjoy playing with them on her own.

Get her started. Each time you want your toddler to spend some time on her own – and you should do this periodically, even if you don't have something pressing on your own agenda – get her set up with an activity. Sometimes, the sheer overwhelmingness of working out what to play with is just too intimidating for a little one.

Time the alone time – and give it time, too. Alternate between time she spends playing by herself and time she spends playing with you (setting a timer may help delineate between the

two). Realistically, those independent streaks may not last long at first, but with patience and perseverance, she'll start to stretch the periods of solo play.

Provide other playmates. Of course you are your toddler's favourite playmate, but that doesn't mean you have to be her only one. Even though her social skills will still be age-appropriately shaky, she's ready (whenever you are) to begin playdates or to join a playgroup.

A Start in Art

"My toddler always grabs my pens and pencils and tries to scribble with them. Is she old enough to try drawing – and, if so, with what?"

If your toddler's old enough to hold a crayon or a pen, she's old enough for her official start in art. So let her unleash her inner Van Gogh by making some tools of the art trade available for her scribbling pleasure.

As for which supplies to supply her with, safety (hers and your home's) will come first. Because she's likely to put whatever she's scribbling with in her mouth, you'll have to make sure it's non-toxic – and, luckily, just about all children's art supplies are. Pencils (which aren't made from lead, by the way) are also non-toxic, but since they could potentially poke a little eye or jab tender skin, your toddler shouldn't be allowed to scribble with them unless she's closely supervised. Ditto for pens.

Speaking of supervision, that's where your home's safety comes in. A shortfall of artistic experience teamed with a surplus of artistic exuberance may lead your toddler's creative impulses off the paper – and onto the walls, the furniture, and the floors. To make sure she doesn't use your home as her canvas, watch her while she creates.

Colour by Number

Whether your little artist is destined to be the next Great Master – or a master of the stick figure and smiley face, each of your toddler's creations is worth a spot in your fridge gallery. There are certain developmental patterns most toddlers follow when it comes to creating art, and here's how they're likely to develop by age:

12 to 15 months. Give your tot a crayon or a paint-loaded brush and you'll get lots of large random arcs, blobs, movement, and unintentional scrawling – a study in pleasure rather than technique. Still, the technique is evolving, along with a growing appreciation of artistic cause and effect: "If I press hard with the brush, I'll get a blob of paint on the paper. If I swoosh softly across the paper, I'll get a wispy line."

15 to 18 months. Now it's time for drawing with a purpose – though that purpose will still be very much open to interpretation. You may not see the forest or the trees in those swirls, but you will see that your toddler's working more intently. Chalk that up to his or her more precise fine motor skills, which become more refined midway through the second year. So instead of those tentative strokes you saw a few months ago, you'll see distinct blocks of colour, stronger marks, and more definitive swirls of . . . is that the sun or a banana?

18 to 24 months. Your toddler's scribbles – which likely fill up more space on the paper now – are becoming slightly more recognisable: whirls for circles, zigzags for lines. To your toddler, every stroke represents something – those black loops may be a dog, that collection of brown and blue streaks, Daddy. To nurture the process and reduce frustration, try to be a supportive patron of the toddler arts. If you can't make heads or tails out of that dog, applaud the use of colours, rather than questioning the apparent lack of legs.

Choose washable supplies (and hide those that aren't), but consider pulling even washable felt tips and crayons out only when you can keep a close eye on scribble sessions – at least until you can trust her to control her artistic impulses.

Practicality matters, too, and the right supplies will enhance the artistic experience all around. Chunky crayons, felt tips, and chalk will be easier for her tiny hands to grasp and manoeuvre than slim ones, and when it comes to crayons and chalk, they'll be harder to break, too. A large sheet of newspaper placed under her paper can make it somewhat less likely that your toddler's masterpiece will stray onto the furniture, and taping the sheet down will keep the scribbling surface from shifting and bunching (and causing frustration). To start drawing the distinction between the paper your toddler's allowed to draw on and the paper she's not (in books, on your desk), point out often: "*This* paper is for drawing."

When your toddler has lapses in artistic judgement, leaving her marker mark on the dining room table, your dresser, the rug, her white T-shirt, her legs, or your legs, pat yourself on the back for remembering to hide the permanent markers, and then redirect her efforts onto a piece of paper (see the next answer for more tips). Want to leave an impression on her about the impression

Music Making

You've crooned to your colicky new-born for hours on end. Lullabied your stubbornly awake baby into sleepy submission. Used a silly song to distract a fidget into the car seat or to banish boredom at the supermarket. But now that your little one has graduated to toddler, it's time to take note of all the benefits music making can offer a growing mind, body, and soul – and to tap into them with a variety of fun musical experiences:

Music moves. Listening to favourite songs at home and in the car is a great way to broaden your tot's sensory environment, but don't relegate music to the background. Young toddlers get the most out of music when they feel it, engage in it, move to it, and make it their own. Give your little one plenty of opportunities to rock, roll, march, tap, clap, sway, spin, and otherwise move to the beat. You'll not only be nurturing a lifelong love of music and dance, but also encouraging the development of coordination, fine motor skills, and large motor skills (and even, accord-ing to some research, helping your child build brain connections that will one day help solve maths problems). Songs with simple hand movements ("Wind the Bobbin Up"), those that get the whole body in motion ("Hokey Cokey"), and those that involve inter-action with you (lap songs like "The Grand Old Duke of York") allow your toddler to own the musical experience. Take participation up a notch by danc-ing with your tot: play some slow music and show him or her how to sway slowly, then rev up the beat and twirl around quickly with your child. Bring out the musical instruments, too (bells, shakers, rhythm sticks, toy drums, a xylophone or keyboard, tambourines, toddler-size cymbals, or a simple pot and wooden spoon) and encourage him or her to play to the beat. No instruments on hand? Use those hands to tap the floor, each other's knees, an unbreakable table – or just to clap to the rhythm.

Music teaches. Any song with lyr-ics builds language skills, but certain

---

she left on the coffee table? Have her "help" clean up her marker mishap.

A certain amount of crayon nib-bling is inevitable at this age, and defi-nitely won't hurt your toddler in any way (though, warning: such colourful snacks can leave a vibrant imprint in her next nappy). Still, it should be dis-couraged. Try to intercept any crayon-to-mouth manoeuvres ("Crayons are for drawing, not eating"), and prepare to repeat the interceptions . . . a lot. If she seems more interested in eating the crayons than creating with them, take a snack break ("Here is some cheese. Cheese is for eating").

"My toddler loves to draw with crayons, but not on paper. Today I walked into his room and found that he'd scribbled on the walls with bright red crayon."

Are your toddler's creative juices overflowing . . . onto the walls? That's because, while he's worked out what crayons are for (drawing), he hasn't quite discerned the differ-ence between surfaces for drawing on (paper) and surfaces not for drawing on (the kitchen cabinets, the coffee table, Daddy's briefcase).

Does that mean you should let your mini-Michelangelo take his crayons (and felt tips, and paints) and transform

songs teach a whole lot more – while making learning fun. There are letter songs (the alphabet song, "Bingo"), counting songs ("One, Two, Buckle My Shoe"), songs that help tots learn about their environment ("The Wheels on the Bus", "Old McDonald", "Twinkle, Twinkle, Little Star"), and songs that speak to emotions ("If You're Happy and You Know It").

Music releases. Is your toddler a little wound up? There's no better release for extra energy (or frustration . . . or anger) than music making and dancing – especially when the beat's up-tempo.

Music soothes. At bedtime, naptime, stressful times, grumpy times – any time your toddler needs a little mellowing out – soft, mellow music can soothe, calm, pacify, relax, offer comfort. Dim the lights to enhance the mood.

Music makes everything more fun. From that trip to the market to the post-playdate clean-up, from getting dressed to going to bed, a song makes the humdrum more fun. Associating a specific chore or routine with a certain

song can also encourage cooperation and ease those tricky transitions (like when it's time to leave the sandpit behind).

Getting the same song request again and again? Variety may be the spice of life, but most toddlers don't have a taste for it yet – and that goes just as much for music play lists as it does for breakfast menus. Listening to familiar music always brings the most pleasure (remember when you used to play your favourite song over and over and barely bothered with the rest of the album?), but especially for your toddler. And through the power of repetition those replays enhance learning – and help boost your little one's verbal skills, too. So spin your toddler's favourite as many times as he or she asks for it (but also try to introduce new songs – and new types of music – once in a while, especially after that favourite has been pretty well mastered). With patience, this broken-record stage will eventually play itself out.

One music caveat: to protect those little ears, make sure you never play music that's too loud to speak over.

your home into his version of the Sistine Chapel? Definitely not. Scribbling murals on the walls may be an artistic impulse, but it isn't acceptable.

Fortunately, it's possible to cultivate his creativity while protecting your property:

Draw the line. When you catch your toddler in the midst of a mural (or when his strokes stray off the paper you've provided), calmly explain that his choice of canvas was a mistake: "That's a beautiful picture you drew, but we don't draw on the walls." As exasperated as you might (understandably)

be, try not to attack his artistic effort ("Look at the terrible mess you made on the wall!"). Remember, he's probably very proud of his work (what's a mess to you is a masterpiece to him) – and he expects you to be proud of him, too. (By the way, weren't you the one who encouraged him to use a crayon in the first place?) Besides, if he enjoys all the attention his bedroom-wall art stirs up, he may be more tempted to reproduce it on the living room wall.

Change the canvas. While his creative juices are still flowing, sit him down and show him that "We draw on paper."

Dance Fever

Most tots don't need much encouragement to get their groove on – after all, they're already in perpetual motion. But dancing does a whole lot more than expend that excess toddler energy (though that's always a plus, especially on those endless, rainy afternoons). It helps hone motor skills and fine-tune coordination and balance, foster self-expression and boost self-confidence, teach body awareness and increase spatial perception (look what my arms and legs can do . . . oops, didn't see that table coming), and tap into your little one's natural affinity for rhythm.

Best of all, toddlers are born dancers – without any inhibitions to hold them back. By their first birthdays, toddlers (even those tots who aren't yet walking) can manage to bob up and down to the beat. Pretty soon, they'll add to their dance moves – wiggling that cute little bottom, spinning in circles, shaking and swaying rhythmically.

So how do you inspire the tiny dancer in your toddler? Just turn on the music to get the dance party started. Experiment with different beats, and then watch how your toddler mixes up moves to match the rhythms (swaying slowly to classical, going wild to rock, clapping along to pop). Make bopping to the beat even more fun for your older toddler by playing dance games like "musical statues" (play the music, get dancing, and then when the music stops everyone has to freeze). Or give your little one a prop to dance with, like a colourful scarf or a scrap of silky fabric to wave around (for safety's sake, no long scarves). Your toddler will get a kick out of watching it twirl and float while moving to the music.

And don't just sit on the sidelines. Toddlers love a dance partner. So bust out your own best moves and challenge your tot to imitate them, or hold hands and dance together.

Have two left feet, no rhythm, or a dance complex you picked up in school? Not to worry – this dance partner won't notice.

The larger the sheet of paper, the better the chance his scribbles will stay on it, rather than drifting onto the floor, table, or a nearby wall. A roll of paper, which can be unrolled as he fills up space, can be particularly satisfying to the toddler artist. Taping the paper to the floor, a table, or an easel will keep it from moving around and frustrating his artistic efforts. Don't hover over him as he works, but do keep an eye on him to be sure he stays on the page.

Wipe the slate clean. To further reinforce the message that walls aren't for drawing on, have him "help" wipe away his unauthorised mural with his own wet cloth or eraser sponge (make sure any cleanser he comes into contact with is nontoxic).

Schedule in art. Make time every day for supervised drawing, so that your toddler has plenty of opportunities to express his artistic vision. When you can't supervise, keep crayons (and other tools of the art trade) out of his reach.

Open a gallery. Display his scribbles proudly on the fridge, at your desk, by your bed, in his room. Appreciation of his "works on paper" will hopefully inspire more of the same – instead of more on the wall.

Of course, if your renegade artist continues to return to the wall despite your redirection, you'll have to move on to Plan B: taking away the crayons. Remind him as you do that colouring on the walls is not allowed. Then, move him swiftly to another activity, waiting a few days before you break out the crayons again.

Playground Trepidation

"Our son refuses to use the slide or swings at the playground. He seems scared of them both and sticks close to the sandpit."

What's keeping your toddler out of the playground action? It could be foresight ("I know that if I let go of the swing, I could fall off – and that would be scary"). Or it could be hindsight ("I remember once I slid down the slide and landed on the ground with a thud – and that hurt"). Or maybe it's simply his nature: some tots are innately more cautious than others (and here's the upside: fewer bruises for him, less stress for you).

Whatever the reason why your toddler rejects a need for speed and clings to terra firma (and the sandpit), respect his fears. Each time you go to the playground, casually offer him the opportunity to try the equipment. Having you go along for the ride (you can hold him securely while you slip down the slide together, or let him cling to you while you swing slowly on the big-kid's swing) may gradually ease his trepidation. So may having you right behind him as he attempts the big climb up the slide ladder. Or having him sit in the swing without pushing (or with just a teensy push, when he's ready). Let him explore the lowest levels of the climbing frame, again with you at his side. If he turns down your suggestions or wants to call

it quits after one trip down the slide or a couple of swings on the swing, don't press him to reconsider. Reassure him that the swings and the slides will be there when he's ready to play on them, and that, in the meantime, the sandpit is a perfectly acceptable place to hang. You can also see if he's willing to take on a smaller and/or indoor play space, which might be less intimidating, at a soft play area, a friend's house, or the waiting room at the doctor's office.

Also be sure you aren't inadvertently standing in the way of his standing up to his fears by being overprotective at the playground or by overreacting to minor falls and other mishaps (a casual "Woopsie daisy!" will reassure him that it's fine to get up and try again . . . that is, if he wants to). Instead, build your toddler's confidence by arming him with the skills necessary to negotiate playground equipment at his own pace – without pushing or hovering (offer him a hand getting up that first step, but don't lift him up).

Even the least risk-taking tots will eventually conquer their playground fears, becoming swingers, sliders, and climbing frame scalers at last. But some kids will always be less adventurous than others, going on to sit out the roller coasters and high diving boards.

For now, sit back on the park bench and relax (which, by the way, the parents of mini-daredevils never can) while your cautious tot calmly and safely scoops sand.

Playground Safety

To make sure your tot's playtime at the playground is as safe as it is fun, check out the playground safety tips on page 426.

Playdate Guidelines

Put two toddlers together and anything can happen – and usually does. From enchanted moments in the play kitchen to tugs-of-war over the plastic shopping trolley, playdate sessions can represent toddler togetherness at its best and worst.

To bring out more of the best and less of the worst in your toddler's playdates:

Don't feel obligated. Here's the first thing you need to know about playdates (and playgroups, for that matter): They're definitely good social practice for your toddler – and a nice change of pace for you – but they're not a must-do. Your toddler picks up plenty of social skills from interacting with you and with other adults and children in his or her life, and will start picking up the rest once preschool starts (before you know it!). If you don't have the time to fit playdates into your schedule – or if you or your toddler are just not that into them – don't feel obligated to pencil them in.

Have schedule savvy. A playdate once or twice a week can be a fun diversion for 1- to 2-year-olds. But playdates every day, or even every other day, may become too much of a bore – especially if there are lots of behaviour expectations attached to the dates (and particularly if the expectations are too high).

Children who attend nursery may be even more prone to social burnout if they're overscheduled with playdates in their free time (though, on the flip side, some may actually prefer group play to solo play, since they're accustomed to a crowd). Unsure how many playdates are enough, and how many are too many? Look no further than your toddler. If your tot seems happy on the playdate circuit (goes cheerfully, isn't stressed out later), then the schedule's just fine. If he or she seems miserable, out of sorts, or uncharacteristically clingy or aggressive before, during, and/or after, try scaling back the social calendar for now.

Keep playdates brief. Most little ones have little tolerance for long periods of play – especially with others. While your toddler's still getting into the social swing, limit sessions to 1 to 1½ hours.

Time wisely. Toddler meltdowns can happen at any time – but there's no point in asking for one. Avoid scheduling playdates at a time when your little one's apt to be grumpy, in need of a nap, overstimulated (say, right after a trip to the toy shop), or soon to become hungry. Ideally, toddlers should be well fed, well rested, and at least moderately mellow when the playdate begins.

Playdate Clinging

"I'm trying to encourage my daughter to interact more with other kids, but when we go on a playdate or to her playgroup, she spends more time clinging to me than playing with the other kids."

Trying to get your not-yet-social butterfly to act more like a butterfly, less like a caterpillar (still safely cocooned behind your legs)? Try the tips for clinging on page 182 and these suggestions for helping your toddler spread her social wings at playdates or playgroup:

Do crowd control. Handling the company of just one other child is challenge enough for some toddlers – handling a larger play crew may approach the impossible.

Make the most out of hosting. Children often have a harder time when the playdate is held at home, since it steps up behaviour expectations, sometimes unfairly. Hosting a playdate isn't easy for a toddler – it means you have to share Mummy or Daddy or your babysitter, your home, your room, your toys, and even your food (oy – those are my crackers!). Be sensitive to this stress factor. Talk up the job of host as an exciting one. Assign fun responsibilities: answering the door (with you), meeting and greeting, doling out toys (having your toddler set aside some "special" toys that won't have to be shared may make sharing the rest slightly less painful), choosing and preparing the snack (in advance), and planning special activities will make your tot feel important, provide a sense of control, and (hopefully) make hosting playdates a little easier.

Supervise, supervise, supervise. One-on-one play may work well for a while, but in case it dissolves into one-on-top-of-one (even with supervision), be ready to distract the combatants with an adult-directed activity.

Start with a snack. Not only is snack time a non-threatening activity (as long as both children receive the same amount of juice and the same number of crackers, cheese cubes, or banana slices), it'll help curb hunger-induced grumpiness. Always check ahead to see if the other child has any food allergies.

Keep your expectations realistic. At this age, even a few minutes of harmonious play or even one instance of sharing can be considered an achievement – anything beyond that is a bonus.

Don't push togetherness. If the children are happy playing in different corners of the room or even in different rooms (each with adult supervision), let them do their own things. You can encourage interaction with the right activities – building with bricks, colouring on a large sheet of paper, Ring a Ring o' Roses – but don't force it. Close encounters of the toddler kind typically aren't very close at all.

Be a home base. Some tots need a lap to crawl into periodically during a playdate, or an occasional reassuring touch or friendly smile that says "I'm here, don't worry". A quick hug may be enough to get a wary toddler back into the action, but if it doesn't, leave your lap open for as long as it's needed.

Prepare for conflict. Because chances are, you're going to get some. Read up on peacekeeping throughout this chapter so you'll know what to do when a fight erupts. And if "sharing" is a major cause of friction, use a timer for taking turns.

Start small. Your tentative tyke may feel more comfortable one-on-one than as one-in-a-crowd. So take social baby steps – consider mastering the mellow playdate before you tackle the bigger group again. Keep visits brief, too, until she's clocked up some social experience and bolstered her confidence.

Go slow. At first, let your toddler play on her own terms – and, if she wants to, on your lap, at your knee, or wedged right next to you. Then try sitting her down near the other children with an appealing activity – a bucket of bricks, a stack of books, a workbench, or a shape sorter. Gradually, edge away from her and over to the parent side of the room. If she chooses to follow, let her. But after a few minutes on your lap, cheerfully return her to the play area, again with a setup of toys. Repeat that manoeuvre until she starts to feel secure enough to separate herself from you.

Remain unruffled. She's tugging on your jeans? So what? She's superglued to your knee? Who cares? Hiding between your legs? No problem. Making it clear to your toddler that her participation in the social scene is no big deal to you will help her relax and enjoy.

Have an open-lap policy. Knowing that she's always welcome on your lap – that she can climb off and climb back on again whenever she needs a reassurance recharge – may give her the social mojo she needs to venture out on her own, at least some of the time. On the other hand, being stingy with your lap – or your hugs – is likely to compound her clinginess (as always, she'll separate best if it's her idea – not yours).

Remember, your butterfly's one of a kind. Some little ones take instantly to the social scene – flitting off without a moment's hesitation (or a second look at Mum or Dad). Others need a bit more time before they're ready to shed their comfort cocoon and launch. Give her the right balance of encouragement and support and your tot will take off socially, sooner or later.

Starting a Playgroup

"I'd like to get some other toddlers (and mums) together for a playgroup for my son. How do I go about setting one up?"

There's something for everyone in a playgroup. For toddlers, it's a chance to practise basic social skills

while enjoying (or at least learning to enjoy) the company and camaraderie of other children. For parents, it's a chance to swap war stories (and cuteness chronicles) with others in the toddler trenches. After all, just seeing and hearing that you're not alone – that your toddler isn't the only one who grabs toys, or the only one who's battling bedtime, or the only one who won't eat anything but cereal – can be remarkably therapeutic. Plus, the parent-to-parent exchange of ideas, insights, and tips on dealing with toddler behavioural eccentricities can be invaluable. Finally, who beyond the world of toddler parents will appreciate the anecdotes you're aching to tell (like that adorable thing your little one did this morning)?

Don't have a group of parents and toddlers in mind, or not sure whether you want to start your own group or join one already in progress? Joining an established one is definitely the easier option, if you can track down a compatible group in your area. Check online resources for local playgroups, or look for postings at the GP's surgery, a nearby community centre, the local library, or your house of worship. Or use those resources to locate parents interested in starting a group with you.

Of course, setting up and maintaining a playgroup isn't child's play – it'll take some effort to get it up and running smoothly. In launching that effort, remember that there are no hard and fast playgroup rules. You and the other parents will have to figure out, as you go along, what works best for everyone involved. But the following guidelines should help you get started:

Figure out format. In most playgroups for the very young, toddlers attend with a parent (or other caregiver), allowing adults to talk while children play. This format also permits parents to (hopefully) discipline their own child when necessary, making peacekeeping (hopefully) less complicated and less political. What it doesn't allow is for parents to get some child-free time off. If this is part of the objective, you might consider a co-op arrangement, which combines a playgroup situation with shared childcare.

Limit the number of players. A group of six toddlers (each accompanied by a parent or caregiver) is probably the ideal – small enough to be accommodated in most homes and large enough to function even if one or two members are absent. Groups of four or five can work well, too, but more than eight can lead to overcrowding, overstimulation, and all-out chaos (not enough toys to go around, not enough room to serve a snack comfortably).

Look for a good match. Temperament and interests may be tricky to synch up, particularly since toddlers tend to fluctuate in those areas from day to day and week to week. But major disparities in development and skills can be avoided by aiming for an age gap of less than six months between the oldest child and the youngest.

Match parents, too. Parents in the group don't have to start out as best friends (although they may end up that way), but all should be compatible, fairly well matched in personality and parenting style. Test the chemistry of potential playgroup parents (and their toddlers) by holding a few trial meetings to see how it goes. Likewise, if you're joining an established group, attend a couple of sessions on a trial basis before signing on.

Decide where to meet. Most groups rotate from home to home. Others meet regularly in one place, such as

---

Have a Little Slugger?

Or a biter . . . or hair puller . . . or shover? The second year is prime time for primal behaviour – especially when toddlers are interacting with equally unevolved peers. For tips on nipping these primitive though age-appropriate habits in the bud, see pages 167 through 174.

---

a community centre. For a change of place, head for a park or playground in pleasant weather, or a child-friendly museum or indoor play area on a rainy day. You can even brave a coffee shop that provides toys and books to play with and a child-friendly vibe (pick an off-peak hour) or a child-centric restaurant.

Decide when to meet. Toddlers are generally jollier at certain times of the day than others. Pick a time when all participants are relatively well rested (not just before naptime) and well fed (not right before mealtime, unless you plan to serve a substantial snack). Avoid the very end of the day if parent and toddler stress levels tend to be high at that time (and they usually are). At first, plan to keep sessions short – an hour or so – so that the children can get acclimated to the group gradually. As they start becoming more comfortable, begin extending the sessions until you reach the children's limit for togetherness, probably about two hours.

Plan to meet regularly. Once you've chosen a time that fits everyone's schedule, stick to it. Change the time only when necessary (a winter storm warning is in effect, for example, or three children are down with a cold). If you start

TWINS

Double the Fun

When you're a toddler twin, life's just one endless playdate. From the time those two pairs of eyes pop open in the morning, until the time they finally surrender to sleep at night, twin tots have a built-in playmate – someone to explore with, tackle new skills with, and of course, have double the fun with (and often, get into twice the trouble with, too). Maybe most importantly, at least as far as their friend-making futures are concerned, twins have someone to practise social skills with – from taking turns to sharing, solving disputes to working as a team – pretty much around the clock. And while all that practice doesn't make perfect (you'll still have your share of tugs-of-war to break up and turn-taking tussles to mediate), it can give twins a real edge in social development. There's even something in it for you: because twins always have someone to play with, they're usually able to keep themselves occupied for much longer stretches than singleton toddlers can – leaving you more time to get other things done (like cleaning up after the double messes they make). Plus, since the two of them can be each other's playdates, you can keep your twins' social calendar full

without all that effort (and driving time).

If you think about it, it's not surprising that twins win when it comes to social skills. Take sharing, for instance – typically the most challenging social stumbling block for 1-year-olds. From day one, literally, twins are used to sharing Mummy and Daddy time, toys, a play space, probably a room, possibly a cot. They share a pushchair, they share the backseat of the car, they share the bath – they even have to share your lap. Every twin also learns early on about taking turns: that someone always has to go first, and it won't always be him or her (something that doesn't usually dawn on singletons until the preschool years). And then there's cooperation. Though twins will still parallel play, they'll also play together (so-called cooperative play) a lot sooner than singletons do. And because they're constantly copying each other (one throws a ball, the other throws a ball; one stacks a brick, the other stacks a brick), they tend to spur each other's development of play skills, too.

That's not to say that your tots won't squabble over coveted toys or coveted lap space, about who goes first on the swing or who gets the first chance to

switching around (2 o'clock on Tuesday one week, 11 o'clock on Wednesday the next) or cancelling casually (because one parent has a business meeting or another has social plans), the group could start losing steam. With irregular meetings (or irregular attendance at a playgroup that meets regularly), children could also lose some of the social momentum they've been building up,

and tentative toddlers could take much longer to feel comfortable separating from their parents and joining the play.

Set basic health and safety rules. For instance, sick children should stay at home. Each playgroup location should be thoroughly childproofed. Only age-appropriate toys and activities should be provided.

push the doll pushchair. And it definitely doesn't mean that they'll be seasoned social pros by age 2 (especially when it comes to practicing those same social skills with non-sibling peers). Even with that social head start, they'll still need their share of gentle coaching. Here's how to provide it:

- Don't undermine "mine". All kids need stuff they can call their own. While it's definitely not necessary to buy two of every toy (or else there goes the head start on sharing), do try to double up on a few special items, or designate certain toys sole ownership by one twin. After all, it's not fair to ask your tots to share every single thing, every single time.

- Play to their differences. Even identical twins can have different interests and different play styles. Nurture those differences in the playroom. Say one's a mini-Monet, and one's a junior David Beckham – encourage both in their favourite play pursuits (with art supplies and activities for one, and sports supplies and activities for the other). They always want to play the same? That's fine, too – when it comes to play, don't forget they're running the show.

- Team them up. They're probably doing plenty of interacting without your intervention (or your effort). But you'll add to the fun – and the social skill building – if you occasionally set them up in group activities. As a party of two, they can roll a ball back and forth, crayon or finger paint on one giant sheet of paper, build a big garage for their cars, scout the park for pretty rocks.

- Team them up with others. Of course it's just as easy – for them and for you – to stick to Team Twin at playtime. But playing with others – who offer different perspectives on play, different interests, different sets of skills – can be socially enriching, too. Plus, they'll eventually have to venture out into more challenging, less safe social territory and get used to playing with children who don't happen to be their siblings (and former womb mates).

- Team them up with you, too. Being part of a twin twosome is wonderful, of course, as is time spent playing with other toddlers the same age. But don't underestimate the value of playing with you. As someone who's older, wiser, and more skilled in just about everything, you add a whole lot to the social equation – and a whole lot of fun to playtime.

Set playgroup protocol. Try to head off conflict and confusion by discussing and deciding on playgroup etiquette in advance. For example: who will clear up after each session (host only, or everyone)? What kind of notice is required if a child won't be attending group? What kinds of behaviour will be considered off-limits? Who will discipline the children (best bet: your child, your discipline) and how quickly will they step in?

Set a toy policy. The best toys to provide for the playgroup set are those that encourage cooperation (theoretically) and/or can be shared (again, theoretically): a bucket of bricks, a toy car and lorry collection, a beach ball or other large lightweight balls, board books, a doll collection, a tea set, pretend food, arts and crafts materials (crayons, paper, Play-Doh and finger paints), dressing-up items, a sandpit, a water table, and so on. Until the children are old enough to start taking turns, you may want to put away riding toys (unless you have enough to go around or you each bring your own) and other one-of-a-kind items. The host parents should also consider putting away "special" toys that their child might not want to see others play with or that might easily be damaged in a toddler tussle. They may even want to keep their child's room off-limits, if there's another place that's practical for play.

Set a food policy. Decide with the other parents what kinds of snacks will be served (for example, crackers, cheese, juice, fruit, milk) and what kinds of snacks will be avoided (for example, sugary biscuits, fizzy and fruit drinks, crisps, and boiled sweets – as well as foods that any of the children are allergic to). Put safety on the list, too – if

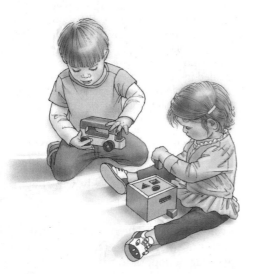

Most young toddlers are still playing side by side (parallel play) instead of with each other. With time and experience, toddler socialising becomes more interactive.

some of the parents are more lax about serving chokables (like grapes, raisins, popcorn, and sausages), there could be conflict (and worse).

Watch, don't hover. While toddlers need constant supervision for safety's sake, too much parental hovering can keep little ones from doing their thing. If you'd like to include a group activity that requires parental participation, balance it with some free time, when the tots can play on their own (probably in their trademark parallel style) and the parents can watch from the sidelines. When disputes come up (and they will), give the children the chance to work out minor disagreements by themselves, but step in and mediate if they come to blows (or bites, or shoves).

Playing with Others

"I've got together with a few other mums to form a playgroup. We have five toddlers all between 12 and 15 months old. They play . . . just not with each other."

Not-so-social socialising is standard for young toddlers – for very valid developmental reasons. Early on in the socialising game, toddlers view fellow toddlers pretty much as objects – objects that move and make noise, but objects nonetheless. Objects whose toys and food are up for grabs; objects that can be pushed aside or pushed around as necessary (and that, curiously, often push back); objects that are interesting to observe, poke, and prod, but not to interact with in any meaningfully cooperative way. Though most toddlers will show at least some empathy for other children at least some of the time (when they see another child crying, they might offer a toy or a pat on the head), they're not yet ready to give up their centre-of-the-universe status – to put the needs, desires, or feelings of other kids ahead of their own. Their naturally egocentric focus keeps playing together – so-called "cooperative play" – mostly beyond their developmental reach until about age 2.

Children are born social beings, but the art of true social interaction is learned – and it's learned gradually. And as with other skills, your toddler will learn best through a combination of practice, exposure, and example. Being part of a family is a vital first step of that social education, and being part of a playgroup (or having regular playdates) is a helpful – if not essential – second step.

Most of all, these still socially primitive toddlers need time to evolve. While you're waiting for those social skills to kick in, expect more of the same at your toddler's playgroup. Parallel (side-by-side) play will be the rule, and cooperative play will be the exception – if it's in the picture at all. The toddlers will enjoy each other's company, but won't cultivate it. Interactions may be mainly limited to pushing and grabbing, biting and hitting. Some children will cling to their parents or caregivers and won't join the group at all. Aggressive children may try to establish dominance over more submissive ones. The concept of sharing won't be understood, never mind practised.

Does all of this mean that playgroup sessions are pointless for your toddler (even if a welcome change of pace for you)? Not at all. It may be difficult to believe, but what you're witnessing as you observe that seemingly antisocial group of 1-year-olds is social change in the making. Your toddler is picking up valuable social experience that he and his playmates will one day be able to put to good use – and it won't be all that long, especially if the group meets regularly, before the play takes a turn for the interactive.

Bad Habit Swapping

"Every time we go to playgroup, my toddler comes home with a new annoying habit that she's picked up from one of the other children. One week it was screeching, the next week it was making blowing noises, the week after that it was banging."

When toddlers step out into the social scene, they learn a lot from their peers by example – unfortunately, not all of it so exemplary. Because they're such excellent mimics, young children pick up habits (the good, the bad, the annoying) easily. Generally, they test each new habit out for a week or two, then drop it as they pick up a new one that's caught their interest. Sometimes, a habit sticks around longer – especially if they find it attracts attention.

So don't pay attention. As always, toddlers typically prefer even negative attention to none at all – so scolding or nagging ("Stop screeching!") tends to encourage a behaviour rather than discourage it. Instead, do your best to ignore what you deplore, or to distract your toddler when she starts pursuing those picked-up habits. When the copycat behaviour is not only annoying but unsafe or unacceptable – hitting or biting, for example – deal with it calmly but promptly (see Chapters 6 and 7 for tips).

It may also help to discuss concerns about unacceptable behaviour (sorry, screeching and blowing noises probably won't qualify) with the other parents in the group so you can form a united front – and some strict policy guidelines – against it.

Being a Pushover

"Everyone else at playgroup grabs toys. My toddler doesn't – he just stands there and lets other kids grab from him."

The meek may inherit the earth, but in a room full of toddlers, they'll always be short on toys.

Although it's part of the typical toddler profile, grabbiness isn't universal among tots. To some, assertive behaviour (as in "I see your toy, I want your toy, I take your toy") just doesn't come naturally. Usually, that's a matter of temperament, not development – some children are more pushy, while others are more passive, even if they have a strong sense of self (sometimes, actually, because they have a strong sense of self). What's more, a more aggressive or more submissive temperament isn't all that predictive of behaviour later in life. Grabby toddlers don't necessarily turn into grabby adults, and easy-going, mild-mannered tots won't necessarily become tomorrow's doormats.

It's important that a toddler know he has rights, not that he needs to be forceful in sticking up for them. As long as your son seems content with himself and his social lot – he doesn't mind having toys snatched and seems just as happy picking up another when one's been grabbed – there's no reason to try to change his ways. It's possible that with time, social practice, and plenty of encouragement and modelling from you, he'll grow more assertive. Of course, it's also possible that he won't. Many successful people speak softly and get along just fine without carrying a big stick. If your son's destined to be among them, accept his gentle ways – even if your personality tends to be more force-forward.

If, however, your toddler seems unsettled by all the grabbing, yet unable to defend himself against the onslaught of tiny hands, come to his rescue. Step in when he's being confronted by an aggressive peer. If, for example, a playmate is trying to wrestle a toy from him, encourage him to take a stand. Until his social and language skills improve, you'll need to show him how it's done and how it's said: "Jack is playing with that toy now." If the toy's been grabbed away, don't grab it back (two social wrongs don't make a right – the idea is to teach him to assert his own rights, not to trample on the rights of others). Instead, ask for it nicely but firmly, and repeatedly if necessary (putting your hand out will help give the other child a clue about what you're asking): "Jack wasn't finished playing with that lorry yet. He would like to have the lorry back, please." If the playmate obliges, say "thank you" – and when your child finishes playing with the toy, encourage him to offer it back to the grabber. If the playmate refuses, don't get into a tug-of-war (remember, your toddler's watching your every move). Instead, find something else for your toddler to play with, and stand by to be sure that this new toy isn't filched as well.

Try this tack whenever your little man appears to be unhappily pushed around – when he's been shoved out of the queue at the slide, had his spade commandeered in the sandpit, or had his riding toy hijacked at the playground. But always give him the chance to handle these incidents by himself before you step in to handle them for him. It's possible that after a year or so of having everyone at home respect his rights and put his needs first, he just doesn't realise yet that it's a toddler jungle out there, so he's still developing the skills he needs to hang in it. Don't worry – he will.

Trouble Taking Turns

"Our toddler doesn't seem to get the idea of 'taking turns'. She won't wait her turn at the playground or at playgroup. And she always pushes her way in and insists on being first."

That's because in the world according to toddlers (where everyone else just revolves around her), she should come first. She – and she alone – should have first or even exclusive use of the slide, the swings, the rocking horse, the shape sorter, the riding toy, the giant teddy bear.

Sounds a little . . . egocentric? It is – but it's also normal and age-appropriate. Young toddlers are typically self-centred, which doesn't mean they're on their way to becoming selfish for life. Like most of her peers, your little me-firster just has a lot of growing up to do before she realises other people have rights, and even longer before she can be counted on to regularly respect those rights. She'll probably figure this out sooner if she's in a nursery situation (where turn-taking is required), or if she meets frequently with a playgroup (where it's encouraged). But she'll also pick it up faster if she learns from the best role model she has – you. Try these tips to teach the fine art of turn-taking – and broaden her view of the world (and the playground) beyond her own little universe:

Take turns together. Because your toddler's likely to feel more secure and less threatened with you than with her peers, she may be more willing to practise turn-taking at home. When you're eating lunch, take turns taking bites of your sandwiches or sips of your drinks. When she's in the bath, take turns splashing each other. When you're reading her a book, take turns turning the pages. For the most cooperative results, turn-taking practice sessions should be fun, not a bore. Attempt it only when your toddler's in a sporting mood – not when she's tired, hungry, or otherwise grumpy. And don't push more practice when she's had enough.

Take turns being first. When taking turns with your toddler, don't always let her go first (guess what message that reinforces?). Instead, try to alternate first turns. She won't go for going second to your first? Don't force her – it's more important for her to get the hang of taking turns in general. Keep trying though.

Turn to a timer. Using a timer as an impartial referee is one of the most effective ways to teach children to take turns. Generally, it's tougher to dispute a clock than a parent. First, try the timer at home, so your toddler starts to grasp the concept: "When the timer rings, it will be my turn to play with the doll." Then bring out the timer trick at playdates or playgroup. Explain: "I am going to set the timer. When the timer rings, your turn will be over and it will be Oliver's turn." It may take several demonstrations and run-throughs before the children accept the timer idea – and let's face it, sometimes acceptance won't be on the cards at all – but with persistence, this turn-taking technique will start gaining traction.

Turn on the patience. Remember that learning to take turns takes time. Your little one can't be expected to regularly cooperate in the give-and-take of turn-taking (or of sharing) with playmates until at least her third birthday.

Difficulty Sharing

"My son never lets anyone touch his favourite stuffed animal. Why does he have such a hard time sharing?"

To a toddler, there is no "yours", "mine", and "ours" – there is only "mine". Not only do toddlers label "mine" those things that are rightfully theirs (their toys, their cot, their chair, their mummy and daddy), but also those things that rightfully belong

Sharing, Caring . . . or Showing Off?

When your little one offers a favourite blanket to a playmate who's crying or shares a piece of biscuit with Daddy when he seems stressed, it's not usually in the spirit of generosity (that's still to be developed) – it's in the spirit of empathy (that's just emerging). Your toddler isn't sharing so much as comforting. Definitely a behaviour to encourage, especially because caring inevitably leads to sharing (in fact, it's hard to share unless you care).

Your toddler may also seem to "offer" a toy or other belonging to a friend or family member, then withdraw it quickly if he or she's actually taken up on the offer. In this scenario, your little one probably had no intention of parting with the possession – he or she was more likely showing it off than offering it up ("Look what I have!" not "Here, you can have it").

to others (a brother's book, Mummy's keys, a friend's toy car). Even things that are supposed to belong to everyone (the bus, the slide at the playground, the flowers in the park) may be viewed as personal property. "Mine" is, for now, a toddler's only article of possession – and among his favourite words. Even if he can't yet say "mine", he shows he means it by clinging fiercely to whatever he believes is his.

What makes sharing so hard for toddlers? Several age-appropriate factors: first, they're starting to grasp the concept of ownership – but haven't yet worked out that it applies to others. Second, hoarding helps them define their autonomy, establish their identity (I have, therefore I am), and set boundaries between themselves and others. Third, jealously guarding possessions – both their own and those of others – offers an important measure of control ("This is mine, and no one can take it away from me") that boosts their emerging sense of self. And fourth, since toddlers can't make sense out of the concept of lending and borrowing, they equate sharing with giving up for good.

Your toddler has trouble sharing not because he's spoiled or selfish, but because he's still evolving as a human being – and at this stage of his evolution, me comes first. It won't be until he's more comfortable with his own sense of self that he'll be comfortable putting his needs and wants after those of others.

Respecting that evolution – and letting it takes its normal and necessary course – can actually help speed the development of generosity. A toddler who's allowed to savour ownership now (by clinging to it for dear life, if he chooses to) won't feel so threatened by parting with property later on. On the other hand, one who's forced to share may be even more reluctant to share.

Sharing doesn't come naturally to toddlers, and it doesn't come at all to most children until they're closer to 3 or 4 years old. Like all social skills, it generally comes faster to children who have more frequent and more regular exposure to others their own age – whether it's in a child care situation or in some form of playgroup (or with their twin; see box, page 308). Still, there are ways to nurture generosity in your toddler now – so that when the time's right, he will both a borrower and lender be. Here's how to begin:

Don't share what's not yours. Your toddler's toys belong to your toddler – in other words, they're not yours to offer up. Always ask permission before handing your toddler's stuff to a playmate. If permission isn't granted, don't insist (though do suggest a different toy to share: "I know you don't want to share Teddy, because he's special. But maybe you can share this stuffed elephant"). Respecting your toddler's property will help him feel better about sharing it . . . eventually.

Don't force sharing. Pushing your child to share implies that you consider his needs less significant than those of others – which can be both damaging to that fledgling sense of self and counterproductive to the sharing agenda. Feeling that possessions are always up for grabs can also make your tot feel insecure at a time in his life when he's craving security most. Plus, forcing a toddler to share doesn't teach generosity – it just teaches him to do as he's told. Finally, instead of showing a toddler that giving feels good (which it should), you're reinforcing that it feels pretty bad.

Introduce ownership – as it applies to others. Your little one needs to learn that some things belong to him (like his favourite stuffed animal), some things belong to other people (a playmate's doll or lorry, or your book), and some things belong to the group or to everybody (toys at nursery, equipment at the playground). Illustrate this concept every chance you get ("That's Daddy's computer" or "That's the swing set, and it belongs to all the children who want to swing on it").

Tackle taking turns. Tough as it is, toddlers also need to learn how to take turns on the slide or wait their turn for an empty swing. Promote these rules regularly (see the previous question for tips on teaching taking turns).

Try a little perspective. Unwillingness to part with a toy lorry for even 15 minutes may seem unreasonable, but from where your toddler stands, it's actually very valid (since for a toddler, this may seem more like 15 hours). Put yourself in your child's trainers: how willing would you be to part with your car, your iPad, your favourite shoes, or a special piece of jewellery, just overnight, even if it were borrowed by a trusted friend? To toddlers, who don't understand that they'll get back what they lend, sharing possessions is even harder.

Try a little understanding. Instead of scolding ("You're not being nice to Luke. Let him play with your car"), empathise, saying "I know it's hard to share your car. It's very special to you."

When You Have to Share

When not sharing isn't an option (you're hosting a playgroup or a playdate, for instance), decide with your toddler which special toys will be put away and which will be shared. Knowing that at least some of his or her possessions will be off-limits to grabby little hands may help your toddler feel more secure about sharing some others (though, realistically, it may not). It may also help to have other tots bring a toy or two of their own, no matter who's hosting, in case the sharing gets tough and the tough get possessive. As the toddlers become better negotiators, they may start swapping, and this will be the beginning of sharing. Whenever possible (the fists have not started flying), let your playdaters work out minor disputes over toys. If sharing happens – whether it was adult-prompted or not – offer up plenty of praise.

Such understanding will help your toddler overcome a reluctance to share sooner. You can also try to help your toddler empathise with playmates: "Ella feels sad when you won't let her play with your puzzle."

Share your love of sharing. Since your toddler learns best by your example, be a model of generosity. Offer a piece of your muffin or a sliver of melon off your plate, a look at your magazine, a chance to try on your boots. Explain that "This is mine, but I like sharing it with you."

Play sharing games, too: "You let me play with your doll, and I'll let you play with my computer." Sharing with you will be less threatening than sharing with peers (he knows you're not going to snatch his teddy bear and run off), and it's good practice for the real thing.

Play the "lend" game. Borrowing and lending are tricky concepts for your toddler, but they're worth exploring with him. Explain that when you lend something, you get it back, and when you borrow something, you have to give it back. Then, because actions speak louder – and more meaningfully – than words, show him what you mean by that. Borrow that beloved teddy bear for a few moments, then return it. Let your toddler borrow your sunglasses, then ask for them back. Point out that when children play on the swings at the playground or play with bricks at a friend's house, they don't keep them. They just "borrow" them for a while. Keep reinforcing, repeating, and illustrating, and in time he'll start to get the idea.

Spin it. Compliment all efforts at sharing, no matter how small or grudging, since that positive enforcement will encourage more of the same. Point out the good that sharing does ("See how happy Evelina is because you shared with her!"). But also try to help your toddler see all the positives that sharing offers him, too: that letting a friend play with one of his cars makes the race more exciting, that giving a pal a turn with his shopping trolley means he may be more likely to get a turn with her doll. With time, experience, and some gentle guidance, your toddler will begin to realise that sharing actually makes playing more fun – and that it is its own reward.

The In-Your-Face Toddler

"When my daughter gets together with other toddlers, she's very in their face. Not in an aggressive way, but she doesn't give the other kids much space – poking and prodding the way she does – and they sometimes get upset."

Young rough players like your daughter don't mean any harm when they squeeze, jab, or poke another child. They're just busy exploring their environment firsthand (or hands first) – and the other children are part of that environment. Boundaries? They only know their own. Feelings? Ditto. Propriety? What's that?

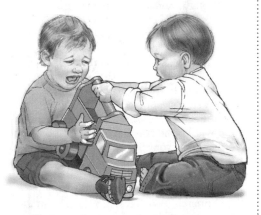

Sharing is rarely a toddler's forté.

No Rough Stuff

Rough-and-tumble play may seem like a great way to have fun with your wee one, but there are several reasons why you might want to proceed with caution, if at all. First, your toddler may take playing cues from you and may mimic your rough stuff when playing with peers. Second, not all children like rough play (just like not all children enjoy cuddling and hugging) – and some find it upsetting.

Rough play can be frightening for some toddlers, and if it's done before bed, it can make it difficult for a little one to unwind and settle down for a good night's sleep (night waking and even nightmares can be triggered by before-bed rough play). And the most compelling case against really rough play: it can be dangerous. A toddler under 2 who is shaken vigorously or thrown up in the air with strong force can suffer serious injury (including retinal detachment and brain damage). Don't worry about any past very rough play (if damage had been done

there would be obvious signs), but do avoid it from now on.

Also unsafe is overexuberantly swinging your tot by the arms ("1-2-3-weee"). Kids love it, it's fun, but it could result in an extremely painful dislocation of the elbow (which can usually be popped quickly back into place by a doctor). Ditto for yanking or tugging a toddler's still growing arm.

Take care, too, when it comes to tickling. While many gigglers love a good parent-induced tickle fest, other toddlers are miserable, especially when the tickling gets rough or goes on too long (they actually find it painful, even if they're reflexively laughing). Watch your toddler's eyes, expression, and body language for signs that he or she wants to continue or to cease and desist. If you sense panic rather than pleasure, stop immediately. If the signs aren't clear, and your toddler is old enough to understand the question, ask directly, "Do you like it when I tickle you?" Tickle away if it's appreciated, give it up if it isn't.

Physical contact also comes in handy when toddlers are trying to communicate what they can't yet express in words. Instead of "Hello, good to see you!" your toddler may greet her friend with a poke in the arm. When she wants a playmate to come to her room to see her new puzzle, she may literally try to drag her pal down the hallway. And when she's ready for a friend to leave, she may just push him unceremoniously out of the door.

She may know exactly what she's trying to do, exactly what she's trying to say, but the problem is, other tots probably won't. From their perspective, she's in their face and invading their space – and that's just not cool. Maybe they'll cry,

maybe they'll seek retribution (a poked eye for a poked eye). Either way it's not likely to end well. What's an in-your-face toddler's parent to do? Try the following:

- Try a gentle touch. Would you like your toddler to be gentler with her pals? Try being gentler with her. Yanking her by the arm when she refuses to leave the playground, grabbing her and plopping her into the car seat when she's balking at being strapped in, pushing her along when she's dawdling, even pinching or poking her playfully can set a rough example. Toddlers are great imitators – especially of their parents' actions – so make an effort to model gentleness. In time, she may model it back.

- Have her try a gentle touch. A gentle touch takes practice for physically exuberant tots. Help her practise by playing a "gentle touch" game: show her how to touch a stuffed animal gently, how to touch you gently. Say "I like when you are gentle with me."

- Discourage the rough stuff. Letting your toddler play rough with you, but not with peers, sends a confusing message. So try to make those boundaries consistent. When she yanks at your ear or bops you in the belly with her head or tugs you hard by the hand, let her know you don't like it (even if it really doesn't bother you): "Please don't do that. It hurts." Explain that certain kinds of contact (hugs, pats, handshakes, high fives) are acceptable and others aren't.

Not-So-Nice Behaviour

"Our son doesn't seem very nice to other kids his own age, and that bothers me."

It's hard to love thy neighbour (in the sandpit, at playgroup) when you're so busy loving yourself. Like every normally egocentric 1-year-old, your toddler's first love – besides you, of course – is "me", and that's completely age-appropriate. Before he can care about others, he has to get himself worked out – which is why he's a little me-occupied right now. Besides, he hasn't even begun to do for himself yet (most of his needs, after all, are filled by you and other obliging adults), so doing unto others isn't exactly on his to-do list.

Toddlers who regularly spend time with other toddlers, as in a nursery situation, or with older siblings, tend to show empathy and sympathy (as well as other more mature social traits) earlier, since the group experience gives them more of a "we're-all-in-the-same-boat-together" perspective than does being the centre of attention at home. Those who don't socialise a whole lot may lag a little in those departments, though only temporarily. Playing nice – and acting nice – is most likely just a couple of years down the road.

Of course, the best way to teach the old do-unto-others credo is to do it yourself. Nice parents inevitably raise nice children. With you showing him the kind way, your little one can't help but respond in kind – at least, once he's outgrown the era of "me".

ALL ABOUT:
Making Friends

As you watch yet another afternoon at the park dissolve into a WWF-worthy pushing and hair-pulling match between your toddler and a playmate, you may be wondering: with friends like these, who needs enemies?

Hang in there. There are more mature friendships (the kind that involve give-and-take, instead of grab-and-pull) in your toddler's future. Just not, realistically, in the very near future. The primitive friendships your toddler is forming now are real, but they're based mainly on proximity and familiarity ("I'm your friend because I see you every week at playgroup"). Empathy, which is the foundation of mature friendships, is only just starting to be glimpsed, and that makes for difficult early social interactions. As in, "Give and take? Nah – I think I'll just take."

Sound hopeless? Far from it. Believe it or not, over the next couple of years your toddler will learn to share and cooperate, to be aware of and sensitive to the feelings of others, to work out disagreements with words instead of aggressive actions – in short, to become friends. Want to help your little one's social evolution along? These top 10 friendship tips can help:

1. Model social behaviour. Your child's first – and most important – social interactions are with you. From those early cooing sessions over the Moses basket to conversations over the dinner table, your toddler learns more about being social from you than from any peer. So try to model the social behaviour you'd like to see (eventually) in your little one. Take turns with the same crayon, or putting pieces in the puzzle, or feeding the doll. Borrow your toddler's stuffed dog for a minute, then return it with a thank-you. Share a cheese stick or a cracker. Play games that have simple rules, and encourage your toddler to follow the rules. Role-play social situations that your toddler may find himself or herself in: asking to play with someone else's toy; lending a toy; taking turns being first at an activity. Let your little one catch you being a good friend to your spouse, too: offering him the last crisp in the packet; sharing the blanket you've been cuddled up with on the sofa; letting him use your smart phone to check the weekend weather.

2. Offer plenty of chances for practice. Children who have plenty of early exposure to other children – in a large family, in a playgroup, in their street, in nursery – tend to be more sociable sooner. If your toddler hasn't spent much time with children his or her own age, consider joining or forming a playgroup, arranging playdates, or making more frequent trips to the local playground or other places where parents and children hang out, like the local library or community centre. A lot of socialising just isn't practical? While it can give your tot a social leg up, it's definitely not developmentally essential, as long as he or she is getting plenty of social experience at home.

3. Give friendship a name. Use the word "friend" often around your toddler when describing a playmate: "Your friend Angelo is coming over to play today." Use the "f" word, too, when talking to your tot about the friends in your life: "I'm talking to my friend Rita on the phone." Then connect your friendships with your toddler's: "My friend is named Rita. Your friend is Amanda." Make up a big deal of friends wherever you spot them – in books, at the park, at the shops ("Those two girls are friends. It's fun to have friends!").

4. Build in cooperation. During playdates and playgroup, choose some activities that naturally promote cooperation – and are even more fun when there's more than one to enjoy them. Brick play, ball playing, music making, dressing-up, hide-and-seek, joint creative projects (scribbling with a large supply of crayons on a large sheet of paper), circle games, and games that require taking turns give budding buddies some basic (if not always successful) experience in interaction. The tots would rather play solo? Parallel play may be an early step in a toddler's social evolution, but don't discount its importance – your little one can learn lots from these noninteractive interactions, too ("Hmmm, I never thought of bouncing my ball. That looks like fun!").

5. Stay nearby, and stay neutral. Even if all seems pretty quiet, keep a constant watch on toddlers at play, and be ready to step in should conflict suddenly break out. But don't anticipate an incident before it actually occurs, and don't step in unless things have started getting physical – learning to be a friend takes practice, not all of it pretty. If adult intervention becomes necessary, avoid taking sides – even if it's clear who's right and who's wrong (remember, they both have a lot to learn). Simply break up the skirmish calmly, and march the troops off to a new activity.

6. Accept your toddler's social style. Each child, like each adult, has a very personal approach to socialising. Some are early to the social party, others make a later entrance. Some are happy to flit around from friend to friend (the more the merrier), others prefer to focus on a single friend. Some barrel into every social situation without a moment's hesitation, others take their tentative time getting ready to make a move, and still others do more observing from the sidelines (or Mum's lap) than active socialising. As long as your child is content with his or her social style, you should be, too.

7. Age up. While social practice with fellow little ones teaches a lot – and most playdates should be with approximate age-mates – your toddler can learn a lot from an older friend, too. So once in a while, let an "old-timer" show your

toddler the social ropes. Invite a willing 4- or 5-year-old for a visit. Your toddler will be mesmerised, of course, by everything the bigger child does – and may even pick up a few pointers on cooperative play. Plus, unless the older child is a sibling (then all bets are off), your toddler is far less likely to be grabby, pushy, or pull-y with someone who has social seniority.

8. Be a booster. Children who like themselves are more likeable to others – and go on to become better friends. Build your child's self-esteem and confidence now, and you'll be building a strong foundation for a lifetime of healthy relationships. On the other hand, be careful not to over-inflate your child's ego by pumping up the praise too much – nobody likes an ego-maniac.

9. Lend a hand, where it's needed. Is a penchant for pushing or a proclivity for being a pushover getting in your toddler's way of having a good time with others? Respecting your little one's social style doesn't mean you can't step in to help when it's holding him or her back. See page 311 for tips on how.

10. Apply no pressure. Pushing the social agenda at an early age doesn't usually help toddlers win friends and influence little people. In fact, it can make tots socially reluctant. Encourage, but don't pressure – and always take your cues from your cutie (he or she has had it after the first playdate of the week? It's time for a social hiatus). Let friend-making take its sweet time and social evolution take its natural course – and remember, it's a process. Ultimately, your toddler will work out that child's play is even more fun when it's played with other children.

CHAPTER 11

Travelling with Your Toddler

....

YOU DON'T HAVE TO LOOK FAR FOR ADVENTURE when you're travelling with a tot. When a toddler gets restless, even a completely relaxed beach holiday can quickly turn wild. Think about it: a tantrum at home . . . well, you can just close the windows and let it take its noisy course. A tantrum at the supermarket . . . a little embarrassing, yes, but you can always fall back on a quick dash to the car or a speedy retreat back home. But a tantrum aloft at 9,000 metres a full two hours from landing, or speeding along the motorway 30 minutes from the next exit, or on a train a day away from your destination, or in a crowded hotel lobby when your room isn't ready yet . . . this is the stuff that parental nightmares are made of. Ditto trying to invent new ways to keep your tot entertained on hour three of a six-hour drive or plane ride – or scrambling to find a familiar snack in an unfamiliar supermarket. Double ditto the daunting task of finding a holiday hotel that truly caters to little guests (and their exhausted parents – calling all babysitters!). Yet the open roads and the friendly skies still beckon (as do doting grandparents or friends eager for your next visit), annual leave days mount up, travel sites promise family fun that doesn't break the bank, and the time does come to get up and go. So go – but not before you've planned, planned, and planned some more.

On the Go with Your Toddler

Little toddlers tend to travel with lots of baggage – and not just the kind you'll have to carry. Here's how to take your show on the road – or up in the air – with as much fun and as little turbulence as possible.

WHEREVER YOU GO

For happier trails, wherever you wander with your tiny traveller:

Check with the doctor. Before heading away from home, make sure your child is in good health and that you have an ample supply of any medicine he or she may need on the road, especially those that might not be readily available locally. Plan for unexpected illness (an allergic reaction, a fever, or a stomach bug) by bringing along a children's antihistamine, a pain reliever, and a rehydration fluid (like Dioralyte).

Some foreign destinations require special immunisations or other health precautions. Health information on travel with children is available from your child's doctor and from the NHS online at www.nhs.uk. General healthy travel info is available at www.travelhealth. co.uk.

Make sleeping arrangements. Whether you're travelling to a hotel or to Grandma's, make sure your tot will have a safe place to rest that sweet, sleepy head every night. Most hotels and resorts can supply a cot for a young toddler, sometimes for a fee – phone ahead to reserve one (and check it over when you get there to make sure it's safe). You can also bring along a portable cot. But the most convenient option on some trips (especially if you're trying to travel light or if you'll be staying at a rental property) may be to rent the toddler gear you'll need, including that cot (as well as a pushchair), from an online or local rental service. It'll be delivered, assembled if necessary, and taken away when your stay is over (all at a price, of course).

If you arrive at your destination and find the cot that's been provided isn't safe, set the cot mattress on the floor (just make sure the bathroom door is closed and the rest of the room is childproofed) or put your little one in bed with you.

Limit your itinerary. One-destination holidays – visiting relatives or a stay at a family-oriented resort, at a beach house, or in a single city – are usually the most successful with toddlers. If you're planning a touring holiday, consider limiting the number of stops so that you're not constantly on the go.

Limit your expectations. The trick to a relatively relaxing holiday with a toddler in tow is to keep expectations low and patience high. True, your toddler may surprise everyone by being agreeable and adaptable, by cheerfully accompanying you on shopping sprees and culture binges, by behaving impeccably on aeroplanes and at four-star restaurants. But your toddler may, more predictably, act like a toddler. Most toddlers will be bored to tears (literally) by long, overscheduled days in museums, boutiques, and with tour groups. So plan accordingly.

Limit the sightseeing. If sightseeing is on your agenda, keep in mind that you likely won't be able to follow the typical tourist routine. You may want to see everything in the guidebook, but chances are your toddler won't. So unless you're lucky enough to be able to bring along a nanny or a family member who will be willing to babysit while you tour, you'll have to alternate adult-interest sightseeing with toddler-interest destinations (zoos, children's museums, beaches, parks, amusement parks). And don't try to crowd too much into any one day. In most cases, one destination in the morning and one in the afternoon will be all your toddler can take . . . and sometimes even that might be a stretch.

Younger toddlers may be fascinated enough by the forms, colours, and shapes at a museum or gallery to allow you to visit for an hour or so, especially if they are comfortably ensconced in a push-chair. Tots closer to 2 years may be more cooperative if you build a game into the visit. Try playing "Can you find it?" Challenge your little sightseer: "Can you find the doggy in the pretty painting?"

For information on attractions that are attractive to toddlers, pick up a local guidebook that focuses on children and/or check the local newspaper online for activities.

Make friends with the mini-fridge. Assuming there's room in your room, try having breakfast in before going out and/or dinner in the room on your return. After all, eating out with a young child can become hard work fast. If your budget doesn't allow for room service (always a thrill for tots – and adults), consider bringing in food. If you have a room with a fridge (or if you can rent one), so much the better. You can stock up on familiar foods and drinks, saving money and stress. Best of all? A kitchenette – or at least, a microwave.

Pack your sense of humour. It's essential to survival when travelling with children. If you're able to have a laugh when things go wrong – and they will – it won't seem half as bad.

TRAVELLING BY CAR

When travelling long distances on the open roads (or the jammed motorways), keep these tips in mind:

Never start without the car seat. It's essential any time you're getting into a vehicle, no matter how long or short the road ahead – and no matter whose vehicle you're getting into (and yes, that goes for taxis and vans, too). If you're renting a car, ask the rental company to supply you with a safe, up-to-date car seat (for a fee) or bring your own.

When there are several travellers on a trip, periodically change seats for everyone but the toddler (moving the car seat around is too cumbersome) to give your little one a change of pace and others in the car a break from entertainment duty.

Load up. Pack all the same stuff you always cram into your car when your toddler's in tow, just lots more of it. It almost goes without saying that you'll need to stock up on favourite snacks and drinks you're not likely to find on the road (a coolbox definitely will come in handy for yogurt, apple slices, cheese, and other perishables). But you'll also want to tote (and prepare to tolerate) toddler-friendly tunes, as well as playthings aplenty. Which toys should you tote? Finger and hand puppets are perfect, as are crayons, books, and miniature music-making toys, which can hold a toddler's attention for long stretches. And keep in mind that now is the time to splurge on or borrow as many unfamiliar toys as possible. They'll keep your tot amused far longer than those same old playthings (though of course, you'll want to bring the favourites, too). Dole out the snacks and toys individually at various times throughout the drive (don't blow through the lot by mile 20). Also be prepared to sing songs, recite rhymes, and play spotting games en route. Young toddlers can try to spot a dog, a cow, a horse, a lorry, a house, a barn, an aeroplane, a bus, a bridge. For more fun activities when you're on the go, see the box on the next page.

Break it up. Those glory days of all-day, all-night driving straight through to your destination, fuelled by adrenalin, black coffee, and the occasional hamburger or bag of crisps, are gone. While it's wise to do as much driving as you can during toddler naptimes, it's also wise to

Fun on the Go

Getting there is half the fun – unless you're a toddler with a bad case of the fidgets and a dislike of seats with straps (after all, little kids aren't exactly made for sitting). What can you do to keep your child happy in a train, plane, or automobile? Plan ahead by packing a few easy kids' travel activities designed for low-effort entertainment so you can make the miles fly by. All you need for these travel activities is loads of imagination and a few simple props. A tray table or a car-seat tray will also come in handy. Try one (or all) the next time your family takes to the rails, the skies, or the road:

Toys on the move. Even young tots are experts at using their hands, and they're working out big-picture concepts like "in and out" and "empty and full". Combine those two emerging skill sets by bringing along two lidded plastic containers, one empty and one filled with toys that'll catch your little one's fancy, like bricks, plastic animals, or squares of brightly coloured cloth. Put the containers next to each other and encourage your pint-size companion to move the objects from one container to the next, then back again. Though this game won't play well in the car, it's a perfect pastime when you're travelling by plane or train.

Book mobile. Small, light, and easy to pack, board books are made for travelling, and they're perfect for distracting a bored toddler on a plane or train (or in the car – if there's a designated driver and an adult or older sib can sit next to your tot in back). Slip a few favourites into your hand luggage and do dramatic readings, complete with funny voices, when your little one gets restless.

Write and erase. One of the most versatile playthings you can pack in your travel activities bag: a mini white board and some dry-erase markers. Your toddler can have a blast simply scribbling and erasing. You can even jump-start his or her artistic imagination by drawing a squiggle or a shape on the board (if you're not the one doing the driving), then having your little one fill in the rest of the picture.

Keep an eye out. Take advantage of the scenery speeding by and make a travel scavenger hunt by using index cards to draw pictures or paste photos of things that are easy to spot on the road, like trees or an 18-wheeler lorry or a tall building. Hand your tiny traveller one card from the pack at a time, and challenge him or her to find the object pictured. Or have the whole family join in the fun by picking a single object for everyone to keep an eye out for, like a cow or a bicycle. When someone spies it, have them shout "toot", "burp", or any buzzword that will have your tot giggling. And don't forget the old favourite, "I Spy", for your older toddler.

take plenty of breaks for exercise, meals, snacks, and other diversions. With kids onboard, two 6-hour days are twice as easy as one monster marathon drive. So if it's needed (and if you can spare the time and money), allow for an overnight stop to space out the trip.

Don't use rest stops only for resting. Sitting in a car for extended periods of time isn't easy for anyone, but it's especially hard for active toddlers. So make sure you break up driving time with plenty of circulation-stimulating breaks. Encourage your tot to stretch

Do as I'm doing. Turn your toddler into a copycat by doing funny things with your hands and arms – blowing a kiss, patting your head – and challenging him or her to mimic what you do. For more of a challenge, create a sequence – chin touch, cheek pat, head nod – and invite your mini monkey to ape along.

Stick 'em up. Draw easy-to-identify shapes (a square, a circle, a triangle, a heart) on small sticky notes and put them on the tray table, the car seat tray, or the window beside your toddler. Then call out a shape and challenge your little one to pull off the right sticky note.

Play with paper. Need a kids' travel activity that's a great quiet-time activity, too? Multitask those magazines you just picked up for the trip by letting your tot play "I Spy" with them, hunting for photos on the pages based on clues you give him or her ("I spy a doggy. Can you find a picture of a dog?").

Create your own travel toys. Boredom has set in at 9,000 metres or halfway between stations? Look no further than that empty water bottle for some DIY toddler entertainment. Just fill halfway with water, drop in a few pennies, then screw the lid on extra tight (so the coins, which are choking hazards, won't fall out). Your tiny tot will have a ball shaking it and watching the water and pennies splash about inside.

Play with your hands. Most young children are fascinated by puppets, but if you don't want to haul any from home, make your own by drawing faces on both your index fingers with eyeliner or a lip pencil. Then have your finger puppets talk to each other. Or use a pen to make a happy face on the back of a paper plate from the train's snack bar (or, if you're on a plane, pull out that air-sickness bag). Have the puppet tell your little one a simple – yet engaging – story.

Freeze dance. Play freeze dance in the car. Turn on some lively music for a minute while you all wriggle and boogie in your seats (except the driver!). When the music stops, freeze in place with a silly face. Your toddler will love the dancing part even if the freezing part is still a little tough to pull off. Bonus: the family will burn off some pent-up energy.

Fun with foil. A few sheets of aluminium foil equals the perfect arts-and-crafts travel activity for kids, since foil is as pliable as Play-Doh but far less messy. By ripping, twisting, folding, and scrunching, your little one can transform foil into funny creations. Make sure there's an adult supervising next to your toddler during this activity so that he or she doesn't rip off a piece and try to swallow it.

Be magnetic. Bring along a small baking sheet and some magnetised alphabet letters. Your toddler will have fun moving the magnets around, and you'll love that the pieces stick to the sheet. Bonus: a rimmed baking sheet makes a great lap tray for containing colouring books and crayons or other small toys, too.

those little legs and burn off some energy with a toy ball (where it's safe to play) or a quick game of follow the leader.

Tweak your schedule. Try leaving really early in the morning, so your tot will sleep through part of the journey – depending on your toddler's sleep tendencies. Big caveat: make sure the driver stays awake. Start out well rested, take turns at the wheel, and pull over as soon as the designated driver becomes drowsy.

Curbing the Queasies

Up in the air, riding the rails, on the road – motion sickness can strike a young tummy any time, anywhere. Even if your toddler has never had a problem with motion sickness before, and especially if he or she has, implement the following tips before and during travel:

Talk to your doctor. If your toddler has experienced serious motion sickness before, talk to the doctor about taking along motion-sickness medication.

Secure Sea-Bands. Sea-Bands (you might remember them from your pregnancy days) are elasticised bracelets that work to curb motion sickness by putting pressure on an acupressure point on the inner wrist. They're inexpensive, easy to use, safe, and comfortable to wear (be sure to purchase the child-size ones).

Keep that tank full (but not too full). A mostly empty tummy is more likely to erupt – a good reason to feed your toddler frequent light snacks when travelling (like crackers). But an overly full tummy may also be prone to overflowing, so don't let your little one eat too much, either.

Skip the acid. Acidic fruit (like oranges) or juice can upset a travelling tummy.

Factor out fats. Greasy and fat-laden foods can also aggravate motion sickness, so think twice about ordering chips with that meal when you're on the road, or serving pasta-and-cheese just before you set out.

Add some air and a view. In a car, fresh air from a partially open window can minimise motion sickness. On a plane, redirecting the overhead air vent is about the best you can do. Watching the horizon can help relieve the quease, so when possible, seat your toddler next to a window, and periodically call attention to sights in the distance. Looking at books or doing anything else that requires focusing close-up may not be the best idea during a queasy moment.

Encourage napping. If your toddler is able to sleep, or at least rest with eyes closed for most of the trip, the chances of motion sickness are greatly reduced.

Have a bag handy. Be prepared for the worst, just in case none of the above do the trick. Pack some large reclosable plastic bags within your reach (but out of your toddler's reach). Also have an extra set of clothing, plenty of wipes (they can be used to clean up your child, clothing, seats, and carpeting), and air freshener handy.

If that queasy feeling does creep up, your little one probably won't know what the sensation is or be able to describe it. Some toddlers just get out of sorts, others clutch their throats with their hands or hold their bellies. Some cough (a reaction to gagging). Some look pale or green-around-the-gills. There may, however, be no obvious symptoms until your child throws up.

If motion sickness strikes your child while you're at the wheel, stop at the first opportunity, clean up as best you can, and try to get your toddler to close his or her eyes and rest for a few minutes before you get back on the road. Applying a wet cloth to your child's forehead may also help, as can getting some fresh air. A sip of cold water or, if you can find one at your stop, an ice lolly can help soothe and rehydrate.

Don't forget cleaning supplies. Make sure you bring loads of nappies, wipes, hand sanitiser, disposable bags for rubbish (and potential car sickness), paper towels for spills, and an extra set of clothes (kept in a reachable spot).

Put safety first. For a safe car trip:

- Make sure everyone in the car is strapped in.

- Don't drive to the point of fatigue (accidents are more likely to occur when the driver is tired).

- Never drive if you've been drinking.

- Don't talk on a mobile phone while driving (even hands free isn't safe).

- Never text, tweet, or e-mail while driving.

- Prohibit smoking in the car.

- Store heavy luggage or potential flying objects in the boot or secured by a cover.

TRAVELLING BY PLANE

Taking flight with your toddler? Keep these plane pointers in mind:

Book early. If you can, purchase your tickets well in advance. On many (though not all) airlines, this allows you to choose the seats you want. Also, print out your boarding passes (if possible) at home before leaving for the airport, or take advantage of mobile boarding passes (if available).

Travel at off-peak times. The less crowded the terminal, the shorter the security lines will be. The less crowded the flight, the more comfortable you will be, the better the service will be, and the fewer passengers your toddler will be able to (potentially) annoy. So check flight loads before you book. Try,

too, to choose flights at times when your toddler ordinarily sleeps (night flights are great for really long trips, naptimes for short trips). Maybe, just maybe, he or she will really sleep for a while on the plane. True, flight delays can foil even the best-booked plans, but it's definitely worth a try.

Consider a nonstop. In most cases, the faster you get from here to there, the better for all. That said, sometimes a very long daytime non-stop may be too much for anyone to handle (your toddler, you, the passengers sitting near you). If you think a long haul flight might put your tot over the top, consider breaking the trip into two shorter ones (you may get a less expensive fare while you're at it). You'll want a layover to be long enough for you to get to the next gate with a minimum of huffing and puffing and have time to get a bite to eat, use the bathroom, take care of nappy changing (it's a lot easier to change a fidgeting toddler in an airport bathroom than on the aeroplane), let your toddler toddle off some energy, watch a few planes take off and land, and – if there is one – visit the airport play centre. But too much time in the terminal can be . . . interminable.

Consider reserving an extra seat. Though on most airlines children under 2 can travel for free (if you keep them on your lap), parents often choose to purchase a seat for their child anyway – and that's a sensible move. Even when confined to an adult's lap only during takeoff, landing, and periods of air turbulence (which can be frequent and unexpected on some flights), a toddler is likely to twist, turn, and wail for release. Paying full fare for a toddler may seem like an extravagance, but it will make sitting, playing, and eating less of a hassle for both of you, and at the same time it will make your child feel more

Passports for Half-Pints

Anyone travelling on an international flight, must present a passport to exit and re-enter the UK – and that goes for tots, too. If your toddler doesn't have a passport yet, you'll need plenty of time to secure one before setting out on an international voyage. All minors under age 16 (including your toddler) must apply in person with both parents or guardians or with a notorised letter from the absent parent. For more information, visit www.passports-office.co.uk.

If you'll be travelling out of the country alone with your toddler (a.k.a. without your child's other parent) you may require special documentation. So be ready to show proof that you have permission from your child's other parent or that you are your child's sole legal guardian.

important (with a safety belt, tray, headphones, and armrests of his or her own). Toddlers buckled into an approved car seat in a separate seat are also far safer in turbulence than those restrained only by a parent's arms. (For more on car seat use in flight, see page 332.)

If you're travelling with another adult and your flight isn't crowded, you may be able to book an aisle and window seat on a three-seat side with an empty seat between. If you specify that you have a lap child, some airlines won't sell that seat unless absolutely necessary. As long as the seat stays unbooked, you've got a free seat for your toddler. If it doesn't, you can be pretty sure the middleman (or woman) will be willing

to trade seats with one of you rather than having a toddler passed back and forth over his or her lap during the entire flight.

Favour the aisle. Children love window seats – but if you're travelling alone with your toddler on your lap, you'll hate not having access to the aisle. So opt for the aisle seat – otherwise you're going to end up trying the patience of those you'll have to keep scrambling over in order to take your restless toddler for a nappy change or for a walk. (Keep in mind, though, that if you bring along a car seat, the flight attendants won't let you place your tot in an aisle seat). Of course, if your family fills the entire row, you can have your aisle and your window, too. When booking a window seat, try to get one that doesn't overlook the wing, which will block most of the view. Also be sure that you aren't inadvertently given the exit row (children aren't allowed to sit there).

Parents often favour bulkhead seats because they provide extra room forward of the seats for a toddler to kick up his or her heels (without annoying the passenger in front) and to play or sleep on the floor when the seat belt sign is off. But these advantages aren't necessarily enough compared with the many disadvantages: trays unfold over your lap, leaving no room for your child; the armrest usually can't be raised (which means your toddler can't spread out across two seats to nap); you're right on top of the TV screen, if there is one; there's no under-seat storage, so even your tot's tiny toy-filled rucksack must be stored overhead during takeoff and landing. If you do opt for the bulkhead, don't let your toddler play on the floor in front of you, despite the extra space, since he or she could be injured if there's unexpected turbulence.

Check in luggage. To avoid having to lug your luggage through a sprawling airport, check everything in but valuables and essentials (your toddler's rucksack of toys, your nappy bag, and a small handbag). To avoid having to lug your toddler, use a luggage trolley with a built-in child seat at the airport or use a lightweight pushchair.

Plan for the security queue. A light umbrella pushchair is your best friend when going through security – it will be easy to fold up at the last second and plop on the X-ray conveyor belt. (You'll probably be allowed to take it right down the gangway and check it in at the gate before you board – it will be waiting for you there after landing.) Slip-on shoes (for you and your toddler) are your next best friends at the security checkpoint – that way, if you're asked to take them off, it won't be a last-minute struggle (but do wear socks so you don't have to walk barefoot on that icky floor). If your toddler can walk solo, he or she will go ahead of you through the scanner with you following close behind (make sure there's nothing in your toddler's pockets). If your child can't walk yet, you'll be able to hold him or her in your arms to go through the screening, but if the alarm sounds, you'll both have to be hand-screened. Don't stress about holding up the queue – nobody expects families with young children to race through security. It may help to try making a game out of the whole thing for your toddler ("Can you put your rucksack in the tray? How about my keys?"). Some airports offer separate security queues for families and others who need extra time.

Think twice about that early boarding. If the airline you're flying does preboards for families, think twice before you take advantage. Yes, boarding before the throngs ensures you much-needed overhead-locker space. But early board can equal early bored, since it means about a half hour extra on the plane – probably not something you want to endure voluntarily with a wriggly toddler who needs constant entertainment.

Find a friendly flight attendant. If you're alone, don't be shy (but do be nice) about asking the flight crew for help. After all, it can be nearly impossible to lift a bag and put it in the overhead locker while holding a toddler. So ask a flight attendant (or fellow passenger) for a hand with one or the other.

Don't expect to be fed. Food on domestic flights has disappeared in economy (you may still find it on international flights) – the best you can expect is a snack for purchase, if that. Phone ahead to find out exactly what will be served and if special children's or toddler's meals are available for purchase (or for free on international flights). Sometimes a snack means nothing more than a drink and a bag of nuts, which, as choking hazards, are off-limits for 4 and under. And no matter what fare's been promised, don't ever board without your own supply of toddler-appropriate snacks. Takeoff delays can result in mealtime delays, food service trolleys can move at a maddeningly slow rate down the aisles, and special meals sometimes don't show up at all (plus, let's face it – they're not all that special).

Since fluids are particularly important when flying (the circulating air in a plane is very dry), be sure to pick up your toddler's favourite drinks in the secure boarding area once you've cleared the security checkpoint. In addition, because of heightened security on planes and in airports, be sure to check the government's website at www.direct.gov.uk for the latest information about bringing other liquids on flights (search travel and transport). There's

Junior Jet Lag

Transitioning between time zones isn't easy for anyone. After all, internal body clocks are much more difficult to reset than external ones. But while an adult is liable to roll over and go back to sleep when that internal alarm goes off at the right time but in the wrong time zone, a toddler isn't. A little Londoner who's used to getting up at 6 A.M. will want to start the day in New York at 1 A.M. local time (which means a rude awakening for Mum and Dad). No matter which direction your trip will be taking you, these tips for travelling time zones may help make the transition smoother:

Reset your toddler's clock only if it'll be worth the effort. If you'll be away from home for only a couple of days, it's probably wise to keep your toddler closer to his or her accustomed schedule. Otherwise, by the time you get onto the new schedule, it'll be time to reset the internal clocks for the return home.

Start to reset before you start out. If you're going west to east, begin trying to get your toddler to bed a little earlier in the evening and up a little earlier in the morning. If you're going east to west, try to push bedtime forward a little more each evening. Begin the reset at least three days before your scheduled departure, so you can adjust gradually.

Reset your watch. As you set off on your trip, set your watch to the time at your destination, and continue adjusting meals and sleep patterns to the new time. If your toddler tends to sleep when in motion, napping a lot as you go and making keeping to any schedule impossible, that's okay, too. The scrambled schedule may so confuse your child's body clock that it won't know day from night – which will probably ease adjusting to the time zone at your destination.

Reset gradually, if you can. If you're driving or travelling by train to your destination, you'll be able to accustom your toddler to the new time one zone at a time.

Reset completely. It's not enough for a traveller to sleep when the locals do. To help reset your toddler's internal clock, you'll also have to work at getting him or her to eat, wake, nap, and play in keeping with the local time. For instance, if you've gone from west to east, start the first day by waking your child at a reasonable hour rather than letting him or her sleep in. Do it gently and be prepared to suffer the grumpy consequences (letting sunlight into the room will help). Breakfast shortly after you get up and continue to stick as closely to the new time as possible for the rest of the day. By the end of the day, exhaustion is sure to have set in and your toddler should be ready for an earlier-than-usual bedtime. Skipping the nap might help a child adjust to an earlier bedtime more

also helpful information about travelling with children, including tips on how to bring along such toddler necessities as mini juice packs when flying the not-quite-as-friendly-as-they-used-to-be skies, at www.babycentre.co.uk.

Bring extra supplies. Carry as many books and plane-friendly toys (but nothing that makes noise or that has lots of pieces that might scatter under seats) as you can fit into your hand luggage and twice as many nappies as you

quickly, but it could also backfire, since an overtired toddler may have a harder time settling down.

Try as you might to reset your toddler's clock, it's possible that it may stay tuned in to home-time, at least for a while. Be ready with some quiet entertainment in case your child wakes in the middle of the night and refuses to go back to sleep. Also have a snack handy in case that tummy clock says "Breakfast, pronto!" (do you really want to be looking for a packet of Weetabix at 4 A.M.?).

See the light. Sunlight appears to play a major role in helping reset biological time clocks. So spend as much time as possible in the bright light outdoors as soon after your arrival as possible. Going west to east through several time zones, you should make a special effort to get out early the next morning; east to west, in the late afternoon. On longer trips through more than three time zones, whether west to east or east to west, making an effort to expose everyone in your family to midday sunshine (rather than early or late) on arrival will make resetting internal clocks easier.

Don't expect to reset your internal clocks overnight. It generally takes at least a few days for anyone to transition between time zones – the more zones, the greater the adjustment (a single zone isn't likely to have much effect). It also takes lots of patience, since your travelling tot is likely to be grumpier than usual while adjusting. During the transition, go easy on your toddler's schedule. Instead of planning major

outings, slow down the pace (chill by the pool, relax in the park). Take it easy again for the first few days on returning home, if possible.

Consider time zones when choosing travel schedule. When you're travelling through more than four time zones, different factors need to be considered. Going west to east, from Los Angeles to London, for example, entails a radical 8-hour change. Many parents find that taking a late-night flight (10 or 11 P.M.) works well. Little ones usually sleep for a good part of the flight, but their sleep is broken up enough, especially when light streams through the windows at dawn, to leave them exhausted the next day. So exhausted that they are usually willing to go to bed earlier than their accustomed bedtime and closer to nightfall in London.

Flying out will be more challenging, since you'll be flying during daylight hours. A couple of naps will help break up the long flight, and arriving in the late afternoon in Los Angeles will (hopefully) mean that your knackered-out tot will be able to settle down for sleep at a reasonable local hour.

In general, be less attached to a schedule while you're away than you are at home – after all, the new schedule is only temporary. Do whatever gets you and your toddler through the day (and as much of the night as possible), even if it means serving up cereal before the dawn's early light. In the end, you may be pleasantly surprised to find that your toddler hardly notices the time change.

could possibly need, endless wipes and hand sanitiser, at least one change of clothing for your child, and an extra shirt for you (forgetting the last item guarantees you'll be thrown up on or drenched in apple juice). Don't forget

an extra layer of clothes for your tot – it can get chilly on a plane.

Put safety first. If your child is occupying a seat, plan to bring an approved car seat aboard. For safety's sake, toddlers should ride in a rear-facing infant seat until they are at least 9 kilogrammes. Tots over a year weighing 9 to 20 kilogrammes can ride in a forward-facing car seat (although they are still safer in a rear-facing seat until they have outgrown the upper weight limit). If you don't want to lug your car seat on the aeroplane (a couple of airlines actually provide seats for pint-size passengers, so ask when you book), consider using an approved harness called CARES (Child Aviation Restraint System). Safe for children 10 to 20 kilogrammes, the harness (which weighs only about 0.5 kilogrammes) wraps around the back of an aeroplane seat and is fitted into place by looping the aeroplane seat belt through two adjustable vertical straps. Your toddler is then strapped into a five-point harness – just like in a car seat. You can buy a CARES harness at kidsflysafe.com.

If your toddler is on your lap, do not belt him or her in with you – serious injury could result from even a mild impact. But do secure your belt around yourself and then hold your toddler around the waist with your hands grasping your wrists during takeoffs and landings. Do not allow your toddler to wander around alone in the aisles or to sleep or play on the floor, because of the risk of injury if the plane should suddenly hit an area of turbulence.

Also carefully review the information on oxygen masks and know where there are extras in case your child doesn't have a seat (and therefore a mask) of his or her own. (There's usually an extra mask provided in every row or section of seats.) Remember, just like they say in the preflight safety announcements, you should put on your own mask first and then attend to your child's. If you try to do it the other way around in a low-oxygen emergency, you could lose consciousness before managing to get either mask on.

Mind those ears. Changes in altitude and air pressure are tough on little ears. Drinking during takeoff and landing can help by encouraging swallowing, which helps release the pressure that builds up in the ears (start as the plane starts speeding down the runway and again when the pilot announces the intitial descent). Let your toddler drink from a cup or a flask with a built-in straw.

One of these popular remedies for popping the ears when pressure builds up in the Eustachian tubes during the flight or on descent may also help:

■ Hot towels. Ask the flight attendant to heat two towels. After checking to be sure they are not too hot (touch them to your inner forearm), place one towel over each of your child's ears. The heat expands the air in the middle ear, relieving the negative pressure on the eardrum.

■ Hot cups. Wet a couple of paper napkins or towels with hot, but not scalding, water (ask the flight attendant to do this; be sure to check that the towels aren't burning hot), wad them into two cups, and hold a cup over each of your child's ears. Again, the heat relieves the pressure.

■ Pain reliever. A dose of paracetamol or ibuprofen may help ease that ache. Don't give other medication unless the GP has recommended it for use during flight.

Blockage of the Eustachian tubes due to nasal congestion from a cold or allergy can make ear pain much worse. If your toddler has been sick, check with the doctor before flying.

If all else fails and your toddler screams all the way up and all the way down, ignore the dirty looks from other passengers (you're likely to see a lot of sympathetic faces, too). And keep in mind – silver lining above those clouds – that the screaming will help reduce the pressure on your toddler's eardrums and ease the pain.

TRAVELLING BY TRAIN

Is your tot ready to go chugging on a choo-choo? Here's what you need to know if a train trip is in your future travel plans:

Book in advance. Ordering train tickets well in advance (online or over the phone) allows you to arrive at the train station with tickets in hand, or to print them out quickly at the station, so you won't have to wait in a long ticket line. If it's possible to make seat reservations, do this in advance, too. Remember, however, that Second (and sometimes even First Class) reservations guarantee a seat for each ticket, but not that those seats are together.

Make timely choices. Peak travel times can be very crowded, especially during holidays, so avoid them if you can. A late-evening train may be a good choice if your toddler is likely to sleep during the trip.

Pack appropriately. For overnight train travel, your carry-on bag should also be an overnight bag, packed with extra clothes, nappies, and all those toddler care basics (like a toothbrush and toothpaste). This should make digging into your neatly packed suitcases unnecessary. Better still, it may make it possible to check your heavy baggage through, giving you less to lug and more room in your compartment or at your seat.

Arrive early. Check ahead to find out what time the train you'll be travelling on ordinarily arrives at the station

Tantrums to Go

Toddlers don't usually need an excuse to throw a tantrum – but they've got plenty of them during the average holiday: disrupted sleep schedules, erratic eating and unfamiliar foods, long periods of enforced sitting, changes in routine, and new surroundings (and that's just for starters). Since tantrums on the road are even tougher to deal with than tantrums at home, you'll definitely want to prevent them when you can.

The prevention protocol? Essentially, it's the same one you use at home. Since being overly tired, hungry, or bored can all trigger tantrums, anticipate and avoid those scenarios when possible. Build naps into your schedule, bring on the snacks when meals will be delayed, and plan toddler pleasing activities. Don't wait until your tot's screaming for attention – become a master of distraction, pulling tricks out of your travel bag to occupy a toddler on the brink. And remember, less is usually more when it comes to travelling toddlers – underscheduling can prevent overstimulation and overtiredness, and possibly prevent a tantrum as well. Building restful time into your schedule – time for reading, listening to music, quiet games, and cuddling – may also prevent explosions.

Too late for prevention? Do the same as you would during a local public tantrum (see page 240).

you'll be departing from. If there is a 10- or 15-minute gap between arrival and departure, try to get there before the train arrives rather than just as it's about to pull out of the station. The

A Travelling Toddler's Tummy

Heading to Africa or Asia – or another exotic locale? Toddlers, like everyone else travelling in a country with unfamiliar (and sometimes unsanitary) food, can be subject to traveller's diarrhoea. Reduce the risk of tummy troubles (which can be more serious for a toddler, especially if they lead to dehydration) by taking these precautions:

- Serve your toddler only pasteurised milk and bottled juices (not fresh squeezed). Yogurt, cheese, and other dairy products should be pasteurised, too. When in doubt, (as when it's unlabelled on a breakfast buffet), leave it.

- Stick to bottled water for drinking and always make sure the top on a bottle is sealed before you open it (carbonated water offers more assurance that the seal hasn't been broken). If you have doubts about the water in a hotel, use bottled water for toothbrushing, too. Forget ice cubes (or anything made with ice, like a smoothie) unless you're certain they're made with purified water.

- If water's suspect, then fresh fruits and vegetables are, too. Don't let your toddler eat any produce that isn't either well cooked or washed in purified water and peeled by you (like a banana).

- All meat, fish, and seafood should be cooked to well done.

- Eat only in restaurants that look as though they follow sanitary food preparation practices (but even in a five-star hotel restaurant, follow the above rules anyway). Local food from those street stalls may smell enticing, but don't succumb.

- Make sure everyone follows sanitation protocol, too. See to it that the entire family faithfully washes hands after toileting (or changing nappies) and before eating. Carry antibacterial wipes or hand gel wherever you go (especially where bathrooms won't be the cleanest).

For information on food and water safety in various parts of the world, visit the World Health Organisation's website, www.who.int. If toddler tummy does strike, see treatment for diarrhoea, page 390.

Toddlers on the road, whether at home or abroad, may also be prone to constipation thanks to changes in diet, schedule, and activity. To avoid clogged pipes, be sure your tiny traveller gets plenty of fruits and vegetables (see safety rules above), whole-grain cereals and breads, and fluids, along with a chance for some active play every day.

---

goal: a better chance of seating the family together. If there are two adults, one should hurry ahead, as soon as the platform number is announced, to save seats for all, while the other struggles down the platform at a snail's pace with your toddler. If you can, grab a window seat (plus the aisle seat) so your toddler can watch the scenery go by.

Derail boredom. Your tot will enjoy watching the scenery and spotting cows out the window for only so long. So carry those toys, books (try to find one about trains), and crayons – and lots of them.

Take advantage of longer stops. Even a 15-minute stop gives you and your toddler a chance to get off the train, stretch your legs, and possibly even wander down to see the engine that's been pulling the train (just be sure someone is watching your luggage and that you reboard in time). If you'll be switching trains and the wait between them will be a long one – as it might be in a hub city – plan to grab a meal, or if you've really got loads of time on your hands and can cope with the logistics, consider taking a trek to a nearby zoo, playground, or park that you've located ahead or on your smart phone.

Bring your own. Even if there's a buffet car, there's no guarantee your toddler will be able or willing to eat what they're serving. So, just as you would when travelling by car or plane, bring your own snacks and drinks.

For safety's sake. Wanderlust can send a tot toddling down the aisle in no time. Because a sudden lurch of the train could slam a small toddler against a seat or another passenger, insist that an adult hand must be held during all strolls on the train.

CHOOSING A FAMILY-FRIENDLY HOTEL

Let's face it – whether you're heading for the beach, the slopes, or the city for your family holiday, where you stay matters . . . and it matters a lot more than it ever did in your pre-toddler holiday days. What you look for in a hotel or resort has changed a lot, too (good-bye couples massages and Jacuzzi baths, hello childproofing kits and cots). Fortunately, you won't have to look far – there are more hotels and resorts offering more family-friendly amenities than ever before. From top-notch kids' menus to fun kids' clubs, there's plenty to keep your toddler happy. But how do you tell which accommodation will be most accommodating to your family? Which

really serve up what they promise – and serve it up with a family-friendly smile (even as your little one upends a bowl of chocolate ice cream onto the restaurant carpet)? Just do your homework before you book your holiday:

Tap into your parent network. Of course, you can find thousands of hotel lists online, but why not narrow the search with trip tips from people you know are in the know (in other words, other parents)? Ask friends with families, but don't stop there. Survey parents in your nursery or playgroups about destination hotels they've enjoyed. If you belong to an online group, post a query asking for recommendations.

Visit travel websites. Didn't get a first-hand recommendation that fit your budget or destination plans? Find virtual inspiration from online sites that feature comprehensive reviews of family-friendly destinations and accommodation across the globe. You can also get the need-to-know nitty-gritty on user-review sites – like whether the rooms are really as big as they look in the pictures, the bathtubs are really clean, the beach is really "just minutes away".

Look for a suite deal. It may be stating the obvious, but suite hotels are ideally suited to families with young children. The extra room is a plus, but so is a kitchenette (where you can whip up less expensive meals or snacks, warm up leftovers, and store drinks).

Find out what "Kids' Club" means. Lots of family holiday resorts offer special clubs or camps that claim they'll keep your little ones entertained while you soak up the sun and sip a piña colada. But to be sure it's really toddler friendly, phone the hotel directly and get specifics. Ask *exactly* what's included in their children's programme (and whether there's a charge for it), how old your child has to be to join (and whether older kids and younger kids play together or in separate groups), how experienced the club's staff are (and whether they're trained in first aid and CPR), and what the ratio of adults to children is. You'll also want to know what activities the programme offers and how safe and age-appropriate they are for a toddler. For example, if water play and beach games are part of the Kids' Club experience, find out how carefully the kids are watched, whether the staff have training in water safety, and what protocol the staff follow for keeping little ones safe in the water.

Ask about the babysitter option. Need a holiday from your family holiday? A ketchup-free dinner-for-two? A romantic stroll down the beach or a midnight dip in the hot tub? Then you'll want to know all about the babysitting services offered by the hotel or resort you're considering: how long babysitters have been employed and whether references are available, how carefully sitters are screened (are background checks routine?), whether they're certified in first aid and CPR, what their fees are and how they are paid (will you be able to add the services to the bill or will you pay directly?). No matter how reliable the service seems, it's always a good idea to spend some time with the sitter before you leave your child in his or her care.

Survey the services. Never gave hotel laundry service – or access to washers and dryers – a second thought before? You should now (before a week's worth of clothes ends up soggy and soiled in three days). What about 24-hour room service (that can come in handy when your jet-lagged toddler wails for breakfast at 4 A.M.)? Childproofed rooms or childproofing kits? Truly safe cots, cot mattresses, and cot sheets?

Double-check that all the amenities advertised on the hotel's website will be open and running when you plan to visit. There's nothing worse than arriving at a destination with a suitcase full of swim nappies only to find that the pool is under construction – or counting on the Kids' Club and finding out it's operational only during high season.

Scout out the dining options. Most restaurants at family resorts and hotels offer a kids' menu, and that's always a good (and usually familiar) place to start. But even better is a buffet, one that will give finicky eaters more choices (and potentially healthier choices, like fresh fruit). Ask, too, whether the kitchen will accommodate special requests (cereal for dinner, plain pasta instead of with sauce) and diet restrictions (if allergies mean no peanuts for your little peanut). You'll also want to double-check if the restaurant has convenient family-dining hours (dinner starting at 5:30, not 7:30).

Choose the right room. Whether it's a sweeping suite or a cupboard-size room, make sure the accommodation you choose addresses your family's needs. Be sure any doors to balconies or outdoors (such as in a scenic but dangerous-for-a-tot poolside room) can be securely locked (and that the lock is out of your toddler's reach). If there's no kitchenette, can you rent a mini-fridge to store your snacks and drinks, or is there a minibar you can empty and refill with your own, more appropriate and less expensive selections? What about a bathtub, so you won't have to try rinsing sand off a squirming tot in the shower? Also, unless you plan on going to bed at 7 P.M. when your child does, make sure there's a balcony, an alcove or, best of all, another room where you and your spouse can hang out without waking up your sleeping beauty.

Toddler-Free Travels

Desperate for an adult-only holiday but worried about how your tot's going to handle you going away? Stop worrying and start packing. Toddlers often handle separations better than their parents do, especially if they're left in familiar, loving, and capable hands (a standard that grandparents, aunts, uncles, and trusted babysitters usually meet easily). Plus, getting your toddler used to parental getaways now will make it easier for you to take those getaways later (and every adult needs adult time – whether it's on his or her own, as a couple, or with friends). Travelling for work or because of a family emergency or other situation, not pleasure? The same exit and re-entry strategies apply. When planning a trip away from your little one, consider the following:

Start short, if you can. Best not to dive into a weeklong Caribbean cruise if this is your maiden tot-free voyage. The very general rules (and there are times when circumstances dictate exceptions to the rules): don't leave children overnight if you haven't left them for several evenings; don't leave them for a weekend if you haven't left them overnight; don't leave them for a week if you haven't left them for a weekend.

Try to schedule sensitively. If at all possible, try not to plan that first child-free trip when there is anything unsettling going on in your toddler's life, like an illness or a new childcare situation.

Pick a sitter, but not just any sitter. It's important to select a sitter who's not only competent, caring, and attentive, but known and liked (preferably loved) by your toddler. Grandparents always top the list, but so do other favourite relatives and friends. Next best is a regular, trusted, beloved babysitter. Another possible option: a swap with the parents of one of your toddler's playmates (they care for your child while you're away, you return the favour while they have a holiday).

Prepare the caregiver. Be sure the person staying with your toddler is familiar with your toddler's regular routine. Consistency is always comforting to toddlers, but even more so during times of change. Relay, too, any of your toddler's little idiosyncrasies, like refusing to eat from any plate but the one with the bunnies, or insisting that a favourite bedtime story be read three times, or having a nightlight on and the stuffed kangaroo standing guard over the cot every evening. Pass along tried-and-true ways to distract and calm your toddler and a list of your toddler's favourite foods, drinks, stories, activities, and toys. Keep in mind, though, that your tot may be a lot more flexible with someone else than with you, and may (toddler's prerogative) opt to change things entirely. Let the sitter know that's fine, too.

In most cases, the sitter should not attempt anything groundbreaking (like weaning from the bottle or dummy) while you're away. The rare exception: a grandparent or sitter your little one is very attached to may be able to accomplish a goal you've had trouble with. But that should only be attempted with your prior agreement, and with a plan you've approved.

Prepare your toddler. Leaving without notice or good-byes is never a good exit strategy, whether you're going

(continued on next page)

(continued from previous page)

out for the night or for the weekend. Short term, you'll avoid the tears – but long term, you may step up separation anxiety (your tot may come to fear any separation, even a brief one). Begin preparing your toddler two or three days before your planned trip rather than weeks ahead (toddlers have trouble understanding the concept of future time, and very early notice could give anxiety too much time to build) or as you're going out the door (which wouldn't allow your toddler time to get used to the idea). Let your toddler know, in simple language, that you're going on a trip, where you're going ("to the country", "to the city"), when you're going to come back, who will be staying with him or her, and where they will be staying (at home? At Aunt Sara's place?). Doesn't mean your toddler won't flip out when you leave on your trip – but it does mean that trust won't be the issue.

Occasionally, a trip comes up suddenly, meaning that a parent will have to go off without first having a chance to prepare a child for the unexpected absence. No worries in that case – paying lots of special attention on the return end of the trip will ensure a happy reunion and a smooth transition for all.

Pack after hours. Pretrip preparation tends to be frantic, and your toddler can pick up on your packing stress. So try to take care of packing and other preparations when your little one's in bed, and keep routines as routine as possible in the day or two before you leave (with lots of together time built into the schedule).

Plan some fun. Try to set up some special activities for while you're away (a trip to the children's museum, going to the petting zoo with Grandpa, cake baking with Uncle Chris), and let your little one know in advance the fun that's in store. Make it clear that it's okay to have fun even when you're not around: "Have lots of fun with Grandma while Mummy and Daddy are on our trip." And don't forget to have some fun yourself. Even if you're going away on business, sneak in an extra-long bath or an in-room film or two.

Keep the parting short and sweet. Of course you're frazzled with last-minute arrangements, sitter instructions, and trying to remember the 300 other things on your pretrip to-do list that you're sure you've forgotten to do. But take a few deep breaths, think some happy thoughts (about the room service you've been dreaming about), and put on your biggest, most believable smile before you leave with your bags. Moods are contagious, and you want your toddler to catch a calm, carefree mood – not an apprehensive, anxious one. It'll definitely help to schedule your exit so you're not faced with a mad dash out of the door (there's nothing like the meter running in the taxi to send stress soaring). Give plenty of cuddles, kisses, and hugs, but try not to get clingy or weepy. Reassure your child that you'll be back soon (to make the time seem more concrete, you can try translating "two days" into "two bedtimes" or "two long sleeps"). Using the same parting phrase you use when going off to work or when dropping your child off at nursery ("Have fun, play well, get dirty", for example – or a special version of that old favourite, "See you later, alligator") may also help make it clear that you will return – just as you always do.

Keep your cool, no matter what. So the parting's not turning out to be sweet? Some kids won't spare the hysterics, while others give Mum and Dad the brush-off (maybe because the whole trip thing has gone right over their heads, a definite possibility at this tender age). Don't take any of it personally or seriously. For more on goodbyes, see page 186.

Start some going-and-coming rituals. Especially if you travel frequently, establishing familiar and happy "going away" and "coming home" traditions can provide comfort and security, easing those transitions for both of you. So initiate some fun rituals to enjoy with your toddler before you leave on a trip: eating ice cream together, reading a book about a parent going on a trip, drawing a picture for your little one to keep until you come home (he or she can scribble one for you to pack). Also set up some rituals that your toddler can associate with your homecoming: decorating the house in preparation for your arrival, visiting a favourite soft play area or the cake shop together soon after you get home. Observe these rituals as best you can (trying to make time for them even if you're harried, dead tired, anxious to pack or unpack, or catch up on messages and e-mail) and your toddler will always have something to look forward to when you leave on a trip – and something to look forward to when you return . . . in addition to you.

Skype with your tyke . . . maybe. The effect of long-distance contact with your toddler while you're away depends on your toddler. Some children get a thrill out of talking to absent parents on the phone or via videoconference – and enjoy looking at images of Mummy and Daddy, even if they're not quite ready to talk back. If your toddler seems to enjoy "visiting" with you long-distance, try calling at the same time each day, if possible. Be upbeat and cheerful (no melancholy "I'm so sad without my baby!"). If your tot seems upset by seeing or hearing you but not being able to be with you (high-tech communication can be pretty confusing to a little one), you may be better off skipping the calls. Have the babysitter pass your greetings along instead.

You can also keep in touch (and give your trip a comfortingly concrete context) by sending colourful postcards or e-mails from wherever you are – even if the postcards won't arrive home until after you do and even if the e-mails aren't opened till hours after you sent them. Give your child a scrapbook to keep the postcards and downloaded photos in and look at them together frequently to provide additional continuity ("Remember when I went to Boston? Then I came back home.").

Accept that the going may be rough when you first get going. Toddlers who are left for the first time – or even the first several times – by their parents can react in a wide variety of ways. Some separate without a problem; others have a harder time. Even toddlers who've had an exceptionally wonderful time with grandparents or the babysitter may have conflicting feelings to express when their parents return. They may be especially clingy, whiny, or out of sorts, have more tantrums than usual, experience increased separation anxiety, refuse even favourite foods, have trouble settling down for bed, or begin waking during the night. They may even give a parent who's returned from a trip the cold shoulder. Remember, transitions of any kind – even happy ones – are tough on toddlers.

No matter how your toddler reacts during your re-entry, practise patience

(continued on next page)

(continued from previous page)

and heap on the attention and reassurance. Mostly reassure yourself that negative reactions are normal (not a sign that you've done something wrong or shouldn't have left at all) – and that they're likely to disappear within a few days.

If your toddler seems very sad or becomes very difficult to handle while you're away, when you return, or both, and this doesn't change as trips become routine, take a look at the childcare situation. Would a different babysitter be a better fit for your toddler? Is there a possibility of neglect or abuse? Are there any other problems that could be causing the behaviour changes? If you can't work out why your toddler's having such a tough time, turn to the doctor for help.

CHAPTER 12

Keeping Your Toddler Healthy

. . . .

NOBODY LIKES BEING SICK. But for your toddler, who has absolutely no patience for being a patient, being sick is especially no fun. Seeing your little one miserable with a stuffy nose or a fever is no fun for you, either (any time your toddler's miserable, you're bound to be miserable, too). All good reasons to keep your toddler healthy through regular checkups and up-to-date vaccinations – and when that plan doesn't quite pan out (the best prevention intentions often aren't a match for determined germs), the next best thing is to beat those bugs and other illnesses promptly and effectively. And this chapter is here to help: it tells you what a parent needs to know about the most common early childhood illnesses and conditions and their treatment, plus information and tips on immunisations, checkups, calling the doctor, fever and other symptoms, how to make the medicine go down, and much more.

What You Can Expect at Checkups

Fewer scheduled checkups are on the calendar in the second year – probably a welcome respite for you and your little one from the first year's busy schedule of visits. Remember to keep making regular visits to the health visitor's clinic to have a check of your toddler's growth (height, weight, head circumference); and to voice any concerns about your child's development, behaviour, eating habits, and health since the last visit. Your health visitor may also schedule an informal check of physical and intellectual development and of hearing and vision. She may ask you to fill out a developmental

Doctor, Doctor

Even if your toddler stays healthy all year (and really, what are the chances of a completely sneeze-free year?), you should still be visiting the health visitor or doctor regularly for routine checkups. To make the most of each visit:

Do your homework. And don't forget to bring it. Keep a running list of questions and concerns (about behaviour, health, eating, sleeping, and so on) to bring along to the checkup. And though having your questions answered (finally!) may be the best part of the checkup for you, don't save them for last, when your toddler has had enough of this doctor's-surgery stuff. Try to ask most questions first, before all that holding still, and preferably even before undressing your child.

Have schedule sense. When you can, book appointments during your toddler's most cooperative time of day. Think first thing in the morning or after a nap – and always after a meal or snack. As a general rule, avoid those busy after-school hours like the plague – extra waiting and a harried staff can definitely make for a less pleasant experience. And if you think you'll need more time than usual (to talk over tantrums, or sleep issues, or developmental concerns, for instance) ask the surgery if you can book a double appointment. Nurse practitioners or physician's assistants may be able to spend more time answering questions than doctors can, so keep that in mind when scheduling. Or see if you can tackle some of the topics with the doctor via e-mail or on the phone.

---

checklist (either before or during the visit), which can help him or her make a more accurate assessment of your little one's progress, as well as screen for delays and other developmental problems. And then there are those immunisation visits (nobody's favourite day, but one of the best ways to keep your toddler healthy; see page 351 for the recommended immunisation schedule).

If you have any pressing questions or have noticed any concerning symptoms between doctor's or health visitor's sessions, be sure to check in by phone (or e-mail, if the office offers that option).

Fear of the Doctor

"The last couple of times we visited the GP we had to drag our son in, literally. He seemed terrified."

So let's recap what happens at the doctor's office. Your toddler is probed, prodded, poked, and occasionally pricked, while holding still – a lot. From his side of the examination table, there's not much to like about those visits. And since he can remember past visits (with his newly improved memory), he can also dread the visit he's about to have.

In other words, his fear of the doctor is completely understandable. Recognising the reasonableness of his feelings – and being patient with your little patient – is the first and most important step you can take to help him overcome his fear. The next steps:

Read up. The more your toddler knows about doctors and doctors' surgeries, the less trepidation he'll be likely to feel when faced with them. Read a simple picture book about visiting the doctor,

Expect the best, but be prepared for the worst. There is no such thing as underpacking for a trip to the doctor. Bring snacks, enough distractions for several rainy days (books, favourite toys, crayons and paper, bubbles), and any favourite comfort object. Pull some out in the waiting room, some during the checkup (here a toy doctor's kit may be just what you need), and keep some in reserve for just after (especially if an injection is on the agenda).

Write it down. Of course, you're planning to ask for answers to your questions, and for advice on all toddler topics. But your little one is fidgeting, maybe crying, and you're flustered, definitely preoccupied, feeling exhausted. How are you supposed to remember all those gems of medical wisdom by the time you get home? By writing it all down – before you forget.

Record it. Yes, the doctor's surgery will keep a record of immunisations, but so should you. Always remember to take your child's "Personal Child Health Record" (their red book) to every checkup or doctor's appointment.

Don't be shy. Those who provide health care for young children are used to providing advice, reassurance, and support to their parents. This is your chance to ask away (or to vent) – so don't choose this moment to keep mum, Mum and Dad.

Trust your instincts. If you feel something isn't right with your child – even if you're not sure what it is – let the doctor know. A parent's intuition is sometimes the keenest diagnostic tool.

Turn off your mobile phone. A phone call or text in the middle of your child's appointment will waste precious time – and, worse, can interrupt a discussion and disrupt the doctor's and your train of thought.

---

offering plenty of comforting commentary along the way. But try not to overexplain or get too complicated or technical. The most pertinent points: the doctor is a nice person whose job is keeping children healthy, and the doctor's office is a safe place.

Let him play doctor. Buy a toy doctor's kit for your toddler, and encourage him to practise playing doctor on you, on friends or older siblings, on his stuffed animals, on himself. Show him how the various toy instruments are used to examine the ears and throat, to listen for a heartbeat, to check for a temperature. Knowing what to expect will help your child feel more in control of the examination, easing anxiety.

Dangle a carrot. Plan a treat for after the doctor's visit – a trip to the playground, the children's museum, or a favourite friend's house. Follow through with the plan no matter how your toddler handles the visit – withholding the treat because he didn't cooperate this time isn't fair and might further undermine his cooperation next time. Make a ritual out of the after-visit treat (going to the bigger playground after every visit, for example) so that your toddler will have at least one happy doctor association.

Don't make any promises you can't keep. Assuring your toddler that the examination won't hurt is likely to make him wary. Simply suggesting the possibility of pain to a highly suggestible toddler could also make him more apt to expect and experience it. And if the examination does hurt, even a tiny bit, there goes your credibility. Also, don't promise "no injection" if you're not entirely sure there won't be one.

You Know Your Child Best

When it comes to your child, you're something of an expert. Unlike the doctors, nurses, and other health-care professionals who see your toddler just a few times a year (and see a whole lot of other children, too), you have a daily window into your little one's world. With that up-close-and-personal parental perspective, you're likely to notice nuances in his or her development that others – those who only get the big picture – might miss.

If you're concerned about something in your toddler's development, or if you just have a nagging feeling that something's not quite right – speak up. Maybe it's nothing (sometimes parents have a way of overthinking – and overreacting – when it comes to their children). But just in case, point it out to the GP at the next visit. If you're not comfortable waiting that long, call the office to discuss your concerns with the doctor, or e-mail the surgery, if that's an option.

Child development experts agree that parents play a crucial role in diagnosing delayed development or developmental disorders (such as autism) early. And early diagnosis is key to the early intervention that can make all the difference in a child's developmental future.

If you notice any of these developmental red flags in your toddler – or if you think you might, but you're not 100 per cent sure – check in with the doctor:

- Your child does not smile or make other warm, joyful expressions, does not share back-and-forth sounds or other facial expressions, and/or does not babble (combining vowels with consonants), wave, or point at things by 12 months of age.

- Your child doesn't speak any single words (including "mama" or "dada") by 16 months.

- Your child doesn't communicate with two-word meaningful phrases (without imitating or repeating) by 24 months.

- Your child loses language or social skills that he or she has already mastered, such as speaking in sentences or interacting with you, at any age. (Don't worry, however, if your child seems to slow down developmentally for a short time due to teething, illness, stress, or a challenging situation, like the arrival of a new sibling – or if he or she stops using one recently mastered skill altogether while busy tackling another.)

Concentrate on comfort. Do everything you can to make your little one feel comfortable at the doctor's surgery. Bring along his favourite blanket to drape over the crackly paper on the examining table. Encourage him to take a favourite stuffed animal or other toy for support during the examination. (Perhaps, time permitting, the doctor will be willing to check the toy animal's ears, nose, eyes – or yours – along with your toddler's.) Or arm him with his doctor's kit, so he can check you while you're waiting. And if you think your toddler will do better on your lap, let him sit there – for as much of the examination as possible. If he cries, let him know it's okay. But also calmly remind him that the better he sits still, the faster the examination will be over – and the sooner that post-visit treat can be enjoyed.

Check your own stress. Anxiety is more contagious than a cold virus. Seeing that you're relaxed and confident about the doctor's visit will help him stay calmer, too – while anxiously anticipating a scene ensures one. When it's time to leave for the doctor's surgery, make the announcement a cheerful "It's time to go visit Dr Ben now", instead of an ominous "You have to go to the doctor's now" or a resigned "Guess we have to go to the doctor now." At the doctor's, show him how calm and comfortable you are. Volunteer to have your heartbeat listened to with the stethoscope first, or your ears checked with the otoscope. And don't gasp or cover your eyes (or your toddler's) when a needle appears. As for anxiety about your child's behaviour – forget it. The doctor and the staff have seen it all before – and more.

Don't forget the applause. Reinforce even minimal cooperation ("Good job!") whenever you can, but don't criticise if he kicks and screams the whole time.

Something else to keep in mind: using the threat of a doctor visit to get your toddler to cooperate is never a

---

Tell It Like It Is

It may be tempting to spring surprises on your toddler (a visit to the dentist for a checkup, to the doctor for an injection), if only to spare yourself a scene – that is, until you arrive at the destination. But honesty's a much better policy. Leaving the house as though you're on your way to the playground, only to detour to the dentist – or promising that there won't be any injections at the doctor, when you know there will be – builds mistrust and generates undue anxiety. Plus, it's likely to result in an even bigger scene once your toddler discovers the truth. Instead, tell it like it is before you leave the house – offering information on a need-to-know basis: just enough to prepare, not enough to step up stress.

---

good idea – and can end up sparking or feeding his fear of the doctor. So don't say "You'd better take your medicine (or eat your broccoli, or put your hat on), or you'll get sick and I'll have to take you to the doctor."

Immunisations

If you're like most parents today, you may have heard of serious childhood diseases like diphtheria, polio, pertussis, mumps, pneumococcal disease, rotavirus – but you probably have only the vaguest idea of what they are. And that's not surprising, thanks to one of the most important – and successful – public health interventions in history: vaccinations. Because of vaccines,

widespread epidemics of such illnesses as smallpox, polio, diphtheria, measles, rubella, and mumps – devastating childhood diseases that were once serious threats to children in this country – are mostly a thing of the past.

But for vaccines to continue protecting children, children have to continue being vaccinated. Of course, no parent likes to see a needle aiming towards his or her child. And you may even be wary of having your child vaccinated because you've heard some negative stories about those injections (misinformation, in case you're wondering). But keeping up with the schedule of recommended immunisations and ensuring that your child receives those toddler doses is by far one of the best strategies to help keep your child (and all the rest of the children in your community) healthy.

RECOMMENDED VACCINATIONS

What's on tap for your tot when it comes to vaccines? Happily, your little one has already received more than half the recommended vaccinations during his or her first year, which means there will be fewer injections on the agenda this year. Plus, you're both pros by now, right?

Here are the ABCs of routine childhood immunisations (for the recommended schedule, see page 351):

Diphtheria, tetanus, acellular pertussis vaccine (DTaP). Your child needs four DTaP injections. DTaP is recommended at 2, 3, and 4 months, and between 3 and 4 years. This combination vaccine protects against three serious diseases: diphtheria, tetanus, and pertussis.

Diphtheria is spread through coughing and sneezing. It begins with a sore throat, fever, and chills, and then a thick covering forms over the back of the throat, blocking airways and making breathing difficult. If it isn't properly treated, the infection causes a toxin to spread in the body that can lead to heart failure or paralysis. About 1 in 10 of those affected will die.

Tetanus is not a contagious disease, but it is an extremely serious one. A person typically becomes infected if tetanus bacteria found in soil or dirt enter the body through a wound or cut. Symptoms include headache, grumpiness, and painful muscle spasms. In some cases, tetanus is fatal.

Pertussis (a.k.a. whooping cough) is a very contagious airborne bacterial infection that causes violent rapid coughing and a loud "whooping" sound upon inhalation. One in ten children who get pertussis develop pneumonia, too. Pertussis can lead to convulsions, brain damage, and even death.

Up to one-third of children who receive DTaP injections have very mild local reactions where the injection was given, such as tenderness, swelling, or redness, usually within two days of getting the injection. Some children are fussy or will lose their appetite for a few hours or perhaps a day or two. A low fever may also occur. These reactions are more likely to occur after the fourth dose than the earlier doses. Occasionally, a child will have a more serious side effect, such as a fever of over 104°F/40°C.

Measles, mumps, rubella (MMR). Children get two doses of MMR, the first between 12 and 13 months, and the second between ages 3 and 4 (though it can be administered at any time as long as it is 28 days after the first). The vaccine prevents (not surprisingly) measles, mumps, and rubella.

Measles is a serious disease with sometimes severe, potentially fatal, complications. Rubella (a.k.a. German measles) is often so mild that its symptoms are missed. But because it can cause birth defects in the foetus of an infected pregnant woman, immunisation in early childhood is recommended – both to protect the future foetuses of girls who are immunised and to reduce the risk of infected children exposing pregnant women to the disease, including their own mothers. Mumps rarely presents

Vaccines:
They're Not Just for Kids

Thought your days of routine vaccinations, boosters, and lines like "this will just pinch a bit" were over, Mum and Dad? Think again. Adults need vaccines, too – not just because you want to be in good shape to take care of your children, but also because you want to do everything you can to lessen their risk of contracting serious illnesses. If you're vaccinated against preventable diseases, you're less likely to get these diseases and, in turn, pass them on to your children – it's as simple as that.

Check with your GP first that it's safe for you to have these injections as he or she will know your medical history.

Influenza (a.k.a. flu) vaccine. If you have had any vaccine as an adult, it's probably this one. That's because the flu injection is recommended for vulnerable groups each year in the autumn or winter – and is widely discussed by the media each flu season. The flu injection helps prevent some strains of the flu, which can be very unpleasant for adults and much more serious (even deadly) to babies, small children, the elderly, and anyone with a chronic medical condition or compromised immune system (including pregnant women).

Tetanus, Diphtheria, and Pertussis (Tdap) vaccine. Tdap is the DTaP formulation for adolescents and adults. If you haven't had a booster for these serious diseases in the past ten years (or weren't immunised as a child), you need one now – not only to protect yourself, but to protect your little one. Pertussis (whooping cough), for instance, is most often passed on to babies by their unvaccinated or not-fully-vaccinated parents. Choose the Tdap vaccine over the frequently offered Td, which doesn't protect against pertussis.

Measles, Mumps, Rubella (MMR) vaccine. While it's likely you're already immunised against these highly contagious diseases, sometimes immunity wears off – and that could be dangerous for you (especially if you plan to get pregnant again) and your not-fully-protected tot. That's because these diseases are still present in other parts of the world, and the prevalence of international travel means these serious illnesses can and do cross borders and oceans often. As they say, an outbreak of infectious disease is only a plane ride away.

Varicella vaccine. If you didn't have chicken pox as a child and you catch it as an adult, it could end up being a very serious case (it's far more severe in adults than in children).

Also recommended for adults with particular risk factors are the hepatitis A vaccine (if you might be exposed to hepatitis A through your work or travels, if you live in a high-incidence area, or if you take blood products to help your blood clot) and the hepatitis B vaccine (if you're a health-care worker, dialysis patient, or someone who travels to countries where the disease is prevalent).

When to Call the Doctor
After an Immunisation

Most reactions to vaccines are mild – nothing that a dose of paracetamol or ibuprofen, some extra cuddling, and a warm bath can't take care of. More severe reactions are exceedingly rare, but as a precaution you should call the doctor right away if your toddler experiences any of the following reactions within two days of an injection (these reactions aren't usually serious):

- High fever (over 104°F/40°C).

- Crying for more than three hours.

- Seizures/convulsions (jerking or staring with a lack of awareness and responsiveness for a brief time – like 20 seconds) – usually febrile (caused by fever) and not serious.

- Seizures or major alterations in consciousness within seven days of injection.

- Listlessness, unresponsiveness, excessive sleepiness.

- An allergic reaction (swelling of mouth, face, or throat; breathing difficulties; immediate rash). Slight swelling and warmth at the injection site is common and nothing to be concerned about (a cool compress should bring relief).

Reporting these symptoms isn't just for your toddler's sake (and yours, since the call will almost certainly bring you peace of mind), but also so that the doctor can report the response to the Medicines and Healthcare products Regulatory Agency (MHRA).

---

a serious problem in childhood, but because it can have severe consequences (such as sterility or deafness) when contracted in adulthood, early immunisation is recommended.

Reactions to the MMR vaccine are generally very mild and don't usually occur until a week or two after the injection. A few children may get a rash or slight fever. In case you were concerned (and you definitely shouldn't be), studies have repeatedly shown no link between the MMR vaccine and autism or other developmental disorders.

Haemophilus influenzae type b vaccine (Hib). Your child should get the Hib vaccine at 2, 3, and 4 months of age, with a fourth dose at 12 to 13 months.

The vaccine is aimed at thwarting the deadly Hib bacteria (which has no relation to influenza, or "flu"), the cause of a wide range of very serious infections in infants and young children. The disease is spread through the air by coughing, sneezing, even breathing – and prior to the introduction of the vaccine, thousands of children contracted serious infections of the blood, the lungs, the joints, and the covering of the brain (meningitis). Hib meningitis frequently led to permanent brain damage and killed hundreds of young children every year.

The Hib vaccine appears to have few, if any, side effects. A very small percentage of children may have fever, redness, and/or tenderness at the site of the injection.

Meningococcal C conjugate (MenC). The MenC vaccine protects against infection by meningococcal group C bacteria, which can cause meningitis and septicaemia. The first MenC vaccinations are given to babies when they are 3 and 4 months old. A third dose is given at 12 to 13 months, which is combined with the Hib vaccine. Babies aged between 5 months and a year who have not had the vaccine need two doses at least one month apart in order to be fully protected. This vaccine has been specifically made to produce high levels of antibodies to protect children against the disease and has led to a 99 per cent reduction in tested cases since it was introduced in 1999.

Bacterial meningitis (group B) is the more serious form of the condition and is common in the UK, so it is important to be aware of the symptoms of meningitis in babies and young children so you can act quickly. Your child might become floppy and unresponsive, or have a stiff body with jerky movements, become irritable and not want to be held. He or she might vomit and have no appetite, have pale and blotchy skin, and a staring expression, or be very sleepy and reluctant to wake up. If you suspect a case of bacterial meningitis, you should phone 999 immediately to request an ambulance.

Pneumococcal conjugate vaccine (PCV). Children should get the PCV vaccine at 2, 4, and between 12 and 13 months.

The PCV vaccine protects against the pneumococcus bacterium, a major cause of serious or invasive illness among children. It is spread through person-to-person contact (touch) and is most common during the winter and early spring. Large studies and clinical trials have shown that the PCV vaccine is extremely effective in preventing the occurrence of certain types of meningitis, pneumonia, blood infections, and other related, sometimes life-threatening infections. Though the vaccine wasn't intended to prevent ear infections, it's somewhat effective in preventing those caused by these same bacteria.

Side effects, such as low-grade fever or redness and tenderness at the injection site, occasionally occur and are not harmful.

Polio vaccine (IPV). Children should receive four injections of inactivated polio vaccine (IPV): the first at 2 months, the second at 3 months, the third at 4 months, and the fourth at 3 to 4 years – except in special circumstances (such as when travelling to countries where polio is still common, in which case the schedule may be moved up).

Polio (a.k.a. infantile paralysis), once a dreaded disease that left thousands of children physically handicapped each year has virtually been eliminated in the UK through immunisation. Polio is caused by a virus that is spread through contact with the faeces of an infected person (such as when changing nappies) or via throat secretions. It can cause severe muscle pain and paralysis within weeks, though some children with the disease experience only mild coldlike symptoms or no symptoms at all.

The IPV is not known to result in any side effects except for a little soreness or redness at the site of the injection and the rare allergic reaction. A child who had a *severe* allergic reaction to the first dose generally won't be given subsequent doses.

Vaccines for Risk Groups

Varicella vaccine (Var). Children who fall into certain risk groups may be offered extra vaccines. A child who has already had chicken pox (a.k.a. varicella) doesn't need to be immunised against it (you usually can't catch it again). The vaccine appears to prevent chicken pox in 70 to 90 per cent of those who are vaccinated once, and a second dose pushes the protection rate close to 100 per cent. The small percentage who do get chicken pox after receiving a single dose of the vaccine usually get a much milder case than if they hadn't been immunised.

Varicella was until recently one of the most common childhood diseases. Highly contagious through coughing, sneezing, and just breathing, chicken pox causes fever, drowsiness, and an itchy blister-like rash all over the body.

Should a Cold Delay an Injection?

A mild illness (a runny nose, an ear infection, a cough, mild diarrhoea, or low fever) is usually not a reason to delay a vaccination. In fact, skipping an injection for a mild illness can result in a child being incompletely immunised. That's because many toddlers (especially those who attend nursery or who have an older sibling) have frequent colds, and finding sniffle-free windows of opportunity to vaccinate them according to the schedule often proves difficult. So don't delay those injections for a mild illness. On the other hand, if your tot is battling a severe illness or has a fever over 101°F/38°C, it's probably best to postpone injections until he or she is feeling better. Do let the doctor or nurse know about any illness your child may have before he or she is vaccinated.

Though usually mild, it occasionally causes more serious problems such as encephalitis (brain inflammation), pneumonia, secondary bacterial infections, and, in rare instances, even death. Those who contract the disease when they are older are much more likely to have severe chicken pox with complications. And the disease can be fatal to high-risk children, such as those with leukemia, immune deficiencies, those who take medications that suppress the immune system (such as steroids), or newborns born to unvaccinated mothers.

The varicella vaccine is very safe. Rarely, there may be redness or soreness at the site of the injection. Some children also get a mild rash (just a handful of spots) a few weeks after being immunised.

Hepatitis B (hep B). This vaccine, given as a series of 3 doses – typically, the first at birth, the second at 1 or 2 months, and the third at 12–13 months – is only recommended for children who are considered at high-risk for contracting Hepatitis B.

Hepatitis B, a chronic liver disease, is spread through contact with the blood or other body fluids of an infected person. Those who become infected with the disease can have serious problems such as cirrhosis (scarring of the liver) or liver cancer. Hepatitis B is not very common in the UK, with new infections occurring in about 7 out of every 100,000 people every year, and usually in adults.

Side effects of the hep B vaccine – slight soreness and fussiness – are not common and pass quickly.

Hepatitis A (hep A). In the UK, most cases of hepatitis A are seen in people who have returned recently from travelling to countries where there is poor sanitation or where disposal of sewage is substandard. If your child needs to

Recommended Immunisation Schedule for Early Childhood

Curious about what injection (if any) is on the schedule at your toddler's next checkup? Here is the recommended timetable for early childhood vaccines (check with the GP about the most current recommendations).

Age	DTaP	IPV	MMR	Hib	PCV	MenC
2 months	✕	✕		✕	✕	
3 months	✕	✕		✕		✕
4 months	✕	✕		✕	✕	✕
12–13 months			✕	✕	✕	✕
3–4 years	✕	✕	✕			

be vaccinated against hep A, three doses will be given: the first dose is given at 12 months of age or older and a booster dose is given at 24 months of age or at least 12 months after the first.

Hepatitis A is a liver disease that affects an estimated 1.5 million people a year worldwide. The virus is spread through personal contact or by eating or drinking contaminated food or water. Symptoms of the illness in children over 6 include fever, loss of appetite, stomach pain, vomiting, and jaundice (yellow skin or eyes). Although hep A infection rarely has the lifelong implications hep B infection often has, it's still a significant contagious illness that can be easily and safely prevented with immunisation in early childhood.

Side effects, such as tenderness at the injection site or a low-grade fever, occasionally occur and are not harmful.

Influenza (flu) vaccine. Influenza, or "flu", is a seasonal illness spread through sneezing, coughing, and even breathing or touching a surface with the virus on it (and then passing the virus from hand to mouth or nose). The influenza virus (there are many different strains, including H1N1) causes fever, sore throat, coughs, headache, chills, and muscle aches. Complications can range from ear and sinus infections to pneumonia and even death. Influenza is different from most other diseases because the viruses are always changing, meaning that immunity acquired one year may not protect against future influenza viruses. That's why a yearly vaccine is developed to protect against the strains of the flu virus that are expected to be most prevalent. Keep in mind, though, that the rules and recommendations for who gets what when may change every year. Check with your GP for this flu season's guidelines.

Better Late Than Never

Never got around to getting your little one vaccinated completely (or at all)? Maybe you were on the fence about vaccinations during the first year and now that you've read more about the risks of skipping vaccinations, you'd like to jump on the immunisation bandwagon. Or maybe your toddler missed a dose or two because you were travelling or he or she had a run of ear infections. The good news is that you can still get your toddler caught up and on schedule. Ask the GP about how you can get your child's immunisations up-to-date.

THE REALITY ABOUT IMMUNISATION MYTHS

Worried about those vaccines headed your tot's way? Though most worries about immunisation are perfectly understandable, they are also, happily, completely unfounded. Don't let the following myths keep you from immunising your child:

Myth: *Giving so many vaccines all at once in a combination vaccine isn't safe.*

Reality: Current vaccines are just as safe and effective when given together as when given separately. There are many combination vaccines that have been used routinely – and safely – for years (MMR, DTaP). More combination vaccines are being used these days, such as one that combines Hib and MenC. But the best part about these combination vaccines is that they mean fewer total injections for your child – something you're both likely to appreciate.

Myth: *If everyone else's children are immunised, mine can't get sick.*

Reality: Some parents believe that they don't have to immunise their own children if everyone else's children are immunised – since there won't be any diseases around to catch. That so-called "herd" theory doesn't hold up. First of all, there's the risk that other parents are subscribing to the same myth as you, which means that their children won't be immunised either, creating the potential for an outbreak of a preventable disease. Second, unvaccinated children put vaccinated (as well as unvaccinated and not fully vaccinated) children at risk for diseases as well. Since vaccines are about 90 per cent effective, the high percentage of immunised individuals limits the spread of disease but doesn't eliminate it completely. So not only might you be hurting your own child, you might also be hurting other children as well. Something else to keep in mind: some diseases, like tetanus, aren't transmitted person-to-person. An unvaccinated child can contract tetanus after being cut by a rusty object or having contaminated soil seep through a scratch – so even universal immunisation of the "herd" wouldn't be protective.

Myth: *Vaccines have wiped out childhood diseases, so my child won't get sick.*

Reality: Wondering why you should bother having your child immunised against diseases that seem to be a thing of the past (after all, when was the last time you heard of someone who had rubella)? The truth is that many of these diseases are still around and can harm children. In fact, in 2011 unvaccinated under-25s in England and Wales who travelled abroad caused a sharp jump in the number of measles cases – 334 cases compared with 33 the previous year. The Health Protection Agency (HPA) sent out letters to some primary schools warning of the risks of not vaccinating children. Similarly, an increase in cases of mumps in 2009 in the 17–25 age group who had missed out on the MMR vaccine led to more warnings from the HPA. Pertussis is definitely still around, causing severe disease and many deaths yearly, sometimes at epidemic proportions.

Myth: *One vaccine in a series gives a child enough protection.*

Reality: Researchers have found that skipping vaccines puts your child at increased risk for contracting the diseases, especially measles and pertussis. So if the recommendations are for a series of four injections, for example, make sure your child receives *all* the necessary injections so he or she is not left unprotected.

Myth: *Multiple vaccines for such young children put them at increased risk for other diseases.*

Reality: There is no evidence that multiple immunisations increase the risk for diabetes, infectious disease, or any other illnesses. Neither is there any evidence that there is a connection between multiple vaccines and allergic diseases such as asthma.

Myth: *There's mercury in vaccines and it's dangerous.*

Reality: The truth is, most of the recommended childhood vaccines (MMR, IPV, varicella, and PCV, for instance) never contained mercury (thimerosal) at all. What's more, since 2001, all routinely recommended vaccines have either been mercury free or (in the case of the flu vaccine, for instance) have contained only extremely small amounts of mercury. How small? Around 12.5 microgrammes per dose – and to put that number into perspective, 170 g of tinned tuna chunks contains, on average, 52.7 microgrammes of mercury. Most important, many studies have proven that this extremely low level of mercury in the form of thimerosal doesn't cause harm and that the type of mercury used in the flu vaccine is expelled from a child's body faster than the mercury found in fish, leaving little chance for buildup in the body. Thimerosal-free flu vaccines are available, too – ask the doctor.

Myth: *Vaccines cause autism or other developmental disorders.*

Reality: Despite numerous large-scale studies that have thoroughly discredited a link between autism and vaccines (including a large study from the US Institute of Medicine based on comprehensive data and evidence gathered over a number of years), it's a controversy that just won't seem to go away – at least as long as Internet rumours keep getting passed around. The entire vaccine–autism scare began in 1998 when a UK doctor published a study (the only one of its kind, in fact – and involving only 12 children) that suggested a possible link between the MMR vaccine and autism. The journal that published the study (*The Lancet*) retracted it in 2004, and in 2010 the General Medical Council found that the doctor responsible for that faulty study actually fudged the data, manipulated the outcomes, and misreported results in his research. In 2011, the journal *BMJ* called the flawed study "an

Taking the Fears, Tears, and Ouches Out of Injections

Has your tot cottoned on to the fact that doctor visits might include an injection – and has that realisation led to lots of pre-visit stress and in-surgery hysterics? Nobody likes getting an injection (or watching their child get one), but these tips may help minimise the fears, tears, and ouches for both of you:

- Be up front. If your toddler asks if there will be an injection at a checkup, remember: honesty is the best policy. Don't say there isn't going to be an injection when you know there is going to be one – this ploy will work only once, then backfire indefinitely. Mistrust isn't something you want your toddler to associate with doctors – or with you, for that matter. Of course, there's no need to bring up the injection unless your tot does, and a young toddler is unlikely to.

- Play doctor. Investing in a toy doctor's kit, complete with toy syringe, can buy loads of doctor-anxiety relief. Having your toddler give pre-tend injections to you and to stuffed animals and dolls can offer control and comfort – and stress reduc-tion when the needle comes his or her way. As your toddler's compre-hension increases, you can explain "Injections keep us from getting sick."

- Pretreat, possibly. The truth is, injections are over in a flash, and the pain your child feels will be minimal and very fleeting. Though they really aren't necessary, there are some topical anaesthetics that can numb the injection site. The problem is they can be a bit of a logistical pain (you have to obtain and apply one in advance and know exactly how much to apply

elaborate fraud". In other words, there was never any credibility in the theory that vaccines cause autism.

For the most up-to-date facts on vaccine safety, as well as the lat-est immunisation recommendations for your child, visit the NHS Choices website at www.nhs.uk/planners/vaccinations. You can download all the information on each vaccine. The doctor, by law, will provide informa-tion whenever an injection is given, but checking it out ahead of time will allow you to read up on vaccine benefits, risks, side effects, and contraindications.

IMMUNISATION PRECAUTIONS

Vaccines are extremely safe, but they're even safer when both par-ents and professionals take the appro-priate precautions:

- Remind your child's doctor about any previous reactions to earlier vaccinations.

- Be sure your child receives a checkup before an immunisation to be certain no serious illness is present that isn't yet apparent. If your child has been

and where on your little one's leg to apply it), and they can sometimes even step up anxiety in a child. EMLA is an anaesthetic cream you'll need a prescription for and that must be applied about an hour before the injection in order to be fully effective (a whole lot of effort for a moment of pain prevention). There's also a somewhat faster-acting cream called Ametop Gel that works its numbing magic in 30 to 45 minutes and is available from the pharmacy. Both medications may trigger some minor skin irritation (redness, itching, and rash, plus some residual numbing). Another option is a cooling spray (the kind you'll find in the first-aid aisle), which may work as effectively as EMLA – unless your toddler is the type to be scared of being sprayed. Check with your doctor to get more info on all anaesthetic options, and to discuss whether any are worth trying, or whether it's better to leave it.

- Prepare to distract. Bring along that favourite blanket, a beloved book, or a treasured teddy to clutch. Having the doctor pretend to give your tot's doll or stuffed animal an injection before turning the needle on your toddler can help ease anxiety, too.

- Blow it. Blowing out during an injection not only distracts, it minimises pain. But it's a skill that must be learned. Practise blowing with your toddler ahead of time, then do it together just before the needle closes in on his or her skin (blow bubbles and you'll be distracting your toddler even more).

- Keep a stiff upper lip. Often, parents dread injections more than their child does. That's normal and easy to understand – after all, no parent wants to see his or her child in pain, even for a quick second. Problem is, it's way too easy to spread the dread to your little one. So be the model of mellow when the needle appears.

showing any signs or symptoms of being sick, let the doctor know.

- Watch your child for any side effects during the three days after immunisation and report severe reactions to the doctor immediately (see page 348). Make a note of any reactions in your child's immunisation or health record.

- Make sure that the vaccine manufacturer's name and the vaccine lot/batch number are noted in your child's chart, along with any reactions you report. Bring your child's

immunisation record to every checkup so that it can be updated.

- Severe reactions should be reported to the Medicines and Healthcare products Regulatory Agency (MHRA) by the doctor. If you believe your child may have been harmed by any vaccine, contact the Vaccine Damage Payments Unit(01722 899944) or e-mail cau-vdpu@dwp.gsi.gov.uk for information. This government programme protects both those who produce vaccines and those who receive them.

Calling the Doctor

New parents tend to call the doctor at the drop of a symptom. But now that you've got a year-plus of experience assessing baby coughs, colds, and fevers, you're a relative professional – which means you'll probably pick up the phone less often. Still, there will be times when nothing but medical advice or reassurance will do. Here's what you'll need to know about calling the doctor.

WHEN TO CALL THE DOCTOR

Deciding which symptoms say "call immediately", which say "call some time today", and which say "wait and see" isn't always easy. And a "call-the-doctor" symptom in one child or in one situation may be a "wait-and-see symptom" in another. That's why you should ask your child's doctor, nurse-practitioner, or health visitor for specific when-to-call recommendations for your child. Jot down these recommendations or make note of them on your phone.

No matter what instructions you've been given, call immediately (or go to Accident & Emergency if the doctor can't be reached) if you feel that there is something very wrong with your child – even if you can't confirm it with the help of this list and even if you can't quite put your finger on what it is. Parents often know best.

If your 1-year-old develops any of the following symptoms, call your doctor as noted. If a symptom that warrants a call during regular surgery hours appears at the weekend, you can wait until Monday to contact the doctor. If a symptom that requires a call within 24 hours appears at the weekend, call within that time frame, even if you have to call the doctor's answering service.

Fever (unless otherwise specified, temperatures given are for rectal readings):

- Over 105°F/40.5°C call immediately.

- Between 104°F/40°C and 105°F/40.5°C call within 24 hours (unless it is accompanied by any "call immediately" signs or symptoms).

- Between 102°F/38.8°C and 103.9°F/39.9°C call during regular surgery hours, unless fever is gone by then.

- Under 102°F/38.8°C, with mild cold or flu symptoms, that lasts for more than three days call during regular surgery hours.

- That lasts more than 48 hours when there are no other detectable signs of illness call during regular surgery hours.

- That suddenly rises after being low-grade (under 102°F/38.8°C) for a couple of days or after having gone away completely, or that suddenly develops in a child who has been sick with a cold or flu (this may indicate a secondary infection, such as an ear infection or strep throat) call within 24 hours, unless the child appears sicker, if something starts hurting (like an ear), or if breathing becomes fast or laboured, in which case, call straight away.

- With onset following a period of exposure to an external heat source, such as the sun on a hot day or the closed interior of a car in hot weather; immediate emergency medical attention is required (see heat illness, page 453).

- That suddenly increases when a child with a moderate fever has been over-dressed or bundled in blankets. This should be treated as heat illness; call straight away.

Fever accompanied by:

- Limpness or unresponsiveness (you can't interest your child in anything); call straight away.

- Convulsions (the body stiffens, eyes roll, limbs flail); call immediately the first time. If your toddler has had convulsions in the past, the convulsions were brief, and your child seems fine afterwards, call within 24 hours, unless the doctor has advised you to do otherwise (see page 366).

- Convulsions that last longer than 5 minutes; call 999 immediately for emergency assistance.

- Inconsolable, out-of-the-ordinary crying that lasts two or three hours; call straight away.

- Crying, as if in pain, when your child is touched or moved; call immediately.

- Whimpering or moaning unrelated to behaviour; call immediately.

- Purple spots anywhere on the skin; call immediately.

- Difficulty breathing; call immediately.

- Severe headache, especially with vomiting. Headache may be hard to identify in a preverbal toddler, but signs might include pained crying (especially when moving head), rubbing or pointing to head, squinting at light; call immediately.

- Excessive drooling and a refusal to swallow liquids; call immediately.

Where Does It Hurt?

How can you tell if your prever-bal toddler has a headache? An earache? A tummy ache? Without illness-describing words in his or her repertoire, it isn't easy. Here are a few clues to a little one's aches and pains:

- Headache. A young child with a headache may grab or rub his or her head (or sometimes bang it), or may just be uncharacter-istically irritable. Serious causes of head pain (like a concussion) are frequently accompanied by vomiting.

- Stomachache. Your little one may bend over and grab his or her belly, and – if a walker – may toddle carefully so as not to shake things up.

- Throat pain. Definitely not easy to spot. There may be discomfort on swallowing or hesitancy to swallow food or drink. Lack of appetite may indicate another illness, too.

- Chest pain. Another tough one. There may be nothing more than unexplained irritability, but your child may hold or rub his or her chest and will likely have a change in breathing pattern – shallow, rapid breaths may be a clue.

- Neck stiffness (the child resists having his or her head moved forward towards the chest); call immediately.

- Suspected burning or pain during urination (this might be difficult to confirm in a young toddler, but might cause a toddler to "hold it in" or to cry when wetting) with or without foul-smelling urine; call as soon as possible.

- Sore throat – again, it can be hard to identify this in a toddler, but signs might include crying with swallowing, refusal to take food or drink; call during regular surgery hours.

- A rash; call during regular surgery hours.

- Repeated vomiting; call within 24 hours; repeated and forceful vomiting, or vomit that contains bright green bile, call straight away.

- Mild dehydration (see page 390 for signs); call during regular surgery hours.

- Severe dehydration (see page 390 for signs); call immediately.

- Uncharacteristic behaviour – excessive grumpiness or crying; excessive sleepiness; lethargy; sleeplessness; sensitivity to light; loss of appetite; ear pulling or clutching; call within 24 hours.

A cough:

- That is mild (not barking or whooping) and lasts more than two weeks; call during regular surgery hours.

- That disturbs sleep at night; call during regular surgery hours.

- That brings up yellowish or greenish phlegm; call during regular surgery hours.

- That brings up blood-tinged phlegm; call immediately.

- That sounds very barky or chesty; call during regular surgery hours.

A cough accompanied by:

- Difficulty breathing; call immediately.

- Wheezing (a whistling sound while breathing out); call during regular surgery hours.

- Retractions (the skin between the ribs appears to be sucked in with each breath); call right away.

- Rapid breathing (see page 360); call during regular surgery hours; if persistent or accompanied by fever, call same day.

Sore throat:

- Following exposure to someone with diagnosed strep infection; call during regular surgery hours (though keep in mind that strep is rare in a child under age 2).

- In a child with a history of chronic lung disease, rheumatic fever, or kidney disease; call within 24 hours.

Sore throat accompanied by:

- Fever over 102°F/38.8°C; call during regular surgery hours.

- Discomfort when swallowing; call during regular surgery hours.

- Severe difficulty swallowing, drooling; call immediately.

No Silly Questions

Have you got a question about a symptom? A treatment plan? A side effect of a medication? Something you read on a website or message board or heard from a friend that conflicts with the doctor's advice? Ask. Remember, as far as health professionals are concerned, there are no silly questions – especially coming from a caring parent.

- White spots or blisters on reddened throat; call during regular surgery hours.

- Swollen, or tender, glands in the neck (see page 360); call during regular surgery hours.

- A rash; call during regular surgery hours.

Bleeding:

Report any of the following symptoms to the doctor immediately:

- Blood in the urine.

- Blood in the stool, except for streaks of blood that you know are from anal fissures (little tears in the anus, usually from straining to pass hard bowel movements).

- Blood in sputum or phlegm.

- Blood leaking from the ears.

General demeanour:

Call immediately if your toddler displays any of the following symptoms:

- Severe lethargy, with or without fever; a semi-awake state from which he or she can't be fully roused; lack of responsiveness.

- Crying or moaning as if in pain when moved or touched.

- Restlessness – your child can't settle down to sleep for more than 30 minutes at a time. Use your judgement here – if you think restlessness is caused by pain, call.

- Continuous crying for more than three hours; high-pitched crying; faint whimpering or moaning unrelated to behaviour.

- Refusal to eat or drink at all for an entire day.

Other:

- Swollen glands (see page 360) that become red, hot, and tender; call within 24 hours.

- Severe pain anywhere in the body, especially in the head or chest (a nonverbal toddler might clutch the affected body part); call immediately.

- Severe abdominal pain that doesn't appear to be related to constipation or lactose intolerance and that lasts more than three hours, or is accompanied by vomiting, call the same day.

- Yellowing of the whites of the eyes or of the skin; call during regular surgery hours.

BEFORE YOU CALL THE DOCTOR

So you've decided that a call to the doctor is necessary (or you think it might be – when in doubt, go with your instinct). To make that call count, it'll help to be as specific as possible when describing your child's symptoms (not always easy when those symptoms have you stressed out). So that you'll be familiar with the information you may need – and the answers to the questions the doctor may have – look over this section before the next sniffle strikes:

Information on your toddler's symptoms. Often, just looking at your toddler will tell you something isn't right. But a physician or nurse needs more of a detailed assessment to make an accurate diagnosis. So before you call to report an illness, check your toddler to assess any of the following that might be relevant to his or her condition:

- **Temperature.** If your toddler's forehead feels cool to the touch (with the back of your hand or your lips), you can assume there's no significant fever; if it feels warm, get a more accurate reading with a thermometer (see page 363).

- **Breathing.** Young children normally take about 20 to 40 breaths per minute. Breathing is more rapid during a period of activity (including crying) than during sleep, and may speed up or slow down during illness. If your toddler is coughing or seems to be breathing rapidly or irregularly, check respiration (rate of breathing). If your toddler's respiration is faster or slower than usual or is outside the normal range, or if his or her chest doesn't seem to rise and fall with each breath, or if breathing appears laboured or raspy (unrelated to a stuffy nose), report that information to the doctor.

- **Respiratory symptoms.** Is your toddler's nose runny or stuffy? Is the discharge watery or thick? Clear, white, yellow, or green? If there's a cough, is it dry, hacking, heavy, crowing, or barking? Is the cough productive – does it bring up any mucus? Has your child vomited mucus during a forceful cough?

- **Behaviour.** Is it pretty much behaviour as usual, or is there a change from the norm? Would you describe your child as sleepy and lethargic; grumpy and irritable; inconsolable; or unresponsive? Can you elicit a smile?

- **Sleeping.** Is your toddler sleeping much more than usual, or is he or she unusually drowsy or difficult to arouse? Or is he or she having more trouble than usual sleeping?

- **Crying.** Is your toddler crying more than usual? Does the cry have a different sound or unusual intensity – is it high-pitched, for instance, or low-pitched?

- **Appetite.** Has there been a sudden change in appetite? Is your toddler refusing fluids and/or solids?

- **Skin.** Does your toddler's skin appear or feel different in any way? Is it red and flushed? White and pale? Bluish or grey? Does it feel moist and warm (sweaty) or moist and cool (clammy)? Or is it unusually dry or wrinkly? Are lips, nostrils, or cheeks excessively dry or cracking? Are there spots or other lesions anywhere on your toddler's skin – under the arms, behind the ears, on the arms, legs, or trunk, or elsewhere? How would you describe their colour, shape, size, texture? Is your child scratching or rubbing them?

- **Mouth.** Are there any red or white spots or patches visible on the gums, inside the cheeks, or on the roof of the mouth or tongue? Any bleeding?

- **Throat.** Is the arch framing the throat reddened? Are there white or red spots or patches?

- **Eyes.** Do your toddler's eyes look different from usual? Do they seem glazed, glassy, vacant, sunken, dull, watery, or reddened? Is there yellowing of the whites? Do they have dark circles under them, or seem partially closed? If there's any discharge, how would you describe its colour, consistency, and quantity? Do you notice any "pimples" on the eyelids? Is your child squinting or unwilling to open his or her eyes in the light?

- **Ears.** Is your toddler pulling or poking at one or both ears? Is there a discharge from either ear? If there is, what does the discharge look like?

- **Lymph glands.** Do the lymph glands in your child's neck seem swollen? (See illustration on the opposite page for how to check them.)

- **Upper digestive system.** Has your toddler been vomiting? How often? Is there a lot of material being vomited, or are your toddler's heaves mostly dry? How would you describe the vomit – mostly clear, mucus-streaked, greenish (bile-stained), pinkish, bloody, like curdled milk, like coffee grounds? Is the vomiting forceful? Does it seem to project a long distance? Does anything specific seem to trigger the vomiting – eating or drinking, for example, or coughing? Do you know, or suspect, that your toddler has ingested a toxic substance? Is there an increase or decrease in saliva? Excessive drooling? Or any apparent difficulty swallowing?

- **Lower digestive system.** Has there been any change in bowel movements? Does your toddler have diarrhoea, with loose, watery, mucousy, or bloody stools? Are the colour and odour of the bowel movements different than usual? Are movements more frequent (how many in the last 24 hours?), sudden, explosive? Or does your toddler seem constipated?

- **Urinary tract.** Does your toddler seem to be urinating more or less frequently? Have nappies been dryer than usual? Is the urine different in colour – dark yellow, for example, or pinkish – or have an unusual odour? Does urination seem to be painful or burning? (This discomfort could cause a toddler to "hold it in" or to cry when wetting.)

- **Abdomen.** Is your toddler's tummy flatter, rounder, more bulging, or firmer than usual? When you press on it gently, or when you bend either knee to the abdomen, does your child seem to be in pain? Where does the pain seem to be – right side or left,

upper or lower abdomen, or all over? Is your little one grabbing or clutching his or her belly, or walking very gingerly or bent over?

- **Motor symptoms.** Has your toddler been experiencing chills, shakes, stiffness, convulsions, or neck stiffness (can he or she bend chin to chest without difficulty)? Does he or she seem to have difficulty in moving any other part of the body? Do balance and coordination seem to be off (more than is usual)?

- **Pain.** Is your child complaining of pain in the arms, legs, abdomen, head, ears, or anywhere else? Or is he or she communicating his or her pain nonverbally – by tugging at an ear, for instance? Any red, tender, or swollen joints?

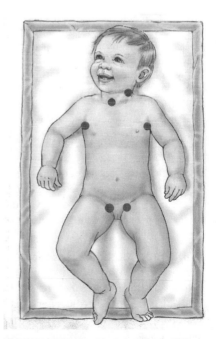

The lymph glands are part of the body's protection against disease. When there is an infection nearby, they often swell and may sometimes become tender and hot. You can feel for them with your fingertips.

Your Toddler's Pain Threshold

Toddlers, like people of every age group, vary in their responses to pain. Some can tolerate a great deal (the curious climber who falls off the slide, gets up without so much as an "ouch", and climbs right back on) and some very little (the fledgling walker who wails with every tumble, even when the landing is cushioned by a plush carpet). It's a good idea to take such differences into account when deciding how sick your toddler is. For example, if a feverish child who is ordinarily a stoic is pulling an ear and rubbing the cheek on the same side, consider an ear infection – even if he or she doesn't seem to be very uncomfortable – and call the doctor. On the other hand, if you've got a very pain-sensitive child, you might be wise not to fly to the phone at each and every whimper. Be wary, however, of the cry-wolf syndrome; keep in mind that the child who complains a lot will sometimes actually be sick.

■ **Other unusual signs.** Do you note any unpleasant odour coming from your child's mouth, nose, ears, vagina, rectum? Is there bleeding from any of these areas?

The progress of the illness so far. No matter what the illness, the symptoms alone won't tell the whole story. You should also be ready to answer these questions:

■ When did the symptoms first appear?

■ What, if anything, triggered the symptoms?

■ What worsens or alleviates the symptoms? Does sitting up decrease the coughing, for example, or does eating increase vomiting? Are symptoms affected by the time of day (are they worse at night)?

■ If pain is a symptom, where exactly is it located (if your child can tell you or if you can figure that out)?

■ Which over-the-counter or home remedies, if any, have you already tried?

■ Has your toddler recently been exposed to a virus or infection – a sibling's stomach virus, the flu at nursery, or conjunctivitis at playgroup?

■ Has your toddler recently been involved in an accident (like a fall), in which an unnoticed injury could have occurred?

■ What, if any, medicines does your toddler regularly take? Has he or she recently begun taking a new medication?

■ Has your toddler recently eaten a new or unusual food or drink or a food or drink that might have been spoiled? Any dairy product or juice that might have been unpasturised ("raw")?

Your child's health history. If the doctor doesn't have your child's chart at hand (which is usually the case when you're calling, especially during non-surgery hours), you'll have to refresh his or her memory about certain relevant details. This information is especially important if the doctor has to prescribe medication:

■ Your child's age and approximate weight.

■ If your toddler has a chronic medical condition and/or is presently taking medication.

- If there is a family history of reactions or allergies to medication.

- If your child has had any previous reactions to medications.

- The telephone and fax numbers of your pharmacy (if a prescription is to be phoned or faxed in).

Your questions. In addition to details of your toddler's symptoms, it will also help to jot down any questions you want to ask (about diet, keeping your toddler away from others, calling back if the symptoms continue, etc.) and to have at hand paper and pen or a hand-held electronic device to write answers down. Keeping an illness "diary" (in your child's health record) will give you an important resource for the future when you are trying to remember which medicines your toddler can't tolerate and how many ear infections there were last year.

Figuring Out Fever

Your typically high-energy tot is sitting listlessly on the floor, barely giving his or her beloved Little People set a second look. Lunch wasn't touched (pasta-and-cheese, no less!), and those chubby cheeks are as flushed as cherry tomatoes. You reach out to touch your tot's forehead, and ouch! – it's hot. Your heart starts to race, and you wonder just how high your toddler's temperature has climbed.

While it's hard to relax when your child is roasting up faster than a Christmas turkey, try to keep your own cool. Not all toddler fevers are panic-worthy, and not all of them warrant a trip to the doctor, or even a call. In fact, fever is actually one of the immune system's most effective allies. It's the body's way of letting you know an infection has settled in and your child's immune system is being called into action, as it should be. Still, it's important to find out how much of a fever your child has so that you (and maybe the doctor) can treat it appropriately.

TAKING YOUR TODDLER'S TEMPERATURE

The fastest and easiest way to determine whether your toddler has a fever is to touch your lips or the back of your hand to his or her forehead, the nape of the neck, or the torso. With a little practice, you will quickly learn to discern the difference between normal and feverish, low fever and high fever, if you haven't already. But your touch can't read a temperature precisely – for that, you'll need to use a thermometer. (Be aware, too, that the lip-touch system may not work at all if either you or your toddler has been outside in the cold or the heat, or in a warm bath, or if you recently sipped a hot or cold drink. A young child's forehead may also feel toasty after waking whether there's fever or not.)

The four parts of the body that can most conveniently reflect core body temperature are the mouth, the rectum, the axilla (armpit), and the ear canal. Since keeping a thermometer in the mouth and under the tongue of a young toddler isn't practical, most doctors don't recommend taking temperatures orally until a child is at least 4 or 5. The tympanic (or infrared auditory canal), temporal artery, and dummy thermometers may be convenient, but they don't always provide accurate readings (see below).

It is recommended that parents do not use glass mercury thermometers. If you still own one, be sure to properly dispose of it (not in the regular rubbish bin – check with your local recycling authority to see how to get rid of it safely). Instead, use a digital thermometer – they're safe, accurate, easy to use, readily available, and relatively inexpensive, and they can be used to take a rectal, oral, or axillary reading (but don't use the same thermometer for oral and rectal). Digital thermometers register temperature quickly (within 20 to 60 seconds), which is an advantage when dealing with a fidgeting toddler. Look for one that has a flexible tip for extra comfort. You can buy disposable covers in chemists, but they aren't really necessary.

Tympanic thermometers are fairly

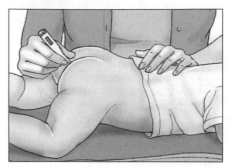

The rectal thermometer is most often used with toddlers.

expensive, and though they provide a reading in just seconds, they can be difficult to position (if you own one, you may want to ask the doctor for a demonstration of proper use). In general, a reading in the ear is less reliable than an axillary one, and neither is as accurate as a rectal reading – still considered the gold standard. Wax in the ear can also interfere with the temperature reading.

Temporal artery thermometers measure temperature with a transducer that rolls across the forehead. They are easy to use and are becoming more widely available, though they are expensive and not as accurate as a rectal thermometer.

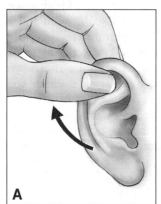
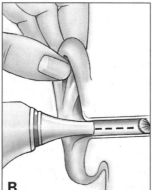
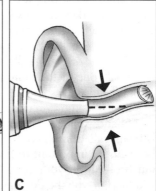

For the tympanic thermometer, the ear must be pulled upward (A) to straighten the ear canal (B) and permit a clear "view". If the canal isn't straightened (C), the angle may distort the reading.

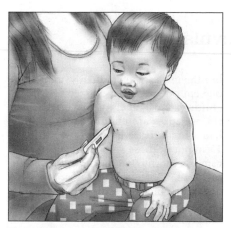

The axillary thermometer is useful when a child has diarrhoea or refuses to allow a rectal thermometer to be inserted.

Taking a rectal temperature. Clean the end of the thermometer with surgical spirit or soap and water and rinse with cool water. Turn the thermometer on and make sure you've erased any old readings from its memory. (Since every digital thermometer is different, be sure to read the instructions *before* you have a half-naked toddler on your lap.) Prepare the thermometer by lubricating the sensor tip with Vaseline. Sit down and place your toddler belly down in your lap with a pillow for comfort (see illustration, facing page). Keep your hand on the lower back to keep your fidgeting toddler stable. If that's uncomfortable, lay him or her tummy down on a flat surface, or tummy up with his or her legs bent in towards the chest, positioned as for nappy changes. To ease anxiety, be gentle, talk reassuringly, and try distraction (with a couple of favourite songs, a toy).

Spread the buttocks with one hand, so you can see the rectal opening. Then slip the thermometer in until about 1.25 to 2.5 cm of the bulb is in the rectum (don't push if you feel resistance). Hold the thermometer in place until it beeps or visually signals that the reading is done (usually 20 to 60 seconds).

Taking an axillary, or underarm, temperature. Use this somewhat less precise method of temperature-taking when your toddler won't lie still for a rectal thermometer or has diarrhoea, which would make the rectal process messy and uncomfortable. Clean the thermometer with surgical spirit or soap and water and rinse with cool water. Place the tip of the thermometer well up into your toddler's armpit (the thermometer should touch only his or her skin, not any clothing) and hold his or her arm down over the thermometer by gently pressing the elbow against his or her side. (A good tip: sit your child on your lap with his or her legs dangling beside you, so that the arm you've placed the thermometer under is pressed firmly against your chest, holding it still.) Hold the thermometer in place until it beeps or visually signals that the reading is done.

Taking a tympanic temperature. Carefully follow the directions that came with the thermometer. Basically, it's just a matter of aiming the instrument correctly into the ear canal.

READING THE THERMOMETER

A rectal temperature is believed to be the most accurate of all readings because it indicates core body temperature, and so it is used as the standard for determining temperature in young children. When the doctor asks what your little one's temperature is, be sure to tell him or her if you've taken an oral, an underarm, or a rectal reading. Ditto for temperature references in this

Febrile Convulsions

It's estimated that 2 to 4 of every 100 young children experience convulsions (their eyes roll back, the body stiffens, the arms and legs twitch and jerk involuntarily) caused simply by a sudden high fever, usually at its onset. Though febrile convulsions are frightening for parents, ordinarily they aren't harmful. Studies show that children who have experienced febrile convulsions show no later neurological or mental impairment. There appears to be a genetic factor in these convulsions (they run in families), but in most instances the major factor is probably the immaturity of the young child's brain. When the brain matures, febrile seizures stop.

If your toddler had febrile convulsions as an infant, he or she has a 30 to 40 per cent greater chance of having an episode as a toddler than does a child who's never had such convulsions, but the majority of children who have one episode never have a second. The children most likely to have recurring seizures are children who have had a first seizure lasting longer than 15 minutes, those whose convulsions came on shortly after the onset of fever, or those whose fevers were not very high at the time of the seizure. Far less often, there's an underlying cause for seizures.

Treatment of a fever does not seem to reduce the incidence of seizures during illness in predisposed children, probably because these convulsions almost always occur at the outset of an illness, just as the fever is rising and before treatment can be given.

If your toddler has a febrile convulsion, keep calm (remember, these kinds of seizures aren't harmful) and take the following steps:

book. Normal rectal temperature averages 98.6°F/37°C, but it can range from 98°F/36.6°C to 100°F/37.7°C .

Not taking a rectal temperature? Normal axillary temperature may average around 97.6°F/36.4°C, but can range from 96°F/35.5°C to 99°F/37.2°C. In other words, a reading of 100.2°F/37.8°C taken in the armpit is equivalent to a rectal reading of 101.2°F/38.4°C to 102.2°F/39°C. Not exactly a precise correlation, but a pretty good approximation. A tympanic thermometer can be adjusted to give a reading that is comparable to a rectal reading.

No matter how you take the temperature, keep in mind that "normal" may vary considerably from person to person and at different times of day. For instance, a normal reading might be lower when your toddler wakes up in the morning, a little higher in the late afternoon.

After reading and recording the temperature, wash the thermometer with cool, soapy water or clean it with surgical spirit. Be careful not to wet the digital display, on/off button, or battery cover. And be sure to read the manufacturer's instructions for proper storage as well.

TREATING A FEVER

An estimated 80 to 90 per cent of all fevers in young children are related to self-limiting viral infections

- Check the clock, so that you can time the duration of the seizure.

- Hold your child gently in your arms or place him or her on a bed or another soft surface, lying on one side, with his or her head lower than the rest of the body, if possible.

- Don't try to forcefully restrain your child in any way.

- Loosen any tight clothing.

- Don't try to give food or drink or put anything into your child's mouth, and remove anything, like a dummy or food, that might be in it. (To remove a bit of food or an object from your toddler's mouth, use a sweep of one hooked finger, rather than a two-finger pincer grasp, which might force the food further into his or her mouth.)

A child may briefly lose consciousness during a seizure, but will usually revive quickly without help. The seizure will probably last only a minute or two.

If your child wants to sleep when the febrile seizure has ended, prop him or her in a side-sleeping position with blankets or a pillow. Then call the doctor (unless this is a repeat incident and the doctor has told you it isn't necessary to call). If you don't reach the doctor immediately, you can give paracetamol to try to lower the temperature while you're waiting. But don't put your child in the bath to try to reduce the fever, because if another seizure occurs, bath water could be inhaled.

If your child isn't breathing normally after the seizure or if the seizure lasts five minutes or more, or if your child isn't responding normally after the seizure, get immediate emergency help by dialing 999 or your local Accident and Emergency number. A trip to A&E will probably be necessary to determine the cause of this kind of complex seizure.

(the kind that get better without treatment). Most experts don't recommend treating fever in toddlers unless it is at least 102°F/38.8°C or unless a fever pain-reliever (paracetamol or ibuprofen) is needed to make a toddler more comfortable (especially at bedtime). Illnesses caused by bacteria will usually (but not always) be treated with antibiotics, which lower temperatures indirectly by wiping out the infection, though paracetamol or ibuprofen may be given as needed for a child's comfort, too.

Unlike infection-related fevers, fever associated with heat-related illness (fever that's triggered by a too-warm environment or overbundling) requires immediate treatment to lower the body temperature (see page 453).

If your child has a fever, take these measures, unless the doctor has recommended a different course of action:

Keep your toddler cool. Dress your feverish child lightly to allow body heat to escape (no more than a nappy or underpants may be needed in hot weather), use only a sheet and/or a light blanket as a covering, and maintain a comfortable room temperature (not so cool that your child has goose bumps). When necessary, use an air conditioner or fan, if you have one, to maintain this room temperature (but keep your toddler out of the path of the air flow or any draughts from an open window).

Typical Body Temperatures

Body Site	Normal Range		Fever	
	(F)	(C)	(F)	(C)
Rectum	98.0° to 100.0°	36.6° to 37.7°	100.5°	38.0
Axillary (underarm)	96.0° to 99.0°	35.5° to 37.2°	99.4°	37.4
Mouth	95.9° to 99.5°	35.5° to 37.5°	99.6°	37.5

Up the fluid intake. Because fever increases water loss through the skin, it's important to be sure a feverish toddler gets an adequate intake of fluids to prevent dehydration. Encourage but don't force your child to take frequent sips of favourite drinks. If your toddler shows any signs of dehydration (see page 390), check with the doctor.

Fever: Just Part of the Picture

In most cases, behaviour is a better gauge of how sick a toddler is than body temperature. A toddler who's lethargic with no fever may be sicker than a child who's running around with a temperature of 102°F/38.8°C. What's more, a young child can be seriously ill with appendicitis and have no fever at all – or have a high fever with just a mild infection. So it's important to base your assessment of your child's condition not only on body temperature, but on the signs and symptoms that go with it as well. See page 356 for tips on when to call the doctor for a toddler with a fever.

Down the fever. The doctor may recommend paracetamol or ibuprofen (see page 378) if your child has a fever of 102°F/38.8°C or higher, seems very uncomfortable or in pain, or is unable to sleep. Be careful not to exceed the recommended dose.

Encourage a slowdown. Your child's body usually knows best, so a very sick child will likely slow down without prompting. Allow moderate activity if your toddler's up to it, but discourage too much running around, which could raise body temperature further.

Feed the fever. The effort of running a fever raises the body's caloric requirements, which means that a feverish child actually needs more calories, not fewer. Don't force food, though.

Don't overtreat. Do not give any medication (other than paracetamol or ibuprofen), except under a doctor's directions. Do not give any medication, including paracetamol, when you suspect heat illness. If your child seems to have more than mild abdominal pain, don't give ibuprofen (paracetamol is fine).

Caring for a Sick Toddler

Is there anything that tugs at your heartstrings like a toddler with a stuffy nose, a fever, a bad cough, or pain – or worse? Fortunately, you don't have to sit there watching your little one suffer. There are plenty of steps you can take to offer your sick sweetie some relief, whether he or she is at home with an illness as mild as the common cold or hospitalised with something much more serious.

AT HOME

Paging Dr Mum or Dr Dad: whether your toddler has a cold, a fever, or a stomach bug, you can help spell relief, even without any medical training. Here's the general protocol for caring for your sick toddler at home:

Rest. It's hard to keep a toddler down – even a sick one. Luckily, it isn't necessary to keep a sick toddler in bed – unless he or she seems to need the rest. In fact, you can almost invariably trust your child to pick up on and comply with his or her body signals. A very sick toddler will readily relinquish playful pursuits in favour of needed rest and relaxation, while a child who is only mildly ill will be reluctant to slow down (just as a child who's on the road to recovery will be eager to pick up the pace). So unless restrictions on activity are "doctor's orders", there's no need to impose any.

Getting out and about. Follow the doctor's advice about when to start venturing outside again with your toddler, and when to schedule a return to nursery or the playdate circuit. In general, it's recommended that a child who's been running a fever of 101°F/38.3°C or greater should stay home until the temperature has stayed below 100.4°F/38°C for 24 hours. A child who has some residual symptoms (such as a cough after a cold) can resume normal activities once the fever's gone, though a child who seems "wiped out" probably could benefit from a little extra time at home, if at all possible.

Eating and drinking. Forget starving colds – both colds and fevers benefit from feeding. If your toddler has a fever, a respiratory infection (such as a cold, influenza, or bronchitis), or a gastrointestinal illness with diarrhoea and/or vomiting, clear fluids and foods with high water content (diluted juices, juicy fruits, soups, and frozen-juice desserts – but not sugar-sweetened fizzy drinks, juices, or fruit squash) will help prevent dehydration. Sometimes, particularly with diarrhoea or vomiting, an oral rehydration solution, such as Dioralyte, may be necessary. Offer fluids frequently throughout the day, especially if your toddler takes no more than a sip at a time. If your toddler's appetite is sluggish, fluids should take priority over solids.

When your toddler's appetite is dampened by illness, it's best to feed small amounts of nutritious food often (to help the immune system fight back). But never force your little one to eat – even if he or she hasn't taken a single bite all day. Do make sure, however, that your toddler gets enough fluids. If you think your child has a serious loss of appetite or an inadequate fluid intake, or if your child has refused food or drink for 24 hours, give the doctor a call.

Medication. See page 373 for more on giving medicine when your child is sick.

When You're Sick

Mummy's got a cold? Daddy's got the flu? Being under the weather is no picnic under the best of circumstances (when you have a comfy bed, a full box of tissues, a DVD, and no responsibilities more pressing than the clicking of the remote control). But it can be particularly trying when you're home alone with an active toddler. One-year-olds generally don't have a whole lot of empathy for a sick parent – especially when that sick parent has been slacking off in the care-and-attention departments.

But when you're down with a cold, you need your rest at least as much as your toddler needs that care and attention, particularly if you'd like to get better fast. If there's any possibility at all of having someone stay at home with you to babysit or of leaving your toddler with a friend or a relative for the day, grab it and go to bed. If not, and you're stuck home alone with your toddler, you can try to enlist cooperation by explaining (in simple toddler terms) why you need to rest – and how much the rest will speed your recovery ("When I feel better, we can play!").

Another approach: appoint your tot "doctor for the day" while you play patient (this will work best with an older toddler who's started to role-play). Besides keeping your toddler occupied, having a job may make him or her more cooperative (you know how little ones love to run the show). Let your toddler go at you with the stethoscope and thermometer from a play doctor's kit; ask him or her to plump your pillows, fluff your blanket, bring you a magazine – even order you to stay in bed. Draw the doctor line at medication dosing, though (toddlers should never touch medications), and while you're at it, don't leave any medication out (even in a childproof bottle) where your toddler can reach it. Have your recovery room stocked with everything you and your child might need: tissues; a flask of warm soup; water; nonperishable snacks and juice packs for your toddler; piles of books, puzzles, crayons and paper, toys, and other amusements. Having the currently healthy parent make your toddler's lunch and leave it in the fridge will save you from having to slave over a jar of jam later on.

When you're sick with a virus your toddler hasn't already had and passed on to you, it's likely he or she will catch it. Still, it makes sense to follow the illness prevention tips on page 387.

TLC. The best medicine for anyone who isn't well, especially a child, is tender loving care. Dose your toddler with it regularly.

IN THE HOSPITAL

Finding out that your toddler has to be hospitalised – whether it's because of an injury or an illness, for just a day or two of testing, or for prolonged treatment – can be stressful, scary, and more than a little overwhelming. But even if the news is sudden, as it most often is with toddlers (you end up going straight from the doctor's surgery to the hospital after discovering that a seemingly minor respiratory infection has progressed to pneumonia, for instance), there are plenty of things you can do to put yourself and your little one more at ease:

■ Make your toddler feel at home at the hospital. For a toddler, the most difficult part of being in the hospital is being away from home and routine. Help make the stay a little easier by bringing along (or collecting as soon as possible) some favourite and familiar items. Check with the hospital to see what's allowed, but possibilities include: your toddler's pyjamas (if the hospital doesn't supply colourful toddler gowns and if a hospital gown won't be required); cot sheets and other comfort items (such as a favourite blanket or stuffed animal); toys (especially those that your toddler can play with quietly in bed); a pad and crayons (if your toddler likes to scribble); framed family photos; favourite music; picture books; a toy doctor's kit (being able to play doctor may help your tiny patient feel more in control); snacks your toddler particularly enjoys – ask the nurses where you can put your toddler's favourite juice, yogurt, or ice lollies (unless there will be diet restrictions). Make yourself at home, too, as much as the hospital will allow.

■ Stay on duty. The most important person at the hospital as far as your toddler and your toddler's care are concerned: you. If at all possible, at least one parent should be on hospital duty around the clock – not only to provide reassurance and comfort as needed, but to afford a sense of security and continuity in the often unpredictable hospital environment. Most working parents are legally allowed to take time off from their jobs to care for sick children (though, unfortunately, they are not always guaranteed pay for the days they miss). If there are two working parents, alternating bed shifts can minimise total missed work time for each and will be less physically and emotionally wearing. If you're a single parent, try to find a friend or relative to relieve you when you need a break, a shower, or some fresh air.

■ Stay involved. A hospital can be a busy, often intimidating, sometimes understaffed place, but even as nurses, doctors, medical students, and other staff swarm purposefully around your toddler, remember that you have an essential purpose, too: to be your child's patient advocate. Ask direct questions and never be afraid of asking too many or asking too often. Be informed and assertive – speak up if you have concerns or reservations about your child's care or condition. In a bustling hospital, a child can be given the wrong medicine or the wrong food, doses of medication can be missed, or something else significant can fall through the cracks. The parent on duty can serve as a vital safety net, making sure that preventable mistakes don't happen. If you speak up but feel your concerns aren't being heard, consult with the doctor, the nurse in charge, or call the Patients Association (0845 608 4455) for advice.

■ Put on a happy face. Anxiety is contagious, so to reassure your toddler about the hospitalisation, you'll need to project a confident, positive attitude. Though it won't always be easy to pull off, being a cheerful, smiling presence at your toddler's side will help put him or her more at ease. When you need to release pent-up fears and tension of your own, leave the room and unload your feelings on a friend or relative who can handle them.

■ Fuel recovery with good nutrition. Hospital food can be dodgy nutrition-wise, so supplement it, if you can,

Preparing for a Hospital Stay

Since most hospitalisations in the second year come suddenly, it's not often that parents have time to prepare themselves or their toddlers. But if you do have any advance notice at all, planning ahead can help make the experience less stressful for you and your little one (you can also take some of these steps when a hospitalisation is sudden – you'll just have to take them at the hospital). Here's how:

Prepare yourself. Learn everything you can about your child's condition and any procedures that are planned. Start with materials the doctor recommends. You'll find plenty of resources online, too, including support from other parents who have experienced or are experiencing similar situations (and support might help more than anything else). Just be aware that not everything you'll read online (or hear from other parents) will be medically valid or applicable to your toddler's situation, so check any information you're not sure about with the doctor. Learn, too, what you should expect at the hospital: ask the doctor as many questions as you can. If there will be surgery, will your child receive general anaesthesia? Can you be present while it is administered? What kinds of after-effects can you expect? Will your little one have to be immobile for a while? Will food be restricted? Will your toddler need an intravenous line? Will pain medication be available? If you're still breastfeeding, will you be able to continue?

Prepare your toddler. Most young toddlers won't understand a thorough prehospitalisation briefing – so there's not much you need to do to prepare your toddler for a hospital stay. If you think your older toddler may benefit from some advance notice and preparation, provide only an age-appropriate explanation – a brief overview with a few details. Explain that a hospital is a place where children go when they are sick (or have hurt themselves), and that there are nice doctors and nurses there to help make them better. If your toddler has questions, answer them honestly, but don't provide more information, or more detail, than is asked for. Looking at picture books and adding a few age-appropriate comments ("Look, there's a girl with a sore leg. There is the doctor to make the girl's sore leg all better!") can help familiarise your toddler with the hospital experience, as can playing "hospital" (secure a couple of surgical masks and a toy medical kit and help your child become familiar with a stethoscope, blood-pressure cuff, and even with play syringes).

with food and snacks brought from home. And though parents rarely think of themselves when they're worried about a sick child, remember that you can't help your little one if you're running on empty or running yourself ragged. So make sure you eat well and take care of yourself, too.

- Be prepared for behaviour changes. Illness, hospitalisation, and the period following them can be rough going for young children. Expect that your toddler may be uncharacteristically clingy, withdrawn, listless, frightened, unhappy – or any combination of these – temporarily. Be patient and understanding through it all. Having someone on their side (as well as at their side) helps little patients recover faster, both physically and emotionally.

ALL ABOUT:
Medication

Sometimes, all you'll need to make a sick toddler all better is cuddles, comfort, and rest. Other times, you'll need to add medication to the mix. But before you dole out any drug – prescription or over-the-counter – to your little one, you'll have to make sure you're using the right medication the right way. Here's what you need to know about medication safety for toddlers.

GETTING MEDICATION INFORMATION

Whether the doctor has suggested an over-the-counter pain reliever or a prescription antibiotic, you'll need to do more than pick it up at the pharmacy. You'll also need to become familiar with what the medication is, what it does, what dose should be given, how

---

Online Medication: A Prescription for Danger?

Chances are you've received an e-mail (or two . . . or three . . .) offering prescription drugs online at discounted prices. Maybe your computer routinely spams them, maybe you move them to a junk folder yourself – or maybe you've been seriously tempted to buy what these sites are selling, especially once you realise how cheap those lower-than-chemist prices are, and particularly if you have a toddler who always seems to be on one antibiotic or another.

Don't give in to temptation – for a couple of important reasons. First, if you're considering buying a medication based on a diagnosis you've made (you're positive it must be another ear infection, so you thought you'd save yourself some time and money by skipping the doctor's visit and prescribing antibiotics for your toddler yourself), you could be unwittingly putting your toddler in danger by prescribing medication that isn't needed or using the wrong prescription drug or the wrong dose. A second risk of ordering from a "discounted" online pharmacy: many of these cheap medications are fakes, placebos, or watered-down versions of the real thing. Not to mention that the questionable websites that sell them are not regulated (it's illegal to sell prescription drugs without a prescription in this country, so most of these websites are based outside the UK). National pharmacy chains (like Boots or Lloyds) do have legitimate websites, but all legitimate sites require a doctor's prescription, certify each prescription before dispensing any medications, have a licensed pharmacist you can speak to (stay away from any site that doesn't), and comply with all of the regulations set by the General Pharmaceutical Council (GPhC).

Herbal Remedies

They've been used for centuries to relieve the symptoms of hundreds of ailments. They're available without a prescription. They're natural. But are herbal remedies really effective and safe, especially when it comes to your little one?

No one knows for sure. What we do know is that some herbs have a medicinal effect (some very powerful prescription drugs are actually derived from herbs), and that any substance that has a medicinal effect should be categorised as a drug. That means the same precautions need to be taken with herbs as with other drugs.

The current weak regulation of herbal remedies in the UK has led to specific safety concerns. Since April 2011, all manufactured herbal medicines are required to have either a traditional herbal registration (THR) or a product licence (PL). To help you identify which products have been registered under the THR scheme, the packaging includes a 9-digit registration number starting with the letters THR. To qualify for a THR, products are required to meet specific standards of safety and quality, and be accompanied by suggested traditional usage, and patient information for the safe use of the product. Some herbal medicines in the UK hold a product licence just like any other medicine. These products are required to demonstrate safety, quality, and efficacy (or effectiveness) and be accompanied by the necessary information for safe usage. On the packaging, these can be identified by the letter PL followed by a 9-digit number.

However, just as you wouldn't give your toddler a medicine without the doctor's approval, you shouldn't give an herbal remedy (aside from those listed below) without a medical okay either – and no, the man in the supplement department of the health food shop doesn't count. Ask the doctor before you dose your tot.

This doesn't mean all alternative medicine therapies are off the table. There are some safe and simple alternative-medicine remedies that are worth trying at home:

Chamomile. If you've got a toddler who can't settle down at night, offer a small cup of chamomile tea (let it cool down first). The tea has a calming effect, and some experts (and many parents) say the herb also relieves an upset tummy and can ease the torment of teething. Some toddlers like it as is, while others will lap it up faster if milk is added.

to give it, how to store it, what side effects might be expected, and more. Hopefully, the prescribing doctor will give you most of the information (and if not, hopefully you'll remember to ask for it). But you should also do some homework at the pharmacy before you bring the medication home. When it comes to medications and your toddler, it pays to be extra careful.

Pharmacists provide an information sheet along with prescription drugs that usually answers most (if not all) of your questions. Prescription drugs – and some over-the-counter drugs – will also come with a manufacturer's package insert or detailed labelling. Check out the information when you pick up the prescription, and if you still have questions or need clarification, ask the pharmacist or the prescribing doctor. Here are some of the questions you may need answered

Peppermint. Like chamomile tea, a lukewarm cup of peppermint tea may help soothe a bellyache. Peppermint can also ease skin itchiness. So if your toddler is itching for relief from a rash or skin irritation, pour a cup of peppermint tea into the water at bathtime (the mint creates a cooling sensation on the skin).

Ginger. Ginger can calm an upset tummy. Mix a quarter of a teaspoon of grated fresh ginger in hot water and add some lemon juice and honey; let it steep and then strain. Your tot's not a fan of teatime? Offer a cake or biscuit made with ginger. It may not be as potent as ginger tea, but it may offer him or her some relief.

Aloe vera. Slice open the thick leaves of an aloe vera plant, and you'll get a clear, gooey gel that's been used for thousands of years to soothe cuts, sunburns, and skin infections. Direct from the plant, dab the gel onto your toddler's skin so that it covers the entire sore area. Not good with plants? You can find pure aloe gels and creams at the chemist or health food shop.

Oats. When it comes to treating skin conditions such as rashes, hives, and eczema, oats may be your best bet. Not only do they seal in moisture and relieve irritation, oats also contain anti-inflammatory and anti-itch properties, which decrease swelling. Simply mix plain, uncooked rolled oats with water to make a paste, and place it on your toddler's itchy skin. You can also fill a cloth bag or sock with half a cup of oats, close it up, and add it to your toddler's bath.

Honey. How sweet it is! Research shows that when your child has a sore throat, a half teaspoon of honey before bed cuts down on nighttime coughing. The syrup coats the throat and eases soreness. Plus, the sweet taste actually increases salivation, which thins mucus and alleviates the urge to cough. (But remember, don't give honey to babies younger than a year old because it can cause infant botulism – a rare, life-threatening illness.) Another use for honey, ironically, is to prevent irritation after a bee sting. If your toddler is stung by a bee, dab some honey onto the sore spot – it will cover the sting and keep the air out to prevent the area from getting irritated. See page 443 for more on how to treat a bee sting.

When giving any alternative medicines to your child, keep in mind that "natural" does not necessarily mean "safe". So talk with your GP before giving your child any complementary or alternative medicine.

---

before you give your toddler a medication (some questions may not apply):

- Does this medication have a generic (less expensive) equivalent? Is it as effective as the brand-name equivalent?

- What is the drug supposed to do?

- How should it be stored?

- Does it have a toddler-friendly taste, or can it be flavoured by the pharmacist?

- What is the appropriate dose?

- How often should the medication be given? Should I wake up my child in the middle of the night for a dose? (This is rarely necessary, fortunately.)

- Should it be given before, with, or after meals?

- Can it be given with milk, juice, or other liquids? Does it interact negatively with any foods?

- If the prescribed medication is to be given three or more times a day, is there an equally effective alternative that can be given just once or twice a day?

- If the dose is spit out or vomited up, should I give another dose?

- What if a dose is missed? Should I give an extra or double dose? What if an extra dose is inadvertently given?

- How soon can I expect to see an improvement? At what point should I contact the doctor if there is no improvement?

- When can the medication be discontinued? Does my toddler have to finish the full prescription?

- What common side effects may be expected?

- What adverse reactions could occur? Which should be reported to the doctor?

- Could the medication have a negative effect on any chronic medical condition my child has?

- If my child is taking any other medication (prescription or over the counter), could there be an adverse interaction?

- Is the prescription refillable?

- What is the shelf life of the medication? If any is left, can it be used again at a later date if the doctor advises the use of the same medication?

GIVING MEDICINE SAFELY

To be sure that your child gains the maximum benefit from medication with the least amount of risk, always observe these rules:

- Do not give your toddler medication of any kind (over-the-counter, his or her own leftover prescription, or anyone else's prescription) without a specific go-ahead from the doctor. In most cases, this will mean getting an okay to medicate each time your child is sick, except when the doctor has given you standing instructions (for example, whenever your child runs a temperature over 102°F/38.8°C, give paracetamol; or when wheezing begins, use the asthma medicine).

- Unless the doctor specifically instructs you otherwise, give a medication only for the reasons listed on the label or information insert.

- Do not give your toddler more than one medication at a time, unless you've checked with the doctor or pharmacist to be sure the combination is safe.

- Check the medication's expiration date. Drugs that have expired are not only less potent, but they may also have undergone chemical changes that can in some cases make them harmful (this applies to prescription medication you may have hanging around from a previous toddler illness, too). Always check the expiration or use-by date before you buy a drug or pick up a prescription. Recheck expiration dates periodically – otherwise you may end up making a pharmacy run in the wee hours of the night.

Don't Give These to Your Toddler

Some of the medications you may be used to reaching for when you're sick or aching can be unsafe for toddlers. These include:

Cough and cold remedies. Studies have shown that children's over-the-counter cough and cold remedies don't stop the sniffles or silence the hacking, and they may even cause young kids to develop serious side effects, such as a rapid heart rate and convulsions. That's why the Paediatric Medicines Advisory Group advises that these drugs not be given to children under age 2, and why cough and cold remedy labels recommend against using these medicines to treat children 4 years old and younger.

Aspirin (and anything containing salicylates). Doctors have been warning parents for years against giving their children aspirin, but the message bears repeating: don't give aspirin (even children's aspirin), or a medication containing aspirin, to children younger than 18, unless it has been specifically prescribed by the doctor for the child. Aspirin has been linked to the onset of Reye's syndrome, a potentially lethal disease in children. Although research comes down hardest on aspirin, NHS Choices advises against giving children any medication that contains any form of salicylate, so read ingredient lists on drug labels carefully.

- Administer medications only according to the directions your child's doctor (or the pharmacist) has given you, or according to label directions on over-the-counter products. If directions on the label – or on the printed pharmacy materials that come with the drug – conflict with the doctor's or pharmacist's instructions, call the doctor or pharmacist to resolve the conflict before giving the medication. Follow suggested dosing information about timing, shaking, and giving with or without food.

- Reread the label before each dose to be sure you have the correct medication and to remind yourself about the proper dose, timing, and other pertinent information. If you're giving it at night, check the label in the light to make sure you haven't grabbed the wrong bottle.

- Measure medications meticulously. Once you've nailed down the correct dose, make sure you dispense that dose precisely. Dispense the medication in the cup or dropper that comes with it, or use a calibrated medicine spoon, dropper, or cup. Don't use spoons from your cutlery – you can't count on them for true measurements. Never increase or decrease a dosage without your doctor's explicit instructions.

- If your child spits out or vomits up part of a dose of pain reliever medicine or vitamins, it's usually sensible to play it safe and not give extra – under-dosing is less risky than over-dosing. If you're giving antibiotics, however, check with the doctor about what to do if your toddler spits out or vomits up part of one or more doses.

Paracetamol or Ibuprofen?

There are many kinds of pain relievers and fever reducers on the market, but only two that should be considered for young children: children's paracetamol (such as Calpol) and children's ibuprofen (such as Nurofen for Children). Generic or store brands of children's paracetamol or ibuprofen can also be used. Both paracetamol and ibuprofen relieve pain or fever, though they work differently in the body and have different side effects (ibuprofen has an anti-inflammatory effect – more effective when there's inflammation, as there is with teething – and is slightly more powerful and longer lasting). The dosing for ibuprofen is every 6 to 8 hours compared to every 4 to 6 hours with paracetamol. There are few side effects to these medications when used properly – and proper use is the critical part. Although paracetamol is considered safe when used as recommended, taking it regularly for more than a week at a time can be dangerous. A large overdose of paracetamol (about 15 times the recommended dose) can cause fatal liver damage, yet another reason why all medicines should be stored out of your toddler's reach.

The biggest drawback to ibuprofen is the potential for stomach irritation. To avoid this side effect, give your toddler the medicine with a meal or drink. As a rule, don't use ibuprofen to treat stomach pain – it can make it worse.

If your child has pain or fever, you may start either medication unless the doctor has recommended otherwise. If one doesn't do the job, try the other one, as long as you make sure to give correct doses; wait until it's safe to give another dose of medication (at least 4 hours with paracetamol; at least 6 hours with ibuprofen), and follow the recommended schedule according to the instructions on the label and advice from the doctor. Never give your child a pain reliever formulated for adults (even in a reduced dose). And when you're not using pain relievers, keep them (like all medications) safely locked away, out of the reach of children. Many tots love the taste of pain relievers, and that can encourage overdosing.

- To prevent choking, don't squeeze your toddler's cheeks, hold his or her nose, or force his or her head back when giving medicine. Dispense it with your child standing or sitting upright, not lying down. Follow up a medication with a drink of water (unless you are instructed otherwise).

- Keep a record of the time each dose is given, so you'll always know when you gave the last one (it's easy to forget). This will minimise the chance of missing a dose or accidentally doubling up.

But don't worry if you're a little late with a scheduled medication. Just get back on schedule with the next dose.

- Always complete a course of antibiotics, as prescribed, even if your toddler seems completely recovered, unless the doctor has specifically told you not to.

- Don't continue giving a medication beyond the time specified in the prescription.

- If your toddler seems to be having an adverse reaction to a medication, stop it temporarily and check with the doctor before resuming use.

- If another caregiver, at home or at nursery, is responsible for giving your child medication during the day, be sure that he or she is familiar with the drug-dispensing protocol.

- Never pretend medicine is a treat. It's a trick that might get the dose down without a fuss, but it could lead to overdosing if your toddler finds the bottle later and helps himself or herself to a snack.

- Store all medications completely out of your toddler's reach at all times, even if you're going to have to pull out a drug often for dosing.

HELPING THE MEDICINE GO DOWN

If you're lucky, your toddler is one of those who actually enjoys (or at least doesn't strongly object to) the medicine-taking ritual – who savours (or tolerates) the taste of those sweet, syrupy liquids, and opens up wide enough to accommodate a double ice-cream cone at the sight of a medicine spoon. If you're not so lucky, your child probably possesses a sixth sense that says "Clamp mouth shut!" when medicine is anywhere in the vicinity. To outwit the tight-lipped:

Check your reaction. Maybe you're feeling bad about forcing your toddler to take a medicine he or she can't stand. Maybe you're anticipating another struggle and you're stressed out about it. Or maybe the artificial grape smell is making you retch. Try not to let on. Instead, be matter of fact about giving medicine; upbeat, even cheerful if you can pull it off. A frown, a wrinkled nose, a look of fear or concern will all give your little one the impression that something unpleasant is about to happen.

Time it right. Unless you're instructed to give the medication with or after meals, plan on serving it up just before a meal or snack time. First, because your child is more likely to accept a dose of medicine when hungry, and second, because if he or she does vomit it right back up, less food will be lost. Have something yummy waiting, though (unless you're not supposed to feed right afterwards).

Switch delivery systems. Delivery can make all the difference. If your toddler has already turned up that button nose at the medicine spoon, try giving the medication in a medicine dropper. You might also ask the pharmacist for a plastic syringe (sans the needle) that squirts out liquid medicine, or a small cup (make sure it offers exact measurements so you can dose properly). Any variation in your approach may distract enough to get a dose in. Don't use a regular spoon, though.

Take the right aim. Taste buds are concentrated on the front and centre of the tongue, so bypass those finicky taste zones by placing the medicine closer to the back of his or her tongue (but not so far back that you stimulate the gag reflex). Or try dropping it between the rear gum and the inside of the cheek, where it will easily glide down the throat with minimal contact with taste buds. (Yes, this requires a bit of skill, and maybe an extra set of hands to keep your toddler still while you perfect your technique.)

Try chilling. Ask the pharmacist whether chilling the medication will affect its potency. If it won't, offer the medicine to your toddler cold – the taste will be less pronounced. Or try numbing those finicky taste buds by having your toddler suck on an ice pop just before taking the medicine.

Hide the flavour. Ask the pharmacy whether a better-tasting flavouring can be added to a yucky-tasting liquid. Medication flavourings come in several fruit flavours from apple to tangerine and are designed to combat the taste and smell of liquid medicines. It may be the answer to your tot's medicine-taking troubles. And your medicine-giving ones.

Hide the medicine, maybe. As a very last resort, ask your doctor if it's okay to sneak the particular medicine into foods or drinks. If you get the thumbs-up on that, stir the medicine into a small amount of fruit juice, a smoothie, or fruit purée (apple purée à la amoxicillin is pretty tasty). But remember, if you do mix the medicine into something else, your toddler needs to eat or drink the whole portion in order to get the full dose.

The Most Common Toddler Illnesses

Is your cutie coming down with a cold or other infection? Don't be surprised. After all, your tot (like almost all toddlers) probably likes to explore his or her world by touching everything in sight. One touch – and then one wipe of the eyes or one finger in the nose – is all it takes for that germ on the supermarket trolley handle to get an open door right into your little one's body. Then bingo – your toddler ends up with a cold or another common illness (remember, that immune system is still a work in progress).

Fortunately, most common toddler illnesses are easily treated and quick to recover from. Here's what you need to know about them the next time your toddler's under the weather.

COMMON COLD

Symptoms. Happily, most common cold symptoms are mild, but they can be annoying. They include:

- Runny nose (discharge is watery at first, then thickens and becomes opaque and sometimes yellowish or even greenish)

- Nasal congestion or stuffiness

- Sneezing

- Sometimes, mild fever

- Sometimes, sore or scratchy throat (not easy to spot in a toddler)

- Dry cough (which may get worse at night, and towards the end of a cold)

- Fatigue, grumpiness

- Loss of appetite

Cause. Contrary to popular belief, colds aren't caused by being cold, going bareheaded in the winter, getting feet wet, exposure to cold draughts, and so on. Colds (also known as upper respiratory infections, or URIs) are caused by rhinoviruses. These viruses are spread via hand-to-hand contact (for example, a child with a cold wipes her snotty nose with her hand and then holds hands with another child, and the infection is passed on); via droplet transmission from sneezes or coughs; or via contact with an object that's been contaminated (such as a toy that's mouthed first by a sick child and then by a healthy child). There are more than 200 viruses known to cause colds – which explains why colds are so "common".

The incubation period for a cold is usually one to four days. A cold is typically most contagious a day or two before symptoms even appear, but can also be passed along when the cold is already underway. Once the really runny nose dries up, a cold is less contagious.

Duration. The common cold usually lasts seven to ten days (day 3 is usually the worst). A residual dry nighttime cough, which may not appear until the end of the cold, may linger longer.

Treatment. There is no known cure for the common cold, but symptoms can be treated, as necessary, with:

- Saline nose drops to soften dried mucus that may be clogging your tot's nostrils.

- Humidification to help clear nasal passages. Run a cool-mist humidifier (which is safer than a warm-mist humidifier should your toddler toddle too close to it) in his or her bedroom at night.

- Moisturising ointment, spread lightly on the rims of the nostrils and under the nose to help prevent chapping and soreness.

- Elevation of the head of the cot (by placing pillows under the head of the mattress) to make breathing easier.

- Paracetamol or ibuprofen for fever reduction if needed (it usually isn't

Good News About That Runny Nose

What could possibly be the upside to your toddler having three colds in 2 months? Well, exposure to germs (and the resulting illnesses) builds up your toddler's immune system, making it stronger in the long run – and helping your tot better fend off the next bug that comes his or her way. In other words, you can think of today's snotty nose as an investment in a healthier (and less snotty) tomorrow.

with a cold). Check with your doctor for guidelines.

- Plenty of fluids, particularly warm ones (chicken soup really is effective in soothing cold symptoms), and a nutritious diet. Be sure to offer vitamin C-rich foods and drinks each day. Frequent small meals may be more appealing than three squares. And despite what you may have heard, it isn't necessary to limit dairy products with a cold. They don't increase mucus production in most people.

Prevention. The number one way to prevent a cold is to wash your child's hands regularly. Can't get to a sink? Hand-sanitising gels or wipes will do in a pinch, though they're not as effective as soap and water in washing away those germs. Keep your child away from anyone with a cold, when possible. Use a disinfectant solution to clean surfaces that may be contaminated with cold germs, and follow other tips for preventing the spread of illness (see page 387). But remember that nothing will

Your Smoking Is Bad for Your Toddler's Health

Children who are regularly exposed to secondhand smoke (and thirdhand smoke – smoke that lingers on clothes and other fibres) are more susceptible to asthma, tonsillitis, respiratory infections, ear infections, and to bacterial and viral infections severe enough to land them in the hospital. On average, they are more likely than other children to be in fair or poor health. They also, as a group, score lower on reasoning-ability and vocabulary tests. Children of smokers appear, too, to have an increased risk of developing lung cancer down the road. In addition to these risks, smoking in front of a young child sets a dangerous example. Children who see someone they love smoke are more likely to become smokers themselves, with all the serious risks for a shortened life span that the habit involves. So kick the habit if you smoke, and don't allow smoking in your home or near your toddler.

entirely protect your child from cold viruses. The average child has six to eight colds a year, and some will have as many as nine or ten – and that's not usually a concern as long as growth and development are normal.

When to call the doctor. Usually, there's no need to contact the doctor for a simple cold, but if your child displays any of the following, a call to the GP is a good idea, if only to put your mind at ease:

- Extreme lethargy
- No appetite
- Difficulty sleeping, extreme restlessness during the night, or pain that causes night waking
- Foul smelling, greenish or yellowish discharge from nose or from coughing
- Wheezing
- Breathing more rapidly than usual
- Chest discomfort
- A cough that's getting worse or continues during the daytime after other symptoms are gone
- Throat pain, trouble swallowing, or a red throat
- Swollen glands in the neck
- Pulling on ears day or night
- Fever over 102°F/38.8°C, or low-grade fever for more than four days
- Symptoms that last longer than 10 days

If your toddler seems to have a continuous cold, a chronically runny nose, or very long-lasting or frequent colds (especially when accompanied by under-eye circles), talk to the doctor about the possibility that allergies might be responsible.

EAR INFECTION

Symptoms. Also known as acute otitis media, an ear infection is when the middle ear (between the outer part of the ear and innermost part of the ear) gets plugged with fluid and becomes infected and inflamed. When examined by the doctor (you won't be able to see this from the outside), the eardrum

Tubes for Toddlers

Sometimes, fluid in a toddler's ears just doesn't seem to clear up, even with treatment – and in some cases the ear infections keep reoccurring, in part because the fluid never really clears up. This means not only too many courses of antibiotics, but a potential for impaired hearing and speech delays. If there is persistent fluid in the middle ear for over three months, recurrent ear infections (usually more than four to five infections in a 12-month period), and/or if hearing (due to persistent fluid) is affected, the doctor may recommend tube insertion. These tiny tubes or grommets (each about the size of two exclamation points side by side) are implanted by a paediatric ear, nose, and throat (ENT) specialist into a small hole in the eardrum (after the fluid is drained). General anaesthesia is used, but the surgery itself takes only a few minutes to perform (usually on an outpatient basis). You can expect your little one to be up and running (or toddling) the next day. The tubes usually fall out on their own 6 to 18 months after insertion, but while they're in place, they prevent fluid and bacteria from building up, reducing the incidence of infections and the risk of hearing loss.

Keep in mind, though, that the doctor will likely not recommend tubes if your child only has lingering middle ear fluid and a minimal amount of hearing loss without recurrent ear infections. That's because placing tubes hasn't been shown to improve speech or language skills in these children, and most doctors prefer the wait-and-see approach before jumping to tubes. The only exception would be toddlers who also have developmental delays slowing down their speech (such as autism). Experts agree that such children do benefit greatly from anything that improves their hearing (and consequently, their speech). Talk to your GP about the risks and benefits of placing tubes in your child's ears.

---

appears pink early in the illness, then turns red and bulging. Symptoms include:

- Pain, often worse at night because lying down changes pressure in the ear (your toddler may complain, or tug, rub, or clutch at an affected ear)

- Fever

- Fatigue

- Grumpiness and irritability

If the infection persists or worsens, the eardrum could perforate (develop a small hole, which usually heals in less than a week). If this happens, pus, often blood-tinged, may spill into (and be seen in) the ear canal. The perforation will relieve the pressure, and thus the pain, but treatment of the infection will help prevent further damage – so it's crucial that you tell the doctor if you suspect a rupture (crust in and around the ear is a telltale sign).

Often, even after treatment, fluid remains in the middle ear, a condition called otitis media with effusion (also known as glue ear). Symptoms include hearing loss (your toddler may fail to respond consistently to sounds, such as your voice). While typically temporary (usually lasting about four to six weeks), the hearing loss can become permanent if the condition continues untreated for many months, especially if there are also frequent bouts of infection.

Cause. Ear infections are often secondary infections brought on by a cold or other upper-respiratory infection (or sometimes allergies), which causes the lining of the Eustachian tube (the tube that connects the middle ear to the nose and the back of the throat) to swell, become congested, and accumulate fluid. The fluid becomes a breeding ground for infection-causing germs. Behind the inflamed eardrum, the buildup of pus and mucus produced by the body in an attempt to respond to the infection causes the pain of earache. Toddlers and preschoolers are more likely than adults to get ear infections because their Eustachian tubes are narrow and short (allowing germs to travel up them more quickly and making it easy for them to become blocked) and horizontal rather than slanted (making drainage poor), and because they get more colds and other respiratory illnesses in general than older children and adults do.

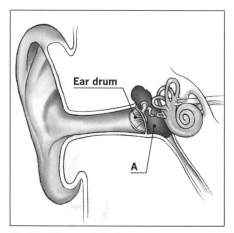

Most toddler ear infections occur in the middle ear, the tiny chamber (A) at the end of the outer ear canal. The eardrum is the wall separating the outer ear and the middle ear.

Duration. Although pain, fever, and other symptoms usually diminish or disappear shortly after treatment is begun, it can take 10 days of antibiotic medication to resolve an acute ear infection. Fluid may remain in the middle ear for much longer.

Treatment. If you suspect an ear infection, call the doctor so that you can get your child's ears checked. If the infection is severe, the doctor will probably prescribe a course of antibiotics (the wait-and-see approach is usually reserved for children over age 2 or 3).

Whether or not your toddler is prescribed antibiotics, your doctor will likely recommend paracetamol or ibuprofen for pain and fever relief. Heat (applied to the ear with a heating pad set on low, warm compresses, or a hot-water bottle filled with warm water) or cold (applied with an ice bag or with ice wrapped in a wet flannel) can also be used to relieve pain. Elevating your child's head (with pillows under the cot mattress) during sleep may also be helpful.

At the end of the course of treatment, the doctor may want to recheck your child's ears. Though the infection may clear quickly on antibiotics, in rare cases the ears remain filled with fluid for three months or more after the infection has cleared up (otitis media with effusion), in which case your GP may refer your child to a specialist to have tubes inserted (see box, previous page), especially if hearing is affected.

Prevention. Here's what you can do to minimise your child's risk:

- Prevent exposure to secondhand smoke, which makes children more vulnerable to ear infections.

- Reduce exposure – as much as possible – to germs, since even common

Some Probiotics with Those Antibiotics?

Unfortunately, no matter how many times you wash those little hands or how much hand sanitiser you dispense, sooner or later, your toddler is going to come down with an infection that requires antibiotics. While antibiotics are wonderful for wiping out bacterial infections, broad-spectrum antibiotics aren't all that clever – they aren't able to differentiate between the infection-causing bacteria and other benign bacteria in the body. Which means that along with the bad bacteria that get wiped out, some good and very important bacteria – especially bacteria found in the digestive tract – are also destroyed. And that can come with a very inconvenient and unpleasant drawback: diarrhoea.

One way to manage antibiotic-related diarrhoea (besides investing in extra-absorbent nappies) is to give your toddler probiotics. Probiotics (live active cultures, like Lactobacillus or Bifidobacterium) are just what they sound like: beneficial (or "pro") bacteria that help to counterbalance the negative effects of antibiotics. Research shows that giving probiotics to children can reduce antibiotic-related diarrhoea by 75 per cent. For this reason, GPs may recommend that children take probiotics whenever they're on antibiotics. Another reason: probiotics prevent the overgrowth of yeast (the culprit in candida nappy rash) that can be triggered by antibiotic use.

But that's not the only thing probiotics can do. They may also combat regular diarrhoea and constipation, sinus and respiratory infections, urinary tract infections, and possibly even asthma and eczema. What's more, probiotics are believed to boost the immune system in general, making it even less likely that your toddler will come down with those illnesses in the first place. Think of probiotics as the reserve team – the reinforcements sent in to bulk up the numbers of helpful bacteria and crowd out the illness-causing bacteria. These good little soldiers also help strengthen the intestinal lining so that bad bugs can't cross into the bloodstream. Probiotics can change the intestinal environment, too, making it more acidic and therefore less hospitable to bad bacteria.

The most obvious source of probiotics is yogurt (be sure to choose brands with live active cultures – it'll say so on the label). Or ask the GP if there's a probiotic supplement that he or she recommends for your toddler. Ask, too, about how frequently that supplement should be given, when it should be administered (probiotics shouldn't be given at the same time as antibiotics), and how it should be stored (often in the fridge).

colds can lead to ear infections. That means steering clear of sick children and washing your hands and your child's hands frequently.

- Stay up to date on your child's immunisations. The pneumococcal vaccine, which is given to prevent serious infections such as pneumonia and meningitis, may also reduce the risk of ear infections.

- Wean your toddler off the bottle by age 1 (or soon after) and discourage drinking from the bottle (particularly non-vented ones) or beaker while lying down. These habits can step up the risk of ear infection (breastfeeding doesn't).

• Consider limiting – or weaning off of – the dummy, the use of which may also increase ear infection risk.

When to call the doctor. Call during regular surgery hours if you suspect an ear infection (it's not an emergency). Call again if your child isn't feeling better after three days (with or without antibiotics) or if the infection seems to get better and then returns (it could be a sign of a chronic ear infection). Call, too, if you notice any hearing loss.

FLU

Symptoms. The flu (short for "influenza") is a contagious viral infection that usually rears its very infectious head between the months of October

and April (a.k.a. flu season). Its symptoms include:

• Fever

• Dry cough

• Sore throat (your toddler may reject food and drink, or seems to be in pain when swallowing)

• Runny or stuffy nose

• Muscle aches and pains

• Headache

• Extreme fatigue, lethargy

• Chills

• Loss of appetite

• Sometimes in young children, vomiting and diarrhoea

Cause. The flu is caused by the influenza virus – and different strains (or, rarely, new strains like the H1N1 virus) circulate each year. Your child can catch the flu by coming into contact with an infected person (especially if that sick someone sneezes or coughs on your toddler) or by touching something (a toy, a beaker) that an infected person has touched. The incubation period for the flu is usually two to five days. If your little one comes down with the flu, symptoms usually last about a week, though some can linger for up to two weeks.

Treatment. Treatment includes fluids and rest. To relieve flu symptoms, humidify the air in your child's room, and give paracetamol or ibuprofen only as needed for pain or high fever (do not give aspirin or any medication containing aspirin or salicylates). An antiviral drug may be prescribed for children with severe symptoms or at high risk of complications, but it needs to be administered in the first 48 hours to be effective.

A Sore Throat

It's very uncommon for toddlers under age 2 to come down with strep throat, a bacterial infection affecting the tonsils and throat, but it can happen. And since toddlers are unlikely to complain of a sore throat (they lack the vocabulary and body awareness), you'll have to look to other strep clues. If your toddler is rejecting food or drink (it could be painful to swallow), has swollen neck glands, has white dots on the tonsils, and is running a fever (some children also vomit with strep), call the doctor – a throat culture may be in order. In the meantime, ease the pain and reduce any fever with paracetamol or ibuprofen, offer plenty of fluids, and use a cool-mist humidifier in your child's bedroom (the moist air will help alleviate the throat pain).

Prevention. Since complications from the flu are more serious in children under age 5, you should do everything you can to prevent your toddler from getting the flu, including washing hands often, steering clear of sick people and consider getting your toddler the flu injection (see page 351) and even the whole family and all childcare providers could be vaccinated, too.

When to call the doctor. If you suspect your child has come down with the flu (just check the symptom list above if you're not sure), call your doctor.

CROUP

Symptoms. Croup (laryngotracheo-bronchitis) is an infection – usually seen in late autumn and winter – that causes the voice box and windpipe to become inflamed, and the airways just below the vocal cords to swell and get very narrow. Symptoms include:

- Laboured or noisy breathing – you may hear a high-pitched breathing sound when your child inhales (called stridor)

Keeping Germs Contained

Germs have a way of getting around, especially around a family with young children (germs are about the only thing toddlers share readily). Here's how you can help to contain germs before they make your whole family sick:

- **Wash those hands.** Hand washing is probably the single most effective way to stop the spread of illness, so make it a house rule – whether family members are healthy or sick. You probably know the drill, but it pays to drill it into your family: wash your hands before touching your mouth, nose, or eyes; before eating and handling food; after nose blowing or coughing, using the toilet, or contact with someone who's sick. No sink around? Keep antibacterial wipes or gels (child-safe ones for your little one) handy when you can't manage frequent washing or when you're out of the house.

- **Put tissues in their place.** Do sick family members tend to leave a trail of dirty tissues behind (or beside)

them? Then they're leaving a trail of germs, too. Make sure tissues are disposed of immediately after use in a covered bin.

- **Separate the sick.** As much as possible (and it won't always be), try to isolate sick family members, at least for the first few days of a contagious illness.

- **Cover those coughs.** If they can't all reliably cough or sneeze into a tissue yet, train your little ones to do it into their elbows, not their hands.

- **Limit sharing.** To each their own in the bathroom (their own cup, or disposable ones; their own toothbrush; their own towel) and at the table (no sharing from the same cup, spoon, fork, bowl, or plate).

- **Mind your surfaces.** Frequently wipe down or spray potentially contaminated "hot spot" surfaces (such as bathroom taps, telephones, toys, keyboards, and door handles) with a disinfectant, especially when someone in the family is sick.

- A harsh, barking cough that sounds like a seal's call (and usually comes on at night)

- Retractions (the skin between the ribs is visibly sucked in with each inhaled breath)

- Sometimes, fever

- Hoarseness

- Stuffy nose (cold-like symptoms may appear first)

- Irritability

Cause. Croup, most common in early childhood, is usually caused by the parainfluenza virus, a respiratory virus, though it can also be caused by other respiratory viruses, including the influenza virus (flu). It's spread the same way other contagious germs are spread: your child can become exposed by coming into contact with another tot who has croup (especially through a cough or sneeze), or by coming into contact with something an infected child has touched (the germs can survive on surfaces, like toys).

Duration. Croup can last several days to a week and may recur.

Treatment. Though the cough may sound scary, these simple measures will usually relieve discomfort in your croupy toddler:

- Steam inhalation. Take your toddler into the bathroom with you, run hot water in the shower, close the bathroom door, and encourage him or her to take deep breaths. Continue, if you can, until the barking noise settles down.

- Cool moist air. On a cool night, take your child out into the fresh air for 15 minutes. Or open the freezer and have him or her breathe in the cold air for several minutes.

- Humidification. Humidifying your toddler's room may help make it easier to breathe.

- Upright position. Try to keep your child in an upright position for a while, since this can make it easier to breathe. You can use extra pillows under the mattress to prop your tot up at night.

- Comfort and support. Do your best to minimise your toddler's crying, since it can make the symptoms worse.

When to call the doctor. If you suspect your toddler has croup, call the doctor, especially if this is the first attack. If it's a repeat occurrence, follow instructions the doctor has given you previously. Also call if:

- The steam or cold air doesn't stop the barky cough.

- Your child lacks colour (if there's a bluish or greyish hue around your child's mouth, nose, or fingernails).

- Your child has difficulty catching his or her breath (especially during the day), or you can see retractions (when the skin between the ribs pulls in with each breath).

- Stridor (a high-pitched, musical sound made when breathing) during the day, or nighttime stridor that isn't promptly relieved by exposure to steam or cold.

If your child's croup seems especially severe, your GP may prescribe a dose of steroids to relieve swelling in the airways and make breathing easier.

CONSTIPATION

Symptoms. Timing isn't everything when it comes to bowel movements – in fact, when it comes to diagnosing constipation, it's a matter of quality, not frequency. A toddler who goes a few days without pooing isn't necessarily clogged up (just as a toddler who goes twice a day doesn't necessarily have diarrhoea). If the stool comes out easily and looks normal (formed but soft), everything's moving along just fine – if at a somewhat slower pace. On the other hand, if your tot is producing small, round, hard stools that seem difficult to pass (face scrunching, extra grunting, and pain with pushing are all clues), the diagnosis is most likely constipation.

Cause. Some toddlers (like some adults) are more prone to constipation than others. But often constipation is linked to not eating enough high-fibre foods, not drinking enough fluids, and not getting enough physical activity. The end result is dry, hard stool that builds up in the lower bowel. Constipation can also develop during or after an illness (because a child isn't eating, drinking, or moving much) and can be a side effect of certain medications. Toilet training can also lead to constipation (the longer poo is held in, the harder and drier it becomes, and the more difficult and painful it is to pass). Often, a cycle of constipation becomes self-perpetuating: the stool is hard and painful to pass, so the child holds it in. The more the child holds it in, the more stool builds up, and the harder and more painful it is to pass.

Treatment. To help get your toddler back on track (or to prevent constipation in the first place), try:

- Fibre. Serve high-fibre foods such as fresh fruits (ripe pears and kiwi are particularly effective), soft-cooked, minced dried fruits (especially raisins, prunes, apricots, and figs), vegetables, and whole grains. Avoid serving refined grains like white bread and rice, which can clog up the works.

- Probiotics. These beneficial bacteria can help get things moving again – and keep them moving. Feed your little one yogurt that contains active cultures, and ask the doctor about whether a probiotic supplement might be a good idea, too.

- Fluids. Make sure your toddler is getting enough fluids (at least a litre a day) – especially if he or she was recently weaned (many tots drink much less after graduating to a cup). Certain fruit juices (such as prune juice or pear juice) are particularly beneficial, as is water, but limit cow's milk to the recommended 500 ml a day, since the calcium salts in it can harden stools.

- Exercise. While there's no need to sign up your toddler for membership at the local health club, do make sure his or her whole day isn't spent in the car seat or pushchair. Moving gets your child's digestive system moving, too.

- Lubrication. Dabbing a bit of Vaseline at the anal opening may help the movement slip out more easily.

- Medication. If all else fails, ask the GP about giving your toddler a stool softener such as Lactulose. If that doesn't work, the GP might recommend a laxative. Don't give any medication – or even a suppository or enema – without the doctor's advice.

When to call the doctor. While an occasional blockage of toddler poo is no big deal, you should call the doctor when:

- Your toddler has not had a bowel movement for four or five days.

- Constipation is accompanied by abdominal pain or vomiting.

- There is blood in or around the stool.

- Constipation is chronic and the dietary treatments described above have been ineffective.

Chronic constipation can be very painful and can affect your child's appetite, sleep, and mood. Some children suffering from constipation also develop anal fissures (cracks or tears in the skin near the anus) that bleed and cause stools to have streaks of blood. The fissure should heal once the constipation clears up.

DIARRHOEA

Symptoms. When your toddler's poo flows a little too freely (loose, watery poos that make an appearance several times a day), you're dealing with diarrhoea. Other symptoms of diarrhoea include poo colour and/or odour that may vary from the usual, mucus in the stool, and/or redness and irritation around the rectum. When diarrhoea continues for several days to a week, dehydration and weight loss can occur. Keep in mind that some children are naturally on a more frequent pattern of elimination than others, and as long as the stool is normal in appearance, that's not considered diarrhoea.

Cause. Diarrhoea occurs most often when your child has a virus, has eaten something irritating to the digestive system, or has gone a little overboard in the fruit department (apple juice is

---

Signs of Dehydration

Children who are losing fluids through diarrhoea and/or vomiting may become dehydrated and require prompt treatment with rehydration fluids (such as Dioralyte). Call the doctor if you note the following in a child who is vomiting, has diarrhoea, has a fever, or has otherwise been ill:

- Dry mucous membranes (you might notice cracked lips).

- Tearless crying.

- Decreased urination. Fewer than six wet nappies in 24 hours or nappies that stay dry for two or three hours should alert you to the possibility that urinary output is abnormally scant (urine may also show up darker on nappies). If your child uses the toilet, this possibility might be signalled by the child using the potty less often and/or by urine that is darker or more yellow than usual.

- Listlessness.

Additional signs appear as dehydration progresses. These signal the need for immediate medical treatment. Do not delay in calling the doctor or getting your child to an emergency room if you note any of the following symptoms. While waiting to reach the doctor or en route to the emergency room, give your toddler rehydration fluids, if possible.

- Coolness and mottling of the skin of the hands and feet.

- Very dry mucous membranes (dry mouth, cracked lips, dry eyes).

- Extreme fussiness or unusual sleepiness.

- No urinary output (nappies are dry) for six or more hours.

a common culprit). An allergy or food intolerance (to milk, for instance) can also cause diarrhoea, as can certain medications (such as antibiotics). Diarrhoea that lasts longer than six weeks (after all the above mentioned culprits have been discontinued) is called intractable and may be linked to an overactive thyroid gland, cystic fibrosis, coeliac disease, enzyme deficiencies, or other disorders.

Method of transmission. Diarrhoea that's caused by microorganisms can be transmitted via the faeces-to-hand-to-mouth route or by contaminated foods. Diarrhoea can also be triggered by excesses of, intolerances of, or allergies to certain foods or drinks.

Duration. An occasional looser-than-normal stool (lasting anywhere from a few hours to several days) is not a cause for concern. Some intractable cases can last indefinitely, unless the underlying cause is found and corrected.

Treatment. To treat diarrhoea:

- Give fluids. Try to get your child to drink at least 90 ml of fluid every waking hour. Milk, white grape juice (probably a better choice than apple juice when there's diarrhoea), or water may be sufficient in mild cases. In severe cases or if there's also vomiting, give your toddler rehydration fluids (such as Dioralyte) to prevent dehydration. If your toddler rejects the rehydration solution, try using a syringe to direct it to the back of the mouth, where the taste will be less noticeable.

- Feed right. Mild diarrhoea tends to improve more quickly when solids are continued. Severe diarrhoea (with or without vomiting) usually calls for rehydration fluid the first day followed by a slow resumption of the normal diet over the next couple of days.

- Medicate. If the diarrhoea is due to an underlying medical problem, the doctor will treat the problem. Antibiotics may be prescribed for bacterial and parasitic infections, but medication is not routinely given to young children for simple diarrhoea. Don't give any medication for diarrhoea unless it's been recommended or prescribed by the doctor.

- Go pro. Research suggests that probiotics can help prevent or treat diarrhoea in children. Feeding your tot yogurts containing live cultures or giving a probiotic supplement (in drops or powder form) – particularly during antibiotic therapy – can help prevent or help treat a case of the runs.

Prevention. Prevent diarrhoea by:

- Limiting foods (such as fruit), beverages (such as juice), and medications that trigger diarrhoea.

- Giving probiotics regularly.

- Following food safety guidelines (see page 123).

- Thoroughly washing hands after bathroom use or after changing nappies.

When to call the doctor. Call the doctor if your toddler:

- Shows signs of dehydration (see box, facing page).

- Is vomiting for longer than 24 hours.

- Refuses fluids.

- Has stools that are bloody or vomit that is greenish, bloody, or looks like coffee grounds.

- Has an abdomen that is bloated or swollen or if there seems to be anything more than mild abdominal discomfort.

URINARY TRACT INFECTION (UTI)

Symptoms. The symptoms of UTI (some of which are hard to recognise in young toddlers) include frequent and painful urination, blood in the urine, pain in the lower abdomen, lethargy, unusual-smelling urine, and/or fever.

Cause. UTIs occur because bacteria enter the urethra (the tube that carries urine from the bladder for excretion), causing infection. Because the urethra is shorter in girls and bacteria can travel up it more easily, girls have UTIs much more often than boys (and when boys do get a UTI, it is more likely the result of a urinary tract abnormality). An inadequate fluid intake could encourage a UTI.

Treatment. The treatment of choice is antibiotics. Ample fluid intake is also encouraged. Real cranberry juice, which seems to prevent bacteria from adhering to the lining of the urinary tract, may be particularly helpful.

Prevention. To prevent UTIs, take extra care when putting nappies on your toddler: wipe front to back and wash your hands before and after changing the nappy. Also, make sure your tot gets adequate amounts of fluid and regular nappy changes and avoid using potentially irritating bubble baths and soaps. Real cranberry juice (choose one without added sugar) contains compounds that prevent bacteria from sticking to the bladder and urethra walls. Citrus juice, like orange juice, on the other hand, may promote UTIs, as do caffeinated and carbonated drinks (not good toddler drinks, anyway).

When to call the doctor. As soon as you notice symptoms of a possible UTI, call the doctor.

The Most Common Chronic Conditions

ALLERGIES

What is it? That runny nose hasn't let up for weeks, that nagging cough is never-ending – and nothing you do can stop those tiny fingers from rubbing those watery, red eyes. At first you were certain your sniffling sweetie had a cold, but now you're wondering: could it be an allergy? Colds and allergies are actually pretty hard to tell apart: both can cause runny noses, sneezing, and coughing, and both can make your toddler miserable. But colds and allergies are very different conditions. While colds are infections caused by rapidly spreading viruses, allergies happen when your toddler's immune system overreacts to a normally innocuous substance.

Common allergenic substances include mould, dust mites, pet dander, pollen, and foods. If your toddler is allergic to something, his or her body will treat that substance like it's an invader. In an effort to fend off the invader, your child's immune system will churn out antibodies that trigger the release of a protein called histamine into the bloodstream. The histamine is what causes allergy symptoms.

It's estimated that about 10 to 20 per cent of children have or will have allergies at some time in their lives, and family history definitely can play a role.

If one parent has allergies, a child has a 25 per cent chance of having them, too. If both parents have allergies, the odds soar to at least 50 per cent. The way allergies are expressed is often different in different family members – one may have hay fever, another asthma, while a third may break out in hives when eating strawberries. An allergen can enter a child's system via inhalation (of pollen or animal dander, for example), ingestion (of nuts, milk, wheat, egg whites, soy products, or other food allergens, as well as medications, like penicillin), injection (or bee sting), or skin contact (jewellery made from nickel, clothing made from wool).

The symptoms of allergies vary depending on what body part or system is being affected:

- The upper respiratory tract (nose and throat): watery, runny nose (officially called allergic rhinitis); sore throat (from the allergy itself, but also as a result of mouth breathing when the nose is stuffy); postnasal drip (mucus dripping from the back of the nose into the throat can trigger a chronic cough); coughing.

- The lower respiratory tract (bronchial tubes and lungs): allergic bronchitis, asthma (see page 397).

- The digestive tract: gassiness; watery, sometimes bloody diarrhoea; vomiting.

- The skin: atopic dermatitis, including eczema (see page 46); hives (a blotchy, itchy, raised red rash); and facial swelling, particularly around the eyes and mouth.

- The eyes: itching, watering, redness, dark circles under the eyes, and other signs of eye inflammation.

- General: irritability.

Is It an Allergy? Or a Cold?

How can you tell whether that runny nose is a cold or an allergy? Take this quick test:

1. How would you describe the consistency and colour of your tot's mucus?
  a. Watery and clear
  b. Thick, cloudy, discoloured

2. If your tot is coughing, how would you characterise the cough?
  a. Dry
  b. Wet

3. Are your toddler's eyes
  a. Itchy and/or watery?
  b. Just fine?

4. Does your toddler have a fever?
  a. No
  b. Yes

If your answers were mostly "b", your toddler likely has a cold (or another respiratory infection). If most of your answers were "a", it might be an allergy you're dealing with.

If you notice any of these symptoms in your toddler, allergies are a possibility – but for testing and a diagnosis (and to determine the allergenic culprit), consider getting a referral from the GP to test for allergies. See the box on page 395 for information on severe allergic reactions.

Management. Once the offending allergen (or allergens) is identified, there are several approaches to treating the allergic child. First, and at the very least, you'll want to try to keep the allergenic substance out of your toddler's environment. Though it often isn't easy (especially in the case of an allergen that's in the air, like pollen), it is a positive first step. Here's what you need to know:

- **Food allergens:** In infants and young children, the foods most likely to trigger an allergic response are egg whites, cow's milk, nuts and peanuts, soy, and wheat. Following close behind at the top of the food allergy list are citrus, shellfish, and other fish. Keep in mind that not every adverse reaction to a food is allergy. Some people (tots included) have food "intolerances" or "idiosyncrasies" – reactions that don't involve the immune system. If a food bothers your child, even if the response isn't allergic, remove the food from your child's diet, but speak to the doctor about ways to gradually reintroduce the offending food, if possible.

  The only way to prevent food allergy reactions is to avoid eating the food (and, in rare cases, touching or even being near the food). That means you'll need to become adept at screening the food your toddler eats and is around, both at home and out of the house, and making sure it's always free of allergens. Some advanced label-reading skills will be invaluable, since milk, eggs, and other allergenic foods are often listed by other names on labels.

  Ask about ingredients at restaurants and when visiting other homes, and be sure that anyone who cares for your child, at home or away, is thoroughly briefed on the feeding protocol. To prevent leaving gaps in your toddler's diet, look for nutritionally equivalent substitutes. Substitute, for instance, oats, rice, and barley for wheat; mangoes, melon, kiwi, broccoli, cauliflower, and sweet red peppers for citrus; other protein sources (poultry, meat, cheese) for eggs; enriched soy milk for cow's milk.

  Researchers are studying whether slow exposure to allergenic foods can actually desensitise children with allergies, making it possible for them to overcome certain allergies. More study on that will need to be done before doctors start prescribing this approach to their allergic patients.

- **Pollens:** Most children do not develop hayfever (a.k.a. allergies to pollen) until the preschool years or later, but some start their sneezy seasons sooner. If you suspect pollen allergy (the clue: persistent symptoms when pollen is in the air and the disappearance of symptoms when the season is over), keep your child indoors as much as possible when the pollen count is high (usually in the morning) and when it is particularly windy during pollen season (spring, late summer, or autumn, depending on the type of pollen). Give daily baths and shampoos to remove pollen, and use an air conditioner in hot weather rather than opening the windows and admitting airborne pollen. Cut grass short to reduce pollen output. Outdoor pets should be bathed frequently, too, since their fur can pick up pollen.

- **Pet dander and other pet allergies:** Dander, the tiny scales sloughed off by the skin of animals, is the most common offender in an animal allergy. But some people are allergic to the saliva or the urine of animals, in which case the litter of cats or of small caged animals can be a problem. Cat dander is more often a problem than dog dander, and long-haired pets cause more problems than short-haired ones. If you suspect or have confirmed that your child is allergic to a pet, try to keep

Life-Threatening Allergies

Most allergy symptoms are just annoying: scratchy throat, runny nose, teary eyes, itchy bumps. But some allergic reactions – primarily anaphylactic responses to a specific food or drug or, rarely, to a bee sting – can be far more severe, even fatal. Serious reactions can include wheezing, hoarseness, and difficulty breathing; flushing of the skin, intense itching or hives, along with swelling of the face, lips, and throat (which can interfere with breathing); vomiting, diarrhoea (sometimes bloody), and abdominal cramps; a sudden drop in blood pressure, dizziness, light-headedness, fainting, loss of consciousness, and cardiopulmonary failure (anaphylactic shock). Such reactions require immediate medical treatment.

If your child is prone to severe reactions, your GP will give you a prescription for injections of epinephrine (a synthetic hormone for emergency treatment of anaphylaxis) in the form of an easy-to-use auto-injector pen (brand name EpiPen Jr). One injection of the EpiPen Jr will usually halt a severe allergic reaction in its tracks, allowing time to get medical attention. Make sure you and all of your toddler's other caretakers always carry it whenever you're out and about and know where the injector is at home and how to use it. Any time the epinephrine is used, your child should still go to the emergency room for follow-up because allergy symptoms can return. (Take the used auto-injector pen with you to A&E for safe disposal.)

Dial 999 immediately if your child has a severe allergic reaction and you do not have epinephrine on hand.

---

your animal and your child in different rooms. It may also help to relegate the animal to the garden, the cellar, or the garage as much as possible (if these are options) and bathe it weekly, get rid of wall-to-wall carpets (if you can), minimise upholstered furniture and other furnishings that retain dander, and use an air purifier with a high-energy particulate filter. In severe cases, the only solution may be to find the pet another home. Animal-hide and animal-hair rugs, carpets, and ornaments should also be avoided. Some children are allergic to birds, so if you can't work out your toddler's problem, consider that it might be your feathered friend. Find it a new home, and opt for synthetic rather than down-filled duvets, pillows, and upholstered furniture.

■ **Household dust:** It isn't the dust that triggers the sneezes in most dust-allergic people, it's the dust mites. These microscopic insect-like creatures can fill the air in your home and may be inhaled, unseen, by everyone in your family. That's no problem for most people, but for someone who is hypersensitive to these substances, it can mean misery. Limit your toddler's exposure, even if you only suspect this allergy, by keeping the rooms he or she spends the most time in (his or her bedroom, especially) as dust-free as possible. Dust often with a specially treated dust cloth, a damp cloth, or a cloth moistened with a bit of furniture polish when your toddler is not in the room; damp-mop floors and thoroughly vacuum rugs and upholstered furniture often. If possible, invest in a vacuum with a special high-filtration dust bag in your present vacuum so that you don't recirculate dust particles back into the air when you vacuum. Avoid carpeting, heavy draperies, chenille bedspreads, and other dust catchers in rooms where your toddler sleeps and plays; wash stuffed toys and blankets or comforters frequently in hot water (over 131°F/55°C seems to do the best killing job – warm water only kills some mites, and cold water only disables the mites' allergy-producing capacity). Wash any curtains, throw rugs, or other such items at least twice a month (or pack them away). Sheathe mattresses and pillows in airtight casings (cot mattresses usually come with airtight covers). Put filters over forced-air vents, and install a central air cleaner, if feasible. And, probably most important, keep humidity in your home moderately low, since dust mites generally can't survive where humidity is below 50 per cent. For suggestions on sprays or powders that can be used to kill mites in your carpeting and upholstery and advice on their safety, check with an allergy specialist.

■ **Moulds:** If your toddler is allergic to moulds, control moisture in your home by using a well-maintained dehumidifier. Provide adequate ventilation and use an exhaust fan vented to the outside to dispose of steam from the kitchen, utility room, and bathrooms. Areas where moulds are likely to grow (rubbish bins, fridges, shower curtains, bathroom tiles, damp corners) should be cleaned meticulously and frequently with a solution of equal parts of bleach and water or an anti-mould agent. Paint cellars and other potentially damp areas with a mould-inhibiting paint. Don't allow clothing or shoes to lie around damp or wet. Limit houseplants and dried flowers to rooms where your child spends little time, and store firewood outside the house. Live Christmas trees can foster mould, so keep yours in the house for only a few days or decorate an artificial tree instead. Outdoors, be sure that drainage around your home or building is good and that leaves and other plant debris are not allowed to pile up. Sunlight helps prevent damp areas from spawning mould, so cut back plants and trees to maximise sun exposure, if possible. If you have a sandpit, keep it covered at night and when it rains. In good weather, let it bake dry in the sunshine.

■ **Bee venom:** Keep a toddler who is allergic to bee venom away, as much as possible, from outdoor areas known to have bee or wasp populations (flower gardens, for instance). See page 428 for how to try to prevent stings and page 443 to treat them.

■ **Miscellaneous allergens:** Many other allergens can be removed, if necessary, from your child's environment: wool blankets (cover them or use cotton or synthetics) and clothing that touches your little one's skin; down or feather pillows (opt for foam or hypoallergenic polyester-filled pillows); tobacco smoke (allow no smoking in the house at all, and keep your toddler out of smoke-filled rooms away from home); perfumes (use unscented wipes and sprays, and avoid wearing cologne or perfume); soaps (use only hypoallergenic types); detergents (switch to a fragrance-free detergent for the washing).

The doctor may recommend antihistamines and prescribe steroids in certain cases to counteract the allergic response and/or reduce swelling. Allergy injections may be given for environmental or seasonal allergies, but usually not until a child is a little older. In severe allergic reactions, an epinephrine injection (see box, page 395) may be needed.

Prognosis. The majority of children who have milk, egg, and wheat allergies outgrow them by the time they're 5. And surprisingly, about 20 per cent of children with a peanut allergy outgrow that, too, by school age. Shellfish allergies, however, usually last a lifetime. Keep in mind that working out if your child is no longer allergic isn't something to experiment with on your own. Your GP can refer your child for a supervised feeding test to determine whether your child has outgrown an allergy.

Some nonfood allergies can also be outgrown, others are lifelong. Sometimes one allergy (to milk, for instance) will seem to be exchanged for another (hay fever).

ASTHMA

What is it? Asthma is a condition in which a person's small breathing tubes (called bronchioles) occasionally become inflamed, swollen, and filled with mucus, often in response to an allergen or other irritation to the airways. Asthma flare-ups can cause shortness of breath, tightness in the chest, coughing, and/or wheezing – and when an attack happens to your toddler, it can be downright frightening for both of you. In young children, sometimes the only symptom may be a recurrent hacking cough that is worse with activity or at night and may sometimes lead to vomiting. But there may also be rapid and/or noisy breathing, retractions (the skin between the ribs is sucked in with each inhaled breath), and chest congestion.

Over 1.1 million children in the UK have asthma. It is more common in young boys than young girls. Certain hereditary and environmental risk factors can predispose a child to

Asthma . . . or Not?

Your toddler has a cold and then starts to wheeze. The wheezing happens each time your little one gets a respiratory infection, and you've started wondering and worrying about whether asthma may be the underlying trigger. The truth is it may be too early to tell. That's because a 1-year-old is too young to take a lung function test – the gold standard method of asthma diagnosis – and because there are so many other conditions that can mirror the symptoms of asthma in a young child. So even if you're convinced your tot is showing all the hallmarks of asthma – for instance, a cold that lingers for many weeks, residual viral inflammation and excess mucus in your toddler's tiny airways that results in coughing and wheezing – your GP may not necessarily diagnose asthma unless the symptoms keep recurring and there is a family history of asthma or allergies.

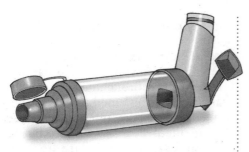

A spacer device (or holding chamber) helps administer asthma medication.

developing asthma, including a family history of asthma or allergies, having eczema or other allergic conditions such as hay fever, living with a smoker, having been exposed to smoke in utero, living in a polluted urban area, low birth weight, and obesity.

There are several factors that can trigger asthma in toddlers, and what causes an asthma flare-up in one person may be different from what causes a flare-up in someone else. Genetics play an important role, but the most common asthma triggers are allergens such as dust, pollen, and pet dander; irritants such as secondhand cigarette smoke, pollution, and paint fumes; infections like a cold or the flu; cold air; exercise; and even intense emotional outbursts (like a temper tantrum).

It's often not easy to diagnose asthma in toddlers because lung-function tests (in which a child blows into a machine that measures how quickly and how much air he or she can exhale) aren't accurate in children younger than 5. That means the doctor will rely heavily on what you reveal about your child's symptoms. So take careful notes about what your toddler's symptoms are, how often they happen, and under what conditions – and bring these notes with you to your appointment.

The doctor will also ask you about your family's medical history (does Mum or Dad have asthma or other allergic conditions?) to try to determine if your toddler is genetically predisposed to developing asthma.

Management. Depending on the nature of your child's asthma, the doctor might prescribe one or both of these medications:

- A quick-relief (short-acting) "rescue" medication called a bronchodilator that quickly opens up your child's airways when they are swelling during an asthma attack.

- A preventive (long-acting) medication, like an anti-inflammatory corticosteroid, which your toddler would need to take daily to keep the airways from getting inflamed in the first place.

Unlike medications that come in a liquid form, which children can swallow, most asthma medications need to be inhaled so they get delivered directly into your toddler's airways. The doctor will prescribe a metered-dose inhaler with an attachable plastic tube (or holding chamber) spacer

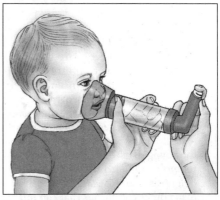

Young toddlers will use a mask when taking asthma medication.

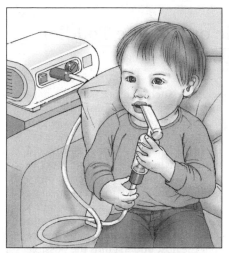

A nebuliser delivers asthma medication in the form of a mist, using either a mask or a mouthpiece.

device (see illustration, facing page) which makes the inhaler easier to use and more effective (the medicine gets farther down the airway). You activate the inhaler (usually by pressing down on the canister) and the correct dose goes into the spacer device. Then your child breathes normally for a few breaths and the medication makes its way into the airways. Since inhalers can be difficult for toddlers to use, you'll probably need to put a little mask over your toddler's mouth and nose that will be attached to the inhaler (older children will use the spacer device with a mouthpiece).

Another option is a nebuliser, which creates a mist from the liquid medicine and delivers it to your young toddler via a mask (or for an older child, via a mouthpiece). The nebuliser is powered by a small air pump that you plug in (which makes it less convenient and portable than the inhaler).

Whether or not your toddler is prescribed medication, there's plenty that you can do to keep those symptoms in check – particularly, helping him or her steer clear of allergens or irritants that cause the asthma to flare up (keeping the house clean and dust-free, for one, and staying away from homes with cats and dogs, for another). Trying as best you can to prevent your little one from catching colds, flu, and other infections that can step up symptoms will help, too (the flu injection is helpful for children with asthma). Probiotics may show promise, also, in helping to manage asthma – and since there's no harm (and there are many other potential benefits) in giving them to your toddler, this is something you may want to ask the doctor about.

Prognosis. While many children with asthma exhibit prolonged remission as they approach adolescence, airway hypersensitivity is lifelong. Symptoms often return in adulthood, though sometimes only mildly and intermittently (only with exercise, for example). But even when asthma continues into adulthood, most asthmatics can keep the condition under control with the right medicines, medical care, and self-care.

COELIAC DISEASE

What is it? Also called coeliac sprue, coeliac disease is an autoimmune digestive disorder in which there is a sensitivity to gluten (found in wheat, rye, and barley). When the gluten comes in contact with the small bowel during digestion, it damages the small intestine and interferes with the absorption of nutrients from food. Coeliac disease can begin any time in childhood or adulthood.

When the Food-Allergic or Coeliac Toddler Steps Out

Parties and playdates don't have to be off limits for toddlers with food allergies, food intolerances, or coeliac disease. But special precautions are necessary when your toddler goes visiting. At first, you'll have to be the one taking all the precautions (pulling out the gluten-free cupcake when the birthday cake is distributed, checking labels before a snack's served). Even as you do, though, it's important to begin teaching your little one how to stay away from the forbidden food or foods (though you'll still have to be the food police until he or she can be trusted to take over that duty). As your toddler becomes more verbal, rehearse such lines as: "I can't have milk, thank you." Point out foods that might contain off-limits ingredients (there's milk in the ice cream, there may be wheat in the muffins and crackers, there could be peanuts in that cereal bar). When it seems appropriate, supply your toddler's meal or snack. When it's not, let your child's host know in advance what foods your child can't have. Either way, be sure that the host understands the possible consequences of eating "just one bite" of such foods, and, if your child could have an anaphylactic reaction when you're not there, that he or she knows exactly what to do.

There is a wide range of symptoms (and some people are asymptomatic), but most infants and young toddlers with coeliac disease have stomach pain, diarrhoea-like stools (or less commonly, constipation) for more than a few weeks, a distended abdomen, and there is failure to thrive. In older toddlers there may be poor appetite, lack of weight gain (or even weight loss), and irritability. Occasionally, the only symptom is failure to thrive.

Evidence suggests the prevalence of coeliac disease across Europe is 1 per cent, but many go undiagnosed. Since coeliac disease is inherited, the odds are increased if either parent or any other siblings have the condition.

If you suspect your toddler may be showing signs of coeliac disease, ask the doctor about testing. A blood test can determine if your toddler has increased levels of certain antibodies related to coeliac disease. If the blood test is positive for the antibodies (or inconclusive), the doctor will likely want to take a biopsy of the small intestine via an endoscope through the mouth and stomach to check for damage to the villi, tiny finger-like projections that line the walls of the intestines.

Management. Once the diagnosis is confirmed, you'll have to keep your toddler on a strict gluten-free diet. Foods with gluten include most grains, pasta, cereal, and many processed foods. But baked goods and pasta made with rice, corn, soy, potato, or other gluten-free flours can easily replace the traditional grains. And happily, most supermarkets carry gluten-free products (check the label, and look for those that are not only gluten free but also whole grain). Plus, there are plenty of "regular" foods that easily fit into a gluten-free diet – like fruits and veggies, eggs, and unprocessed meat and poultry. There is also some preliminary research that suggests probiotics could be beneficial in managing coeliac disease.

As with food allergies (see page 393), you'll have to carefully monitor your tot's diet – particularly when he or she is out and about (at playdates, birthday parties, nursery). Support systems (online and in your community) are helpful, too, as you learn to cope with your toddler's condition. You can also get more information from NHS Choices (www.nhs.uk), and Coeliac UK (coeliac.org.uk).

Prognosis. The good news is that a gluten-free diet will keep your child symptom free for life.

SEIZURES AND EPILEPSY

What is it? A seizure is a sudden, temporary, involuntary alteration in physical movement or consciousness caused by abnormal electrical discharges in the brain. The severity and type of seizure, as well as how much and what part of the body is affected, vary depending on the portion of the brain involved. Seizures can range from involuntary convulsions of the entire body to a sudden and brief lapse of awareness of the environment. Epilepsy is a chronic (often inherited) disorder of the brain that causes recurrent seizures. An epileptic seizure is a temporary malfunction and does not mean the brain is deteriorating in any way.

Seizures occur in about 1 in every 25 children. They can affect children at different times in their lives and in different ways and can even be outgrown. Not all seizures are epileptic. Febrile seizures (see page 366), for example, are not – and the older a child is when the first febrile seizure occurs, the less likely he or she is to have another.

Management. The first step is diagnosis. Report a first seizure to your child's doctor, including such details as what preceded it, what your child looked like during it, and how long it lasted. Keep in mind that it's often difficult for an observer to be sure a child really is having a seizure, especially when the seizure is very brief or "absent" (when the child goes into a vacant stare for a few moments, but there is no shaking).

Happily, most seizures will stop on their own and do not require medical attention. Epileptic and other seizures are usually handled alike (see page 446). If epilepsy is diagnosed, medication or a combination of medications, carefully monitored, can often control or reduce the incidence of seizures.

Prognosis. After two seizure-free years, a child is generally no longer considered epileptic and medication may be gradually tapered off and then stopped. And more good news: the likelihood that a child will continue to have seizures drops each year as he or she gets older. For support and more information, contact the Epilepsy Society (epilepsysociety.org.uk).

HEARING LOSS OR IMPAIRMENT

What is it? There are many degrees of hearing impairment or hearing loss, and not all children with hearing loss are considered deaf. The child who is deaf has a profound hearing loss and can't understand speech through hearing alone, even with the use of a hearing aid.

There are two main types of hearing loss in young children:

- Conductive hearing loss. With this type of hearing loss, there may be an abnormality in the structure of the

Hearing Tests

Since a hearing deficit can affect so many aspects of a young child's development, early diagnosis and treatment is key. The most common hearing tests for toddlers under 2 are:

- Behavioural audiometry and play audiometry. In these tests, an audiologist teaches, and then looks for behavioural responses to, increasingly softer sounds.

- Otoacoustic emissions test. This test measures sound waves produced in the inner ear by placing a thin probe inside the ear canal and measuring the child's response to clicks or tones. It's based on the fact that the human ear not only hears sounds but also makes sounds in response to what it hears.

- Auditory brainstem response test. This test measures how the brain responds to sound, and is performed by placing electrodes on a child's head and earphones that play clicks or tones over the ears.

If tests show a hearing loss, further tests are recommended to confirm what type and degree of hearing impairment a child has.

ear canal or there may be fluid or structural abnormality in the middle ear (the space just beyond the eardrum). As a consequence, sound is not conducted efficiently through the ear canal and/or middle ear, making sound extremely low or inaudible.

- Sensorineural hearing loss. With this type of hearing loss, there is damage to the inner ear or to the nerve pathways from the inner ear to the brain. Usually present at birth, this type of hearing impairment is most often an inherited condition. It can also be caused by maternal infection before birth, or by certain medications taken by a mum-to-be.

In the UK around 840 babies are born with some hearing loss each year. Some will have hearing loss in only one ear (but even that can lead to problems with language and speech). Most newborns are given hearing tests soon after birth. If your child did not receive a hearing test as a newborn or if you suspect hearing loss now (even a child who "passed" the hearing test as an infant can develop hearing loss; see page 31 for those signs), speak to the GP about getting a hearing test for your child (see box). Since hearing deficits are more common among graduates of the Special Care Baby Unit, toddlers who were premature babies should be screened more carefully.

Management. It is important to diagnose a hearing loss early and to determine the level of impairment, which can range from mild to profound. Treatment of hearing loss, beginning as soon as a diagnosis is made, is very important to maximise a child's future hearing, learning, and language development. Treatment depends on the cause and may include:

- Medication (such as antihistamines or antibiotics), if the hearing loss is due to fluid in the ear. If there is no improvement over a 3-month period and the fluid persists, the doctor may recommend inserting tubes (see page 383). Happily, children who develop language delays due to temporary hearing loss from fluid in the ears will catch up to their peers language-wise by school age.

- Hearing aids. If a hearing loss is due to a malformation of the middle or inner ear, hearing aids (which amplify sounds) may be able to restore hearing to normal (or almost normal) levels. Hearing aids can also help with conductive hearing loss, as well as some types of sensorineural hearing loss. There are many types of devices, and the type used will depend on the child's age and the type of hearing loss.

- Surgery. Cochlear implants (electronic devices that are surgically placed in the bone behind the ear), possibly in conjunction with amplifying hearing aids, can make a huge impact by restoring limited hearing and improving the ability of totally deaf children to learn spoken language. The earlier a child receives the cochlear implants (preferably between age 1 and age 3), the better. Other surgical options, depending on the situation, include eardrum repair and repair of the tiny bones in the middle ear.

- Education. An education programme should be begun as soon as significant or sustained hearing loss is diagnosed, and may include: teaching a child to use devices that assist in learning to hear and/or to speak; cued speech, in which a system of manual cues is used to supplement speech (or lip) reading; a total communication programme, which uses a combination of speech reading, signing, and finger spelling and may also emphasise listening skills and speech production. Speech and language therapy (as well as counselling and training for parents) will also be part of the education process. The GP and hearing specialist can work together with you to help find the treatment programme that best meets your child's needs.

Prognosis. With proper treatment, children with hearing impairments can have successful, completely fulfilling lives. Some may eventually hear and speak, while others will learn to communicate through signing. Whether a child with a hearing impairment attends mainstream school depends on the individual child and the approach of the schools in your area to the education of deaf children.

CHAPTER 13

Second Year Safety

REMEMBER THE GOOD OLD DAYS, when you could plunk your not-yet-mobile child just about anywhere and trust that he or she would stay put – and stay relatively safe? Well, those days were officially over the moment your little one pulled to standing, and they've disappeared completely now that cruising and crawling have given way (or soon will) to walking . . . and running. And while these fledgling feats on two feet have provided your toddler with a brand-new, exciting perspective on the world (so much more to see! to touch! to pull down!), it's also given you a new – and somewhat scary – perspective on his or her safety. Fortunately, though toddlers-on-the-go may be accidents-waiting-to-happen, there are plenty of steps you can take to keep those accidents from happening. Most accidents (and accidental injuries) are, in fact, preventable. With a little know-how, a few childproofing gadgets here and there, some smart proactive injury-preventative manoeuvres, and a lot of vigilance, you can significantly reduce the odds of bumps, bruises, and worse.

Safety in the Home

Now that your toddler is toddling, your childproofing efforts will literally have to reach new heights. But it's not enough to merely pack away your fragile vases and heirloom candlesticks. There's still the toilet to contend with (a porcelain wishing well!), not to mention the stairs (a child-size climbing wall!), plus that jumble of computer wires in the home office (a toddler jump rope!). Clearly, you'll have to step up your child-proofing campaign to make sure your wily little one can't step, or climb, or reach into trouble. Here's a complete top-to-bottom how-to.

Being Careful Doesn't Mean Being Obsessive

All parents worry. And a certain amount of worry is healthy – it keeps parents on their toes, watchful, thoughtful, careful. But it's easy for any caring parent to cross the line from a healthy amount of worry to an obsessive amount (especially after reading this safety chapter, not to mention the first-aid chapter that follows), turning those carefree early childhood years into stressful ones.

It makes sense to be vigilant enough to keep your toddler safe – but not so much that you keep your toddler from being a toddler: curious, active, adventurous, inquisitive. Children pick up on parental anxiety, and a child who gets the impression that danger's lurking behind every corner may figure it's not worth turning those corners – and that could slow development. Growing requires taking calculated chances, and children whose parents have made them afraid of taking any chances may have a tougher time moving ahead.

So don't stop being vigilant, but try to keep safety concerns sensible and keep worry in perspective.

CHILDPROOFING AROUND THE HOME

Tour your home looking for potential trouble spots (for a toddler's eye view, get down on your knees), and make changes as necessary:

Windows. Children love looking out of the window. To make sure your child's perch at the window is safe, install metal window guards that attach to the sides of the window frame and have bars no more than 10 cm apart. Or install a locking device on double-hung windows that prevents the lower window from opening more than 10 cm. However you child-secure your windows, make sure that you can open these windows quickly in an emergency, as in case of fire. Fire brigade officials recommend that you use releasable window guards (which will allow for an escape in the event of a fire but still provide protection against falling) on at least one window in every room.

As an extra precaution, never place furniture that your toddler can climb on in front of a window. And if you have a window seat, make sure the window it's under is always locked or is protected by a window guard.

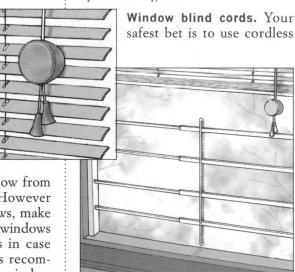

Window blind cords. Your safest bet is to use cordless

Window guards and cord stops (for Venetian or roller blind cords) make windows safer for toddlers.

window coverings throughout the house, especially in your toddler's bedroom. If you have blinds with cords and you can't replace them, then it's absolutely vital to keep those cords (which are strangulation hazards) out of your toddler's reach. Tie up cords on wall hooks so your toddler can't become entangled. Eliminate looped pull cords and install cord stops on all horizontal blinds and corded shades, which can be found at Safe Tots (www.safetots.co.uk).

Never place a cot, bed, other furniture, or a large toy that a child can climb on within reach of window coverings.

Doors. Since toddlers are quite capable of slipping out a door without anyone taking notice, keep all exterior doors, sliding doors, and screen doors locked at all times. Stick decorations or hang prisms on large glass doors so that toddlers (or anyone else) will be less likely to walk into them.

When it comes to interior doors, it's a good idea to seal off high-hazard rooms such as the bathroom (which

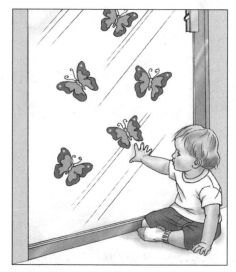

A glass door can look like an open door. Affix decorations to prevent dangerous collisions.

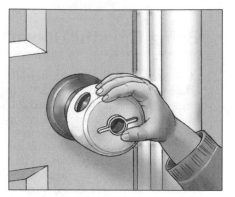

A doork handle cover, which makes it difficult for a toddler to turn the handle, can keep your child from leaving a safe area and entering an unsafe one.

contains water dangers and electrical appliances like hair dryers), the office (which may have computer wires and staplers), and the garage with hard-to-turn plastic door handle covers. Or install a lock high above your child's reach.

Install doorstops and door holders (that hold the door open) to protect fingers and hands from getting caught in slamming doors or door hinges.

Install safety gates at doorways to unsafe areas and always keep an eye on your toddler to make sure he or she doesn't scale the gates (see box, facing page).

Stairs. Prevent your wobbly walking tot from tumbling down a flight of stairs by installing sturdy safety gates at the top of the stairs *and* at the bottom. Consider putting the lower gate three steps from the bottom, so your child has a small, safe area to practise stair-climbing (a skill vital to keeping your tot safe in the future).

Keep steps clear of toys, shoes, and anything else that could trip up your toddler (or anyone else). Carpeting on the stairs may improve footing and help minimise injury in case a fall does occur. A plush, well-padded carpet or a thick

Safety Gates

Sometimes the only way to keep your toddler away from danger is to make it inaccessible – and that's why safety gates can be indispensable. Use them to keep your toddler in a room that's safe, or out of a room that's not, and at both the top and bottom of stairs.

Gates can be portable (these usually have to be released and completely removed for anyone to get through the doorway) or permanent (these usually stay in place, but swing open after unlatching), depending on your needs. Both varieties are generally adjustable to fit different door-frame sizes and can vary from 60 to 80 cm in height. If you are installing a permanent gate, be sure to screw it into wooden wall studs or use drywall anchors to prevent its toppling under the pressure of an eager-to-escape toddler or a child rolling along on a riding toy (drywall or plaster alone won't hold the screws securely). If you use a portable gate with an expandable pressure bar, be sure your little climber can't get a toe-hold on the bar, and don't use pressure gates at the top of stairs (opt for a gate that's secured to the wall, so your toddler won't be able to push it down and fall). Choose new models with plexiglass or fine mesh (if the mesh is flexible, it will be even harder for your toddler to climb on the gate) or with vertical bars (no more than 5.5 cm apart). Avoid using a hand-me-down gate, because older models are often unsafe. Any gate you use should be sturdy, with a smooth nontoxic finish, no parts that can catch little fingers, no sharp parts, and no small parts that can break off and be mouthed. Follow installation directions exactly. Gates are not useful once a toddler is over 86 cm tall or over 2 years old (by then a tot can usually work out how to get past them), except perhaps in the middle of the night, when a gate may discourage midnight wandering.

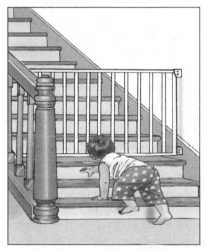

A gate at the top and bottom of the stairs will prevent falls. Leave the three lowest steps ungated so your toddler can practise stair-climbing skills.

nonslip rug at the foot of each staircase should also cut down on bumps and bruises.

Railings and balconies. Be sure that balusters (the upright posts) aren't loose and that the distance between these posts on stairs or balconies is always less than 12.5 cm, so a toddler can't get stuck or slide through (a 10-cm gap is safer for infants). If the gap is wider, consider a temporary safety "wall" (usually available at shops that sell child safety equipment) of plastic or firm mesh along the length of the stairway or balcony.

Your toddler's cot. One-year-olds don't usually have the height or climbing skills

Safe Heights

The "safety line" in your house will move ever higher as your toddler gets older, taller, more mobile, and more resourceful. Anything above the head of a child who's only mastered crawling is usually safely out of reach. The early walker can often reach the edge of the dining table, end tables, and low dressers. The young climber can clamber up a chair or other furniture to get to something higher. The competent walker–climber can push a chair (or a box, or a pile of books) over to the kitchen counter, the washing machine, and anything else seemingly out of reach – and scale it before you can turn around. Childproof and supervise accordingly.

necessary to scale the sides of a cot – but that doesn't mean they absolutely can't. So adjust the mattress to its lowest position and remove bulky toys, pillows, bumper cushions, and anything else that could be used as a stepping-stone to freedom. To soften a fall should your toddler manage an escape, place a plush rug, an exercise mat, or a couple of cushions next to the cot. Also be sure not to string any toys (such as a cot gym) across the top of the cot. Don't place a cot next to a window, near a heating vent or radiator, close to a floor lamp, or within reach of a heavy piece of furniture.

Your toddler's portable cot or playpen. A playpen or portable cot (if you use one) should have fine mesh sides (less than 0.5 cm openings) or vertical slats less than 5.5 cm apart. Always be sure the playpen or cot is fully open before putting your toddler in it, and never leave it partly opened – it could close up on a child who climbs into it.

Your toddler's bed. When it's time to graduate from the cot (don't rush – it's safest to wait until at least age 2½ to 3, or until your child is a minimum of 89 cm tall) install safety rails on both sides of your little one's bed and place it at least 0.6 m from windows, heating vents, radiators, wall lamps, or window blind cords. Never buy a bunk bed for a toddler or allow your toddler to sleep in the upper bunk of someone else's bunk bed.

Toy chests. In general, open shelves and bins are safer for toy storage. But if you still prefer to use a chest, look for one that has a lightweight lift-off lid or a safety-hinged lid – one that doesn't snap closed automatically when released. The hinge should allow the lid to remain open at any angle to which it is lifted. If you have an old toy chest that doesn't meet these requirements, remove the lid permanently. There should also be airholes in the body of the box (drill a couple on each side if there aren't) just in case a toddler climbs in and becomes trapped. Like all furniture children spend a lot of time around, a toy chest should have rounded corners or corner padding.

Unstable furnishings. Put away lightweight, rickety, or unstable chairs, tables, or other furniture that might topple if leaned on or pulled up on until your toddler is sure-footed enough not to need furniture for support. Climbers, too, need to be protected from furniture they can pull down easily.

Heavy furniture. Bracket heavy furniture (dressers, bookcases, entertainment units, shelves, and so on) to the wall with safety straps, L-brackets, screws, or even heavy-duty Velcro to prevent it from tipping over onto a toddler. Place heavy items on the bottom shelves of bookcases instead of up high so the unit is bottom heavy – and therefore more stable. Don't place items that are tempting to children (toys, stuffed animals, keys, remotes) on high shelves or on top of a cabinet, because your tot may want to climb up to retrieve them.

Heavy knickknacks and bookends. Place them where your child can't reach them and pull them over. Always overestimate the strength and ingenuity of a toddler.

Dresser drawers. Open drawers are an open invitation to climbers. Keep dresser and cabinet drawers closed so your child will be less likely to climb into them, possibly upending an unstable dresser. Place heavier items in lower dresser drawers if possible, to keep the dresser bottom heavy and less likely to tip over.

Loose handles on furniture or cabinets. Secure any loose handles that are small enough to be swallowed, cause choking, or get stuck in your toddler's mouth.

Sharp edges or corners. The sleek coffee table with the glass top was so chic last year, but now that your toddler is walking, it's looking more dangerous than stylish. Cushion sharp table corners and edges with bumpers that can soften the impact if your toddler knocks into them. The same bumpers work on any sharp edges throughout the house, such as fireplace hearths and low windowsills.

Floors. To minimise falls, keep clutter out of high-traffic areas; put away toys, wipe up spills, and pick up papers and magazines promptly; and be sure to repair loose or damaged floor tiles and carpeting so your new walker doesn't get all tripped up. Remember, bare feet offer more traction on any floor.

Rugs. Be sure they have nonslip backings and don't place them at the top of stairs or allow them to remain rumpled. Rubber matting or two-sided adhesive tape under small rugs and runners help make them slip-resistant.

Electrical cords. Move them behind furniture so that your toddler will be less tempted to mouth or chew on them (risking electric shock) or tug at them (pulling computers, lamps, or other heavy items down). If necessary, fasten the cords to the wall or floor with electrical tape or specially designed gadgets or place all your wires in a wire-and-cable protective cover. Do not use nails or staples and do not run cords under carpets, where they can overheat. Don't leave an appliance cord plugged into a socket when the cord itself is disconnected from the appliance – not only could this cause a major shock if the cord becomes wet, but serious mouth burns can result if it is mouthed.

Electrical sockets. It's important to cover electrical sockets to prevent your child from inserting an object or probing its mysteries with a drooly finger. But the small plug-in caps can easily end up in your toddler's mouth. Instead, use

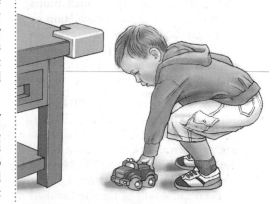

Bumpers on the sharp edges of furniture help prevent bumps and bruises.

Mechanical Fascination

A toddler's burning curiosity about everything – but especially about everything with an on/off switch, buttons to push, cords to pull – is one of the many traits that makes these little creatures so fascinating. But it's also one of the many traits that puts toddlers at risk. A tot's curiosity still outpaces his or her good sense and judgement by a long shot – and will continue to do so for years to come.

So keep dangerous electronics – sockets, the kitchen range and oven, the blow-dryer – completely inaccessible to curious fingers and mouths by child-proofing thoroughly. Then, find plenty of safe, supervised opportunities for your toddler to satisfy that fascination about the way things work. Let your toddler turn on the iPod or TV for you, switch on the lights or slide the dimmer from low to high, push the buttons that control the ceiling fan, "turn" the pages on your e-reader, almost tap computer keys, or manipulate the mouse to make letters, numbers, or pictures appear on the screen. If you can, visit a children's museum that has hands-on science exhibits that encourage pressing, pulling, pushing, experimenting, and exploring. Most of all, always remember what fuels that burning curiosity: your toddler has a lot to learn – and it's his or her job to learn it.

---

removable caps that cover both sockets (and that are too big to be a choking hazard) or replace the socket cover itself with a cover that has a sliding safety latch. Or place heavy furniture in front of sockets. If you use multiple-socket power strips, look for ones that are child-safe or have childproof cases.

Lamps and light fixtures. Don't place a lamp where a toddler could touch a hot bulb (choose cool-touch bulbs if you can), and don't leave a lamp or other light fixture without a bulb within your toddler's reach – probing an empty socket might be irresistible to your child, and it's very unsafe.

Fireplaces, heaters, stoves, AGAs and radiators. Put up protective grills, covers, or other barriers to keep small fingers away from fire and hot surfaces. Remember, too, that most of these surfaces stay very hot long after the heat has been turned off or the fire has died down.

Ashtrays. There are plenty of reasons not to allow smoking in your home, ever. Here's another one: a toddler who reaches into a used ashtray can get hold of a hot butt or sample a mouthful of ashes and butts. Always keep ashtrays out of your toddler's reach.

Rubbish containers. Because rubbish is always tempting to toddlers (and is rarely safe for them to touch or mouth), it may be easier to switch from open wastebaskets and recycling containers to ones that are covered and inaccessible to curious little hands.

Exercise equipment. Great for getting you in shape, but potentially dangerous for your toddler. Don't let your toddler near bikes, elliptical machines, rowing machines, treadmills, weights, and weight machines, and if possible keep rooms that store them inaccessible to your little one. Safety risks come with every piece of exercise equipment, and most are extremely tempting to curious tots (especially those with moving parts). Keep equipment unplugged when not in use by an adult (and make sure to keep the plug away and out of reach) so that it can't be turned on by a toddler. Be sure, too, that any safety straps or other long straps on exercise equipment are tied up and completely out of reach for a toddler (they could pose a strangulation risk). Ditto if you exercise with a jump rope; always store it out of reach of your toddler.

Tablecloths. Best to leave your table bare when there's a toddler afoot (or crawling around). Plan B: use short tablecloths with little or no overhang so your toddler can't pull them (and everything on the table) down, or hold longer tablecloths securely in place (with clasps designed to keep outdoor cloths from blowing away in windy weather). If you do set the table with a long, unsecured tablecloth or you encounter one on a visit, make sure your toddler is carefully supervised. Placemats can be a good alternative to long tablecloths, but remember that an intrepid toddler can pull down a placemat, too – so if it's set (with china or hot coffee, for instance), be sure your toddler is carefully supervised and kept away from the table.

Houseplants. Keep them out of reach, where your child can't pull them down or sample the leaves or dirt. Best to keep poisonous plants out of your home entirely (see box, below).

Painted surfaces. Many homes built before 1992 still harbour paint with high lead concentrations beneath layers of newer applications. As paint cracks or flakes, microscopic lead-containing particles are shed. These can end up in household dust and on a child's hands,

---

Red Light Greenery

Even toddlers who spurn greens at the dinner table have been known to chomp on a handful or two of leaves off the house and garden plants, as well as sample some potting soil. Problem is, some common plants are poisonous, or at the very least cause an upset stomach when eaten. So keep all plants out of reach and farm out potentially harmful plants to friends who don't have small children, at least until your toddler is more mindful of what belongs in his or her mouth. And just in case, know the names of all your plants (so if your toddler does take a nibble of one you'll be able to identify the plant in question to the doctor).

The following is a list of some (but not all) of the more common poisonous houseplants:

Amaryllis	English ivy	Oleander
Arrowhead vine	Flamingo flower	Oxalis
Azalea	Foxglove	Peace lily
Caladium	Holly	Philodendron
Clivia	Ivy	Poinsettia
Devil's ivy	Jerusalem cherry	Umbrella tree
Dumb cane	Mistletoe	
Elephant ears	Myrtle	

Lead Can Lead to Trouble

Lead is a major, proven environmental danger, especially for the very young. Large doses of lead can cause severe brain damage in children – even relatively small doses can reduce IQ, retard growth, and damage the kidneys, as well as cause learning and behaviour problems and hearing and attention deficits. Doctors can do a finger-prick test for lead, so if you think your toddler should be screened, ask the doctor – particularly if you live in a high-risk area or in a pre-1970s home or building which may have lead pipes; if your water supply might be contaminated with lead; if a sibling, housemate, or playmate has been diagnosed with high levels of lead in the blood; if you or another adult in your home has a job or hobby involving lead exposure; or you live near an industrial site that is likely to release lead into the air, soil, or water (a battery plant or a lead smelter, for example).

If testing shows high lead levels in your child's blood, it may be helpful to consult with a specialist in treating this problem. The use of iron and calcium supplementation may be recommended to minimise lead absorption into the body, and if blood levels are high, medication (chelation therapy) may be prescribed to remove the lead and prevent the damage it can cause.

You can find out if the water supplied to your house contains high levels of lead because your water company takes regular samples. However, if there are lead pipes on your property it is up to you to replace them.

---

toys, clothing – and eventually, of course, in the mouth. Check with the Lead Paint Safety Association (LiPSA), www.lipsa.org.uk for information on testing the paint in your home for lead. If testing shows evidence of lead, it'll need to be either completely removed by a professional trained in hazardous waste removal or covered with an approved sealant.

But lead paint doesn't just lurk on painted walls. Older toys, some new imported toys, and furniture can also contain lead-based paint. Keep up-to-date with furniture and toy recalls by going online to the Trading Standards Institute (www.tradingstandards.gov.uk).

Hazardous objects. Keep all hazardous household objects out of the reach of your toddler by storing them in drawers, cabinets, chests, or wardrobes with childproof latches; on absolutely out-of-reach shelves (you'd be amazed at how high some toddlers can manage to climb); or behind closed doors your toddler can't open. Be sure your child can't get at hazardous items that you're using when you turn your back, and always put away these dangerous items as soon as you've finished with them:

- Sharp implements such as knives, scissors, needles and pins, letter openers, razors and razor blades (don't leave these on the side of the bath or sink or dispose of them in a bin your toddler could get into), and wire hangers.

- Pens, pencils, and other pointed writing implements. When you let your toddler scribble with a pencil or pen, make sure he or she is seated and closely supervised – or substitute chunky nontoxic crayons or fat washable markers.

- Assorted small items, including thimbles, buttons, marbles, coins, safety pins, and anything else a child might possibly swallow or choke on.

- Lightweight or filmy plastic bags, such as produce bags, dry-cleaning bags, and packaging on new clothing, pillows, and other items. These can suffocate a young child if placed over the face. Remove clothing from dry-cleaning bags and new items from their plastic wrapping as soon as you get them home, then safely recycle or dispose of the plastic.

- Incendiary articles, such as matches and matchbooks, lighters, and unextinguished cigarettes.

- Tools of a trade or hobby: toxic paints, paint thinners, sewing and knitting supplies (including thread and yarn), woodworking equipment, and so on.

- Toys meant for older children. Keep building sets with small pieces or dolls with small accessories; large tricycles, bikes, and scooters; miniature cars and lorries; and anything with sharp corners, small or breakable parts, or electrical connections out of the reach of children under 3. Whistles can also be a hazard – a young child could choke on a tiny toy whistle and on the small ball inside any whistle if it comes loose.

- Button batteries. The disk-shaped type used in watches, calculators, hearing aids, and cameras are easy to swallow and can release hazardous chemicals into a child's oesophagus or stomach. Store new, unused batteries in an inaccessible place in their original packaging rather than loose. Keep in mind that "dead" batteries are as hazardous as fresh ones; dispose of them promptly and safely. Know what

No Gun Is a Safe Gun

Accidents involving young children and the tools, knives or even guns they find at home are too common and too often tragic. They're also completely preventable. Not by hiding the tools or weapons (children are capable of seeking and finding, or inadvertently discovering, just about anything their parents try to hide). Not by locking them up (all it takes is forgetting to secure the lock just once). Not by teaching children to stay away from tools or weapons (curiosity can easily erase parental warnings and overwhelm a toddler's underdeveloped impulse control). But by keeping tools in a secure garage and any kind of weapon or firearm out of the home.

Toddlers are impulsive and incurably inquisitive, perfectly capable of pulling a trigger on a gun, but not capable of comprehending the possible consequences of that seemingly innocent action. Keeping a gun or other weapon in the home, whether you think your toddler can get to it or not, leaves open the very real possibility of tragedy.

If you live on a farm and must keep a gun at home, keep it locked up, inaccessible, and unloaded; store the bullets in a separate locked location (children can work out how to load a gun); and buy a trigger lock or other device to prevent accidental discharge.

kind of batteries you are using. If your toddler swallows one, call 999 or take your child to A&E immediately. Keep regular batteries inaccessible to your toddler as well.

Happy Christmas Without the Hazards

It might be the season for merriment and Christmas magic, but to make sure it's as safe as it is festive, keep these safety tips in mind no matter which festival you're celebrating:

- Don't take a holiday from safety. Assess Christmas decorations for safety as you would any other household objects (examine for breakability, small parts, toxicity, size – tiny tree ornaments or dreidels, for example, are unsafe), or hang them high, out of the reach of young children. Avoid decorations that resemble sweets or food and might tempt your toddler to taste.

- Light safely. Be sure any decorative lights you use are CE-approved and are installed according to instructions. Check wires from lights used in previous years to be sure they are not frayed.

- Get that glow the safe way. Place lighted candles where children can't reach them and away from curtains and paper decorations. Keep nearby windows closed, so a breeze won't fan the flames. Never leave lighted candles on a table draped with a cloth that a toddler can pull off, and be sure to blow out the candles carefully before going to bed or leaving the house. Keep carved pumpkins unlit, or light them with a glow stick instead of a candle.

- Give the gift of safety. Don't leave potentially unsafe gifts under a tree or arranged anywhere else accessible to your toddler. Be sure gift-wrapping bows or ribbons are out of your toddler's reach, and clear away all wrapping, bags, and gift decorations promptly after the gifts are opened.

- Treat your toddler safely. Whether it's Halloween, Easter, or another festival that features sweets prominently, make sure you bring only safe treats into your home (nothing hard, gooey, sticky, or nut-filled, and no chewing gum) – just in case your tot finds a way to dip into the stash.

- Toddler-proof your tree. When trimming a tree, make sure your toddler can't pull down on the hanging lights or branches and topple it over (best to let your little one have access to the tree only when you're supervising closely). And in the interest of fire safety, purchase the freshest tree you can find (the needles should bend, not break), then have about 5 cm sawed off the trunk and set it up in a water-filled tree stand (but make sure your toddler can't get to the water). Or opt for a live tree you can later plant or donate to a local park (though keep your toddler away from the soil).

- Plant safely. Watch out for poisonous Christmas plants. See page 411 for a list.

- Leave fireworks to the pros. Don't try to create your own fireworks display. Even fireworks labelled BS⁷114, the British Standard that all fireworks should meet, are potentially dangerous, as are sparklers. More children than adults get hurt by fireworks so it is recommended that you never use fireworks or sparklers at home, especially near children. Get your fireworks fix at public events.

- Fake food. Apples, pears, oranges, and any other fake food made of wax, papier-mâché, rubber, or any other substance that isn't safe for children tempted to taste them (a candle that smells and looks like an apple pie, a child's rubber that smells and looks like a strawberry).

- Cleaning materials and other household products.

- Glass, china, or other breakables.

- Lightbulbs. Small bulbs, such as those in nightlights, are particularly easy for the toddler to mouth and break. Use an LED nightlight (it won't get hot) or a nightlight made specifically for infants and children (the bulb won't be accessible).

- Jewellery. Most risky: beads and pearls (which can be pulled off the strand and swallowed), and small items like rings, earrings, and pins. Some inexpensive imported children's jewellery may also contain toxic metals (like cadmium), which means that mouthing them could be dangerous.

- Mothballs. They're toxic as well as chokable. Opt instead for cedar or lavender blocks (not small balls, which can be mouthed). If you do use mothballs, store them in an area not accessible to your toddler, and air clothing and blankets out thoroughly (until the odour has dissipated) before using these articles.

- Shoe polish. If your child gets into it, the results can be messy. If your child eats it, it can cause digestive problems.

- Perfumes, toiletries, cosmetics of all kinds. They are potentially toxic.

- Vitamins, medicines, and herbal remedies, both topical and oral.

- Matches and lighters. Even very young children may be able to work out how to use a lighter. If you carry matches or a lighter in your bag, be sure that your bag, too, is always out of reach. Avoid igniting a lighter in front of your toddler and never allow him or her to light one under your supervision – that could literally inspire your tot to play with fire.

- Guns or weapons (see box, page 413).

- Strings, cords, ribbons, belts, measuring tapes, or anything else that could get wrapped around a child's neck.

CHILDPROOFING THE KITCHEN

The kitchen is the happy hub of most homes, and chances are your toddler spends plenty of time in yours. To ensure that your kitchen is as toddler-safe as it is busy, take the following precautions:

- Rearrange storage areas. Try to move anything that's off-limits to young children to upper cabinets and drawers – this includes glass and china breakables, food wrap boxes with serrated edges, sharp knives, utensils with slim handles that can poke an eye, skewers, graters, peelers, utensils and appliances with intricate gears that can pinch little fingers (like an eggbeater, nutcracker, tin opener), cleaning products, alcoholic beverages, medicines, anything in a breakable container, or potentially dangerous foods (nuts, hot chillis, bay leaves). Keep chairs, stepladders, and stools away from cabinets to discourage climbing (a little one can also get a leg up on an open cabinet shelf). Keep child-safe pots and pans, wooden and plastic utensils, tinned goods, paper

Poison Control

Every week, 500 under-5s are rushed to A&E because it's thought they have accidentally ingested a hazardous substance – and that's not surprising. Children, particularly very young ones, often explore their environment orally – which means that anything they pick up may go right into their mouths. They don't stop to consider whether a substance or object is safe or edible – or whether it's toxic. Their unsophisticated taste buds and sense of smell don't warn them that a substance is dangerous because it tastes or smells bad.

If your toddler ever ingests something you think might be harmful, (or you suspect that he or she might have), call 999 immediately.

To protect your toddler from accidental poisoning, follow these rules:

■ Lock all potentially poisonous substances out of reach and out of sight of your toddler. Even crawlers can climb up on low chairs, stools, or cushions to get to items left on tables or counters.

■ Follow all safety rules for administering medicines (see page 376). Never call medicine "sweets" or take medicine in front of your child.

■ Purchase products that have child-proof packaging, when possible – but don't rely on it to keep your toddler from getting them open. Store them safely away.

■ Make a habit of closing all containers tightly and returning hazardous substances to safe storage immediately after each use. Don't put a hazardous cleanser or a bottle of dishwasher detergent down even for a moment while you answer the phone or the door.

■ Store food and nonfood items separately and never store nonedibles in empty food containers (bleach in an apple-juice bottle, for example). Children learn very early where their food comes from, and will assume that what they see in a food

goods, unopened food packages that don't present a hazard when opened, and tea towels and cloths in the more accessible lower cabinets and drawers.

■ Install child-guard locks on drawers or cabinets that house dangerous items or items you don't want your toddler to touch, even if you believe these cabinets are inaccessible to your toddler. If your toddler works out how to unlock the safety locks (some clever toddlers do), consider installing a gate to keep your toddler out of the kitchen when you can't supervise

closely. Or, if you have an especially wily child, try doubling the protection by installing two locks per drawer or door, one at the top and one at the bottom or one on each side, since it would be very difficult for a toddler to open both locks at the same time. What your toddler cares to go after and to what lengths (and heights) he or she will go to get it will change over time (and depend on your toddler), so your storage arrangement may have to change as well. Reassess as needed – and always overestimate your toddler's resourcefulness, strength, and skill.

container is edible, without wondering why the "juice" isn't golden or the "jam" isn't purple.

- Never leave alcoholic drinks within your toddler's reach, and keep all wine and spirit bottles in a locked cabinet or bar (if you store any bottles in the fridge, make sure they're kept at the back of the highest shelf). Keep a close watch on your toddler at parties, where half-finished drinks might be left around, and never offer (or let anyone else offer) "just a sip" of an alcoholic drink for fun. Any amount of alcohol, no matter how small, can be harmful to your little one.

- Always choose the less hazardous household product over the one with a long list of warnings and precautions. But also be aware that even "green" products can be unsafe, so keep those out of your toddler's reach as well.

- When discarding potentially poisonous substances, empty them down the toilet – unless they can harm the septic system or pipes, in which case follow label directions for disposal. Rinse the containers before discarding (unless the label instructs otherwise) and put them out in a tightly covered recycling bin or wheelie bin immediately.

- To help everyone in your household automatically think "danger" on seeing a potentially poisonous product, put "poison" stickers on them. If you can't locate commercially printed labels (some websites can provide poison labels, www.keysigns.co.uk), simply put an "X" of black tape on each product (without covering instructions or warnings). Explain to your family that this mark means "danger". Regularly reinforce the message, and eventually your child will also come to understand that these products are unsafe.

- Be alert for repeat poisonings. A child who has ingested a poison once is statistically likely to make the same mistake again within the year.

- Set aside at least one easy-open cabinet (a child's fingers are less likely to be caught in a cabinet than in a drawer) for your toddler to explore. Some sturdy pots and pans, wide-handled wooden spoons, strainers, a colander, tea towels, plastic bowls, and containers with lids can provide hours of safe yet satisfying entertainment. If this cabinet is away from major kitchen work areas (not too close to the stove or the sink), your toddler will be less likely to be underfoot when enjoying it.

- Use the back rings of the stove for cooking, when possible, and always turn the handles of pots towards the rear so they can't be reached and pulled over by a curious child. If you'd like to be extra careful, you can install a stove guard (see illustration, page 419) that prevents small children from reaching even the sides of pots that are on the stove. If gas or electric ring controls are on the front of the stove, snap on commercial stove-knob covers. Appliance locks can keep conventional and microwave ovens inaccessible. Remember

Not a Do-It-Yourselfer?

Just don't have the time, the inclination, or the confidence to totproof your home (and feeling pretty overwhelmed about doing it, anyway, after reading over this chapter)? Hire a professional to do the job for you. Childproofing services do it all – from fire and electrical safety to locks of every variety. They'll investigate your home for potential dangers and take all the appropriate precautions for you – securing furniture, cabinets, and doors; installing window guards, gates, and alarms; scanning for choking, poisoning, and burn hazards; checking wiring; safeguarding your pool or pond; and more. Does peace of mind come with a price? Definitely – these services can be expensive. Visit www.babysafehomes.co.uk for more information.

that the outsides of some ovens (and of other appliances, such as toasters, coffeemakers, and slow cookers) can get hot enough to cause burns and that they can stay hot long after they've been turned off – so keep them out of reach or keep your toddler away when you use these appliances.

- Keep the dishwasher locked between uses, and be careful when you're loading and unloading – it takes only a second for a toddler to grab something sharp or breakable. Add detergent just before you wash the load, and close the door promptly. Particularly tempting to tots: brightly coloured dishwasher pellets.

- Keep sponges out of reach. One bite of a sponge can turn into a choking hazard.

- Keep the fridge off-limits by installing an appliance lock. Hang that precious artwork with large fridge magnets, since small ones can be pulled down and mouthed (a choking hazard).

- Don't let your child sit on a countertop. Besides the potential for a tumble, those curious fingers could quickly end up reaching for something they shouldn't (like a knife or a toaster).

- To avoid spills that burn, don't carry your wriggling toddler and a hot drink or plate at the same time. Be careful, too, not to leave a hot cup or a hot plate at the edge of a table or counter, near your toddler's place at the table, or anyplace else where small hands can reach it.

- Keep rubbish and recycling in tightly covered containers that your child can't open and rummage through or under the sink behind a securely locked door.

- Clean up all spills promptly – they make for slippery floors.

- Store kitchen detergents, scouring powders, silver polishes, and all other potentially toxic kitchen supplies out of your toddler's reach (see box, page 416).

- Keep your toddler away from toothpicks, skewers, and any other pointy objects; they can be accidentally or intentionally poked in eyes, nose, ears, and elsewhere, with serious results. If you're using a knife, make sure your toddler can't reach it when you put it down.

- Don't leave a cleaning or utility bucket or other container of water

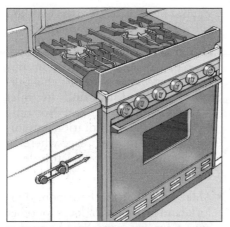

Protect your toddler with safety devices such as cabinet locks and a stove guard.

standing around and within reach of your toddler. A toddler can drown in about 5 cm of water.

CHILDPROOFING THE BATHROOM

The bathroom is full of fascination for a curious toddler (all that water, for one thing), but it's also full of potential risk – which means your toddler should always be closely supervised in it. One way to keep your little one from wandering into the bathroom when you're not looking is to put a hook and eye or other latch or lock high up on the bathroom door, and to keep it latched when not in use. (Once your child is using the toilet, the lock will have to go.) But don't count on locks – inevitably, there will be times when the door will be left open. Make your bathroom toddler-safe, too, by taking the following precautions:

- If the bath isn't nonslip, apply non-slip decorations or use a rubber bathmat.

- Use nonslip bath rugs on the floor to minimise falls and to cushion your toddler when falls do occur.

- Lock all bathroom drawers and cabinets, including the medicine cabinet – you can't assume any of them are out of reach for a climbing toddler. Among the many bathroom staples you should keep behind locked doors: medications (including over-the-counter ones), vitamins, mouthwash, toothpaste, hair products, skin products, cosmetics, sharp grooming implements (razors, scissors, tweezers, clippers), and bathroom cleaning products (including the toilet bowl brush and the plunger).

- Keep the edge of the bath, the top of the cabinets, and the back of the toilet clear of anything your toddler shouldn't touch or mouth (including soaps, shampoos, razors). Place those on a high shelf between uses instead.

- Never use a hair dryer or other electrical appliance near your toddler when he or she is in the bath or playing with water. Always unplug and safely store the hair dryer, hair straighteners, and other small electrical appliances when they're not being used. Some of the potential risks if you leave them plugged in: electric shock when a child dunks a hair dryer in the toilet or nibbles on the cord; a burn when he or she flicks on the switch on a curling or flat iron; skin irritation from trying to "shave" with an electric razor. Even unplugging appliances won't be enough if your child has good manual dexterity or if hair straighteners or a hair dryer is still hot (they can cause burns for several minutes after they've been turned off). And the cords themselves present a strangulation hazard.

■ To prevent severe or lethal shocks, make sure all sockets in the bathroom (and kitchen) are RCD-protected and conform to Building Regulations 2008.

■ Keep the hot water temperature in your home set no higher than 120°F/48.8°C to help minimise accidental scalding. Young children have thin skin, so water at 140°F/60°C can give a child a third-degree burn – serious enough to require a skin graft – in just three seconds. If you can't adjust the heat setting (if you live in a block of flats, for example), install an antiscald safety device (available from plumbing supply shops) in the bath, which will slow water to a trickle if it reaches a dangerously high temperature. For additional safety, always turn on the cold tap before the hot and turn off the hot tap before the cold. And routinely test bath water temperature with your elbow or whole hand, swishing it around to make sure the temperature is even throughout, before letting your toddler climb in. If you're planning to install new bathroom fixtures, a tap with a single control – which you can set at a comfortable temperature and allow your toddler to turn on and off – is safer than separate hot and cold taps.

■ Consider a protective cover for the bath spout to prevent bumps or burns should a child fall against it.

■ Never leave your toddler in the bath unattended, even in a bath seat (these aren't recommended, anyway, since kids can topple over in them), even for a moment. This rule should be strictly observed until your child is at least 5 years old.

■ Never leave any amount of water in the bath when it's not in use; a small child at play can fall into the bath and drown in about 5 cm of water.

■ When the toilet isn't being used, keep the lid closed with suction cups or a safety lock made for this purpose. Most toddlers find the toilet a fascinating play space. Not only is this kind of exploration unsanitary, but it's another place where an energetic toddler could topple in headfirst.

■ Make sure that the bathroom door lock (and interior door locks for other rooms, for that matter) can be opened from the outside, and stash a tool or key for opening it above the door frame.

■ Don't bring your toddler into a sauna or steam room. A young child's body isn't adept yet at heat regulation. Hot tubs and Jacuzzis are also unsafe for young children.

Dressing for Safety

Cuteness counts, but safety is the most important feature to consider when choosing your little one's clothes. Use only flame-retardant sleepwear, and be sure that trouser cuffs aren't too long or pyjama feet too floppy. If your toddler walks around the house in socks, be sure they have nonslip bottoms. Soles of slippers and shoes that are slippery smooth should be roughed up by rubbing with sandpaper. Avoid long play scarves or sashes that can trip up your child (or pose a strangulation risk), as well as strings or ties longer than 15 cm.

CHILDPROOFING THE UTILITY ROOM

When you have a toddler, you've got dirty clothes – and lots of them. But while your washer, dryer, detergent, stain remover, and other laundry products may be indispensable to you, they can be dangerous in the wrong little hands. To reduce the risks:

- Limit access to the laundry room or area. If it has a separate door, keep it closed and locked. If not, secure the area with a gate, if possible.

- Keep the washer and dryer doors closed when you're not loading or unloading.

- Keep bleach, detergents, and other laundry products in a locked cabinet and store them promptly again after using. When containers are empty, rinse them thoroughly, then place them in a toddler-inaccessible recycling or rubbish bin.

CHILDPROOFING THE GARAGE

Not surprisingly, most family garages (and greenhouses, workshops, sheds, and hobby areas) are crammed full of toxic products, sharp objects, and other potential hazards, so:

- If your garage is attached to your house, keep the door between the two locked at all times. If the garage is separate, keep the garage door closed. Keep any vehicles in the garage locked, too.

- If you have an automatic garage door, be sure that it's one that automatically reverses or stops if it hits an obstacle (such as a child). Recent changes in safety regulations require that your door be fitted with a self-learning safety protection system or a pressure sensitive safety sensor switch across the lower edge of the door. Check your garage door periodically by lowering it on a heavy cardboard box or another expendable item to be sure the safety features are still operating; if not, disconnect the door operator until it's been repaired or replaced. The inside button for the door operator should be too high for your toddler to reach, and any remote controls should be kept where children can't get to them. Another reason to keep the car locked: that will lock the remote.

- Store paints, paint thinners, turpentine, pesticides, weed killers, fertiliser, antifreeze, windscreen washer fluid, and other car-care products in an out-of-reach cabinet. (A locked cabinet installed as high up on the wall as possible can work well.) All hazardous products should be stored in their original containers, so that there is no mistaking their contents, and the directions for their use and safety warnings should be visible. If you aren't sure of what's in a particular container, dispose of it as you would hazardous waste.

- As an extra precaution, don't let your toddler loose in the garage (or a workshop or other dangerous space), even for a moment. Carry your toddler to and from the car.

CHILDPROOFING TODDLER TOYS

Toys and tots are a natural combination, and most toys meant for tots are safe. Still, when filling your toddler's toy box, you'll need to consider not only which playthings are fun and

Detecting Trouble

To keep your family safe from fire, be sure to install smoke detectors (at least one on every floor – better yet, one in each bedroom) and test them monthly to make sure they're in working order. Replace the batteries on battery-operated models at least once a year (pick an easy-to-remember date, such as your birthday or when daylight saving time changes).

Install and regularly test carbon monoxide detectors as well (they'll warn you of increasing levels of this odourless but treacherous gas).

educational, but also which are completely safe.

Check all toys for:

- Age-appropriateness. For safety's sake, stick to the label recommendations on toys you buy (or borrow) for your toddler. And keep the toys of any older siblings away from your toddler if they don't meet the standards listed below.

- Safe size. How small is too small? Avoid any toy that can fit completely into your toddler's mouth or that has any small parts that can (use the toilet paper roll test; see illustration). Also be sure that a larger toy can't be squeezed or moulded into a smaller, potentially dangerous size, or that a small piece can't be bitten or pulled off. Wondering if it's okay to bring on the small parts if your little one seems to have moved beyond mouthing objects? Play it safe and keep those small parts away – you never know when that oral impulse will strike once again (or the impulse to stick

an object somewhere else it doesn't belong, like in an ear or up the nose or rectum), if only out of boredom or curiosity.

- Sturdy construction. A flimsy toy won't last long and could also shatter or fall apart, producing dangerously small or sharp parts that could injure your toddler.

- Safe finish. Paint, if any, should be nontoxic, lead free, and durable; the finish should be unlikely to peel or splinter.

- Safe ingredients. Art supplies, which end up in the mouth and on the skin as often as they do on paper, should be nontoxic (look for notification of this on the label). Look for water-based felt tips and paints; white glues or pastes; and nontoxic crayons.

Avoid all toys with:

- Removable or loose small parts: button eyes on teddy bears, shoes on dolls, tiny toy "people" or characters, small beads, tiny building bricks, easily detachable squeakers in or on squeeze toys, and any other toys or parts small

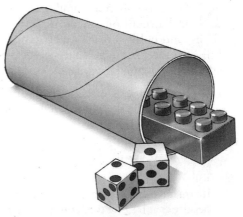

Anything that can fit through a toilet paper roll can present a choking hazard to young toddlers.

Certifiably Safe

Pushchairs, booster seats, safety gates, cots, and a variety of other equipment designed for children must conform to the British Standards Institution and carry a BSI number. Look for this certification when making purchases (or borrowing them). To learn more, visit www.bsigroup.com.

enough to swallow, choke on, or be poked into an ear or a nostril.

- Strings, ribbons, or cords longer than 15 cm. Toys that come with strings attached pose a strangulation risk. Avoid these toys or remove or trim the strings before letting your toddler play with them.

- Springs, gears, or hinges that can catch little fingers or hair.

- Sharp points or edges. Watch out for sticks picked up outdoors – fun to play with, but too easy to poke an eye with if they're pointy. Pencils and pens should be scribbled with only under supervision.

- High noise levels. Toys that produce sounds of 100 decibels or more (such as cap guns, motorised vehicles, and very loud squeeze toys) can damage a toddler's hearing – and even prolonged exposure to toys that emit 85 decibels of sound can be harmful. There are voluntary maximum decibel standards for toy makers to follow, but not all manufacturers stick to the standards. And since there's no decibel labelling on toys, it's not easy for parents to know whether a toy their child is playing with exceeds safe sound limits or not. So to protect

your little one's hearing, experts recommend that you listen: don't buy toys that sound too loud in the shop (you can't speak normally over the noise), and make sure the volume on toys you already own is on the softest setting, or remove the batteries from loud toys.

- Heating elements or electrical connections. Battery-operated toys are okay as long as the batteries are completely inaccessible to curious fingers. Small button batteries are a choking and swallowing risk, and all batteries are dangerous if a toddler chews on them.

- Sponge-like construction. Toddlers are often tempted to chew on balls and other items made of spongy material (like paint sponges) and can gag or even choke on them or on pieces bitten off of them.

- Decorations or other small stickers. Should your toddler manage to

There's No Substitute for Supervision

You've latched and locked, capped off and padded, checked and rechecked. All the hazards you can think of are taken care of. Time to relax? Not really. Though you've taken the first and extremely crucial step in keeping your toddler safe by childproofing his or her surroundings, you're not off the hook yet. Constant adult supervision is as important as childproofing when you've got a toddler under 2. So keep your home safely childproofed for your little explorer, but also keep him or her within eye- or earshot at all times.

Indoor Pest Control

Ants. Flies. Mice. Woodworm. Bedbugs. Unwelcome pests are unavoidable in virtually every flat and house – at least occasionally. And you'll want to keep them out of your home or get rid of them once they enter. But how do you do this without using substances hazardous to your toddler? Try:

Sticky insect or rodent traps. Not reliant on killer chemicals, these snare crawling insects in enclosed boxes (roach traps) or containers (ant traps), flies on old-fashioned flypaper (with no added insecticide), and mice on sticky rectangles. Because human skin can stick to their surfaces (the separation can sometimes be painful), these traps must be kept out of the reach of children or put out after they are in bed at night and taken up before they are up and about in the morning. From a purely humane standpoint, these traps have the disadvantage of prolonging the death of their victims.

Baited traps. These traps do contain a poison, but it gives off no chemical fumes and is enclosed in the trap, making it more difficult for a toddler to reach. Still, place the traps out of reach of your child.

Box traps. The tenderhearted can catch rodents in box traps and then release them in fields or woods far from residential areas, though this isn't always easy or practical. Because trapped rodents can bite, the traps should be kept out of the reach of children and carefully monitored or put out only when children are not around.

Safe use of chemical pesticides. Virtually all chemical pesticides – including boric acid – are highly toxic, not just to pests but to people as well. If you opt to use them, do not spread them (or store them) where young children can get to them or on food-preparation surfaces. Always use the least toxic or most "green" substance available for the job. If you use a spray, keep your child out of the house while spraying and for the rest of the day, if possible. Better still, have the spraying done while you're on holiday or otherwise away from home for a time. When you return, open all the windows for a few hours to air out your home.

To find information on the safest pest control, contact: Pest Control Direct, 01323 846845, pestcontroldirect. co.uk; Pest Control Services, direct. gov.uk; or Environmental Protection, environmental-protection.org.uk.

remove a very small sticker (not a very difficult task) and mouth it, it becomes a choking risk.

- Projectile parts. Toy bows and arrows, dart guns, and so on, are inappropriate for young children, as they put eyes at risk. Also stay away from high-powered water pistols, which can do a lot of damage, too.

- Latex balloons. Little ones love balloons of all shapes, sizes, and varieties. And as long as they're fully inflated, all balloons are safe for tots to enjoy. The problem is, a toddler can choke on a deflated latex balloon, fragments of a balloon that's popped, or a slowly deflating balloon left lying around. And once a toddler has inhaled a balloon, there may not be much anyone can do – even the Heimlich manoeuvre (abdominal thrusts) may not work. If you bring latex balloons into your home, closely supervise their use. Don't allow young children to try to blow them up, play with them unsupervised, or chew on them. Deflate and dispose of them carefully and promptly after the party's over. Better still, use Mylar balloons.

- Damaged toys. Check your toddler's toys periodically for wear and tear – exposed stuffing bursting from the seam of a teddy bear, cracked plastic on a push toy, splinters on a wooden toy, or anything else that could make a once-safe plaything hazardous. Repair or discard those that are unsafe.

Calling All Recalls

Wondering if the toddler toys, furnishings, and gear you have at home are safe for your tot to use? Find out which products have a history of safety problems and keep up-to-date on the latest recalls by calling Trading Standards 08454 040506, www.tradingstandards.gov.uk.

Safety When Out and About

So you've childproofed every inch of your house or flat, which – along with all that watching and supervising – will keep your toddler as safe as possible at home. But what about when you step out of your home? Injuries can happen in your own back garden or someone else's, at the local playground or on the street. You can't childproof the whole world (though there will be times when you'll wish you could), but you can easily prevent most outside-the-home accidents.

OUTDOOR SAFETY

Keep these safety tips in mind when you're outdoors with your toddler:

- Never let a toddler play outdoors alone, or snooze in a pushchair outside alone.

- If possible, enclose a small area of the garden (if you have one) for toddler play. Use fencing that is continuous or has less than 10 cm between its slats and that a toddler couldn't possibly scale. Equip the space with playthings and be sure it doesn't contain any hazardous plants (see page 411), rocks, or potentially harmful debris. Even in a safe outdoor space, a child under age 2 should be supervised.

- Never leave your toddler alone on the driveway or in an area where he or she might be able to access the driveway. Always walk around (and look under) your car to check for children before you back out.

- Don't mow the lawn when your child is in the garden. Even if you try to clear all debris from your route before you begin, a pebble or other missed

A Safe Place to Play

Swings, slides, climbing frames – what could be more fun for a toddler than spending time at a playground? To make sure that the fun stays safe, be sure that any playground equipment your toddler plays on, at home or away, meets the following standards:

- Be sure it is age-appropriate. Best for home use are adjustable units that are appropriate now and will grow with your child. For toddlers, equipment should be no higher than 1.8 m at its topmost point; play platforms should be no more than 1.2 m high, have guardrails, and be easy to get down from. A slide should have no more than a 30-degree incline, and the platform should be as wide as the slide and at least 56 cm deep; if the slide is more than 1.2 m high, it should have raised sides.

- Be sure that it's safe. Outdoor play equipment should be sturdily constructed, correctly assembled (follow the manufacturer's directions exactly), firmly anchored in concrete (which should be covered with soft earth or padding), and installed at least 1.8 m from fences or walls. All screws and bolts should be capped to prevent injuries from rough or sharp edges; check for loose caps periodically. Avoid S-type hooks on swings (the chains can pop out of them with vigorous swinging). If there's a climbing rope, it should be anchored at both ends. Swing seats should be bucket-type, of soft, shock-absorbent materials (such as plastic, canvas, or rubber rather than wood or metal) to prevent serious head injuries, and at least 61 cm apart and 76 cm from support posts. All rings and other openings should be designed to avoid head

object (such as a nail) could become a dangerous projectile. Store the mower, and all other gardening tools, safely out of your toddler's reach. And don't carry your little one with you on a riding mower – it's just as dangerous.

- Be sure that porch and deck railings are sturdy (check them regularly for deterioration or damage) and spaced so that young children can't stick their heads through or fall through the sides. Any outdoor area with a precipitous drop should be inaccessible to young children.

- Check public play areas before letting your toddler loose. Be alert for dog droppings, broken glass, and anything else potentially harmful.

- Don't allow your toddler to play in deep grasses or anywhere poison ivy or stinging nettles might lurk, or where – out of sight – he or she might snack on some poisonous plant. This is also the kind of locale where ticks may be biting.

- If you have a sandpit, keep it covered when it's not in use (to keep out animal droppings, leaves, blowing rubbish, and so on). If the sand gets wet, let it dry out in the sun before covering. When filling the sandpit, be sure to use play sand or sifted ordinary beach sand.

- If you have an outdoor fireplace, fire pit, or barbecue grill, make sure to keep your toddler away from it while

entrapment (smaller than 9 cm or larger than 23 cm). Metal should be painted or galvanised to prevent rust; wooden equipment should be weather-treated to prevent rotting and checked periodically for splinters.

- Be sure that play equipment is in good repair; check regularly for broken parts, loose bolts, missing protective caps, worn bearings, exposed mechanisms that could catch fingers, eroded metal (which could cause cuts), splintered or deteriorated wood. Repair home equipment immediately; if that's not possible, remove any damaged parts or make the play area off-limits until repairs are made. If park equipment is in poor repair, report the problems to your local parks department, and avoid that playground until the equipment is fixed.

- Be sure that surfaces under play equipment are soft. Remove rocks and tree roots that are exposed or just under the surface of the play area, then spread with a layer of play sand, sawdust, wood chips, or mulch that's 30 cm deep, composition rubber mats, or other shock-absorbent material. Do not use concrete, packed earth, or grass, which are all dangerously hard; serious injury is possible on such surfaces should a young child take a fall from as little as 30 cm up. The surfacing material should extend roughly 1.8 m beyond the play area.

- Be sure that children using play equipment aren't wearing capes, floppy sleeves, flowing dressing-up clothes, scarves, hoodies with long strings, or any other clothing that might get caught or entangled.

- Any play equipment is only as safe as the supervision a child playing on it receives. So be sure to watch your toddler carefully and from close range.

it's in use. The fire should be attended by an adult from the moment it's lit until it's been doused and is completely cool. With a charcoal grill, supervise until the coals, if any, have cooled and been disposed of (remember that coals that aren't doused with water stay hot for a long time after the fire itself is out). If you use a tabletop grill, be sure to set it on a stable surface that your toddler can't reach or overturn. If you have a propane grill, make sure your child can't access the controls, gas tubing, or tank valve.

- If your older toddler has a tricycle, be sure that he or she always wears a specially designed toddler bike helmet when riding – even in the driveway, on the pavement, or in the park. What's more, getting into the helmet habit will not only protect your toddler now but in future years of daring sports to come (and they're coming!). If you ride a bike, set a safety-conscious example: always wear a helmet yourself.

- If you live in a suburban or rural area, be on the alert for wild animals; stray dogs or cats, foxes, and bats can all carry diseases. An infected animal may behave in an abnormal way, and may be more approachable by humans than a healthy one. Keep rubbish bin lids closed to discourage foraging visitors, and don't leave pet food outside.

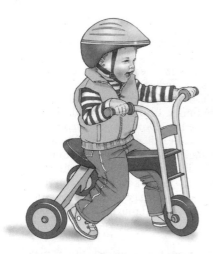

Make bike helmets mandatory for everyone who rides, even a toddler on a scooter.

- In hot weather, always check metal parts on playground equipment, pushchairs and car seats, and outdoor furniture before letting your toddler come in contact with them. Metal can get hot enough, especially in a scorching sun, to burn a child severely with just a few seconds of contact. Tarmac or asphalt can also get hot in the sun, so don't let your toddler play barefoot on it on very hot days.

SAFETY AROUND INSECTS

With their jam-smeared cheeks, fruit-sticky fingers, bright-coloured clothing, and quick, unpredictable movements, toddlers make appealing insect targets. Easy ones, too, given their curiosity, penchant for playing in the dirt, mud, and grass, and lack of insect savvy (a young child doesn't usually know enough to steer clear of bees, to come inside when the flies are biting, or to avoid areas where ticks lurk or mosquitoes congregate).

Though most insect stings and bites are harmless (if often uncomfortable), they can occasionally transmit disease or cause a severe allergic reaction. So it's wise to be wary, and to provide your toddler with as much insect protection as possible. Here's how:

Protect against all insects. Though wearing lots of clothing isn't very practical in hot weather, it does offer the best insect protection. When insects are swarming, dress your toddler in clothes that cover as much skin as possible: a hat, long sleeves, long trousers tucked into socks, and closed shoes. Clothes that are white, pastel, sub-dued green, or khaki are less attractive to insects than those that are brightly hued, dark, and/or flowered. Since insects are attracted to scents, opt for unscented detergents, shampoos and soaps, nappy wipes, lotions, and sunscreens during insect seasons, and don't plant brightly coloured or fragrant flowers in play areas if you can avoid it. Skin or clothes that are smeared with food will also attract insects, so try to leave the house with a clean toddler in a clean set of clothes. Since it's difficult to avoid an insect that's flying around inside a car, keep your windows and sunroof closed while your car is parked.

Insect repellents can be used to deter mosquitoes, biting flies, fleas, and ticks. Use only those designed especially for children, choosing from these types:

- Repellents with DEET. Formulations containing a chemical called DEET offer the best defence against biting insects. It is widely used and is one of the few registered pesticides applied directly to human skin although it is a toxic compound, which can be partially absorbed into the blood-stream. Your safest bet is to stick with 10 per cent unless you're in a particularly buggy area. And it is best not to use a DEET product that contains sunscreen. It may seem like a handy combination, but the DEET can make the sun-protection factor (SPF) less effective, and the need to reapply the sunscreen can result in overexposure to the DEET. Apply sunscreen first, then spray the bug spray.

- Repellents with essential oils from plants. Purified forms of plants like citronella, cedar, and soybean can help ward off insects and are effective. Protection usually lasts less than a couple of hours, so they need to be reapplied often.

- Repellents with permethrin. Permethrin is a chemical that kills ticks and fleas (but not mosquitoes or other flying insects) on contact, so it can help protect against Lyme disease and other tick-borne illnesses. It's effective when applied to clothing or to outdoor gear like sleeping bags and tents – not on skin. Protection lasts for several washings.

Whichever type of product you use for your toddler, be sure to wash off any repellent once you are back indoors.

Protect against bees and wasps. Keep your toddler out of areas bees favour (such as fields of clover or wildflowers, around fruit trees, or near rubbish bins) whenever possible. If you discover a beehive or wasp's nest in or near your home, have it removed by a professional. When bees are buzzing around, avoid serving your toddler sticky, sweet snacks, such as fruit and fruit juice, outside. When you do, wipe fingers and face promptly with unscented wipes to remove all traces

of the snack. (If your toddler has had an allergic reaction to bee stings, see page 443.)

Protect against mosquitoes. Since mosquitoes breed in water, fill in puddles, drain rain barrels, and empty birdbaths on your property. In summer, keep your toddler indoors at dusk, when mosquitoes are out in large numbers, and make sure doors and windows are kept closed. An insect repellent can also be used.

Protect against wood ticks. Wood ticks normally live on deer and can carry Lyme disease, so it's especially important to protect your toddler from their bite. When you know your toddler will be playing or hiking in areas where wood ticks are prevalent (you can check with the local travel information on their prevalence), cover as much of your child's body area as possible with clothing and apply an insect repellent as described above. Check skin and clothing for ticks when out in infested areas and on returning home; also be sure to check pets, since their fur can pick up ticks and pass them on to family members. It takes about 36 to 48 hours for a tick to transmit a full-blown case of Lyme disease; the sooner you remove a tick (see page 443), the less likely it is that infection will occur. A good habit: check your child for ticks nightly at bath time during tick season.

Protect against spiders. Although spiders in the UK are not usually dangerous, they can still bite. Keep children out of warm, dry, dark places (such as wardrobes, attics, unfinished cellars, garages, storage sheds, under outdoor stairs), where spiders spend most of their time. Carefully check for spiders on clothing, shoes and boots, and other items that have been taken out of storage, and remove spiderwebs when you find them.

OUTDOOR WATER SAFETY

When you combine water and a toddler, you get both fun and risk. Reduce the risk without reducing the fun by taking these precautions:

- Keep paddling pools and any other water catchments (ponds, birdbaths) inaccessible to unsupervised toddlers, even if the water is only about 5 cm deep. When not in use, keep wading pools overturned, stored away, or covered, so they don't fill with rainwater.

- It's especially difficult to keep a very young – and vulnerable – child safe when there's a swimming pool in the garden. Swimming pools should be fenced in on all sides. The fence should be at least 1.5 m high and its vertical posts should be no more than 10 cm apart and difficult to climb. Entrances to the pool should be kept locked at all times; gates should open away from the pool and be self-closing, with a self-latching lock that is well out of reach of children. An alarm that signals that the gate has been opened offers additional protection.

- Make sure the pool has an approved safety drain cover with an anti-entrapment device. Never allow your child to use a pool with a missing drain cover until the drain is replaced with an anti-entrapment drain cover.

- If possible, install an automatic pool cover – but don't rely on it instead of a fence, and never leave it partly in place (a toddler could slip beneath it unnoticed). Always drain a pool cover

that's filled with rainwater as soon as possible.

- If you have an above-ground pool that's less than 1.2 m tall, fence it in. Steps and/or ladders to an above-ground pool should be inaccessible to children or removed when the pool is not in use.

- Be sure there are no trees, chairs, benches, tables, or anything else around that your toddler can climb to get over a pool fence or into an above-ground pool.

- Remove toys from the pool and pool area when not in use – they can attract a toddler towards the water. Don't allow riding toys or tricycles near the pool.

- Supervise your toddler every second. Children should never be allowed to enter the pool area without a supervising adult, and an adult (with knowledge of CPR and rescue techniques) must continue to be present and supervising every moment as long as any children are there. It only takes a few seconds for a child to fall into a pool and go under. Constant supervision is necessary even if your toddler is splashing in a plastic paddling pool.

- Just in case, know how you will respond to a water emergency. Learn CPR and make sure that anyone who cares for your child or will be supervising him or her in the pool does, too. Have a rescue pole and life preserver on each side of the pool and CPR directions posted explaining the steps to be taken. When using the pool, keep a phone handy for emergencies.

- If you install a floating pool alarm, don't depend on it exclusively. These alarms don't go off until the child is already in the water – far too late for comfort. The best safeguards are those that keep children away from the pool entirely or warn you before they get into the water.

- Be sure any pool your toddler plays or swims in (other than a child's paddling pool that is emptied daily) is properly chlorinated. Too little as well as too much chlorine (you can smell it) can be hazardous. Even properly chlorinated pool water may cause problems for the child with asthma and allergies.

- Use swim nappies on your toddler in the pool.

- If you have a Jacuzzi or hot tub, keep curious children out of it with a rigid, lockable cover; a fence is also a good idea.

- At the beach, spread your towel close to the lifeguard station if there is one – it's usually set up on the safest area of beach. Even so, supervise your toddler constantly.

- Keep everyone in the family away from pools or other bodies of water during thunderstorms.

- If you take your family boating, outfit all children (even infants and toddlers) in child-size life jackets. Keep in mind, though, that life jackets are not a substitute for parental (or another responsible adult's) supervision. On a boat, there should be at least one adult swimmer for every child nonswimmer.

For more on safety when swimming, see page 82.

SAFETY IN THE SNOW

To adults, a winter snow accumulates with hundreds of headaches – walks and driveways to be salted and

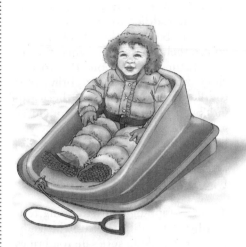

For safe toddler sleigh rides, try a sleigh with sides, back, and a seat belt.

shovelled, slippery roads to negotiate, muddy boots and soggy snowsuits to deal with. To children, snowdrifts represent a pile of pleasures – snow angels to be made, snowballs to be thrown, snow sculptures to create, snow-covered hills begging to be sledded down. To keep your child's winter wonderland safe:

Ensure safe sledding. Your 1-year-old won't be hitting the slopes this early (even the sledding slopes), but he or she may enjoy a sleigh ride (being pulled on a sled). For toddlers, a sled with a seat and seat belt is safest. If you don't have one of those, your toddler should ride nestled between the legs of an adult or much older child.

Ban snow consumption. Even before it's driven on, snow may not be as pure as it looks. Even rural snow can be contaminated by animal urine or faeces or by chemical pollutants. So while you won't always be able to keep your toddler from sampling a handful of the white stuff (remember how good it tastes?), it's wise to stop snow eating when you spot it.

Know when to call it quits. Don't wait for your toddler to start complaining about being cold (little ones often ignore their thermostats when they're having fun). When you start to feel chilly outdoors, it's time to bring your toddler in. Also retreat to the warm indoors if your child's clothes or gloves get wet. Mix wet with freezing, and you have a recipe for frostbite.

CAR SAFETY

From strapping your strapping toddler the right way into the right car seat to making sure safe road rules are always followed, travelling by car with a toddler isn't exactly easy riding. Keeping these tips in mind will help you keep your most precious cargo safe:

Car seat safety. After a year-plus of practice, you're probably a pro at negotiating the straps, harnesses, and buckles of the car seat system you're currently using. But as your toddler grows, you'll definitely be facing some new car seat challenges – and maybe even, soon, a new car seat.

Working out what you need to know about your growing child's car seat safety needs can be confusing. In fact, it can be so confusing that often car seats are installed or used incorrectly. To make sure your toddler is protected:

- Choose the right seat and seat position. It's recommended that toddlers stay rear facing until age 2 – or until a child outgrows the weight limit (usually around 16kg) for the particular rear-facing toddler car seat. Experts say that a rear-facing child safety seat provides much more effective protection of a young child in a car crash. In a rear-facing car seat, a child's head, neck, and spine are better supported,

Sunny and Mild? Not in the Car

It may be hard to believe, but a car sitting in the sun can quickly turn into an oven. Even on a mild day, temperatures can rise from 70°F/21°C to 125°F/51°C and beyond in a matter of minutes, putting a child who's sitting in a parked car at risk of heatstroke, dehydration, and, far too quickly, death. Never leave your little one in a car unattended, not even for a quick moment, no matter what the weather.

making the risk of serious injury much less likely. Research shows that children under age 2 are 75 per cent less likely to be severely or fatally injured in a crash if they are riding rear-facing.

The majority of tots don't hit that upper weight limit until after age 2, but if you have a real chunky monkey, you may need to turn him or her forward-facing earlier than age 2. Got a tot who is small for his or her age? You might need to keep your little one rear-facing past age 2. In other words, the "age 2" recommendation is not a deadline, but rather a guideline to help parents decide when to make the transition. Still not sure? Check with your paediatrician.

Once your little one hits age 2 or the upper weight limit, you can turn a convertible seat to face forward and use it until your child turns 4 and weighs between 18 and 25kg. Or you can switch to a forward-facing seat that, once your child outgrows the car seat part of it (again, around 18 and 25 kg, depending on the seat), transitions to a booster seat.

A Safe Drive

Driving around with your toddler doesn't only mean strapping into a car seat. Whether you're putting your tot in the pushchair, shopping trolley, bicycle seat or trailer, or back carrier, keep these safety tips in mind:

A pushchair. To keep your toddler safe in the pushchair:

- Use a pushchair that has a broad base, is free of nooks and joints that could catch and injure small fingers, and is sturdy enough not to tip over if a child moves around in it.

- If your pushchair tips when the handles are overloaded, make sure they never are.

- When opening or folding the pushchair, be sure your toddler isn't standing close to the mechanisms. A finger could get caught.

- Be sure the pushchair is fully opened and securely locked into position before putting your toddler into it.

- Be sure to strap your child securely into the seat before you start pushing.

- Never place hot drinks in the cup holder of the pushchair above your toddler. One bump could send the liquid flying onto your toddler's head.

Supermarket trolley. Here's how to keep your little one safe while cruising the supermarket aisles:

- Always make sure the trolley's safety belt or harness is securely fastened around your child no matter where he or she is sitting (in the seating area near the handle or in a special themed trolley "car" in the front).

- Don't let your toddler climb on, ride outside, or stand inside the trolley.

Back carrier. Make sure the carrier you're using can accommodate a strapping toddler (some are designed only for babies). And speaking of strapping, make sure your toddler is secured in the carrier (back carriers often have safety straps or safety harnesses). Be careful when you bend over (so that your child won't fall out) or walk through low doorways or under low-hanging branches (a tall toddler's head may be higher than yours when riding in a back carrier).

Bicycle-mounted child seat or trailer. These are best used off-road only (on bike paths, for instance). A trailer is the safest because it's close to the ground (choose one that's brightly coloured for better visibility and add a flag). If you use a mounted seat, choose one for the back of the bike (front-mounted carriers are less safe and can be distracting). Either way, remember to use a toddler-size helmet on your child and keep him or her strapped in at all times. And wear a helmet yourself.

- Install the car seat properly by following the manufacturer's instructions. The best – and safest – place for the car seat is the middle of the backseat. If you're not up for working out the installation of the seat yourself, check with your local police station or check the installation instructions online. For a list of manufacturers' contact details visit www.childcarseats.org.uk.

- ISOFIX (International Standards Organisation FIX) is a new standard for car seat installation that's being adopted by car seat and vehicle manufacturers worldwide. The system operates through ISOFIX points on the back of the child car seat that plug into ISOFIX fittings in the car, creating a solid link between your child's car seat and your car.

  The best way to find out if your car has ISOFIX fittings is to contact your vehicle manufacturer or the dealership that you purchased it from. Or you can consult your car's manual, which should clearly indicate the ISOFIX fitting points. Look in your car for the two lower anchorages (telltale "staple-like" protrusions) that would be located in between the vehicle seat back and bottom cushions.

  No matter which system you use, make sure that when you install the seat (or when you have it installed), it's secure – you can't move it more than 2.5 cm from side to side.

- Belt up. Even the safest seat won't work well if you don't secure your child correctly. Make sure the harness is snug without being too tight (you should be able to fit no more than two fingers between the strap and your child). When the seat is in a rear-facing position, the harness straps should be in the slots that are at or below your child's shoulders. If the seat is facing forward, use slots that are above the child's shoulder level. Adjust the harness and clip to accommodate puffy clothing (though it's a good idea to take off big winter jackets so that your tot can have a safely snug fit in his or her seat). Then make sure everyone else in the car is securely strapped in, including you. After all, children get into the habit of being strapped in by watching you do it, too.

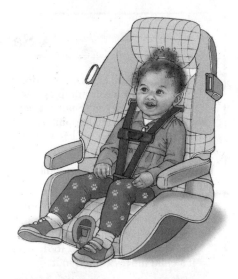

Children should stay rear-facing in their car seats until age 2 or until they outgrow the weight limit (usually around 16 kg). Once they are over 16 kg they can start facing forward.

- Don't neglect car safety when you travel. Take along an appropriate car seat if you're planning any vehicle time, even if you'll be taking a taxi or hotel van. Many car hire companies offer car seat hire too, which could be a good option if you don't want to haul your own seat from home and won't be needing once en route to your destination (say, you'll be keeping your toddler on your lap in flight). Make sure any car seat you hire is the right kind for a young toddler.

General car safety. Belting up may be the first rule of car safety, but it isn't the only one. For a safer ride:

- Never leave a child in an auto unattended, not even for a moment. A number of things can happen – many of them frightening. For example: a toddler playing around in a car could set it rolling off on its own, into someone or something; a stranger could take off with the car and/or the toddler; or the temperature in the car could dip or rise dangerously.

- Always wait until all the car doors are locked and everyone in the car is properly strapped in before you start driving. Make no exceptions to this rule, even if you're just going for a quick trip from one shop to another on the other side of the high street. (For tips on how to keep your toddler happy while strapped in, see page 215.)

- Don't allow your toddler to control the car's power windows (control them yourself from the driver's seat, keeping them locked, if possible). And never roll up the windows without first checking to be sure no one is leaning out and no hand, finger, or other body part is in the way.

- Don't permit the use of pens, pencils, or other sharp objects in a moving car or any other vehicle, or allow play with toys or other objects that can block the driver's vision – a balloon, for example. And don't leave loose objects lying around; they can go flying forward if you have to stop short.

- Don't try to argue with or discipline a child while you're driving; if you're distracted by a behaviour, pull over, then deal with it.

- Never use a mobile phone while you're driving, even a hands-free one (studies show that drivers are distracted even when they're using a hands-free mobile phone). And never, ever text while driving.

- Never allow your child to play behind a parked car or near a car that is not locked.

- Never let your child ride in the back of a lorry or van, whether it's open or enclosed. Children can be injured during such an unprotected drive with just a short stop. Before letting your child ride in a jump seat, and before buying a van or lorry, check with the manufacturer on safety features (ask, for example: where would a child's head impact in a crash? Will seat belts hold a car seat?).

ALL ABOUT:
Teaching Your Toddler to Be Safe

Injuries are much more likely to happen to those who are susceptible to them. And, of course, toddlers – with their eagerness to try new things, their shaky motor skills, their relative immaturity, and their serious lack of judgement – easily fall (often literally) into that category. Your goal as a parent is to reduce this susceptibility as much as you can.

Since you can't count on your toddler to have the good sense or skills to keep himself or herself safe, for now you'll have to rely on careful supervision and thorough childproofing to fill in that vulnerability gap. But that doesn't mean it's too soon to begin the safety training that will eventually allow your child to stay out of harm's way even when a responsible adult isn't by his or her side. In fact, now's the perfect time for your toddler to start learning to live by the safety rules.

Start by building and using a vocabulary of warning words which your toddler will come to associate with dangerous objects, substances, and situations ("ouch", "sore", "hot", "sharp"), and phrases ("Don't touch", "That's dangerous", "Be careful", "That's an ouch", "That could give you a bang"). The red flags may seem to sail right over your little one's head at first, like everything else you're trying to teach. But in time and with consistent repetition, your child's brain will begin to store and process this vital information – until one day, it becomes clear that your lessons have taken hold. Teach your toddler now about the following:

Sharp or pointy implements. Whenever you use a knife, scissors, razor, letter opener, or other sharp implement, be sure to remind your toddler that it's sharp, that it's not a toy, and that only Mummy and Daddy (or other grownups) are allowed to use it. Illustrate more tangibly by touching the point of the implement, saying "Ouch", and pulling your finger away quickly in mock pain. Demonstrate that you always carry scissors point down, holding the blades, and that you never run with any sharp object (you'll be modelling the safety protocol you'll eventually want your child to follow). As your child grows older and gains better small-motor control, teach cutting with a pair of child's safety scissors and teach how to use a knife with a butter knife. Eventually, some time in the school years, you can advance your child to supervised use of the "adult" versions.

Hot stuff. By this time, if you've already begun introducing the concept, your toddler will probably understand (albeit in a very basic way) what "hot" means, that the warning "hot!" means don't touch, and that something that's hot can cause pain. If you haven't taught this yet, start now. Illustrate the concept by letting your toddler touch something warm but not hot enough to burn, such as your coffee cup. Continue pointing out what's hot and shouldn't be touched (the cooker, a lit match or candle, a radiator or heater, a fireplace, the hot-water tap). Be particularly careful to provide the "hot, don't touch" warning when you bring something new into your home – a new toaster, or a lightbulb in the new table lamp.

Steps. True, it's necessary to protect a new walker from serious falls by securely gating all staircases in the home. But it's also necessary to help your child learn how to navigate steps safely. The child who has no experience with steps, who knows nothing about them except that they are off-limits, is at the greatest risk of a tumble the first time an open stairway is discovered. So put a gate at the top of every stairway of more than three steps in your home – going down stairs is much trickier for the beginner than going up, and thus much more dangerous. Downstairs, put the gate three steps up from the bottom so that your child can practise going up and down under controlled conditions. Show your toddler how to hold on to the rail while climbing up or down the stairs.

When your toddler becomes proficient, open the gate occasionally so that he or she can tackle the full flight as you stand or crouch a step or two below, ready to provide support if necessary. Or hold your child's hand as you walk up together. Once going up is mastered, help your child learn how to come down safely. Many toddlers crawl down feet first on their tummies at first, others bump down on their bottoms. As they become more proficient, they start walking down one step at a time. Continue to keep the gates in place, fastening them when you're not able to stand by, until your child is a very reliable step climber (somewhere around 2 years old). Even then, putting a gate at the head of the stairs is still a good idea (especially at night if your toddler is prone to wandering).

If there aren't any stairs in your home, find a set (at the home of a friend, a relative, or at some other accessible location) and let your child do some practising with you close at hand.

Electrical hazards. Electrical sockets, cords, and appliances all hold great appeal for curious toddlers. And it's not enough to use distraction every time you catch your child on the way to probing an unprotected socket, or to hide all the visible cords in your home; it's also necessary to repeatedly remind the toddler of their "ouch" potential.

Baths, pools, and other watery attractions. Water play is fun and educational, so encourage it. But also encourage a healthy respect for water. Teach your toddler basic water safety rules, including: it's dangerous (and prohibited) to get into water (the bath, a swimming pool, a pond, or any other body of water) unless a parent or another grown-up is with you. But, remember, you can't sufficiently "waterproof" a young child, not even with arm bands and swimming lessons (see page 82), so never leave a toddler alone near water, even for a moment.

Choking hazards. When your child puts something in his or her mouth that doesn't belong there (a coin, a pencil, a brick), take it away and explain simply, "Don't put that in your mouth. It can give you a hurt." Teach your child that it isn't safe to run with a lollipop, teething ring, food, pencil, dummy, or toy in his or her mouth (a face-first fall could force any of these down the throat), and that food should only be eaten when he or she is seated.

Poisonous substances. You're always meticulous about locking away household cleansers, medicines, and other hazardous substances. But at a party, one of the guests leaves his vodka and orange juice on the coffee table. Or you're at your parents' house and your father, who's been trying to clear a clogged sink, leaves the drain cleaner on the bathroom counter. You're asking for trouble if you haven't begun to teach your toddler the rules of substance safety. Repeat these messages, over and over and over again:

- Don't eat or drink anything unless your parent or another grown-up you know well gives it to you. This is a difficult concept for a young child to grasp, but repetition will make it stick . . . eventually.

- Medicine and vitamin pills are not sweets, though they are sometimes flavoured to taste that way. Don't eat or drink them unless your parent or another grown-up you know well gives them to you.

- Don't put anything in your mouth that isn't food; this, too, will bear a lot of repeating.

- Only grown-ups are allowed to use cleaning products and dishwasher detergent. Repeat this every time you scrub the bath, wipe down the countertops, or load the dishwasher.

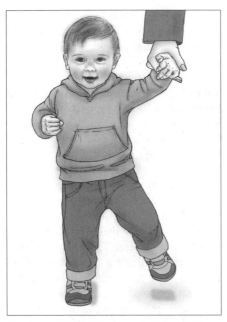

Teach your toddler to always hold an adult's hand when crossing a street.

Street hazards. Begin teaching street sense now. Every time you cross a street with your toddler, explain about "stop, look, and listen", about crossing at the corner, and about waiting for the green man. If there are driveways in your neighbourhood, be sure to explain that it's necessary to stop, look, and listen before crossing them, too. Explain that drivers can't see little children, so they have to hold the hand of someone big, and insist that your toddler always hold your hand (or the hand of another adult) when crossing. Make no exceptions. Teach your child never to step into the street without an adult, even if there's no traffic. Point out the kerb as the line a child must never go beyond on his or her own.

It's a good idea to hold hands even on the quietest pavement, too, but many toddlers revel in the freedom of walking on their own. If you permit this (and you probably will want to, at least some of the time), keep up with and keep a sharp eye on your child – an instant is all it takes for a child to dart into the path of an oncoming car.

Make sure, too, that your toddler knows not to leave home without you or another adult he or she knows well. Toddlers have been known to toddle, on their own, out the front door and straight into trouble.

It's also important to teach your toddler not to touch rubbish in the street – newspaper, broken glass, cigarette butts, food wrappers. But don't make your child neurotic about touching anything at all – it's okay to touch flowers (gently, without eating or picking them), trees, shop windows, street lamps, post boxes, and so on. (If you like, carry wipes to clean your tot's hands before eating – or thumb sucking.)

Car safety. Be certain that your toddler not only becomes accustomed to being strapped into a car seat, but understands why it's essential ("You can get hurt if you don't belt up"). Also explain in simple terms the reason for other car safety rules: why it's not safe to throw toys around, why children must not play with door locks or window buttons.

Playground safety. A toddler who is old enough to play in a playground is old enough to begin learning playground safety rules. Teach swing safety: never twist a swing (even if it's empty), push an empty swing, share a swing meant for one, or walk in front of or behind a moving swing. Address slide safety, too: never climb up the slide from the bottom (always use the ladder) or go down headfirst; always wait until the child ahead of you is off the slide before going down; and, when you reach the bottom of the slide, move out of the way immediately.

Pet safety. Teach your child how to interact safely with pets – your own as well as those of others – and to keep away from strange animals. See page 202 for more.

Insect safety. Teach your toddler to avoid bees, and to stay still when one approaches. Warn your child, too, not to provoke spiders or play with spider-webs. Spiders in the UK are not poisonous, but this lesson will be useful when you travel abroad.

CHAPTER 14

Treating Toddler Injuries

Y OU'VE TAKEN ALL THE CHILDPROOFING PRECAUTIONS YOU CAN, plus a few extra ones – just to be on the extra-safe side. You've mastered the eyes-behind-your-back manoeuvre so you can watch your wily toddler's every move from clear across the room. You've even taught – or tried to teach – your little one to stay away from electrical sockets, hot stoves, and other hazards at home and away. Still, with a toddler on the loose, injuries – big and small – are bound to happen once in a while. And though you can't prevent them all, you can prepare for them – and that preparation can make all the difference. This chapter will give you all the information you need to handle a toddler injury: from small bumps and bruises to burns and more (including CPR and what to do if your child is choking). A grey bar has been added to the top of these pages, making this chapter easy to locate in an emergency.

Preparing for Emergencies

B ecause quick action after an injury is often critical, don't wait until your child dunks a hand in your hot tea or takes a swig of laundry detergent to look up what to do in an emergency. Before an accident happens is the best time to familiarise yourself with the procedures for dealing with and treating common injuries. Take a look at the protocol for handling less common injuries (snakebites, for instance) when you're more likely to encounter them (you're about to go on a camping trip abroad).

But don't stop there. It's one thing to read about injury treatment – it's another thing to apply your skills when an emergency strikes. So reinforce what you learn in this chapter by taking a course in child safety techniques, cardiopulmonary resuscitation (CPR), and basic first-aid techniques. Courses are available at many community centres and hospitals or through the Resuscitation Council; check online or with your child's doctor for options. Keep your skills current and ready to use with periodic refresher courses (or resources from the British Heart Foundation). See that anyone else who cares for your toddler is also fully prepared to deal with emergencies – from minor to major.

To further prepare yourself for emergencies:

- Discuss with your toddler's doctor what the best course of action would be in the event of a non-life-threatening injury as well as a serious emergency: when to call the doctor's surgery, when to go to Accident & Emergency (A&E), and when to do both; when to call 999, and when to follow some other protocol. For minor injuries, the A&E – with its long waits and priority given to life-threatening conditions – may not be the best place to go.

- Keep your first-aid supplies (see page 459) in a childproof, easily manageable kit or box so it can be moved as a whole, as needed. Keep a phone easily accessible so that it can be used at the site of an injury in or near your home.

- Always keep handy (and accessible to anyone who cares for your child):

  □ Emergency phone numbers. The doctor's surgery; the hospital Accident & Emergency of your choice; your pharmacy; the Emergency Services, which can be accessed by dialing 999; your workplace numbers, as well as the number of a close relative, friend,

or neighbour who can be called on in an emergency.

  □ Personal information (updated regularly). Your child's age, approximate weight, immunisation record, medications, allergies, and/or chronic illnesses, if any. In an emergency, these should be supplied to the paramedics and/or taken to the hospital or A&E.

  □ Location information. Home address (include nearby streets and landmarks, if necessary), flat number, telephone number – for use by babysitters or other caregivers calling for emergency help.

  □ A pad and pen. For taking instructions from the doctor or 999 Emergency Services.

- Be sure there's a clearly distinguishable number on your house and a light that makes the number visible after dark.

- Know the quickest route to A&E or other emergency medical facility your child's doctor recommends.

- If you live in a city, keep some cash reserved in a safe place in case you need to call a taxi to get to A&E or the doctor's surgery in an emergency. (If you're very anxious, or you're busy caring for your injured child, it's best if you don't drive.) Let any caregiver or babysitter who stays with your child know where that emergency money is, too.

- If you tend to be an over-reactor, try to learn how to respond calmly to your little one's illnesses and injuries. Practise with everyday bumps and bruises, so if a serious injury ever occurs you'll be better equipped to keep your cool. Taking a few deep breaths will help you relax and focus no matter what you're facing. Try to remember that your expression, tone of voice, and general demeanour will affect your toddler's reaction to an injury, too. If you panic, your child is more likely to panic – and less likely to be able to cooperate. (It almost goes without saying: an uncooperative child is more difficult to treat.)

- To help you both stay calm when there's been an injury, big or small, divert your child's attention by engaging at least three of his or her senses. Stand where your child can see you, speak calmly so he or she can hear you, and touch a part of the body that doesn't seem to be injured.

First Aid for the Toddler

Following are the most common injuries, what you should know about them, how to treat (and not treat) them, and when to seek medical care for them. Types of injuries are listed alphabetically, with individual injuries numbered for easy cross-reference.

ABDOMINAL INJURIES

1. Internal bleeding. A blow to a toddler's abdomen could result in internal injury. The signs of such injury include: bruising or other discolouration of the abdomen, vomited or coughed-up blood that is dark or bright red and has the consistency of coffee grounds (this could also be a sign that a caustic substance has been swallowed), blood (it may be dark or bright red) in the stool or urine, and shock (cold, clammy, pale skin; weak, rapid pulse; chills; confusion; and possibly, nausea, vomiting, and/or shallow breathing). Seek emergency medical assistance (call 999). If the child appears to be in shock, treat immediately (#48). Do not give food or drink.

2. Cuts or lacerations of the abdomen. Treat as for other cuts (#51, #52). With a major laceration, intestines may protrude. Don't try to put them back into the abdomen. Instead, cover them with a clean, moistened flannel or nappy and get emergency medical assistance immediately (call 999).

BITES

3. Animal bites. Try to avoid moving the affected part. Call the doctor immediately. Then wash the wound gently with soap and water. Do not apply antiseptic or anything else. Control bleeding (#51, #52, #53) as needed, and apply a sterile bandage. Outside the UK, dogs, cats, bats, and foxes that bite may be rabid, especially if they attack unprovoked. Infection (redness, tenderness, swelling) is common with cat bites and may require antibiotics.

While low-risk dog bites (bites from a dog that is known not to have rabies) usually do not require antibiotics unless an infection develops, it's still important to consult your child's doctor for any animal bite, both to decide whether antibiotics are needed and for post-exposure rabies protection (keep in mind that while rabies in humans is extremely rare, it is almost always fatal if not treated). Call the doctor immediately if redness, swelling, and tenderness develop at the site of the bite – these are signs of infection.

4. Human bites. If your child is bitten by another child, don't worry unless the skin is broken. If it is, wash the bite area thoroughly with mild soap and cool water. Don't rub the wound or apply any spray or ointment (antibiotic or otherwise). Simply cover the bite with a sterile dressing and call the doctor. Use pressure to stem bleeding (#52), if necessary. Antibiotics will likely be prescribed to prevent infection.

5. Insect bites. Treat insect stings or bites as follows:

- Apply calamine lotion or another anti-itching medication to itchy bites, such as those caused by mosquitoes.

- Remove ticks promptly, using blunt tweezers or your fingertips protected by a tissue, paper towel, or rubber glove. Grab the bug as close to the child's skin as possible and pull upward, steadily and evenly. Don't twist, jerk, squeeze, crush, or puncture the tick.

- If your child is stung by a honeybee, scrape off the stinger by scraping it horizontally using the edge of a blunt butter knife, your fingernail, or a credit card, or gently remove it with tweezers or your fingers. Try not to pinch the stinger because doing so could inject more venom into the wound. Then treat as below.

- Wash the site of a minor bee, wasp, ant, spider, or tick bite with soap and water. Then apply ice wrapped in a towel or cold compresses if there appears to be swelling or pain.

- If there seems to be extreme pain after a spider bite, apply cold compresses and call 999 for emergency advice. If possible, describe the spider's appearance; it might be poisonous. If you know the bite is poisonous – from a black widow or brown recluse spider, a tarantula, or a scorpion, for example – get emergency treatment (call 999) immediately, even before symptoms appear.

- Watch for signs of hypersensitivity, such as severe pain or swelling or any degree of shortness of breath following a bee, wasp, or hornet sting. Most children react to an insect sting with short-lived (less than 24 hours) redness, swelling, and pain in a 5 cm area at the site of the sting. But 20 per cent have a much more severe local reaction – with extensive swelling and tenderness covering an area 10 cm or more in diameter that doesn't peak until three to seven days after the sting. Those who experience such symptoms with a first sting usually develop hypersensitivities (or allergies) to the venom, in which case a subsequent sting could be fatal without immediate emergency treatment. Life-threatening anaphylactic reactions (which are uncommon) usually begin within 5 to 10 minutes of the sting. They may include swelling of the face and/or tongue; signs of swelling of the throat, such as tickling, gagging, difficulty swallowing, or voice change; bronchospasm (chest tightness, coughing, wheezing, or difficulty breathing); a drop in blood pressure, causing dizziness or fainting; and/or cardiovascular collapse. Fatal outcomes in children are extremely rare, but do seek medical help immediately if you notice any systemic reaction (affecting body parts and/or systems other than the site of the sting). Should your child have a life-threatening systemic reaction, call 999 immediately.

After any systemic reaction, a skin test, and possibly other testing, will probably be performed to determine sensitivity to insect venom. If it is determined that your child is at risk of a life-threatening episode from an insect sting, it'll probably be recommended that an EpiPen (see page 395) be taken along on all outings during bee season.

6. Snake bites. Young children are rarely bitten by poisonous snakes, but such a bite is very dangerous. The UK is not home to many snakes, mostly due to its temperate climate. It does, however, support three types of native snake – the adder, the grass snake, and the smooth snake – and all three are protected by law. The adder, which can be found all over the mainland, but not in Northern Ireland, is the only indigenous poisonous snake. Adders very rarely attack but their venom is quite strong and because of a toddler's small size, even a tiny amount of venom can be fatal. Following a poisonous snake bite, it is important to keep the child and the affected part as still as possible. If the bite is on a limb, immobilise the limb with a splint, and keep it below the level of the heart. Use a cool compress if available to relieve pain, but do not apply ice or give any medication without medical advice. Get prompt medical help and be ready to identify or describe the variety of snake if possible. If you won't be able to get medical help within an hour, apply a loose constricting band (a belt, tie, or hair tie loose enough for you to slip a finger under) 5 cm above the bite to slow circulation. (Do not tie such a tourniquet around a finger or toe, or around the neck, head, or trunk.) Check the pulse beneath the tourniquet frequently to be sure circulation is not cut off, and loosen it if the limb begins to swell. Make a note of the time the tourniquet was tied. Sucking out the venom by mouth (and spitting it out) may be helpful if done immediately. But do not make an incision of any kind, unless you are four or five hours from help and severe symptoms occur. If the child is not breathing and/ or the heart has stopped begin rescue techniques (page 464). Treat for shock (#48) if necessary.

Treat nonpoisonous snake bites as puncture wounds (#54), and notify the doctor.

7. Marine animal stings. The stings of marine animals are usually not serious, but occasionally a child can have a severe reaction. Medical treatment should be sought immediately after a marine sting. First-aid treatment varies with the type of marine animal involved, but, in general, any clinging fragments of the stinger should be carefully brushed away with a nappy, a credit card, or piece of clothing (to protect your own fingers). Heavy bleeding (#52), shock (#48), or cessation of breathing (see page 466) should be treated immediately, and if necessary, call 999. (Don't worry about light bleeding; it may help purge the toxins.) If possible, the site of the sting of a stingray, weever fish, fireworm, stonefish, or sea urchin should be soaked in hot water (to break down the toxins) for 30 minutes or until medical help arrives. The toxins from the sting of a jellyfish or Portuguese man o' war can be counteracted by applying regular white vinegar or surgical spirit on the sting (pack a couple of alcohol pads in your beach bag, just in case). Unseasoned meat tenderiser, baking soda, ammonia, and lemon or lime juice can also help prevent pain.

BLEEDING

see #51, #52, #53

BLEEDING, INTERNAL

see #1

BROKEN BONES OR FRACTURES

8. Possible broken arms, legs, or fingers. For young toddlers, "broken" bones are usually just bent or buckled, not snapped, so a break may be more difficult to detect visually. Signs of a break can include: inability to move or put weight on the part, severe pain (persistent crying could be a clue, or an extreme reaction of pain when the area is tapped), numbness or tingling (neither of which a young child is likely to be able to report), swelling, discolouration, and/or deformity (though this could also indicate a dislocation, #17). If a fracture is suspected, don't try to straighten it out. Try to immobilise the injured part by splinting it in the position it's in with a ruler, a magazine, a book, or another firm object, padded with a soft cloth to protect the skin. Or use a small, firm pillow as a splint. Fasten the splint securely with bandages, strips of cloth, scarves, or neckties, but not so tightly that circulation is restricted. If no potential splint is handy, try to splint the injured limb with your arm. Check regularly to be sure the splint or its wrapping isn't cutting off circulation. Apply an ice pack to reduce swelling. Take your child to the doctor or A&E even if you only suspect a break.

9. Compound fractures. If bone protrudes through the skin, don't touch the bone. Cover the injury, if possible, with sterile gauze or with a clean nappy, control bleeding, if necessary, with pressure (#52), and get emergency medical assistance (call 999).

10. Possible neck or back injury. If a neck or back injury is suspected, don't move the child at all. Call 999 for emergency medical assistance. (If you must move the child away from a life-threatening situation, such as a fire or road traffic, splint the back, neck, and head with a board, a chair cushion, or your arm. Move the child without bending or twisting the head, neck, or back). Cover and keep the child comfortable while waiting for help and, if possible, put some heavy objects, such as books, around the child's head to help immobilise it. Don't give any food or drink. Treat severe bleeding (#53), shock (#48), or absence of breathing and/or pulse (see page 465) immediately.

BRUISES, SKIN

see #49

BURNS

> **IMPORTANT:** If a child's clothing is on fire, use a coat, blanket, rug, throw, or even your own body to smother the flames.

11. Limited burns from heat (first-degree). Immerse burned fingers, hands, feet, toes, arms, or legs in cool – not cold – water (50°F/10°C to 60°F/15°C); apply cool compresses to burns of the trunk or face. Continue until your child doesn't seem to be in pain any more – usually 15 minutes to half an hour. Do not apply ice, butter, or burn ointments (all of which could compound skin damage) and don't attempt to break any blisters that form. After soaking, gently pat burned area dry with a soft towel and cover with a gauze pad, a cloth bandage, or another nonadhesive bandage. If redness and pain persist for more than a few hours, call the doctor. Call the doctor immediately for: burns that look raw, that blister (second-degree burns), or are white or charred looking (third-degree burns); any burns on the face, hands, feet, or genitals; or burns that are the size of your child's hand or larger.

12. Extensive burns from heat. Call 999 for emergency medical assistance. Keep the child lying flat. Remove any clothing from the burn area that does not adhere to the wound (cut it away as necessary, but don't pull). Apply cool, wet compresses (you can use a flannel) to the injured area (but not to more than 25 per cent of the body at one time). Keep the child comfortably warm, with burned extremities higher than the heart. Do not apply pressure, ointments, butter or other fats, powder, or boric-acid soaks to burned areas. If the child is conscious and doesn't have severe burns in the mouth, offer sips of fluid to prevent dehydration.

13. Chemical burns. Caustic substances (such as lye, drain cleaner, and other acids) can cause serious burns. Using a clean, soft cloth, gently brush off dry chemical matter from the skin (wear rubber gloves or use a towel or clean nappy to protect your hands) and remove any contaminated clothing. Immediately bathe the skin with large amounts of water. Call the doctor for further advice. Get immediate medical assistance (call 999) if there is difficult or painful breathing, which could indicate lung injury from inhalation of caustic fumes. (If a chemical has been swallowed, see #44.)

14. Electrical burns. Immediately disconnect the power source, if possible, or separate the child from the source using a dry, nonmetallic object such as a wooden broom, wooden ladder, rope, cushion, chair, or even a large book – but not with your bare hands. If the child is not breathing and/or has no pulse, initiate rescue techniques (page 465) and call

999. All electrical burns should be evaluated by a physician, so call your toddler's doctor as soon as possible.

15. Sunburn. If your toddler gets a sunburn, treat it by applying cool tap-water compresses for 10 to 15 minutes, three or four times a day, until redness subsides – the evaporating water helps to cool the skin. In between these treatments, apply a sunburn relief spray made just for kids or a mild moisturising cream. Don't use petroleum jelly (Vaseline) on a burn because it seals in heat and seals out air, which is needed for healing. A children's pain reliever such as paracetamol may reduce the discomfort, but if there's swelling, ibuprofen (which is an anti-inflammatory) is a better choice. Antihistamines shouldn't be given unless they're prescribed by the doctor. When sunburn is severe – there is blistering, pain, nausea, or chills – call the doctor immediately.

CHEMICAL BURNS

see #13

CHOKING

see page 469

COLD INJURIES

see Frostbite and Frostnip, #31, Hypothermia, #35

CONVULSIONS

16. Symptoms of a seizure or convulsion include: collapse, eyes rolling upward, foaming at the mouth, stiffening of the body followed by uncontrolled jerking movements, and in the most serious cases, breathing difficulty. Brief convulsions are not uncommon with high fevers (see page 366 for how to deal with febrile seizures). For nonfebrile seizures: clear the immediate area around the child or move the child to the middle of a bed or carpeted area to prevent injury. Loosen clothing around the neck and torso, and lay the child on one side with the head lower than the hips (elevate the hips with a pillow). Don't restrain, but do stand by ready to prevent injury. Don't put *anything* in the child's mouth, including food, drink, breast, or bottle. Call the doctor.

If the child isn't breathing or has no pulse, begin rescue techniques (see page 465) immediately. If someone else is with you, have them call 999; if you're alone, wait until breathing has started again to call, or call if breathing hasn't resumed within a few minutes. Also call 999 if the seizure lasts more than two or three minutes, seems very severe, or is followed by one or more repeat seizures.

IMPORTANT: Seizures may be caused by the ingestion of prescription medicines or other poisons, so check the immediate vicinity for any sign that your child may have got into a bottle of pills or another hazardous substance. If it is determined that your child has swallowed something hazardous, see #44.

CUTS

see #51, #52

DISLOCATION

17. Elbow dislocations (also known as nursemaid's elbow) are common among toddlers because their joints are relatively loose (in fact, it's pretty easy to accidentally dislocate a little one's elbow by tugging an arm a little too hard or swinging the child by the arms).

When the elbow joint is stretched, nearby soft tissue can slip into it and become trapped, causing severe pain and immobilising the lower arm. A visible deformity of the arm and/or the inability of the child to move it, usually combined with inconsolable crying, are typical indications of an elbow dislocation. A quick trip to the doctor's surgery or the A&E, where an experienced professional can easily reposition the dislocated part, will provide virtually instant relief. If pain seems severe, apply an ice pack and splint before leaving.

DOG BITES

see #3

DROWNING (SUBMERSION INJURY)

18. Even a child who quickly revives after being taken from the water unconscious should get medical evaluation. For the child who remains unconscious, have someone else call 999 for emergency medical assistance, if possible, while you begin rescue techniques (see page 465). If no one is available to phone for help, call later. Don't stop CPR until the child revives or help arrives, no matter how long that takes. If there is vomiting, turn the child to one side to prevent choking. If you suspect the toddler has a back or neck injury, immobilise these parts (see #10). Keep the child warm and dry.

EAR INJURIES

19. Foreign object in the ear. Try to get the toddler to shake the object out by turning the ear down and shaking his or her head gently. If that doesn't work, try these techniques:

- For a live insect, use a lighted torch to try to lure it out.

- For a metal object, hold a strong magnet at the ear canal to draw the object out (but don't insert the magnet in the ear).

- For a plastic or wooden object that can easily be seen and is not deeply embedded in the ear, dab a drop of quick-drying glue on a straightened paper clip and touch it to the object (don't touch the ear). Don't probe into the ear where you can't see. Wait for the glue to dry, then pull the clip out, hopefully with the object attached. Don't attempt this if there's no one around to help hold your child still, or if you don't have a steady hand.

If you're not comfortable attempting the above techniques, or you don't have the necessary equipment to try them, or you try them and they fail, don't try to dig the object out with your fingers or with an instrument. Instead, take your child to the doctor's surgery or A&E.

20. Damage to the ear. If a pointed object has been pushed into the ear or if your toddler shows signs of ear injury (bleeding from the ear canal, sudden difficulty hearing, a swollen earlobe, or substantial pain), call the doctor.

ELECTRIC SHOCK

21. Break contact with the electrical source by turning off the power, if possible, or separate the child from the current by using a dry, nonmetallic object such as a wooden broom, wooden ladder, robe, cushion, chair, rubber boot, or even a large book. If the child is in contact with water, do not touch the water yourself. Once

the child has been separated from the power source, call 999. If the child isn't breathing and/or has no pulse, begin rescue techniques (see page 465) immediately.

EYE INJURIES

IMPORTANT: Don't apply pressure to an injured eye, touch the eye with your fingers, or administer medications without a physician's advice. Keep the child from rubbing the eye by holding a small cup or glass over it or, if necessary, by restraining the child's hands.

22. Foreign object in the eye. If you can see the object (a lash or grain of sand, for instance), wash your hands and use a moist cotton ball to gently attempt to remove the object from the eye, while someone else holds the toddler still (attempt this only in the corner of the eye, beneath the lower lid, or on the white of the eye; stay away from the pupil). Or try pulling the upper lid down over the lower lid for a few seconds. If that doesn't work, try to wash the object out by pouring a stream of tepid (body temperature) water into the eye while someone holds the child still, if necessary. Don't worry about your child crying – tears may help wash the object out of the eye.

If after these attempts you can still see the object or if the child still seems uncomfortable, the object may have become embedded or may have scratched the eye. Don't try to remove an embedded object yourself – proceed to the doctor's surgery or A&E. Cover the eye with a small cup, a sterile gauze pad taped loosely in place, or with a few clean tissues or a clean handkerchief held on gently by hand, to alleviate some of the discomfort en route. Do not apply any pressure.

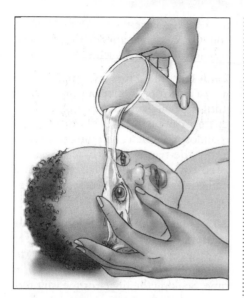

Giving your toddler an eye bath won't be easy, but it's necessary to wash away a corrosive substance.

23. Corrosive substance in the eye. Flush your toddler's eye immediately and thoroughly with plain lukewarm water for about 15 minutes while holding the eye open with your fingers (see illustration). You might have an easier time doing this effectively in the shower, but you can also pour water from a jug, cup, or bottle. If only one eye is involved, keep the chemical runoff out of the other eye by turning the child's head so that the unaffected eye is higher than the affected one. Do not use drops or ointments. Keep the child from rubbing the eye or eyes. Call the doctor for advice. Depending on the substance, the doctor may recommend a follow-up with an ophthalmologist (eye doctor) to be safe.

24. Injury to the eye with a pointed or sharp object. Keep the child in a semi-reclining position while you seek help. If the object is still in the eye, do not try to remove it. If it isn't, cover the eye lightly with a small cup, gauze

pad, clean flannel, or tissue, but do not apply pressure. In either case, get emergency medical assistance immediately (call 999). Though such injuries often look worse than they actually are, it's wise to consult an ophthalmologist or your child's doctor any time the eye is scratched or punctured, even slightly.

25. Injury to the eye with a blunt object. Keep the child lying face up. Cover the injured eye with an ice pack or cold compress for about 15 minutes; repeat every hour as needed to reduce pain and swelling. Consult the doctor if there is bleeding in the eye, if the eye blackens, if the child seems to be having difficulty seeing or keeps rubbing the eye a lot, if the object hit the eye at high speed, or if the child seems to be having continued eye pain.

FAINTING

26. Check for breathing and pulse. If they are absent, begin CPR immediately (see page 465). If you detect breathing,

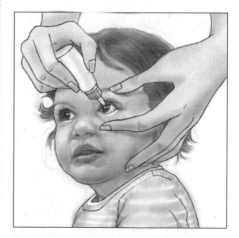

To administer drops, keep the eye open with two fingers of one hand while steadying your toddler's head with the other three fingers. Don't use drops of any kind in your toddler's eye unless they've been recommended or prescribed by the doctor.

keep the child lying flat, head slightly lower than the rest of the body, lightly covered for warmth if necessary. Loosen clothing around the neck. Turn the child's head to one side and clear the mouth of any food or objects. Call the doctor immediately.

FINGER AND TOE INJURIES

27. Bruises. Young children, ever curious, are particularly prone to painful bruises from catching fingers in drawers and doors. For such a bruise, soak the finger in cold water (add a couple of ice cubes to keep it cool). As much as an hour of soaking is recommended, with a break every 10 minutes (long enough for the finger to rewarm) to avoid frostbite. Of course, few toddlers will sit still for that long, though you may be able to treat your child for a few minutes by using distraction. A stubbed toe will also benefit from soaking, but again often isn't practical with a young child. Bruised fingers and toes will swell less if they are kept elevated.

If the injured finger or toe becomes very swollen very quickly, is misshapen, or can't be extended or straightened, call the doctor. It may be broken (see #8). Call the doctor immediately if the bruise is from a wringer-type injury or from catching a hand or foot in the spokes of a moving wheel. In these kinds of "crush" injuries, there may be more damage than is visible or apparent.

28. Bleeding under the nail. When a finger or toe is badly bruised, a blood clot may form under the nail, causing painful pressure. If blood oozes out from under the nail, press on the nail to encourage the flow, which will help to relieve the pressure. Soak the injury in ice water if your child will cooperate. If the pain continues, a hole may have to be made in the nail to relieve the pressure. Contact your GP, who can either do the job or tell you how to do it yourself.

29. A torn nail. For a small tear, secure with a piece of adhesive tape or a plaster until the nail grows to the point where the tear can be trimmed. For a tear that is almost complete, carefully trim away along the tear line with scissors and keep covered with a plaster until the nail is long enough to protect the finger or toe tip.

30. A detached nail. If your toddler injures a fingernail to the point that it detaches or almost detaches, don't try to pull it off – just let it fall off by itself in time. Soaking the finger or toe isn't recommended, since moisture can increase the risk of fungal infections. Do make sure, though, to keep the nail area clean. An antibiotic ointment can be applied but isn't always necessary (ask the GP). Keep the nail bed covered with a fresh plaster until the nail starts growing back in (after that you can leave it uncovered). It usually takes four to six months for a nail to grow all the way back. If at any point you notice redness, heat, and swelling, it could mean the area is infected, and you should call your child's doctor.

FOREIGN OBJECTS

in the ear, see #19; in the eye, see #22; in the nose, see #42; in the mouth or throat, see #40

FRACTURES

see #8, #9, #10

FROSTBITE AND FROSTNIP

31. Frostbite is uncommon in the UK, but young children are more susceptible, particularly on their fingers, toes, ears, nose, and cheeks. In frostbite, the affected part becomes very cold to the touch and turns white or yellowish grey. In severe frostbite, the skin is cold, waxy, pale, and hard. If you notice any signs of frostbite in your toddler, immediately try to warm the frosty parts against your body – open your coat and shirt and tuck the parts inside next to your skin (under your arm is best). You can also breathe warm air on your child's skin. As soon as possible, get to a doctor or A&E. If that isn't feasible immediately, get your child indoors and begin a gradual rewarming process. Don't massage the damaged parts or put them right next to a radiator, stove, open fire, or heat lamp – the damaged skin may burn. Don't try to "quick-thaw" in hot water, either, since this can further damage the skin. Instead, soak affected fingers and toes directly in tepid water (about 102°F/38.8°C – just a little warmer than normal body temperature and just slightly warm to the touch). For parts that can't be soaked, such as the nose, ears, and cheeks, very gently apply warm compresses (flannels or towels soaked in water slightly warm to the touch). Continue the soaks until colour returns to the skin – usually in 30 to 60 minutes (add warm water to the soaks as needed to maintain tepid temperature). Also give sips of warm (not hot) fluids. As frostbitten skin rewarms it becomes red and slightly swollen, and it may blister. Gently pat the skin dry. If your child's injury hasn't yet been seen by a doctor, it is important to get medical attention now.

Once the injured parts have been warmed, and if you have to go out again to take the child to the doctor (or any-where else), be especially careful to keep the affected areas warm (wrapped in a blanket) en route, since refreezing of thawed tissues can cause additional damage.

Much more common than frostbite (and much less serious) is frostnip (also referred to as first degree frostbite). In frostnip, the affected body part is cold and pale, but rewarming (as for frost-bite) takes less time and causes less pain and swelling. As with frostbite, avoid dry heat and avoid refreezing. Though an A&E visit isn't necessary, a visit to the GP makes sense.

After prolonged exposure to cold, a child's body temperature may drop below normal levels. This is a medical emergency known as hypothermia (see #35). Don't waste any time getting a tod-dler who seems unusually cold to the touch to the nearest A&E. Keep your child warm next to your body en route.

HEAD INJURIES

IMPORTANT: Head injuries are usually more serious if a child falls onto a hard surface from a height equal to or greater than his or her own height, or is hit with a heavy object. Blows to the side of the head may do more damage than those to the front or back of the head.

32. Cuts and bruises to the scalp. Because of the profusion of blood ves-sels in the scalp, heavy bleeding is com-mon with cuts to the head, even tiny ones, and bruises there tend to swell up to egg size very quickly. Treat as you would any cut (#51, #52) or bruise (#49). Check with the doctor for all but very minor scalp wounds.

33. Possibly serious head trauma. Every toddler experiences an occasional minor bump on the head – and usually all that's needed treatment-wise are a cuddle and a couple of make-it-better kisses. However, after a severe blow to the head, it's wise to keep a close eye on the child for the first six hours.

Symptoms may occur immediately or not show up for several days – so continue to watch a child who has had a serious head injury even if he or she initially seems fine. Call the doctor or summon emergency medical assistance immediately (call 999) if your toddler shows any of these signs following a severe head injury:

- Loss of consciousness (though a brief period of drowsiness – no more than two or three hours – is common and nothing to worry about).

- Headache that persists for more than an hour (a difficult symptom to discern in a young toddler, who may just cry, whimper, and possibly hold or rub his or her head), that seems to get worse over time, that interferes with normal activity and/or sleep, or that isn't relieved by paracetamol or ibuprofen (a better choice if there's swelling).

- Difficulty being roused. Check every hour or two during daytime naps, and two or three times during the night for the first day following the injury to be sure the child is responsive. If you can't rouse a sleeping child, immediately check for breathing (see page 466).

- More than one or two episodes of vomiting.

- Oozing of blood or watery fluid (not mucus) from the ears or nose.

- Black-and-blue areas appearing around the eyes or behind the ears.

- A depression or indentation in the skull.

- Difficulty walking or clumsiness (beyond usual toddler clumsiness), or the inability to move an arm, a leg, or another body part.

- Disorientation (the child may seem not to know where he or she is, who

you are), slurred speech, extreme irritability, or other abnormal behaviour.

- Unusual lack of balance that persists longer than an hour after the injury (a sign of dizziness).

- Convulsions (see #16).

- Unequal pupil size, or pupils that don't respond to the light of a penlight by shrinking or to the removal of light by growing larger (see illustration).

- Unusual paleness that persists for more than an hour or so.

While waiting for help, keep your child lying quietly with his or her head turned to one side. Do not move the child if you suspect a neck injury, unless not doing so would be dangerous. Treat for shock (#48), if necessary. Begin rescue techniques (see page 465) if your child stops breathing or doesn't have a pulse. (Once your child has recovered, don't offer any food or drink until you talk to the doctor.)

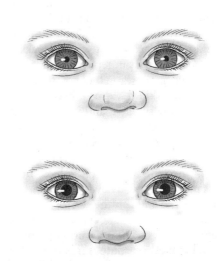

Pupils should constrict (get smaller; top) in response to a light, and dilate (expand; bottom) when the light is removed.

HEAT INJURIES

34. Heat exhaustion, or mild hyperthermia (high body temperature), is the most common form of heat injury. Signs may include: profuse sweating, thirst, headache, muscle cramps, dizziness or light-headedness, and/or nausea (a toddler may be cranky, refuse food, or indicate a need to vomit). Body temperature may rise to 101°F/38.3°C to 105°F/40.5°C. Treat heat exhaustion by bringing the child into a cool environment (air-conditioned, if possible) and giving cold beverages (such as diluted fruit juice) to drink. Cool compresses applied to the body and a fan may also help. If the child doesn't quickly return to normal, vomits after drinking, or has a high fever, call the doctor.

Heatstroke, or severe hyperthermia, is less common and more serious. It typically comes on suddenly after overheating, as when a child has been playing in hot, glaring sunshine or has been enclosed in a car in warm weather. Signs to watch for include hot and dry (or occasionally, moist) skin, very high fever (sometimes over 106°F/41°C), diarrhoea, agitation or lethargy, confusion, convulsions, and loss of consciousness. If you suspect heatstroke, wrap your toddler in a large towel that has been soaked in cold water (dump ice cubes or a bag of frozen peas in the sink while it's filling with cold tap water, then add the towel) and summon immediate emergency medical help (call 999), or rush the child to the nearest A&E. If the towel becomes warm, repeat with a freshly chilled one.

HYPERTHERMIA

see #34

HYPOTHERMIA

35. After prolonged exposure to cold, when heat loss exceeds heat production, a child's body temperature may drop below normal levels. A child with hypothermia may seem unusually cold to the touch, be pale and have blue lips, shiver, be lethargic, move stiffly, and/or have trouble speaking. In severe hypothermia, shivering ceases and there is loss of muscle control and a decline in consciousness. Hypothermia is a medical emergency. Don't waste any time in getting a child who appears to have hypothermia to the nearest A&E (call 999 if you have no quick transportation). Remove any wet clothing, wrap the child in heavy blankets, and turn on the car heater en route to the hospital. If you are awaiting emergency medical help at home, tuck your toddler under an electric blanket, if you have one, or in a very warm bath (not hot enough to burn, of course). If your child is alert, offer warm beverages, such as heated milk or (diluted) juices.

INSECT BITES OR STINGS

see #5

LIP, SPLIT OR CUT

see #36, #37

MOUTH INJURIES

36. Split lip. Few toddlers escape their second year without at least one cut on the lip. Fortunately, these cuts usually look a lot worse than they are and heal a lot more quickly than you'd think. To ease pain and control bleeding, apply an ice pack. Or let your child suck on an ice lolly or a large ice cube (switch to a fresh ice cube before the first becomes small enough to choke on). If the cut gapes open or if the bleeding doesn't stop in 10 to 15 minutes, call the doctor. Also call if you suspect a lip injury may have been caused by chewing on an electrical cord.

37. Cuts inside the lip or mouth. Such injuries are also common in young children. To relieve pain and control bleeding inside the lip or cheek, give the child an ice lolly or a large ice cube to suck on (switch to a fresh ice cube before the first becomes small enough to choke on). To stop bleeding of the tongue that doesn't stop spontaneously, apply pressure to the cut with a piece of gauze, a clean flannel, or a cloth nappy. Call the doctor if the injury is in the back of the throat or on the soft palate (the rear of the upper mouth), if there is a puncture wound from a sharp object (such as a pencil or a stick), or if the bleeding doesn't stop within 10 to 15 minutes.

38. Knocked-out tooth. There is little chance that a dentist will try to reimplant a dislodged baby tooth (such implantations rarely hold), so there's no need to try preserving the tooth. The dentist will, however, want to see it to be sure it's whole, as fragments left in the gum could be expelled and then inhaled or choked on, or the area could become infected. So take the tooth along to the dentist – or to the doctor if you are unable to reach a dentist.

39. Broken tooth. Clean dirt or debris carefully from the mouth with warm water and gauze or a clean cloth. Check thoroughly to be sure there are no broken parts of the tooth still in the child's mouth. Place cold compresses on the face in the area of the injured tooth to minimise swelling. Call the child's dentist as soon as possible for further

instructions. If your child doesn't have a dentist yet, call the doctor for a recommendation.

40. Foreign object in the mouth or throat. Removing a foreign object from the mouth that can't be grasped easily is tricky. Unless done carefully, the effort can push the object in even farther. To remove a soft object (such as a piece of tissue paper or bread), pinch the child's cheeks to open the mouth, and use a tweezer to take the object out. For anything else, try a finger swipe: curl your finger and swipe quickly at the object with a sideways motion. Do not attempt a finger swipe, however, if you can't see the object. If a foreign object is lodged in your child's throat, see choking rescue procedures, beginning on page 469.

NOSE INJURIES

41. Nosebleeds. With the child in an upright position or leaning slightly forward, pinch both nostrils gently between your thumb and index finger for 10 minutes. (Not to worry – the child will automatically switch to mouth breathing.) Try to calm your child, because crying will increase the blood flow. If bleeding persists, pinch for 10 minutes more and/or apply cold compresses or ice wrapped in a dampened flannel to the nose to constrict the blood vessels. If this doesn't work and bleeding continues, call the doctor – keeping the child upright while you do. Frequent nosebleeds, even if easily stopped, should be reported to your child's doctor. Sometimes, adding humidity to the air in your home with a humidifier will reduce the frequency of nosebleeds.

42. Foreign object in the nose. Difficulty breathing through the nose and/or a foul-smelling, possibly bloody nasal discharge may be a sign that something has been pushed up the nose. Keep the child calm and encourage mouth breathing. Remove the object with your fingers if you can reach it easily, but don't probe or use tweezers (or anything else) that could injure the nose if the child were to move unexpectedly, or that could push the object farther into the nasal canal. If you can't remove the object, try to get your child to blow through the nose (have him or her try to move a feather or tiny piece of paper on your hand with each nose blow). If this fails, take the child to the doctor or A&E.

43. A blow to the nose. If there is bleeding, keep the child upright and leaning forward to reduce the swallowing of blood and the risk of choking on it. Use an ice pack or cold compresses to reduce swelling. If swelling persists, see the doctor to be sure the nose isn't broken.

POISONING

44. Swallowed poisons. Any non-food substance is a potential poison. The more common symptoms of poisoning include: lethargy, agitation, or other behaviour that deviates from your child's norm; racing, irregular pulse and/or rapid breathing; difficulty breathing; diarrhoea or vomiting; excessive watering of the eyes, sweating, or drooling; hot, dry skin and mouth; dilated (wide open) or constricted (pinpoint) pupils; flickering, sideways eye movements; tremors or convulsions.

If your toddler has some of these

Poison Guidelines You Should Know

Here's the first thing you should know: **never, ever try to treat a poisoning without professional advice.** Not with home remedies, not with over-the-counter remedies, not with remedies suggested on a product label. If you think your child has eaten something toxic, try to stay calm and call a doctor immediately. The doctor will need all pertinent information in order to advise you, so be ready to provide: what your child had to eat and drink before or since the incident, what toxic substance was apparently ingested and approximately how much, whether anyone has already tried to treat your child and how (treatment of any kind isn't advisable without medical advice). You will also need to tell the doctor how much your child weighs.

Forcing your child to throw up is not recommended. If your child has swallowed a caustic substance it could be extremely dangerous for them to vomit, so always get medical advice first.

Inactivated charcoal is often used in hospital emergency departments as an antidote in cases of poisoning. Large doses are used to prevent the poison being absorbed from the stomach. Although inactivated charcoal tablets are available to buy from pharmacies, these are for the treatment of indigestion and flatulence only and should not be used at home to treat poisoning, so don't keep charcoal tablets in your first-aid kit. In some cases of poisoning your doctor may recommend that you give your child milk to drink, **but only do this if the doctor has advised it**. The safest antidote to poisoning is to call your doctor, call 999, or take your child to A&E.

symptoms and there's no other obvious explanation for them, or if you have evidence that your toddler has definitely ingested a questionable substance (you saw it happen) or possibly has (you found your child with an open bottle of pills or hazardous liquid, found spilled liquid on clothing or loose pills on the floor, smelled a toxic chemical on his or her breath), immediately call (or have someone else call) 999 or the hospital A&E for instructions. Call promptly for suspected poisoning even if there are no symptoms – they may not appear for hours. When calling, be ready to provide: the name of the product ingested, along with the ingredients and package information, if available (if part of a plant was eaten, supply the name, or at least a description, of the plant); the time the poisoning is believed to have occurred; how much of the substance was ingested (give an estimate if you don't know for sure); any symptoms that have appeared; and any treatment already tried. Have a pad and pen handy for writing down exact instructions.

If your child has severe throat pain, excessive drooling, breathing difficulty, convulsions, or excessive drowsiness after the ingestion (or suspected ingestion) of a dangerous substance, call 999 for emergency medical assistance. Begin emergency treatment immediately if the child is unconscious. Place your toddler face up on a table or another firm surface and check for breathing (see page 466). If there is no sign of breathing and/or pulse, begin rescue techniques promptly.

Do not try to treat a poisoning on your own, and don't follow the directions on a product label. Get explicit medical advice before giving anything by mouth (including food or drink, or anything to induce vomiting). The wrong treatment can do harm.

45. Noxious fumes or gases. Fumes from petrol, car exhaust, some poisonous chemicals, and dense smoke from fires can all be harmful. Symptoms of carbon monoxide poisoning include: headache, dizziness, coughing, nausea, drowsiness, irregular breathing, and unconsciousness. Promptly get a child who has been exposed to hazardous fumes to fresh air (open the windows or take the child outside). If the child is not breathing and/or doesn't have a pulse, begin rescue techniques (see page 465) at once. If possible, have someone else call 999. If no one else is around, call 999 yourself after two minutes of resuscitation efforts – then return immediately to CPR, and continue until a pulse and breathing are established or until help arrives. Unless an ambulance is on its way, transport the child to a medical facility promptly. Have someone else drive if you must continue CPR or if you were also exposed to the fumes and your judgement and reflexes may be impaired. Even if you should succeed in re-establishing breathing, immediate medical attention will be necessary.

POISON PLANTS

46. At some point, most children will come into contact with plants that can cause a skin reaction (called contact dermatitis). The most common culprits are chrysanthemums, sunflowers, daffodils, tulips, and primula. The main symptoms of irritation are redness, burning, stinging, and soreness of the affected areas of skin. These will occur within 48 hours of coming into contact with the plant. Make sure you wash any clothing that has touched the plant, including the pushchair, and wipe down your child's shoes thoroughly. To help ease discomfort until the rash disappears, use calamine lotion or an emollient (moisturiser) to ease the irritation. You can cut your toddler's nails to minimise scratching. If the rash is causing a great deal of discomfort because of its location (around the eyes or genitals), it is best to call the doctor.

Some children may experience an allergic reaction to plants. The symptoms are usually redness, itching, and scaling of the affected areas of skin. There is often a delay of many hours to several days before symptoms develop following contact with the plant. If your child has an allergic reaction, other areas of skin that were not in direct contact with the plant may develop a rash. Call the doctor or take your child to A&E if you suspect your child has had an allergic reaction.

PUNCTURE WOUNDS

see #54

SCALDS

see #11, 12, 13

SCRAPES

see #50

SEIZURES

see #16

SEVERED LIMB OR DIGIT

47. Such serious injuries are rare, but knowing what to do when one occurs can mean the difference between saving and losing an arm, leg, finger, or toe. Take these steps, as needed, immediately:

- Try to control bleeding. Apply heavy pressure to the wound with several gauze pads, a fresh sanitary towel, or a clean nappy or flannel. If bleeding continues, increase pressure. Don't worry about doing damage by pressing too hard. Do not apply a tourniquet without medical advice.

- Treat shock if it is present (#48).

- Check for breathing and a pulse and begin rescue techniques (see page 465), as needed.

- Preserve the severed limb or digit. As soon as possible, wrap it in a wet clean cloth or sponge and place it in a plastic bag. Tie the bag shut and place it in another bag filled with ice (do not use dry ice). Do not place the severed part directly on ice and don't immerse it in water or antiseptics.

- Get help. Call or have someone else call 999 for immediate emergency medical assistance or rush to the A&E, calling ahead so they can prepare for your arrival. Be sure to take along the ice-packed limb, finger, or toe – surgeons may attempt to reattach it. During transport, keep pressure on the wound and continue other basic life-support procedures, if necessary.

SHOCK

48. Shock can develop in severe injuries or illnesses. Signs include cold, clammy, pale skin; rapid, weak pulse; chills; convulsions; nausea or vomiting; excessive thirst; and/or shallow breathing. Call 999 immediately for emergency medical assistance. Until help arrives, position the child on his or her back. Loosen any restrictive clothing, elevate the legs on a pillow or a folded blanket or garment to help direct blood to the brain, and cover the child lightly to prevent chilling or loss of body heat. If breathing seems laboured, raise the child's head and shoulders very slightly. Do not give food or water.

SKIN WOUNDS

IMPORTANT: Exposure to tetanus is a possibility whenever the skin is broken. If your toddler gets an open skin wound, check to be sure tetanus immunisation (part of the DTaP vaccine) is up-to-date. Also be alert for signs of possible infection (swelling, warmth, tenderness, and reddening of the surrounding area, oozing of pus from the wound), and call the doctor if they develop.

49. Bruises or black-and-blue marks. If the injury is painful, apply cold compresses, an ice pack, or cloth-wrapped ice (do not apply ice directly to the skin) to reduce bruising and swelling. Half an hour of soaking is ideal, but unlikely to be accomplished with an active toddler, and not necessary for a minor bump. If the skin is broken, treat the bruise as you would an abrasion (#50) or cut (#51, #52). Call the doctor immediately if the bruise is from a wringer-type injury (for instance, from catching a hand or foot in the spokes of a moving wheel), no matter how minor it looks. Bruises that seem to appear from "out of nowhere" or that coincide with a fever should also be seen by a doctor.

50. Scrapes or abrasions. In such injuries, most common on the knees and elbows, the top layer (or layers) of skin is scraped off, leaving the underlying area red, raw, and tender. There is usually slight bleeding from the more deeply abraded areas. Using gauze, cotton, or a clean flannel, gently sponge off the wound with soap and water to remove dirt and other foreign matter. If this tactic is resisted, try soaking the wound in the bathtub. Apply pressure if the bleeding doesn't stop on its own. Apply a spray or cream antiseptic, if your toddler's doctor generally recommends one, then cover with a sterile nonstick bandage that is loose enough to allow air to reach the wound. If there is no bleeding, no bandage is necessary. Most scrapes heal quickly.

51. Small cuts. Wash the area with clean water and soap, then hold the cut under running water to flush out dirt and foreign matter. Some doctors recommend applying an antiseptic spray before taping on a nonstick bandage. A butterfly bandage will keep a small cut closed while it heals. Remove the bandage after 24 hours and expose the cut to air; rebandage only as necessary to keep the wound clean and dry. Check with the doctor about any cuts that show signs of infection (redness, swelling, warmth, and/or oozing of pus or a white fluid).

52. Large cuts. With a gauze pad, a fresh nappy, a sanitary towel, a clean flannel – or, if you have nothing else available, your bare finger – apply pressure to try to stop the bleeding; at the same time, elevate the injured part above the level of the heart, if possible. If bleeding persists after 15 minutes of pressure, add more gauze pads or cloth and increase the pressure. (Don't worry about doing damage with too much pressure.) If the wound gapes open, appears deep, is jagged; if blood is spurting or flowing profusely; or if bleeding doesn't stop within half an hour, call the doctor for instructions or take the child to A&E. If necessary, keep the pressure on until help arrives or you get the child to the doctor or A&E. If there are other injuries, try to tie or bandage the pressure pack in place so that your hands

Stocking the Medicine Cabinet

Toddlers have a tendency to get sick or injured late at night, early in the morning, or whenever it's least convenient to run to the shops for medical supplies. Be sure your medicine chest is well stocked so you will have those necessary supplies handy in case of an emergency, and replace as needed and when they expire. It should include:

- Calpol (children's paracetamol) or ibuprofen (Nurofen for Children); see page 378

- An antihistamine for allergic reactions (if recommended by doctor)

- Saline nasal spray or drops for stuffiness due to colds

- Calamine lotion or moisturiser for mosquito bites and itchy rashes

- Rehydration fluid (Dioralyte) for dehydration caused by diarrhoea, vomiting, fever, or any other problem

- Surgical spirit or alcohol pads, for cleaning thermometers, and so on

- Antiseptic spray

- Antibiotic spray or ointment (if recommended by doctor)

- Petroleum jelly, for lubricating a rectal thermometer

- A digital thermometer (see page 363)

- A medicine spoon, syringe, or dropper

- Sterile adhesive strips, gauze pads, butterfly bandages, and plasters

- A roll of gauze

- Sterile cotton balls

- Scissors with rounded tips for cutting tape and bandages

- Tweezers for removing splinters, ticks, or assorted small foreign objects

- And in your freezer: ice packs, refreezable or refillable (a friendly animal shape may encourage more cooperation). In a pinch, you can use a package of frozen vegetables or fruit.

---

can be free to attend to them. Apply a sterile nonstick bandage to the wound when the bleeding stops, loose enough so that it doesn't interfere with circulation. Do not put anything else on the wound, not even an antiseptic, without medical advice. If the cut is deep and/or large and on the face or the palm of the hand, stitches may be needed. If the cut is on the face, consider having a plastic surgeon take a look at it.

53. Massive bleeding. Get immediate emergency medical assistance by calling 999 or rushing to the nearest A&E if a limb is severed (#47) and/or blood is gushing or pumping out of a wound. In the meantime, apply pressure to the wound with gauze pads, a fresh nappy or sanitary towel, or a clean flannel or towel. Increase the packing and pressure if bleeding doesn't stop. Do not use a tourniquet without medical advice as it can sometimes do more harm than good. Maintain pressure until help arrives.

54. Puncture wounds. Soak a small puncture wound (one caused by a

Making Bumps Better

When it comes to being treated for injuries, toddlers aren't usually the most cooperative patients – and it's really no wonder. After all, for the average 1-year-old, being held still for treatment adds insult to injury. Plus, tots don't connect being treated with feeling better, so promising that soaking a burn or icing a bruise will bring relief doesn't usually make a compelling case for cooperation. For better results, try distraction. A favourite music box, DVD, or CD, a toy dog that yaps and wags its tail, a choo-choo train that can travel across the coffee table, or a parent or sibling who can dance, jump up and down, or sing silly songs can help make the difference between a treatment mission accomplished . . . or abandoned.

Kid-friendly first-aid supplies may also help ease treatment. Look for ice packs and plasters with interesting designs and shapes (you can find ice packs shaped like rabbits, plasters with dinosaurs and character designs and even in the shape of kisses).

How much you have to push the treatment agenda depends on how bad the injury is. Treatment probably won't be necessary for a paper cut, but it's essential for a scraped knee filled with playground pebbles and dirt. A slight bump on the head may not require holding a squirming toddler down while you apply an ice pack. A severe burn, however, will certainly require cold soaks, even if your pint-size patient kicks, screams, and thrashes during the entire treatment. In most cases, try to treat injuries at least briefly – even a few minutes of ice on a bruise will reduce the bleeding under the skin. But drop the treatment protocol if it's clearly not worth the struggle.

---

drawing pin, needle, pen, pencil, nail) in comfortably hot, soapy water for 15 minutes. Then consult the doctor about what to do next. For deeper, larger punctures – from a knife or a stick, for example – take your child to the doctor or A&E immediately. (If there is extensive bleeding, see #53.) If the object still protrudes from the wound, do not remove it, as this could lead to increased bleeding or other damage. Pad or otherwise stabilise the object, if necessary, to keep it from moving around. Keep your child as calm and still as possible to prevent thrashing that might make the injury worse.

55. Splinters or slivers. Wash the area with clean water and soap, then numb it with an ice pack or ice cube. If the sliver is completely embedded, try to work it loose with a sewing needle that has been sterilised with alcohol or in the flame of a match. If one end of the sliver is clearly visible, try to remove it with tweezers (also sterilised by alcohol or flame). Don't try to remove it with your fingernails or your teeth. Wash the site again after you have removed the splinter. If the splinter is not easily removed, try soaking in warm, soapy water for 15 minutes, three times a day for a couple of days, which may help it work its way out or make it easier to remove. Consult the doctor if the splinter remains embedded or if the area becomes infected (indicated by redness, heat, swelling). Also call the doctor if the splinter is deeply embedded or very large and your toddler's tetanus vaccinations (part of the DTaP injections) are not up to date, or if the splinter is metal or glass. Some splinters that are embedded just end up being absorbed into the skin and that's fine (depending on the type of splinter). In that case, trying to remove the splinter can do more harm than good.

SNAKE BITES

see #6

SPIDER BITES

see #5

SPLINTERS

see #55

SPRAINS

56. A sprain is an injury to the ligaments, which are the tough, fibrous tissues that connect bones to other bones. Because during childhood the ligaments are strong in comparison to bones and cartilage, injury to them is less likely than it is in adulthood, when bones become stronger. Still, occasionally a young child will sprain an ankle or, less frequently, a wrist or knee. The symptoms (pain, swelling, inability to use the affected joint or, if it's an ankle or knee that's injured, to walk on it) are similar to those for a broken bone, so a sprain often requires medical expertise, and sometimes an X-ray, to differentiate it from a fracture. Call the doctor if your child displays such symptoms. If there is a possibility of a fracture, see #8. To treat a sprain initially, use the traditional RICE treatment:

- *Rest.* Rest the injured limb. If the sprain involves a leg, keep the child off it as much as possible for the first couple of days, or until the child seems able to walk without pain.

- *Ice.* Apply an ice pack to the injured joint.

- *Compression.* Wrap it snugly (but not so tightly that you restrict circulation) in an elastic bandage.

- *Elevation.* Elevate the injured limb as much as possible, resting it on a plump pillow or a large stuffed animal friend.

Check back with the doctor if a sprain hasn't healed after two weeks or if it has got worse.

SUNBURN

see #15

SWALLOWED FOREIGN OBJECTS

57. Coins, marbles, and other small objects. If a child has swallowed a small object and doesn't seem to be in any discomfort, check with the doctor for advice. It's usually best to wait for the object to travel through the digestive tract (which usually takes about two to three days). Size definitely matters: small coins, for instance, such as pennies and 5-pence pieces, typically pass through without a problem, while larger coins may not. If the doctor suggests a wait-and-see approach, check bowel movements for the object until it turns up. No matter what has been swallowed, if the child has difficulty swallowing or seems to have chest pain (changes in breathing might be a clue), or if chest pain or throat pain (the child refuses to drink or eat), wheezing, drooling, gagging, vomiting, or difficulty swallowing develop later, the object may have lodged in the oesophagus. Immediately call the doctor or take the child to the

Objects in All the Wrong Places

Toddlers love exploring uncharted territory – especially when it's their own bodies. So many mysterious and fascinating orifices, and so many fingers, toys, crayons, and coins that can be plunged deep into them. With temptation so great, and opportunity so near, there may be times when – despite your best efforts to keep your toddler safe – objects end up in all the wrong places. Here's what you need to know:

Swallowed objects. Check with the doctor for advice. As long as your toddler doesn't seem to be having difficulty breathing or swallowing, isn't coughing or choking, and doesn't seem to be in any pain, usually the best course is to observe his or her stools over the next few days (unless the object is a button battery, see #58 or a sharp object, see #59, in which case get medical attention immediately). Most often, swallowed coins or other small objects exit via that route. If your child develops a fever over the next few days, or if the object hasn't shown up in a bowel movement after four or five days, check with the doctor again. An X-ray to find just where the object is lodged may be in order. In some cases, removal – with the help of an endoscope (a flexible instrument inserted down the oesophagus that allows doctors to see what's inside) – may be necessary.

Any time, however, your toddler ingests a foreign object and is coughing, has difficulty swallowing, has changes in breathing, or seems to be in pain immediately call the doctor or 999, or take him or her to the A&E. (For how to handle choking on an inhaled object, see page 469.)

Objects poked in orifices. Any opening that promises to lead somewhere is enticing to a curious young toddler. Enticing, but not risk free. Shoving an object into the ear can damage the eardrum; into the nose can cause bleeding and even infection; into the mouth, choking or poisoning; into the vagina or rectum, infection.

If you find your toddler putting an object in any body opening, explain that this is dangerous and comment on the proper use of the object ("Peas are for eating, not for putting in your nose"). Take it away if the behaviour is continued or if the object is one that your child shouldn't be playing with at all (chopsticks or a marble, for example).

Sometimes a child will insert a foreign object into the nose, ears, or, less often, the vagina or rectum without an adult being the wiser. Suspect the possibility that such an object might have become stuck if you note a foul odour or an unexplained discharge (bloody or not) from the orifice, or if your child begins complaining about pain in the area. For instructions on how to safely remove an inserted foreign object that you can't get a grip on and how to treat any resultant injury, see #19, #40, #42. Call the doctor or take your child to A&E if your efforts to remove the object are unsuccessful.

A&E. If the child is coughing or seems to have difficulty breathing, the object may have been inhaled rather than swallowed; treat as a choking incident (see page 469).

58. Button batteries. If your child swallows a button battery of any kind, call the doctor and head to A&E immediately. The danger: the battery can become lodged in the digestive tract – anywhere from the oesophagus to the intestines – and once there can start to burn through the organs, leading to serious injury and even death. Prompt medical attention (within hours) is necessary.

59. Sharp objects. Get prompt medical attention if a swallowed object is sharp (a pin or needle, a fish bone, a toy with sharp edges). It may have to be removed in the A&E.

TEETH, INJURY TO

see #38, #39

TICK BITES

see #5

TOE INJURIES

see #27, #28, #29, #30

TONGUE, INJURY TO

see #37

First Aid for Toddlers: Choking and Breathing Emergencies

The instructions that follow should serve only to reinforce what you learn in a CPR course for young children. (The training you receive at a class, which may vary somewhat from the protocol described here, should be the basis for your actions when a choking or breathing emergency occurs). Participating in a formal course is the best way to ensure that you'll be able to carry out these life support procedures correctly and according to the latest guidelines. Periodically review the guidelines below, and/or the materials you receive from course instructors.

Resuscitation efforts should be attempted when a child has stopped breathing or is struggling to breathe (gasping, wheezing, flushed or bluish skin colour). If your child is struggling to breathe, have someone call 999 immediately. Meanwhile, keep your child's body temperature normal (cool or warm him as needed), keep him or her calm, and have him or her rest in the position that seems most comfortable and easiest to breathe in.

To determine if resuscitation is necessary, survey your toddler's condition with the Check, Call, Care method recommended by the British Red Cross.

CHECK, CALL, CARE

1. CHECK THE SCENE, THEN THE TODDLER
Try to rouse a toddler who appears to be unconscious by tapping his shoulder and shouting his name: "Matthew! Are you okay, Matthew?"

CPR: The Most Important Skill You'll Hopefully Never Need

Never got around to learning CPR when your little one was a baby? Now that your baby has graduated to toddler, there's more reason than ever to learn.

Chances are you'll never need to apply a single lesson learned in a first-aid class – but more than any safety information you could read in a book, pick up online, or even hear from the GP, a first-aid course will arm you with the skills you would need to save your child's life should the improbable – and unthinkable – actually happen.

A child CPR lesson will provide you with invaluable hands-on instruction from a qualified teacher, showing you exactly what steps you'd need to take in an emergency. And since the best way to learn is through doing, you'll get to practise the skills you're learning on a child-size mannequin: where to place your hands for compressions, how hard and where to strike a child's back when trying to dislodge something stuck in the windpipe, how far back to tilt a child's head to give rescue breaths, and so much more.

The cost for a CPR class varies, around £25 to £50 through the British Red Cross. You can go to redcross firstaidtraining.co.uk to find classes in your area, or contact your local hospital to see if classes are offered there.

If you can't get to a class, because of either location or time constraints, the British Heart Foundation publishes a free booklet in English called *How to Save a Life*, which teaches how to put someone in the recovery position and give CPR. You can also get more information from www.nhs.uk and searching for CPR. This site takes you through the procedure for CPR on children step by step.

2. CALL

If you get no response, have anyone else present call 999 for emergency medical assistance while you continue to Step 3 without delay. If you are alone, provide about 2 minutes of care, then call 999. If you can, periodically call out to try to attract help from neighbours or passers-by. If, however, you are unfamiliar with CPR or feel overwhelmed and panicked, go to the nearest phone immediately – with your child, if there are no signs of head, neck, or back injury. Better still, if a phone is available, bring it to your child's side and call 999. The emergency services operator will be able to guide you as to the best course of action.

IMPORTANT: The person calling for emergency assistance should stay on the phone as long as necessary to give complete information to the emergency services operator. This should include: the name, age, and approximate weight of the child; any allergies, chronic illnesses, or medications taken; and present location (address, cross streets, flat number, best route if there is more than one). Ideally this information should be kept accessible at home and away. Also tell the emergency services operator the condition (is the child conscious?

breathing? bleeding? in shock? is there a pulse?), cause of condition (for example, fall, poison, drowning), and the telephone number where you can be reached. Tell the person calling for help not to hang up until the emergency services operator has concluded questioning and to report back to you after completing the call.

3. CARE

Move the child, if necessary, to a firm, flat surface. Quickly position the child face up, head level with heart, and proceed with the A-B-C survey below.

If there is a possibility of a head, neck, or back injury – as there may be following a bad fall or car accident – go to Step B to look, listen, and feel for breathing before moving the child. If breathing is present, leave the child where he or she is unless there is immediate danger (from traffic, fire, an imminent explosion) at the current site. If breathing is absent and rescue breathing cannot be accomplished in the child's present position, roll the child as a unit to a face-up position, so that head, neck, and body are moved as one, without twisting, rolling, or tilting the head.

A-B-C

A. OPEN THE AIRWAY
Push down on your toddler's forehead while pulling up on the bony part of the jaw with 2 or 3 fingers of your hand to lift the chin (neutral-plus position; see illustration this page). If there is a possibility of a head, neck, or back injury, try to minimise movement of the head and neck when opening the airway.

Which Comes First

The order of rescue techniques detailed here is A-B-C (Airway-Breathing-Circulation/ Compressions). Some countries will advise a different order but this method is considered most effective in the UK.

IMPORTANT: The airway of an unconscious child may be blocked by a relaxed tongue or by a foreign object. It must be cleared before the child can resume breathing.

Even if the child resumes breathing immediately, get medical help. Any child who has stopped breathing (even briefly), has been unconscious, or has nearly drowned requires prompt medical evaluation.

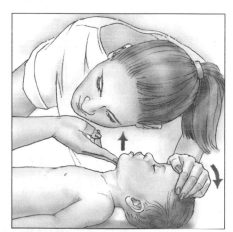

NEUTRAL-PLUS POSITION
Push down on your toddler's forehead while pulling up on the bony part of the jaw with two or three fingers of your hand to lift the chin.

B. CHECK FOR BREATHING

- **B-1.** After opening the airways, look, listen, and feel for no more than 10 seconds to determine if the child is breathing. Can you see the chest and abdomen rising and falling? Can you hear or feel the passage of air when you place your ear near the child's nose and mouth?

If normal breathing has resumed, maintain an open airway in the neutral-plus position as you continue to look for other life-threatening conditions.

ACTIVATE EMERGENCY MEDICAL SYSTEM. If breathing has resumed and no one has yet called for help, call 999 now.

If the child regains consciousness and has no injuries that make moving inadvisable, turn him or her on one side. Coughing when the child starts to breathe independently may be an attempt to expel an obstruction. *Do not attempt to interfere with the coughing.*

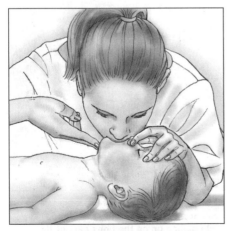

RESCUE BREATHING
Cover your child's mouth completely with your mouth and pinch his or her nose shut with the fingers of the hand on his or her forehead.

If breathing hasn't resumed or if the child is struggling to breathe and has bluish lips and/or a weak, muffled cry, you must get air into the lungs immediately. Maintain an open airway by keeping the child's head in the neutral-plus position (chin pointed up slightly) with your hand on the forehead and continue with rescue breathing below.

IMPORTANT: If emergency medical assistance has not yet been summoned and you are alone, continue trying to attract neighbours or passers-by as you work.

If vomiting should occur at any point, turn the child on one side and clear the mouth of vomit with a finger sweep (hook your finger to sweep it out). Reposition the child to the neutral-plus position and resume rescue procedures. If there is a possibility of neck or back injury, be very careful to turn the child as a unit, carefully supporting head, neck, and back as you do. Do not allow the head to roll, twist, or tilt.

- **B-2.** Pinch the child's nose shut with the thumb and forefinger of the hand that is maintaining the airway opening with the head tilt. Take a breath through your mouth, and then make a complete seal around the child's mouth with your mouth (see rescue breathing illustration, left).

- **B-3.** Blow five initial rescue breaths into the child's mouth. Pause between rescue breaths (so you can lift your head and breathe in again, and to let air flow out of the child's mouth). Observe with each breath whether the child's chest rises. If it does, allow it to fall again before beginning another breath. After five successfully delivered breaths (as evident from the rising chest), move on to Step C.

■ **B-4.** If the child's chest doesn't rise and fall with each breath that you administer, your breaths may have been too weak or the child's airway may be blocked. Try to open the airway again by readjusting the child's head (tilt the chin upward a bit more) and give two more breaths. If the chest still does not rise with each breath, it is possible the airway is obstructed by food or by a foreign object – in which case, move quickly to dislodge it, using the procedure described on page 469 in "First Aid for a Choking Toddler." If the chest does rise, indicating the airway is open, move on to Step C.

C. CHECK <u>CIRCULATION</u>

■ **C-1.** As soon as you've determined that the airway is clear, as shown by the successful delivery of five breaths, check for a pulse at the carotid artery using your index and middle fingers for no more than 10 seconds. (The

carotid pulse is located on the side of the neck, under the jaw, between the trachea and the neck muscles, see illustrations, below).

■ **C-2.** If you can't locate a pulse, proceed with chest compressions (CPR) immediately (see next page). If you find a pulse, the child's heart is beating and chest compressions are not necessary. But if the child is still not breathing (even with a pulse, you'll need to continue giving breaths (see Rescue Breathing box, next page) until breathing resumes.

ACTIVATE EMERGENCY MEDICAL SYSTEM NOW. If you're alone, give care for about two minutes before calling 999. If a phone is close by, bring it to the child's side. If not, and the child is small enough and there is no evidence of head or neck injury, carry the child to the nearest phone, supporting the head, neck, and torso.

Continue rescue breathing as you go. Quickly and clearly report

FINDING THE CAROTID PULSE

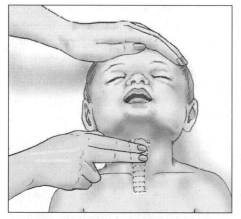

To locate the carotid pulse, place your index and middle fingers on the child's Adam's apple while maintaining a head tilt with the other hand.

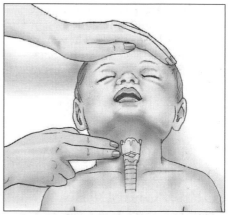

Slide your fingers to the side into the groove next to the windpipe, near the jaw and locate the pulse.

Rescue Breathing

After you've opened the airway (Step A), demonstrated that you can get five successful breaths into the child (Step B), and found a pulse (Step C), but the child still has not resumed breathing independently, proceed as follows. (If the child has no pulse, go straight to CPR, see below):

1. Give rescue breaths into the toddler's mouth as described in B-3, at the rate of roughly 1 breath every 3 seconds (or 20 breaths per minute). Watch to be sure the child's chest rises and falls with each breath.

2. After about 2 minutes, recheck for evidence of breathing, body movement, and pulse for no longer than 10 seconds to make sure the heart is still beating effectively. If there is no pulse, go to chest compressions (CPR, see below). If the child had begun to breathe independently, continue to maintain an open airway and check breathing and pulse frequently while waiting for help to arrive, keeping the child warm and as quiet as possible. If there is a pulse or movement but no breathing, continue rescue breathing, checking for pulse about every 2 minutes.

to the emergency services operator, "My child isn't breathing," and give all pertinent information the operator requests. Don't hang up until the operator does. If possible, continue rescue breathing while the operator is speaking; if that's not possible, return to rescue breathing immediately after hanging up.

IMPORTANT: Continue rescue breathing until the child begins to breathe on his or her own, the location you are in becomes unsafe, you are too exhausted to continue, or another trained responder takes over for you.

CARDIOPULMONARY RESCUSCITATION (CPR): CHILDREN OVER ONE YEAR

1. Position the child. The child should be lying face up on a firm, flat surface. There should be no pillow under the child's head, and the head should be level with the heart or lower and in a neutral-plus position (see illustration, page 465).

2. Position your hands. Locate the correct hand position by placing the heel of one hand on the child's sternum (breast-bone), at the centre of his or her chest. Your fingers should be raised so that only the heel of your hand is touching the child. Place your other hand directly on top of the first hand, interlacing your fingers if it helps you keep your fingers from resting on the chest. Alternatively, you can use a one-handed technique by placing one hand on the child's chest and the other hand on the forehead to maintain an open airway. Position your body correctly by kneeling beside the child, placing your hands in the correct position, and straightening your arms and locking your elbows, so that your shoulders are directly over your hand.

IMPORTANT: Do not apply pressure to the tip of the sternum (xiphoid process). Doing so could cause internal damage.

3. Begin compressions. Compress the chest smoothly to a depth of about one third of the chest using the heel of the dominant hand. Lift your hand without breaking contact, allowing the chest to fully return to its normal position, but maintain contact with the chest. Each compression should take about 1 to 1½ seconds. Repeat, performing 30 compressions (keeping your elbows locked).

4. Pause and breathe. After giving 30 compressions, remove your compression hand or hands from the chest, open the airway, and give two rescue breaths. After giving the breaths, place your hand or hands on the chest in the same position as before and continue compressions. Keep repeating cycles of 30 compressions and two rescue breaths.

> **ACTIVATE EMERGENCY MEDICAL SYSTEM NOW.** If you are alone, provide care for about two minutes before calling 999. If a phone is close by, bring it to the child's side. If not, and the child is small enough and there is no evidence of head or neck injury, carry him or her to the phone, supporting the head, neck, and torso. Continue rescue breathing

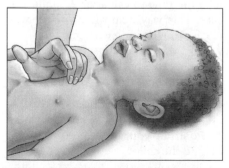

HAND POSITION FOR CHEST COMPRESSION
Place the heel of one hand on the child's sternum (breastbone) at the centre of the chest with your fingers pointing upward. Be sure only the heel of your hand is touching the child's chest.

as you go. Quickly and clearly report to the emergency services operator, "My child isn't breathing and has no pulse," and give all pertinent information the operator requests. Don't hang up until the operator does. If possible, continue compressions while the operator is speaking; if that's not possible, return to CPR immediately after hanging up.

IMPORTANT: Continue CPR until an automated external defibrillator (AED) becomes available, emergency medical assistance arrives, or your child regains a pulse.

FIRST AID FOR A CHOKING TODDLER

Coughing is nature's way of trying to clear the airways or dislodge an obstruction. A child (or anyone else) who is choking on food or a foreign object and who can breathe, cry, and cough forcefully should be encouraged to keep coughing. But if the child continues to cough for more than two or three minutes, call 999 for emergency medical assistance. If the cough becomes ineffective (it's silent) or the child is struggling for breath, making high-pitched crowing sounds, unable to speak or cry, and/or starting to turn blue (usually starting around the lips and fingernails), begin the following rescue procedure.

Start these rescue efforts immediately if the child is conscious and not breathing and if attempts to open the airway have been unsuccessful.

IMPORTANT: An airway obstruction may also occur with such infections as croup or epiglottitis.

ABDOMINAL THRUSTS AND BACK BLOWS FOR CONSCIOUS CHILD

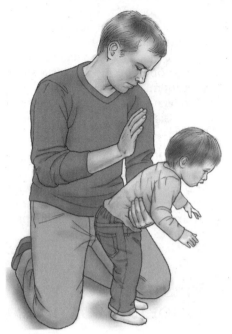

Kneel behind your child, bend him or her over your arm, and give back blows.

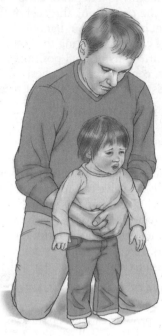

Then straighten your child and give quick abdominal thrusts. Continue back blows and abdominal thrusts until the object is dislodged.

A child who is struggling to breathe and seems ill – has fever and possibly congestion, hoarseness, drooling, lethargy, or limpness – needs immediate medical attention at an emergency care facility. Do not waste time in a dangerous and futile attempt to relieve the problem yourself: call 999.

1. Get help. If someone else is present, have them call 999 for emergency medical assistance. If you're alone, provide care for about two minutes before calling 999. If you are unfamiliar with rescue procedures – or if you panic and forget them – take the child with you to the phone (or bring a phone to the child's side) and call 999 for emergency

medical assistance immediately. It's usually recommended that even if you're familiar with rescue procedures, you take the time to call after 2 minutes of care. That way, help will be on the way in case the situation worsens.

If the child is conscious, a combination of five back blows followed by five abdominal thrusts as follows provides an effective way to clear the airway obstruction:

2. Position yourself. Stand or kneel behind the child.

3. Administer back blows. Provide support by placing one arm diagonally across the child's chest and lean the child forward. Firmly strike the child between the shoulder blades with the heel of your other hand five times, then continue to Step 4.

4. Administer abdominal thrusts. Stand or kneel behind the child and wrap your arms around his or her waist. Make a fist with one hand and place the thumb side against the middle of the child's abdomen, just above the navel, and well below the lower tip of the breastbone. Grab your fist with your other hand and give five quick, upward thrusts into the abdomen. Each thrust should be a separate, distinct movement.

Continue alternating back blows (#3 above) and abdominal thrusts (#4 above) until the object is dislodged and the child can breathe or cough forcefully, or becomes unconscious.

If the child is unconscious, proceed this way:

1. Rescue breaths. Place the child face up on a firm, flat surface (a floor or a table). Tilt the child's head as on page 465. Attempt two rescue breaths. If the chest does not rise, retilt the head and try two rescue breaths again.

Note: If the child was choking and conscious but then became unconscious, skip Step 1 and go right to Step 2, chest compressions.

2. Chest compressions. If the chest does not rise, give 30 chest compressions (see page 468). Check the mouth and look for an object. If a foreign body is visible, use a finger sweep with a hooked finger to remove it. If you can't see anything, try two rescue breaths. If breaths do not go in, repeat chest compressions, foreign body check, and then two rescue breaths.

Continue repeating this sequence until the airway is clear and the child is conscious and breathing normally or until emergency medical assistance arrives.

IMPORTANT: Even if your child recovers quickly from a choking incident, medical attention will be required. Call the doctor or the A&E immediately.

CHAPTER 15

Developmental Disorders

YOUR CHILD, LIKE EVERY OTHER CHILD, IS UNIQUE – with a rate of development all his or her own. Some tots walk sooner than other little ones, while other toddlers speak a mile a minute months before their peers say word one. And because there's a very wide range of normal when it comes to just about every developmental achievement, toddlers typically fall all over that right-on-schedule spectrum. But sometimes, a toddler's not right on schedule, at least not consistently, and instead shows signs of a true developmental delay that calls for therapy or other interventions. Developmental disorders, which can vary greatly in severity, include autism, intellectual disabilities, sensory processing disorders, congenital disorders and syndromes, or other developmental delays. If you have a hunch your child isn't developing normally, don't keep it to yourself – share your concerns with the doctor. Remember, you know your child best, and can pick up on nuances in behaviour that others might miss. And don't wait, either. An early diagnosis and early intervention (or early reassurance that all is well after all) can make a tremendous difference.

What You May Be Wondering About

AUTISM SPECTRUM DISORDERS

What is it? Autism Spectrum Disorders (ASD) are a group of conditions that affect a child's behavioural, social, and communication skills. Affected children have difficulty with social interactions, trouble with verbal and nonverbal communication, and exhibit repetitive behaviours or narrow, obsessive interests. Symptoms within the autistic spectrum can range from mild to severe.

It's estimated that 1 in every 100 children will be diagnosed with autism or another disorder in the spectrum (such as Asperger's syndrome or Pervasive Developmental Disorder; PDD). The numbers seem to be rising significantly, but some experts say that the statistics don't tell the whole story. They suggest that the increased rate may largely be due to more children being diagnosed (thanks to heightened awareness of the disorder, its symptoms, and treatments) and to the fact that a wider range of developmental disorders is now being labelled part of the autism spectrum.

It is unclear what causes autism, though studies have shown that genetics play an important role in the disorder. It is also unclear whether it is one disorder, several disorders, or many disorders with similar manifestations. Boys are four times more likely than girls to be affected, and if one sibling has ASD, the other siblings have nearly a 19 per cent risk of developing it. Some researchers also suspect chromosomal abnormalities may contribute to autism. Other studies point to abnormal brain growth in autistic children, and there is some evidence that environmental factors may play a role as well. One thing that is known for sure – and has been proven by large-scale studies again and again – there is absolutely no evidence of any relationship between autism and receiving childhood vaccines.

While the causes of autism remain mysterious, the signs don't necessarily come out of nowhere. Most parents of autistic children are recognising language delays and other symptoms by about 18 months of age, and children can usually be diagnosed between the ages of 2 and 3, but there are red flags that parents can look out for much earlier. According to NHS Choices, some early, more subtle signs of ASD may be noticeable as early as 12 months. They include:

- Child doesn't turn when you say his or her name.

- Child doesn't turn to look when you point and say "Look at . . ." or doesn't point to show you an interesting object or event.

- Lack of back-and-forth communication with parent.

- Delay in smiling.

- Failure to make eye contact with people.

Other signs of possible ASD that warrant evaluation by the GP include:

- No babbling, or pointing or other gestures, by 12 months.

- No single words by 16 months.

- No two-word spontaneous phrases by 24 months.

- Loss of language or social skills at any time during toddler/preschool years.

There is a wide range of symptoms among children with ASD and no two children will have exactly the same symptoms. Children may have all or only some of the typical ASD symptoms and at varying degrees of severity. Those symptoms can include:

Communication symptoms

- Delays in language: doesn't say single words by 15 to 16 months or two-word phrases by 24 months.

- Poorly developed language skills and a lack of desire to communicate with others.

Down's Syndrome

Every year, about 1 in 1,000 children are born with Down's syndrome, a chromosomal abnormality that produces a set of signs and symptoms, the characteristics of which may vary depending on the type of chromosomal abnormality. Usually they include oval-shaped eyes, an oversize tongue, and a short neck. Children with Down's syndrome may also have a flat back of the head, small ears (sometimes folded a little at the top); a flat, wide nose; short, wide hands; short stature; poor muscle tone; and a sweet, loving, and lovable personality. Children with Down's syndrome may have near normal IQs, while most others have mild to moderate intellectual disability and delayed development.

Early specialised education programmes can dramatically improve the learning and performance of Down's syndrome children, with some approaching the normal range. Most children with Down's syndrome have untapped potential, and intervention begun as soon as the condition is diagnosed can uncover and make the most of their abilities, leaving fewer than 10 per cent severely intellectually disabled. Many children with Down's syndrome can be mainstreamed in school and go on to live productive lives.

- Repetition of words without attaching any meaning to those words.

- Doesn't respond to name being called but will respond to other sounds (such as the wail of an ambulance or a dog's bark).

Social symptoms

- Greater-than-typical difficulties with social interactions, sometimes even with parents (doesn't respond to verbal or physical cues from others and may be socially withdrawn).

- Inability to interpret nonverbal communication (such as an angry voice or a big smile).

- Trouble making eye contact with others (but may gaze into space for hours on end).

- Doesn't point to objects.

- Doesn't have appropriate facial expressions.

- Shows no empathy.

- Never snuggles when picked up (instead arches his or her back the majority of the time).

Behavioural symptoms

- Ritualised behaviour beyond what's typical for a toddler.

- Fascination with parts of objects, such as a tag on a shirt.

- Plays with toys in unusual ways; doesn't use toys for pretend play.

- Tends to engage very little in imitative play and shows little imagination.

- Inappropriate behaviour (for example, smells everything encountered).

- Head banging and self-biting to the point of injury (as opposed to the kind of harmless head banging that many toddlers use to unwind before sleep or when stressed).

- Endless screaming and other kinds of frenzied behaviour, such as frequent and intense tantrums (well beyond what's typical for a toddler).

- Dislikes loud noises, but is mesmerised by many visual stimuli (a moving fan, for example).

- Obsessively repeats activities.

- Rocks, sways, and spins body, twirls fingers, or flaps hands.

- May have some gifted skills (like early reading or excellent math skills), but often without understanding their meaning.

- Extra sensitivity or lack of sensitivity to stimuli such as smells, sounds, touch, lights.

If you've noticed these types of symptoms in your toddler – or if your child has exhibited early warning signs – talk to your GP. He or she can use a standardised screening test to see if your toddler might be affected by ASD and need an evaluation by a developmental specialist.

Management. There is no known cure for autism spectrum disorders, but early intervention – with therapy to help foster normal development (as much as possible) and promote language development, social interaction, and learning – can make a remarkable difference in a child's future. There are a variety of treatment approaches that may modify the condition; some are scientifically based, and others are alternative therapies. What works for one child may not work for another, so therapy should be individualised.

Among the treatments that have shown some success are:

- Applied Behavioural Analysis (ABA, which uses positive reinforcement and other principles to build communication).

- TEACCH (a programme that focuses on communication and social interactions).

- Speech and language therapy (skills training designed to improve your child's language and social interaction).

- Medication to treat specific symptoms (usually reserved for older children).

- Motivation (finding an area of interest to the child, such as music or art or science, and trying to connect socially and physically through it).

Alternative treatments have not been studied enough to prove whether they are safe and effective. For instance, some parents say a gluten-/casein-free diet (GFCF) works, but so far, studies haven't backed up those anecdotal claims. That said, most doctors agree that if parents are willing to try a GFCF diet, there's probably no harm and possibly some benefit. Other dietary alternative therapies (omega-3 fatty acids; vitamin supplements; probiotics; cutting out food additives, like artificial colours) also have not been proven yet to be successful in treating ASD, though some of those may come with other health benefits. Some so-called treatments are downright dangerous (large doses of vitamins, for instance, or chelation therapy or colonics). Sorting out nontraditional therapies touted on websites and message boards may be particularly difficult for parents, especially when you're willing to try anything. For that reason, make sure that any treatment you decide to try has been green-lighted (and is supervised) by your child's GP or developmental specialist.

Helping Your Child

Though the future well-being of a child with a chronic or developmental condition depends a lot on the quality of professional care he or she receives, it depends even more on you, the parent. So:

Know what the condition is. Early diagnosis of the condition and early intervention are extremely important. If you have any doubt about the accuracy of a diagnosis or if your child's doctor is unable to come up with a diagnosis at all, consider getting a second opinion.

Find the best help you can. For many childhood conditions, the expertise of a specialist may be needed to make an accurate diagnosis and to recommend treatment. In some cases, the treatment can be supervised by your child's doctor, with or without consultation with a specialist – in other cases, it's best supervised by a specialist or subspecialist. A specialist affiliated with a children's hospital or a major medical centre is most likely to have the resources available to offer the most up-to-date care.

Be sure to listen. Pay careful attention to what the doctors, therapists, and others involved with your child's care have to say. If you have questions, ask them. If you don't understand the answers, ask for clarification. Request written materials, diagrams, and a list of sources that can help you learn more. Be careful, though, who you listen to. While there are plenty of reliable resources online to help parents of children with any condition, far from everything you'll read or hear will be scientifically valid – and some may be just plain wrong or even dangerous. If you come across any information about treatments or therapies that conflicts with what you've been told by the doctor or therapists caring for your child, but you're curious about them, definitely ask.

Be sure you're being heard. Are the professionals paying attention to you? Do they take your concerns and your input seriously? They should – after all, you know your child better than anyone else and your role is vital in caring for your child. Make sure the lines of communication between you and each care provider stay open all the time, not just during crisis periods.

Be persistent. If you feel strongly that something just isn't right with your toddler, but you can't seem to get an explanation, keep trying. Keep in mind, though, that the answer may turn out to be that there's nothing wrong with your child after all (and if you keep receiving that same answer from various specialists, it's important to accept it). Likewise, be persistent in asking questions and seeking answers if you feel the treatment your child is receiving isn't working or isn't the most up-to-date, if your child's doctor (or doctors) aren't keeping you informed,

Prognosis. How much autism will affect a child's life and future success is difficult to predict during the toddler period, and it varies with the degree of autism and the seriousness of related conditions. But with extensive, intensive intervention by both parents and professionals (25-plus hours a week year round), and with a multifaceted approach (possibly including medical treatment, psychological counselling, speech therapy,

or if you simply have the nagging feeling that more could be done. If your child isn't responding to therapy as expected – speak up.

Become an expert. In time, most parents of children with chronic or developmental conditions really start to know their stuff – well enough to hold their own in any conversation with a professional in the field. The sooner you begin your education, the better for your toddler – when you know what you're talking about, you can ask educated questions and make sound judgements about doctors, therapies, and interventions, helping to ensure the best treatment as soon as possible. And the better for you – you'll feel more in control of the situation and will have less fear of the unknown.

Keep up with the latest treatments and technology. New medical procedures, new therapies, and new technology are developed all the time that can help improve the quality of life of a child with a chronic condition or developmental disorder. Read up about them at reputable sources online, but remember that some new treatments are reported before they've actually passed scientific scrutiny.

Keep a record. Keep all of your child's medical reports, test results, appointments, treatments, medications, doctors, therapists, and so on in a file (ask for copies of everything). Emergency numbers and other pertinent information about your child's condition should be posted at every home phone, carried by anyone who cares for your child, and available to caregivers at nursery.

Stay positive. Sometimes, it'll be challenging – but try not to waste time or energy blaming yourself for your child's condition (after all, you didn't do anything to cause it) or feeling sorry for yourself or your child. An upbeat, positive attitude will help you both move on and move ahead. That said, there will be times when both you and your spouse will need to vent, to be talked up or talked down. You'll definitely be an invaluable source of support for each other, but sometimes you'll also need a healthy perspective from outside the bubble. You can find that in other parents who are going through the same experience with their children. Find a message board or support group that can fill the empathy gap.

Stay realistic. As important as it is to keep a positive attitude, it's also smart to stay realistic. Though you should investigate every avenue when it comes to treatment and management, acceptance of what can't be changed (at least not yet) is important, too.

Become financially savvy. Many of the interventions mentioned take a lot of time and labour, and can cost a significant amount of money. Some local education authorities (LEAs) provide partial (or sometimes total) funding towards specialist education and training, but this varies widely from LEA to LEA. If you would like more advice on what funding is available, and how to request it, visit the National Autism Society, www.autism.org.uk.

physical therapy, and special education), many children improve their communication and social skills significantly. Though some people with autism require life-long protective care, others make remarkable progress and are able to be mainstreamed in school, go on to university, and hold jobs later in life. Improved treatment may continue to better the outlook for today's autistic children.

Keep in mind: the earlier your child is able to begin treatment and interventions, the better the prognosis, so early diagnosis is crucial. If you suspect there is something wrong with your child, talk to your GP right away. Your GP may use a brief screening test, such as the checklist for autism in toddlers (CHAT). CHAT consists of a series of questions, such as "Does your child take an interest in other children?", "Does your child engage in pretend play?", and "Does your child ever bring objects to show you?". Your GP may also carry out a series of exercises with your child, such as asking your child to point out certain objects, or asking him or her to engage in imaginative play. If the results of the CHAT screening suggest that your child may have an ASD, you will be referred to a health professional who specialises in diagnosing ASD. They will make a more in-depth assessment.

For more information, contact the National Autism Society (www.autism. org.uk).

Sensory Processing Disorder (SPD)

What is it? Sensory Processing Disorder refers to a group of signs and symptoms stemming from a child's difficulty integrating information that comes in through the senses – hearing, seeing, smelling, tasting, and touching. It is slowly gaining acceptance as a diagnosis among medical professionals. Children with SPD often exhibit an over- or undersensitivity to stimuli – they receive signals from their senses, but aren't able to organise and interpret those signals and respond appropriately. Some toddlers with SPD may not enjoy being touched, while others like to touch everything. Some kids have trouble with balance, while others like to spin around all the time, and others have problems with coordination. Some children can't handle loud sounds and are overstimulated by certain sights. Some find wearing clothes, especially those made with rough, scratchy, or itchy fabrics, unbearable. Many children with SPD have pronounced food aversions.

Most symptoms of SPD sound like variations of "normal" toddler behaviours, but in children with SPD, the signs and symptoms are chronic and severe enough to interfere with daily functioning. In many cases – but far from all – SPD symptoms are part of a larger picture of Autistic Spectrum Disorders. It is thought that SPD has a genetic component to it and possibly an environmental cause as well (as with autism) – but the research on the condition is still in its early stages.

Many completely normal toddlers seem to be sense sensitive at least some of the time (they get unduly upset about bunched-up socks, turn their noses up at anything that isn't bland-tasting, become easily overstimulated at a birthday party). But if you suspect that your toddler's over- or undersensitivity to any of the senses is extreme – especially if it disrupts normal functioning – bring up your concerns with your child's doctor.

Management. Usually a mixture of occupational, physical, and speech/language therapy that involves activities and games in a sensory-rich environment, guided by a knowledgeable therapist, with the goal of teaching children how to respond appropriately to external stimuli and become more comfortable when they encounter sensations that disturb them or become more alert to sensations they usually don't notice. These types of therapies have been shown to make a difference for some children with SPD, though the clinical evidence is still sparse.

For hypersensitive children (those who overreact to stimuli), treatment might include a slow and gradual introduction to various sensory stimuli, such as keeping the lighting low, touching the child gently, rocking the child – and other activities designed to help the child better handle stimuli that upsets them. For hyposensitive children (those who underreact to stimuli), the approach is reversed. Treatment can involve teaching the child how to be aware of his or her body and body parts and how sensory stimuli affect the body (the child might be asked to wear a weighted vest, for instance, or to lift, push, pull until he or she becomes more alert to the feel of his or her body).

Prognosis. Children with SPD usually grow into adults with SPD, but therapy (early and as needed throughout life or when encountering new situations – like university, for example) can help them learn how to handle the senses more appropriately. Counselling that increases self-awareness and understanding can also allow these children to grow up knowing which strategies can help them cope in new situations.

For more information on SPD, check out the Sensory Integration Network (www.sensoryintegration.org.uk).

Developmental Delays

What are they? As much as they try not to, most parents will compare the development of their child to that of other children in playgroup or nursery. And most of the time, even children who seem somewhat behind the curve when it comes to gross or fine motor skills end up catching up eventually. But occasionally, a child truly falls behind – and

Finding Help

Your child may be eligible for several types of support from social services, but before any department can help you, it must carry out an assessment of what your child's care needs are. Once the assessment has been completed, the local authority has to make a decision about whether or not it will provide or arrange services for you. It does this by comparing your assessed care needs with eligibility criteria that it has set for the relevant care services. There are no national eligibility criteria for care services so each local authority sets its own, which vary around the country. They do, however, receive guidance from the Department of Health.

Social services have a duty in law to assess both you as a carer and the needs of your child. However, when it comes to providing services, the responsibility of social services will differ. If social services agree that the needs of your child are sufficiently high, they are obliged to provide services to meet those needs. Bear in mind that not all services will be provided free of charge, but there are grants available for some.

that's when a developmental delay is diagnosed.

There are a number of different types of developmental disorders that can affect toddlers in the second year, including (but not limited to):

- Fine motor disorders. Children with poor fine motor control may have difficulty holding a spoon or fork. Or they may be unable to grasp a crayon correctly and use it to draw by age 2. Later on, these children will have difficulty writing.

- Gross motor disorders. Some toddlers are consistently behind other children in every gross motor skill. They may have difficulty controlling their large muscles – making it hard to stay balanced and coordinated.

- Oral motor disorders. Some toddlers have trouble controlling the muscles in their mouths – making eating difficult (they'll refuse to eat foods unless they're puréed) and sometimes contributing to excessive drooling beyond the age of 18 months. The biggest risks faced by children with an oral motor disorder are trouble gaining weight (if they don't eat, they won't grow well) and, eventually, difficulty articulating language.

- Language delays. Though screeened for at regular checkups, language delays aren't usually apparent until after the second birthday.

The GP will screen for developmental delays at each visit, but if you sense that something is wrong, don't hesitate to bring it up. Often, parental instinct trumps medical awareness. The earlier therapy is started, the better for your child.

Management. If you or the doctor notice some motor delays in your toddler, neurological examinations that look at your child's muscle tone, strength, reflexes, and coordination will be conducted. The GP will also likely conduct a developmental assessment. If a developmental delay is considered likely, you'll be referred to an early childhood intervention programme so that a treatment plan can be developed. Often, such a plan will consist of occupational, physical, and speech/language therapy (if a language delay is noticed). If necessary, your child might require further evaluation by a paediatric neurologist, a speech and language specialist, and/or a developmental paediatrician.

Prognosis. Treatment begun early (or as soon as a disorder is diagnosed) can be very effective. For more information on developmental delays, look up Carers Direct on the NHS Choices website (www.nhs.uk).

ALL ABOUT:
Living with Your Special Child

Since every child is different, even children who share the same physical or emotional challenge are never exactly alike. But though no two special-needs children are the same, some basic needs are common to all of them – and to their families:

Unconditional love. Even a child who doesn't seem to respond to displays of love and affection needs them and benefits from them. So heap on the hugs and kisses. Squeeze that little hand gently. Make the kind of eye contact that shows you care even when it isn't reciprocated.

Normalcy. This is a tall but important order for a family with a special-needs child. Strive for a normal family life in as many ways as possible and make every effort to treat your special-needs child as you would any child. Nurture his or her self-esteem, encourage without pushing, and don't withhold discipline. Set limits according to your child's abilities, but be sure there are limits. Being overindulgent, overpermissive, or overprotective with a child with special needs won't help – and may actually slow – his or her development.

Remember that, like all toddlers, a special-needs child is likely to want to "do it myself". Instead of always jumping in and taking over, give your child the chance to try to handle things independently whenever possible. When doing it "myself" leads to mistakes (it inevitably will – even for young children with no disabilities), encourage your toddler to learn from the mistakes and try to do better the next time. And no matter what the final result, be sure to reinforce the effort.

Most special-needs toddlers are also prone to other typical toddler behaviours – including tantrums, negativity, self-centredness, and separation anxiety. Try to respond to these behaviours just as you would with any toddler, but with the extra sensitivity your toddler needs (check the index for individual behaviours and tips on coping with them).

And as much as is possible, don't let your child's condition prevent him or her (or you) from living as normal a life as possible, in as many ways as possible – playing with toys, going out, making friends, meeting new people.

Clarification. Explain your child's situation to siblings, grandparents, other family members, and close friends. The more they understand, the more supportive they can be.

Appreciation. Every child, even the most severely challenged, needs to feel appreciated – so let your child know that he or she is. Look beyond special needs for qualities and character traits that make your child special – a beautiful smile or endearing dimples, a kind heart, a way with animals, an indomitable spirit. This appreciation can improve your outlook as well as your child's, and it can give your family the strength it will need to overcome any obstacles that lie ahead.

You, too, will benefit from a little appreciation. Since you're unlikely to get all you need from your child (toddlers aren't usually big on acknowledging their parents' efforts), look to your spouse, other close relatives and friends, or a support group or message board to build you up when you're feeling underappreciated.

Relief. To be effective nurturers and caregivers, all parents need a break once in a while. But because the demands on parents of children with special needs can be so overwhelming, your need for relief is even greater. Assuming you can find someone to care for your little one, try your best to build some "me" time into your week – go to the cinema, relax in the bath, see friends, go to the gym. And never feel guilty about taking time off. You'll return refreshed, more relaxed, and better able to help your child.

Fun. A sense of humour – and an appreciation for simple pleasures – always makes family life happier and less stressful, but it's especially helpful when a family member has special needs. Taking a lighter approach to life can make your child's special needs seem easier to deal with and can help you think more positively (which can be contagious). When the going gets tough, try a little laughter, a little silliness, a little playfulness to get you going again.

Helping the Healthy Sibs

How does growing up in a household with a special-needs sibling affect healthy children? On average, having a special-needs sibling makes children more patient, adaptable, and understanding, as well as better at getting along with all kinds of people. Although being a healthy sibling in a household with a special-needs child is never easy, it can be an enriching, character-building experience. To improve the odds that your healthy children will benefit from the experience:

Involve them. Explain to them in language they can understand just what their sibling's situation is and how the family can work together to take care of him or her and each other. Find small tasks appropriate to their ages. For example, a preschooler can learn simple skills that can help engage an autistic sibling; a teenager can help with physical therapy or other treatment. Try to leave pressure and guilt out of the equation, though.

Reassure them. For older children, make it clear that the primary responsibility for caring for their sibling will fall on you, not on them. When the healthy sibling is a preschooler, simply say "Yes, Jacob has a problem, but it's not your fault. You didn't do it." In fact, all your children (the special-needs one included) need to be reassured that they are not responsible.

Your healthy children may also need reassurance that the illness or disability is not contagious – that you can't catch it the way you catch a cold, and that if they do come down with a cold or flu, it won't make them look or act like their sibling.

Make time for them. Though much of your time may be taken up by caring for your special-needs child, your other children need attention, too. Stretch your time as far as you can to make sure that each of your children gets some one-on-one with a parent every day. Do whatever works for your family. One option: stagger bedtimes so that each child can have a chance to talk over his or her day without vying for attention. Or plan a special outing once a week for each child – even if it means asking a relative or friend for coverage or hiring someone to stay with your special-needs child.

Try to be a positive model. Your attitude towards your special-needs child is almost certain to rub off on your other children, so do your best to stay positive. If you have a hard time thinking positively, get professional help to better handle any negative feelings you may have.

Don't scapegoat. Often it's easier (and less guilt provoking) to take your anger, frustration, and exhaustion out

Early intervention. Virtually every condition can be improved with early intervention. Try to make sure your child gets the best available professional diagnosis and treatment as early as possible. For even greater benefit, get the training you need so you can extend

that intervention to the time your child spends at home.

Parent support groups. Thousands of groups are active around the country and online. Caring for a special-needs child can be physically demanding and

on your healthy children than on your special-needs child ("I have enough trouble – I don't need any from you!"). But kid-gloving your special-needs child and treating your well children as scapegoats isn't fair, and it can lead to resentment and hostility. If you find yourself frequently taking your feelings out on your family, get some professional help.

Be understanding. Healthy siblings often have mixed feelings: "I am worried (or sad, or scared) about my sister.", "I wish I didn't have a sister – my parents have no time for me." This kind of ambivalence is normal and completely understandable (even parents are susceptible to it), and you need to make sure your children know that it is. Encourage them to share their feelings by picking up on nonverbal clues (a look of sorrow, or anger, or concern) and asking about them ("Do you feel sad? . . . angry? . . . worried? . . . stressed? . . . embarrassed?").

Some well children, feeling the stress, develop the same "symptoms" as their special-needs sibling (of course, never assume the symptoms are sympathetic until you've checked with the doctor). And some may intentionally try to mimic behaviour. Most often this is an attempt to either attract attention (after all, that's how the sibling gets it) or to somehow feel at one with the sibling ("I want to know how Ana feels"). Provide some extra attention, lend an understanding ear, and the imitation is almost certain to disappear.

Watch for warning signs. Children who have trouble coping with the stresses generated by having a special-needs sibling may become depressed and withdrawn, or start acting out (having frequent tantrums, for instance, or resisting bedtime). Try to devote some extra time and attention when such signs appear. If that doesn't help, discuss the problem with your children's doctor. Individual or family counselling also may be helpful.

Don't stoke up the pressure. Raising expectations for your healthy children or expecting them to be extra good or extra accomplished in order to compensate for their sibling isn't fair. Encourage all your children to be the best they can be, but don't ask for more than that. Also, let your kids be kids – avoid overburdening a well child with responsibilities or emotional baggage, even if you really need their help. Turn to other adults for help instead.

Provide outside support. Arranging for your well children to join a support group, in which they can share feelings and thoughts with other children in similar situations, can be extremely valuable. If you're unable to locate a local group (check with your child's doctor, the hospital, local adult support groups), consider starting one or finding one for children online.

emotionally draining – and connecting with parents who share your concerns (in person or online) can be very therapeutic. It can allow you to vent your feelings of frustration, anger, and resentment in a healthy way and to an empathetic audience, rather than bottling them up or

taking them out on your child, on yourself, or on the rest of the family. The swapping of various experiences, insights, and coping strategies can also be invaluable.

Relationship support. While just-the-two-of-you time between spouses is always hard to find when there's a young child in the house, it's harder still when the young child has special needs. Yet having a special-needs child doesn't automatically put a relationship at risk – in fact, it's just as likely to strengthen it. Give your twosome every chance of success by supporting each other emotionally, sharing responsibilities (no one parent should have to go it alone), setting aside time to spend as a couple (very difficult, but very important), and keeping the lines of communication open so that you can share your feelings – both positive and negative.

Sibling support. Siblings can have a hard time when so much attention is necessarily paid to the special-needs child. See the box on page 482 for tips on helping siblings cope.

Coping strategies. With help from professionals, support groups (local or online), or others who've already tackled the same issues, learn how to cope with your child's special needs, how to meet your needs and the needs of other family members, how to organise your time, and how to forgive yourself for not being perfect (remember, no parent is – and you're up against more than the average parent is).

A thick skin. There will be those who don't get what you and your little one are up against, and they're bound to say things that get you down. Try to let those comments bounce off you (after all, you can't educate everybody) – even if it just means giving the old smile-and-nod. But also, try to be as open and matter-of-fact about your child's condition as you can (or feel comfortable being), especially with family and friends, so that you don't give anyone, including your child, the impression that you're embarrassed or upset by it.

Proudly point out the special traits of your special-needs child, as well.

Acceptance. Many disabilities and chronic conditions can be controlled or even greatly improved, but most aren't completely curable. So while you should never stop trying to bring out the very best in your little one, it's also important to accept the realities of the condition and the limitations it comes with. To reach that acceptance, you'll probably have to struggle with some other challenging feelings, including anger, grief, and guilt. You may also, at first, find yourself focusing too hard on your child's weaknesses and too little on his or her strengths, and that's only natural. But the more accepting you are of your child, the more self-accepting he or she will grow up to be. Try to focus any frustration or anger you understandably have on the disorder, where it belongs – not on your little one or other family members.

Encouragement. Accepting your child's limitations doesn't mean that you shouldn't make every effort to help your child reach his or her greatest potential. Encourage and nurture intellectual and physical growth and the development of skills of all kinds (including social skills).

Hope. Acceptance also doesn't mean that you've given up hope. For the vast majority of special-needs children, love, support, a positive attitude, and appropriate therapy can improve the prognosis, sometimes dramatically. For many, new research on the horizon may even bring the cure you hope for. Some research suggests that hope itself may also influence a child's (or anyone's) success in life – so keep hoping.

Index

N